Gait Analysis

Theory and Application

Gait Analysis

Theory and Application

Rebecca L. Craik, PhD, PT

Physical Therapy Department
Beaver College
Glenside, Pennsylvania

Carol A. Oatis, PT, PhD

Physical Therapy Department
Beaver College
Glenside, Pennsylvania

with 190 *illustrations*

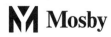

St. Louis Baltimore Boston Carlsbad Chicago Naples New York Philadelphia Portland
London Madrid Mexico City Singapore Sydney Tokyo Toronto Wiesbaden

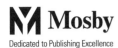

Mosby
Dedicated to Publishing Excellence

**A Times Mirror
Company**

Executive Editor: Martha Sasser
Associate Developmental Editor: Kellie F. White
Production and Editing: Carlisle Publishers Services
Book Designer: Tara Bazata
Cover Design: Sailer & Cook

Printed in the United States of America
Composition by Carlisle Communications, Ltd.
Printing/binding by Maple-Vail Book Manufacturing Group

Mosby–Year Book, Inc.
11830 Westline Industrial Drive
St. Louis, Missouri 63146

Library of Congress Cataloging-in-Publication Data

Craik, Rebecca L.
    Gait analysis : theory and application / Rebecca L. Craik and Carol
A. Oatis. — 1st ed.
        p.   cm.
    Includes bibliographical references and index.
    ISBN 0-8016-6964-2
    1. Gait in humans.   2. Gait disorders.   I. Oatis, Carol A.
II. Title.
QP310.W3C73   1994
612.7′6—dc20   94-34441
                                                       CIP

94 95 96 97 98 / 9 8 7 6 5 4 3 2 1

CONTRIBUTORS

Scott Z. Barnes, MSEM
Department of Biomedical Engineering
Ohio State University
Columbus, Ohio

Clare C. Bassile, EdD, PT
Department of Movement Science
Columbia Teachers College;
Columbia Presbyterian Medical Center
New York, New York

Necip Berme, PhD
Department of Mechanical Engineering
Ohio State University
Columbus, Ohio

Lin Bo, PhD
Biomechanics Corporation of America
Melville, New York

Connie Bock, EdM, PT
Columbia Teachers College
New York, New York

Jane E. Clark, PhD
Department of Kinesiology
University of Maryland
College Park, Maryland

Rebecca L. Craik, PhD, PT
Physical Therapy Department
Beaver College
Glenside, Pennsylvania

Anthony Delitto, PhD, PT
Department of Physical Therapy
University of Pittsburgh
Pittsburgh, Pennsylvania

Francine Dumas, MSc, PT
Program in Physiotherapy
Lavel University;
Neurobiology Research Center
Hospital de l'Enfant Jesus
Quebec, PQ
Canada

Lisa Dutterer, MS, PT
Department of Rehabilitation Medicine
Hospital of the University of Pennsylvania
   Medical System
Philadelphia, Pennsylvania

Martha E. Eastlack, MS, PT
Program in Physical Therapy
School of Life and Health Sciences
University of Delaware
Newark, Delaware

Janice J. Eng, PhD
Department of Kinesiology
University of Waterloo
Waterloo, Ontario
Canada

Alberto Esquenazi, MD
Gait and Motion Analysis Laboratory
Moss Rehabilitation Hospital;
Department of Rehabilitation Medicine
Temple University Hospital
Philadelphia, Pennsylvania

Hans Forrsberg, MD
Department of Pediatrics
Motor Control Laboratories
Karolinska Institute
Stockholm, Sweden

Joseph R. Higgins, PhD

Department of Physical Education
San Francisco State University
San Francisco, California

Susan Higgins, PhD

Department of Physical Education
San Francisco State University
San Francisco, California

Howard J. Hillstromm, PhD

Gait Study Center
Pennsylvania College of Podiatric Medicine
Philadelphia, Pennsylvania

Barbara Hirai

Gait and Motion Analysis Laboratory
Moss Rehabilitation Hospital
Philadelphia, Pennsylvania

Milad G Ishac, MSc

Department of Kinesiology
University of Waterloo
Waterloo, Ontario
Canada

Loretta M. Knutson, PhD, PT

Department of Physical Therapy
Creighton University
Omaha, Nebraska

Daniel G. Koff, MS

Innovative Technical Consulting
Sebastopol, California

David E. Krebs, PhD, PT

Massachusetts General Hospital
Institute of Health Professions;
Department of Mechanical Engineering
Massachusetts Institute of Technology;
Department of Orthopedics
Harvard Medical School
Boston, Massachusetts

Charles T. Leonard, PT, PhD

Program in Physical Therapy
The University of Montana
Missoula, Montana

Francine Malouin, PhD, PT

Physiotherapy Department Laval University;
Neurobiology Research Center
Hospital de l'Enfant Jesus
Quebec, PQ
Canada

Joseph M. Mansour, PhD

Department of Mechanical and Aerospace
    Engineering
Case Western Reserve University
Cleveland, Ohio

Irene S. McClay, PhD, PT

Physical Therapy Department
School of Life and Health Sciences
University of Delaware
Newark, Delaware

Carol A. Oatis, PT, PhD

Program in Physical Therapy
Beaver College
Glenside, Pennsylvania

Aftab E. Patla, PhD

Department of Kinesiology
University of Waterloo
Waterloo, Ontario
Canada

Carol L. Richards, PhD, PT

Physiotherapy Department
Laval University;
Neurobiology Research Center
Hospital de l'Enfant Jesus
Quebec, PQ
Canada

Mary M. Rodgers, PhD, PT

Department of Physical Therapy
University of Maryland
Baltimore, Maryland

Lisa Selby-Silverstein, PhD, PT, NCS

Department of Physical Therapy
Thomas Jefferson University
Philadelphia, Pennsylvania

Rami Seliktar, PhD
Department of Mechanical Engineering
Drexel University
Philadelphia, Pennsylvania

Lynn Snyder-Mackler, PT, ScD
Program in Physical Therapy
School of Life and Health Sciences
University of Delaware
Newark, Delaware

Gary L. Soderberg, PT, PhD
Department of Physical Therapy
Creighton University
Omaha, Nebraska

Michael J. Strube, PhD
Department of Psychology
Washington University
St. Louis, Missouri

Daniel Tardif, BSc
Neurobiology Research Center
Hospital de l'Enfant Jesus
Quebec, PQ
Canada

James D. Tomlinson, MS, PT
Department of Physical Therapy
Beaver College
Glenside, Pennsylvania

Ronald J. Triolo, PhD
Department of Orthopedic Surgery
Department of Bioengineering
Case Western Reserve University;
Department of Orthopedics
Cleveland Clinics
Cleveland, Ohio

James P. Walsh, PhD
College of Podiatric Medicine
Philadelphia, Pennsylvania

David A. Winter, PhD
Department of Kinesiology
University of Waterloo
Waterloo, Ontario
Canada

Ge Wu, PhD
Center for Locomotion Studies
Pennsylvania State University
University Park, Pennsylvania

To the memory of

Mary Patricia (Mary Pat) Murray, PT, PhD

whose pioneering work in human locomotion is familiar to anyone who studies gait. Her work not only contributed to our basic understanding of human locomotion but demonstrated clearly the benefits of focusing the disciplines of physical therapy, engineering, and medicine together on the dilemmas of human walking. We are grateful to her example and hope that this work furthers that spirit of collaboration that will bring us all to a richer understanding of human locomotion.

PREFACE

Each of us is intrigued by some aspect of human walking. Yet while many different disciplines study normal human locomotion, we rarely approach this study from a transdisciplinary perspective. One of the reasons for such a parochial approach to the study of human locomotion is our different conceptual frameworks and the vocabulary we use to describe walking. Although we are interested in understanding how the human system produces the elegant behavior of walking and the factors that lead to decline in performance, each discipline has adopted a unique set of terms to define the theory and measurement of human walking. We designed this book to cut across disciplinary boundaries in order to stimulate and facilitate discussion.

The content provides a comprehensive review of current understanding of gait analysis. The book has been developed to teach the reader about the theories upon which gait measurements are based, basic characteristics of human walking, and technologies available to measure gait performance. Application of this knowledge is demonstrated through examples that involve the evaluation of both nondisabled and disabled walking performance.

The text is divided into four parts. Part I illustrates how different disciplines approach a walking disorder using different conceptual frameworks. Part II provides a detailed review of several theories developed to explain how walking is produced. A mathematical model, a neural control model, a motor learning model, and a dynamical systems model are each presented. Part III addresses the variables used to measure walking performance. The theoretical basis from which the variables were derived is presented, the technology available to perform the measurement is reviewed, and operational definitions and normative data are provided for many of the variables used to describe gait. Chapters address measurement theory, footfall measures, joint kinematics, kinet-ics, and EMG. Part IV applies gait analysis methods and theory to human examples of locomotion. Goals of assessment are reviewed, and each subsequent chapter is an example of the analyses applied to meet a particular goal.

The book is intended for use as a textbook for students learning about movement analysis, biomechanics, or clinical assessment. The book has been designed so that a variety of different disciplines can use selected chapters to teach discipline-specific information. The other chapters can then serve as examples of application. The chapters are written so that even the reader who lacks a sophisticated mathematics background can pass over the equations and glean the essential issues and problems central to each theory.

The book should be useful for entry-level clinicians interested in gait analysis. Engineering students interested in biomechanics, measurement theory, and gait analysis technology can use this book as an entry-level text. Movement science students can use all aspects of the book for entry-level teaching. The content should also be interesting to experienced scientists who wish to approach the analysis of movement from a global perspective. Neuroscientists may wish to use this book to learn about measures of functional performance and to integrate this information with knowledge of the nervous system. Biomechanists may use this book to learn about other disciplines, motor control models, and the clinical needs for movement analysis.

It is our hope that we will help the reader integrate current knowledge about human walking performance with measurement theory, gait analysis technology, and clinical application. We have come away from this task with an enriched perspective about human locomotion. It is obvious that no discipline has figured out how human locomotion occurs or identified the sensitive and specific variables that should be used to describe the behavior. Maybe it is time for a collective effort.

Rebecca L. Craik, PhD, PT
Carol A. Oatis, PT, PhD

ACKNOWLEDGMENTS

This book would not have happened without the able assistance and support of our colleagues, students, friends, and families. In addition to these VIPs we would like to thank some people specifically. Without David Marshall of Mosby, and his gentle nudging, the book would still be a dream rather than a reality. Kellie White, also at Mosby, took up the job of nudging when David moved on in the company. She worried with us when authors pushed our deadlines to the limit and developed creative strategies to ensure that the project stayed on time. When we thought that we had no words left, she pushed us on to complete the glossary. Finally, we thank the authors, who took on their charge with enthusiasm and exceeded our expectations with their contributions. We thank each of you for your patience and encouragement.

Rebecca L. Craik, PhD, PT
Carol A. Oatis, PT, PhD

CONTENTS

Part IV   Applications

Gait Analysis

Theory and Application

P A R T   I

CASE REPORT

♦ This section illustrates how the various theories developed to explain gait are used to explain a particular walking pattern. To introduce and facilitate this linkage, a case study of an unusual walking pattern of a toddler is presented. The case study is followed by an explanation for the walking pattern using four different conceptual frameworks, a biomechanical perspective, a neural control perspective, a motor learning perspective and a dynamical systems perspective.

CHAPTER 1

ELIZABETH: A CASE STUDY

James D. Tomlinson

KEY TERMS

Creeping

Cruising

Fracture

Immobilization

Toddler gait

Elizabeth is a child who had an unremarkable prenatal and perinatal course and was developing normally, meeting major developmental milestones, when she fell down a flight of stairs. Home videotapes informally recorded the events before and after the accident.

Elizabeth began ambulating without external support and with unbounded parental delight at about 9 months. By ten months of age she was using upright ambulation as a primary mode of mobility with a "typical" toddler gait pattern. At 10½ months, she fell down a flight of carpeted stairs. After she calmed down, no obvious injury could be found but she would not bear weight on the right lower extremity. Radiographs made in the emergency room showed a ripple in the distal lateral cortex of the tibia. The fracture did not involve the epiphyseal plate of the tibia. A long-leg plaster cast was applied by an orthopedic resident in the emergency room. The cast maintained the ankle in approximately 45° of plantar-flexion and the knee in approximately 30° of flexion. The cast remained in place 23 days.

Elizabeth adjusted to life with the cast quickly; the parents, somewhat more slowly. Initially she was unable to crawl, creep, or walk with the cast. Within a week she was able to creep on her hands and left knee with the right leg abducted and externally rotated to accommodate the cast. Two weeks after the accident she was able to ambulate short distances with the right leg abducted and externally rotated. She spent minimal time in stance on the right and had minimal weight shift to the right. At the end of the immobilization period she was relatively efficient ambulating with this gait pattern.

On the 23rd day of immobilization the cast was removed at home. Elizabeth was given a bath immediately after cast removal during which she explored the right leg. The parents (both are physical therapists) grossly compared the ROM (range of motion) of the left and right legs during the bath and found no remarkable deficit on the right. She appeared able to actively move the right ankle and knee through full ROM.

Her behavior during the 15 to 20 minutes immediately after the bath was videotaped. Elizabeth experimented with using her right leg while absorbed in "Sesame Street." During this period she played in multiple sitting, kneeling, half-kneeling, and modified plantigrade positions at the bottom stair. She was observed with the foot, ankle, and knee in various positions while weight-bearing and nonweight-bearing. Initially, the foot and ankle positioning varied greatly; She would place the foot flat on the floor while weight shifted over it with the knee either flexed or extended. The right knee buckled inconsistently in weight-bearing positions during this period. She would also contact the floor with the foot in an inverted position and the ankle plantarflexed before weight-bearing. On these occasions the foot and ankle apparently were not stabilized and did not support her as she shifted weight over the right foot. She appeared frustrated when she tried to get from one place to another with the right lower extremity not providing reliable support. The parents were concerned about lack of support from the right lower extremity but found no evidence of grossly altered force production capability in activities such as kicking during diaper changes and play within the first few hours after cast removal.

By the afternoon of the same day she began to maintain the right lower extremity in the position in which the limb had been immobilized (hip abduction, external rotation, knee flexion, and ankle plantarflexion) for creeping, cruising, and walking. This pattern persisted for 10 days, much to the parents' dismay. During this time she fell less frequently and the right hip abduction decreased, but she continued to weight shift minimally to the right and had minimal single support time on the right. The ankle and knee angles were held constant throughout the gait cycle. On the afternoon of the tenth day she was noted to have the foot flat on the floor occasionally and the gait pattern was less asymmetric although there was still less weight shifting to the right and less single-support time on the right. The next morning she again ambulated with the right lower extremity held in the position of immobilization. After a day of playing at day care she interspersed steps where the foot was flat on the floor, the knee was more extended, and the hip was less externally rotated with steps where the limb was maintained in the immobilized position. This transition period lasted several days. Approximately 2 weeks after the cast was removed her gait pattern became relatively symmetric. Over the next 2 weeks, she used the right lower extremity in the immobilized position only occasionally, and the characteristics of her gait pattern approached normal for a 12-month-old child.

CHAPTER 2

EPIGENETIC DEVELOPMENT OF HUMAN LOCOMOTOR CONTROL

Hans Forssberg

KEY TERMS

Canalized development

Central pattern generator (CPG)

Flexibility

Plantigrade determinants

Plantigrade gait

The history of Elizabeth illustrates, first, the flexibility of her locomotor control system and its ability to adapt the locomotor activity to the restricted movement, and second, the epigenetic development of a strongly canalized behavior. Before briefly discussing Elizabeth's case, this chapter offers a brief explanation of the epigenetic process followed by a somewhat longer review of the neural control mechanisms for locomotion and the development of these mechanisms in humans.

Epigenetic development was named by Waddington[23,24] who described how phenotypic characteristics arise during development through a complex series of interactions between genetic programs and environmental signals. He suggested that environmental signals act upon the genome in order to trigger the expression of morphological and behavioral characteristics at different times during development. Some characteristics are tightly constrained—species-typical processes that are expressed even during abnormal environments—while others are less tightly constrained and provide the basis for substantial individual variation among members of the same species. The former category follows a strongly canalized development, and to this category belong vital functions, crucial for fitness, i.e., for survival and reproduction of genes. Locomotion development is a vital function, strongly canalized into species-specific locomotor patterns.

From nonhuman mammals we have learned how the central nervous system (CNS) is organized to generate and control locomotor movements. The basic locomotor rhythm is produced by neural networks in the spinal cord producing alternating activity in flexor and extensor muscles. Sensory afferents from the limbs provide a powerful influence on the spinal locomotor network and modify its activity.[1] This modulation plays an important role in adapting the locomotor activity to the external environment. Indeed, cats can walk properly after a complete spinal cord transection by adapting walking speed and correcting for mechanical perturbations.[10,11] Although the neural network's several functional properties for locomotion are well known, its architecture is fairly unclear. There could be separate networks for each joint of a single limb or one common neural network for several rhythmic behaviors of the limb, e.g., walking, paw shaking, paw squeezing, and scratching.[19] The final pattern of the motor activity would then depend on how the network is activated. A diversity of behaviors can be induced from one simple neural network through activation or modulation by various neuropeptides.[13]

Even though spinal mechanisms can adapt the locomotion in a feedback mode, supraspinal mechanisms are required to achieve a purposeful locomotor behavior according to the goal. Goal-directed locomotion necessitates controlling speed, maintaining equilibrium, and coordinating visuomotor processes (i.e., steering, foot placement, avoidance of obstacles, etc.). Several subsystems in the brain stem control the spinal locomotor networks via reticulospinal pathways.[17] These brain stem networks can initiate, determine the speed, and halt the locomotor activity. Other brain stem networks modulate muscle tone in the limbs influencing the mode of locomotion.[16] In turn, these brain stem networks are controlled by inputs from the motor cortex and basal ganglia.[12] Circuits in the motor cortex, activated from visual cortex, are involved in fast corrections of the ongoing locomotor movements in order to avoid obstacles.[2,7] Spinocerebellar tracts provide the cerebellum with sensory information from the moving limb and with information about activity in the spinal locomotor network.*[3] In turn, the cerebellum modulates the activity in descending brain stem pathways, including rubro-, reticulo-, and vestibulospinal tracts. Hence, based on research from nonhuman mammals, control of locomotion is distributed across several neural networks, organized at higher and lower levels, with parallel pathways (ascending and descending) providing for integration among different subsystems.

The bipedal, plantigrade gait in adult humans is unique. No other living animal has a similar locomotor pattern. Several plantigrade determinants† reduce the energy expenditure during walking. The prominent heel strike at touch-down and the push-off during the end of stance are of special interest. In quadrupeds and nonhuman primates, the calf muscles are active before touch-down and cease activity before the stance phase ends. The main propulsive force occurs at the end of the

---

*This type of information of central activity is called efference copy or corollary discharge. It can act as internal cues coordinating the activity of various neural networks. It also provides information for the detection of errors in the motor performance (e.g., by comparison of the efference copy and the actual sensory input).

†Plantigrade determinants:

1. Foot movement	heel strike
2. Knee movement	flexion of supporting leg
3. Intralimb coordination	joint movements out of phase
4. Pelvic movement	rotation, tilt, translation
5. Muscle activity	specific temporal pattern

(See references 9a, 9b.)

stance and is due to increased activity of the quadriceps muscles.[15] In humans, active dorsiflexion during the end of swing is accomplished by the pretibial muscles. The calf muscles contract first during the stance phase and produce the main propulsive force during the end of the stance phase.[4] The importance of the calf muscles for forward propulsion in humans is reflected by a comparatively larger size and the design of the human foot, with a longitudinal arch acting as a spring during push-off.[8] The multijoint foot of the monkey dorsiflexes during stance and cannot store energy during the stance phase. Hence, during the evolution of plantigrade gait, both the musculoskeletal system and the locomotion generating circuits have been modified.

Although human locomotion is unique, it does share several common characteristics with locomotion of other animals. Indeed, comparative studies suggest an evolution from paired fins in fishes to limbs in terrestrial animals and a corresponding transformation of the neural networks controlling locomotion from swimming to walking.[5] In this perspective, humans have likely maintained a similar neural organization to that of other mammals, even though an important transformation of the locomotor pattern has occurred.

The development of locomotion control varies considerably between species. In carnivores, development has to be completed in utero in order for the newborn animal to escape predators a few hours after birth. In other species, as in humans, the development takes several months or even years to occur. In the first case, the locomotor competence has to be genetically determined (strongly canalized and not requiring environmental triggering). In latter cases, environmental influence may play a larger role forming the movement patterns as suggested by the growing individual "practicing" during development.

The ontogeny of human locomotion can be divided into several stages. The first locomotor-like behavior occurs in utero when the human fetus is 10 to 12 gestational weeks[6] and can be elicited after birth when the child is held erect over a horizontal surface and slowly pulled forwards.[20] The stepping movements usually diminish during the first postnatal months, but may be present until onset of supported locomotion, which emerges at 7 to 9 months of age. During this stage, children can voluntary elicit stepping and support body weight, but need support to maintain equilibrium. Between 9 and 18 months, independent walking usually emerges, mainly reflecting the development of the postural control system.

Kinematic and EMG studies demonstrate that infants have an immature locomotor pattern during the early developmental phases; however, some modifications of the pattern emerge before independent walking.[22] In fact, all the plantigrade determinants are lacking. Flexor and extensor muscles are co-activated, producing synchronized flexion and extension movements in all joints. The calf muscles are activated during the end of the swing phase, plantar flexing the foot before ground contact. This, in combination with a backward rotation of the leg in the end of swing, places the foot flat on ground or on the toes. There is no push-off. In contrast, the leg is moved forward by a synchronized flexion in all joints.

The transformation to a plantigrade gait occurs when the child starts supported locomotion and continues until about 4 years of age. There is a successive phase shift of the calf muscle activity with age. As a consequence, the heel is placed first on the ground at 18 to 24 months,[21] but a prominent heel strike, including an active dorsiflexion until heel strike, does not occur until after 2 years.[9] Meanwhile the muscle activation pattern is shaped[18, 14] to produce desynchronized joint movements characteristic for the plantigrade gait.

Let us return to Elizabeth. She had followed the canalized locomotor development typical for humans and started to walk without support, indicating that her equilibrium system had matured to a certain level. Nothing is known about her locomotor pattern, but she had probably started the gradual process of plantigrade transformation. The injury and subsequent cast suddenly halted the normal locomotor development and prevented her from using ordinary locomotor movements. In this situation Elizabeth tried various movement strategies in her creeping and walking. However, the cast influenced the movement, changing the range of joint movements and the load of the leg, and ordinary movements could no longer be accurately performed. In this situation, Elizabeth adopted a strategy in which various small modifications of the locomotor pattern were tried until the most efficient pattern was achieved. During this phase, sensory mechanisms played a significant role, directly influencing the central networks to modify the pattern, but also monitoring the most efficient movement pattern.

This capacity to modify the locomotor pattern when the movement is constrained is present in all mammals and can be partly managed by an interaction of sensory and motor mechanisms at a spinal level.[1,10,11] It is likely, however, that supraspinal systems are involved in this process as well. The capacity to modify the locomotor pattern is not unrestricted, at least not in nonhuman mammals. In studies attempting to investigate how radical changes of the locomotor pattern could be performed in intact cats, the tendon from the lateral gastrocnemius muscle was transferred to the distal end of the tendon of the anterior tibialis muscle (the TA muscle was removed).[25] The cats adapted very well to this situation and could walk, run, jump, and climb without remarkable impairments. However, when the locomotor pattern was analyzed in more detail, it was seen that the lateral gastrocnemius muscle (now functioning as a flexor) was still active in conjunction with the extensors and not together with the flexors, and the ankle joint had an aberrant movement pattern. The normal-looking movements were accomplished by compensatory mechanisms in the other joints of the same leg as well as in the contralateral leg. Hence, there is evidence for plasticity of the locomotor system that can accommodate reversed movement direction in one joint and still produce apparently normal movement. Some parts of the locomotor activity are more rigid, such as the alternating activation of flexor and extensor muscles.

The retained "new" movement pattern several days after Elizabeth's cast was removed indicates that the adapted locomotor pattern was internalized and memorized somewhere in the motor control system. The mechanism behind this learning effect and at what level it occurs is unknown, as is motor learning in general. However, the gradual return to the "old" locomotor pattern brings us back to the epigenetic development described in the beginning of the chapter. When the environmental influence guiding the development in an atypical direction is abolished, the development will again be "canalized" into the species-specific locomotor pattern.

In summary, the story about Elizabeth demonstrates some general principles of the locomotor control system. The first is its flexibility, which allowed Elizabeth to adapt her locomotion and find a new motor pattern when her movements were restrained. The neurophysiological basis for this adaptation has been discussed in some detail. A second point is that the retained "new" movement pattern for several days after the cast was removed indicated this pattern was internalized (learned) within the motor system. Finally, the gradual return to the species-specific locomotion development illustrates a canalized epigenetic development.

REFERENCES

1. Andersson O et al: Peripheral feedback mechanisms acting on the central pattern generators for locomotion in fish and cat, *Can J Physiol Pharmacol* 59:713, 1981.
2. Armstrong DM: The supraspinal control of mammalianlocomotion, *J Physiol* 405:1, 1988.
3. Arshavsky YI, Orlovsky GN: Role of the cerebellum in the control of rhythmic movements. In Grillner S et al, editors: *Neurobiology of vertebrate locomotion,* Stockholm, 1985, MacMillan.
4. Bresler B, Franker JP: The forces and moments in the leg during level walking, *Trans Am Soc Mech Eng* 72:27, 1950.
5. Cohen AH: Evolution of the vertebrate central pattern generator for locomotion. In Cohen AH, Rossignol S, Grillner S, editors: *Neural Control of Rhythmic Movements in Vertebrates,* New York, 1988, John Wiley & Sons.
6. de Vries JIP, Visser GHA, Prechtl HFR: Fetal motility in the first half of pregnancy. In Prechtl HFR, editor: *Continuity of neural functions from prenatal to postnatal life clinics,* Oxford, 1984, Spastics International Medical Publications.
7. Drew T: Motor cortical cell discharge during voluntary gait modification, *Brain Res* 457:181, 1988.
8. Elftman H, Manter J: Chimpanzee and human feet in bipedal walking, *Am J Phys Anthropol* 20:69, 1935.
9a. Forssberg H: A developmental model of human locomotion. In Grillner S et al, editors: *Neurobiology of vertebrate locomotion,* Stockholm, 1986, MacMillan.
9b. Forssberg H: Ontogenetic development of human locomotor control: infant stepping, supported locomation and transition to independent walk, *Exp Brain Res* 57:480-493, 1985.
10. Forssberg H, Grillner S, Halbertsma J: The locomotion of the spinal cat. 1. Coordination within a hindlimb, *Acta Physiol Scand* 108:269, 1980.
11. Forssberg H, Grillner S, Rossignol S: Phasic gain control of reflexes from the dorsum of the paw during spinal locomotion, *Brain Res* 132:121, 1977.
12. Garcia-Rill E: The basal ganglia and the locomotor regions, *Brain Res Rev* 11:47, 1986.
13. Harris-Warrick RM, Marder E: Modulation of neural networks for behavior, *Annu Rev Neurosci* 14:39, 1991.
14. Leonard CT, Hirschfeld H, Forssberg H: Development of independent walking in children with cerebral palsy, *Dev Med Child Neurol* 33:567, 1991.
15. Manter JT: The dynamics of quadrupedal walking, *J Exp Biol* 15:522, 1938.
16. Mori S: Contribution of postural muscle tone to full expression of posture and locomotor movements: multi-faceted analysis of it's setting brainstemspinal cord mechanisms in the cat, *Jpn J Physiol* 39:785, 1989.
17. Noga BR, Kriellaars DJ, Jordan LM: The effect of selective brainstem or spinal cord lesions on treadmill locomotion evoked by stimulation of the mesencephalic or pontomedullary locomotor regions, *J Neurosci* 11:1691, 1991.

18. Okamoto T, Goto Y: Human infant pre-independent and independent walking. In Kondo S, editor: *Primate morphophysiology, locomotor analyses and human bipedalism,* Tokyo, 1985, University of Tokyo Press.

19. Pearson KG, Rossignol S: Fictive motor patterns in chronic spinal cats, *J Neurophysiol* 66:1874, 1991.

20. Peiper A: *Cerebral function in infancy and childhood,* New York, 1963, Consultants Bureau.

21. Sutherland DH et al: The development of mature gait, *J Bone Joint Surg* [Am] 62:336, 1980.

22. Thelen E, Whitley-Cooke D: Relationship between newborn stepping and later walking: a new interpretation, *Dev Med Child Neurol* 29:380, 1987.

23. Waddington CH: The theory of evolution today. In Koestler A, Smythies RD, editors: *Beyond reductionism,* New York, 1968, Macmillan.

24. Waddington CH, Prechtl HFR: Vestibulo-ocular response and its state dependency in newborn infants, *Neuropediatrics* 1:11, 1969.

25. Forssberg H, Svartengren G: Hardwired locomotor network in cat revealed by a retained motor pattern to gastrocnemius after muscle transposition, *Neuroscience letters* 41:283-288, 1983.

CHAPTER 3

A Biomechanical Perspective

Irene S. McClay

Key Terms

Cocontraction

Ground reaction forces

Joint movements

Kinetics

Range of motion

Strength

Stride characteristics

As movement scientists, we realize that the body cannot be viewed simply from a biomechanic, neurophysiologic, or motor control standpoint. Movement occurs as a result of the integration of all of these systems working in concert. However, one might accuse the biomechanists of being peripheralists, disconnecting the brain from the rest of the body and disregarding the effects of central control. The neuroscientists might then be charged with being centralists, focusing the majority of their attention on the brain. For the sake of interest, we have been asked to take these independent viewpoints as we attempt to predict the consequences of immobilization on Elizabeth's gait pattern.

From a pure biomechanics perspective, the factors that dictate movement are our inherent structure and alignment, available joint range of motion, and overall muscle strength. We are equipped with these biomechanical tools to produce our kinematics (movement patterns) and kinetics (forces and torques which generate these movement patterns). The child presented in this case study was reported as developing normally. Therefore, we will assume that she possessed normal structure and alignment, range of motion, and strength prior to her immobilization. However, we cannot make the same assumption following her 3.3-week period of immobilization.

There is a body of literature that reports the investigated effects of immobilization on both muscle strength and muscle length. Studies have shown that in the cat soleus muscle the number of sarcomeres in series decreases by 40% following four weeks of immobilization in a shortened position.[6] These authors also reported that muscles were stiffer and more resistant to passive stretch. In support of the peripheralists view, they concluded that the control center for these adaptations was in the muscle itself, as similar adaptive changes were found in immobilized muscles whose nerve had been severed. Along with decrease in overall resting length of the muscle, immobilization in a shortened position has been found to negatively effect the force-generating capacity of the muscle. Muscle mass reportedly decreased by as much as 50%, while maximum tetanic contraction decreased 75 to 80%.[4] Immobilization in a lengthened position has significant but less dramatic results with muscle mass decreasing by 15% and maximum tetanic contraction decreasing by 40%. Although these studies were performed on otherwise healthy animals, the findings suggest that the immobilization of the limb of the child in this case study will likely result in both strength and range of motion deficits. Let us now consider how these changes in Elizabeth's basic biomechanic system might translate into alterations in her movement mechanics.

The cast was applied with the knee fixed in approximately 30° of knee flexion and the ankle in 45° of plantarflexion. This would certainly limit her locomotor mobility, thus leading to compensatory movement patterns. During creeping and eventually walking, the lower limb was held in external rotation and abduction throughout the immobilization period. These positions would allow a functional shortening of the limb, providing easier progression over the foot during stance and clearance of the foot during swing. Bearing in mind the previously noted studies, one would expect to see decreases in both strength and resting length of the ankle plantarflexors and the knee flexors as a result of the position in which the leg was casted. Tightness might also be seen in the external rotators and abductors of the hip given the continual posturing of this extremity. Once the cast was removed, one would likely see the gait pattern influenced by these acquired biomechanical deficits. The following is the biomechanist's prediction of this child's resultant gait pattern. Table 3-1 summarizes the phases of gait to be discussed and their descriptions.

TABLE **3-1**   Phases of gait

Abbreviation	Name	Description
FS	Foot strike	Initial contact
FS-FF	Foot strike-foot flat	Loading phase
FF-HO	Foot flat-heel off	Midstance
HO-TO	Heel off-toe off	Propulsive phase
TO	Toe off	Preswing
SW	Swing	Noncontact phase

KINEMATICS

Figure 3-1 demonstrates a comparison of normal kinematics of the hip, knee, and ankle for 1-year-old children[5] during walking to the suggested predicted patterns. Normally, at FS (foot strike),

---

FIGURE 3-1 Comparison of the kinematic profiles for sagittal plane motion of **A**, the hip, **B**, knee, and **C**, ankle joints during walking. The solid line represents typical patterns for normal 1-year-old children (Sutherland et al,[5] 1980). The dotted line represents the predicted patterns of the child in this case study.

A

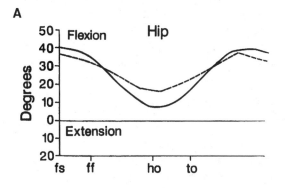

B

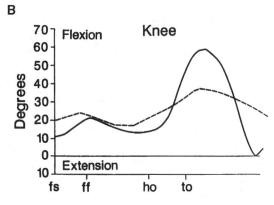

C

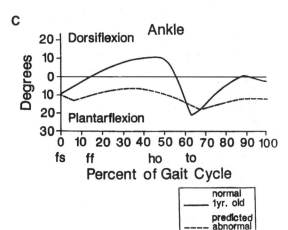

the subtalar joint is inverted approximately 5°, the ankle is in 10° of plantarflexion, the knee is flexed approximately 10°, and the hip is flexed 35°. For Elizabeth, initial contact on the right will probably be made with the ball of the foot due to the decreased range of motion at the ankle joint. The increased plantarflexed position of the ankle joint may also be associated with increased subtalar joint supination[3] and subsequently place the calcaneus in an excessively inverted posture at foot strike. This may cause an instability of the foot as the child begins to bear weight upon it in the next phase of gait. Dorsiflexion will be decreased throughout this phase. The knee will demonstrate increased knee flexion at initial contact and the hip will be abducted and externally rotated due to the tightness of these associated muscles. Greater than normal hip flexion may also be apparent if further functional shortening of the limb is necessary.

During FS-FF (footstrike-footflat), the subtalar joint typically begins to evert. The ankle joint moves into dorsiflexion as the tibia moves anteriorly. The knee begins to flex while the hip begins to extend. As Elizabeth begins to bear weight on this extremity during the period of FS-FF, a decrease in weight shift to the right will be noted. She will be favoring her stronger side, bearing the majority of her weight on her left leg. The child will likely be using the right limb in a strut fashion due to the limited range at the knee and ankle and decreases in muscle strength (knee extensors and plantarflexors), which provides support during this phase. If Elizabeth allowed knee flexion to occur during this period, the moment arm of the ground reaction force vector to the knee joint axis would increase resulting in a greater external flexor torque (Figure 3-2). This places greater demands upon the quadriceps muscle to maintain an upright posture. With full range of motion at the knee, a common compensatory pattern for weakness in the quadriceps is to ambulate on an extended knee. However, assuming Elizabeth has knee flexor tightness, her right knee will be held in a flexed posture throughout contact. In fact, the entire right lower limb will exhibit a fairly fixed posture throughout this loading phase. Cocontraction will likely dominate at the ankle, knee, and hip joints to stabilize them throughout the contact phase. The abducted gait pattern does have the advantage of increasing Elizabeth's overall stability, which is accomplished by increasing her base of support and bringing her center of gravity closer to the ground. However, the abducted gait may also lead to greater mediolateral sway of the center of mass, which would decrease gait efficiency.

FIGURE 3-2 The effect of knee flexion on the moment arm of the vertical ground reaction force (VGRF). Increased knee flexion with its larger moment arm results in a greater external flexion moment that must be resisted by the quadriceps muscle.

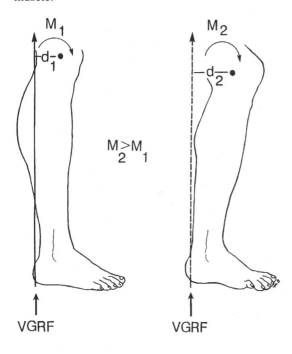

During the early part of FF-HO (foot flat-heel off), the foot normally is continuing to pronate and the ankle dorsiflexes. These joints then reverse their motion as they begin to supinate and plantarflex in preparation for pushoff. The knee follows a similar pattern whereby it is initially flexed and then extends in the last half of this phase. The hip extends throughout this entire period. Due to her range limitations, this child will exhibit decreased dorsiflexion throughout this interval. In fact, HO (heel off) will most likely occur sooner than normal, shortening the relative duration of this phase. The hip and knee will also have decreased excursion for the same reasons as described for the previous phase of gait. Therefore, this portion of gait will be characterized as a continuation of the loading phase whereby limited weight shift will occur and minimal excursion of all joints will be seen. As with the previous phases, the hip will remain in external rotation, placing the foot in a more abducted posture. This facilitates the progression of the leg over the foot, which would otherwise be more difficult given the plantarflexed position of the ankle.

Normally, the next part of the gait cycle is dynamic, with propulsion dominating between HO-TO (heel off-toe off), which requires active concentric action of the gastrocnemius and soleus complex to move the ankle joint from its dorsiflexed position to a plantarflexed position. (The quadriceps and hip extensors are normally quiescent during this time.) This period begins with the foot in a greater amount of plantarflexion than on her unaffected side, thereby decreasing the effective range through which these muscles can act. The combination of the decreased range and decreased strength at this joint results in an ineffective push-off.

Swing is normally characterized by ankle dorsiflexion and hip and knee flexion. A common swing phase compensatory pattern for a plantarflexed ankle involves increased hip and knee flexion providing a functional shortening of the extremity. However, Elizabeth will likely carry through the abducted posture of the hip throughout swing, which is another compensatory strategy. If this mechanism does not provide full compensation, she may either vault over the contralateral side or hike the ipsilateral hip for added clearance. As she prepares for contact, the hip and knee will have greater than normal flexion, and the ankle will be plantarflexed. The cycle would then repeat itself.

Elizabeth's stride characteristics will also be affected. Walking is characterized as having both a single and double support phase of contact. Her stance time on the right will be reduced as she attempts to minimize time spent on this extremity. Most notably, her single support phase will be reduced because she may not be able to fully support her body weight for more than a brief moment. This will result in a decreased stride length on the left. In addition, her cadence will be decreased as a result of the mechanical restraints described previously that hinder her forward progression over the right lower limb. As a consequence, overall walking velocity will also be diminished.

KINETICS

Ground Reaction Forces

Ground reaction forces (GRFs) are the equal and opposite reaction to the forces being applied to the ground. Figure 3-3 exhibits a comparison of normal GRF patterns of two-year-olds during walking[1] to the suggested predicted patterns. Normally, in the vertical direction, there is an initial rise to peak as the subject bears weight onto the support

FIGURE 3-3 Comparison of the vertical, anteroposterior and mediolateral ground reaction forces during walking. The solid line represents typical patterns for normal 2-year-old children (Beck et al, 1981). The dotted line represents the predicted patterns of the child in this case study.

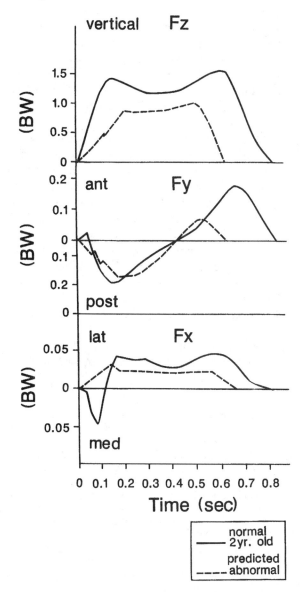

peak), which is associated with propulsion as the foot plantarflexes during pushoff.

With the deficits noted previously, the following abnormalities in the VGRFs would likely be exhibited. Because Elizabeth hesitates to load her right lower limb, the first rise to peak may not be as smooth as normally seen. In addition, the peak will likely be lower since she may not bear full weight on this extremity. The next dip will also be diminished because she was predicted to maintain a fairly fixed posture of the knee and ankle during this phase, thereby lacking the normal mechanisms for the unloading phase. The following rise to peak will also be attenuated due to the lack of active plantarflexion and knee and hip extension noted.

Normal anteroposterior GRFs (APGRFs) are characteristically biphasic with peak values of 0.1 to 0.2 bw. Initially at contact, the center of mass (com), which is moving forward, is behind the foot. The foot applies an anterior force resulting in a braking force by the ground. As the com is approximately over the foot, the APGRFs become 0 crossing the horizontal axis. During propulsion, as the com progresses in front of the foot and the plantarflexors apply their downward and backwardly directed force, the APGRF is directed anteriorly producing a propulsive phase. The impulse-momentum relationship states that the change in velocity is related to the total impulse (integration of the force-time curve). Therefore, if the braking phase impulse is equal to the propulsive phase impulse, total impulse is 0 and velocity is constant. If the braking phase impulse is greater than the propulsive phase impulse, then velocity, over that contact period, decreases. The reverse would be true if the propulsive phase impulse were greater.

Due to the previously noted difficulties in progressing over her lower limb, Elizabeth will spend more time in braking than in propulsion. The initial rise to peak in this dimension of the force may be less smooth than normal. In addition, her deficits in active plantarflexion will greatly reduce the propulsive component of the APGRFs. As in the VGRF, the overall peak forces will be less (due to her lack of complete weight shift); however, the braking phase impulse will probably be greater than the propulsive phase impulse, which results in a decrease in the com velocity during this contact. She may compensate for this reduced velocity by increasing her propulsive phase on her other leg.

Mediolateral GRFs (MLGRFs) are the smallest component of the GRFs and are considered the most variable. Peak forces in the mediolateral

limb. This peak is sometimes called the impact peak and is usually in the range of 1.5 bodyweights (bw). The peak is followed by a period of unweighting as the knee flexes, ankle dorsiflexes, and foot pronates. The vertical GRF (VGRF) dips below bw during this phase, followed by another rise to peak (similar in magnitude to the impact directions are approximately 0.05 bw. As the foot contacts the ground, the hip adducts to bring the foot in medially, creating a medially applied force. Therefore the GRF is laterally directed initially. It is necessary, however, to shift the weight to the opposite side in preparation for the contralateral contact. This requires a laterally applied force by the foot with a resultant medially applied GRF, which typically persists throughout the majority of contact.

Elizabeth's abducted gait pattern will presumably result in an initial laterally applied force to which the ground will respond with a medially directed force. She may have to shift further to the right to apply yet more of a lateral force in order to create a greater medially applied force that will yield the needed change of velocity of her center of mass towards the contralateral foot. As an alternative strategy, she may elect to "pull" medially with the contralateral foot in order to produce the same change in velocity of the com, producing measurable changes in the contralateral GRFs. Overall peak values of the MLGRFs are also expected to decrease because of the unloading on this side.

Joint Moments

Joint moments are typically estimated through equations of inverse dynamics via integration of the segmental kinematics and the ground reaction forces. They are the body's internal response to the external moments being applied to it. A complete description of how torque patterns might be affected will not be addressed here. However, expected overall peak torques would be less at all joints owing to the lower ground reaction forces expected. In addition, the predicted co-contraction that maintains the limb in a fixed posture throughout contact would result in lower net joint moments (if the opposing moments are equal, the net moment would actually be 0). Cocontraction can, however, result in greater joint contact forces,[7] which, if continued over prolonged periods of time, might cause overloading of the articulating surfaces.

NORMALIZATION OF GAIT

Based upon the type of injury Elizabeth sustained, her deficits should soon begin to resolve (barring any complications from the immobilization). She will begin to regain the biomechanical tools (range and strength) necessary for normal movement. Just as muscles atrophy and weaken in response to disuse, the same muscles will hypertrophy and gain strength with increased use.[2] As muscles increase their force of contraction and joint movement is no longer being externally restricted, greater passive stretches to the antagonistic muscles should occur and result in an increased range of motion. (This may also be helped along by her parents through passive range of motion activities.) These initial changes should set off a chain of events leading to normalization of her gait pattern.

As strength gradually increases, Elizabeth will gain the ability to support her weight on her right side. As her dorsiflexion range of motion increases, she will no longer need to abduct and externally rotate the hip in order to advance over her right foot. This will decrease her mediolateral sway making for a more mechanically efficient gait pattern. A positive biomechanical loop will then be developed whereby she will become stronger and able to produce a more normal gait pattern. This will place greater demands on the joints of the lower extremity, which will lead to further range of motion and strength increases, increasing the demands on the joints. This process should continue until she has returned to her preimmobilization status.

REFERENCES

1. Beck RJ et al: Changes in the gait patterns of growing children, *J Bone Joint Surg* 63-A(9):1452, 1981.
2. Lieber RC, editor: *Skeletal muscle structure and function,* Baltimore, 1992, Williams & Wilkins.
3. Lundberg A et al: Kinematics of the ankle and foot complex: plantarflexion and dorsiflexion, *Foot Ankle* 9(4):194, 1989.
4. Simard CP, Spector SA, Edgerton VR: Contractile properties of rat hindlimb muscles immobilized at different lengths, *Exp Neurol* 77:467, 1992.
5. Sutherland DH et al: The development of mature gait, *Bone Joint Surg* 62-A(3):336, 1980.
6. Williams P, Goldspink G: The effect of immobilization on the longitudinal growth of striated muscle fibers, *J Anat* 127:459, 1973.
7. Winter D: *Biomechanics and motor control of human movement,* ed 2, New York, 1990, John Wiley & Sons.

CHAPTER 4

THE EMERGENCE OF GAIT

Susan Higgins
Joseph R. Higgins

KEY TERMS

Adaptation

Arm swing

Leg lift

Motor skill

Self-organization

Toddler gait pattern

Total body response

The case study of Elizabeth offers many interesting examples of what we view as an emergent movement pattern subject to the constraints and opportunities afforded by the child's morphological and developmental status. Elizabeth's evolving gait illustrates the pervasive influence of goal-directedness on the individual's capacity to exploit available resources toward achieving the end—in this case, to locomote.

Before understanding what happened to Elizabeth before and after her injury, we need to explore a few concepts about problem solving and the emergence of movement. This perspective views movements as dynamic, evolving solutions to motor problems having functional significance to the mover. The individual is viewed as actively engaging in the process of accomplishing goals through the use of movement as the problem-solving tool.

THE DEVELOPMENT OF COMPETENCE IN THE YOUNG CHILD

We view the development of motor skill as synonymous with the development of competence—gaining control over one's ability to interact meaningfully with the environment through movement. The development of competence is a lifelong process reflected in ever-evolving behavioral products—movements—that have varying degrees of usefulness to the individual in solving problems. And, it is a process of social significance strongly influenced by social phenomenon. (See, for example, a recent issue of *Human Movement Science,*[19] devoted to the social dynamics of development.)

The process of development is characterized by change—in motor control, in morphology, in strategy, and in one's view of the world—stemming from a unique interplay of genetic and experiential history. Each change has multiplicative consequences on functional behavior and redefines the relationship of the individual to the world.

The development of motor skill throughout life is viewed as a struggle to gain control over available resources that are pertinent to effective interaction with the external surrounds.[18] These resources may be viewed as any characteristic of the individual or the environment that can serve as a tool for problem solving, or as Reed says, that can be incorporated into a biological process.[24]

As characteristics of the individual, resources might be viewed as fundamental functional synergies, structural or physiological characteristics, and cognitive or perceptual processes. As charac-

teristics of the environment, resources might be viewed as the structural and relational characteristics of objects in the physical environment, the field of external forces, and the affordances of sociocultural milieu. Resources may remain relatively stable or change as a function of growth, development, and/or trauma, or, as a function of changes in the external surround. Similarly, that which constitutes a resource and the relative utility of resources may change as the individual, task, or environment changes (Higgins[18] provides further discussion). Clearly, as movers, we must come to know and understand our resources, as well as how they are related to each other and to our purposes for specific tasks or classes of action. We must come to know their utility and develop the cognitive/perceptual skill and the motor control necessary to exploit them toward our purposes. In Elizabeth's case, she had recently emerged from a period of intense exploration of the personal and environmental resources that support (or indeed compel) standing, balancing, and walking.

A gain in competence in motor skill implies an increase in compliance or fit between the individual and the environment through the well-orchestrated organization of resources. We view a large part of skill development as the on going learning and redefining of the relative utility of resources, and, as the acquisition of the means to bring them under control and to adapt them to the activity at hand (see Arend[1] for examples). Our primary means of acquiring this understanding and control is through the movement experiences that underlie our exploratory and performatory activity in the physical and social world.

As part and parcel of the processes underlying the development of motor skill, the individual must be able to extract information about her/himself, the environment, and self-as-agent in the environment. The individual learns what is constant and what can vary about the way self and environment are related. And, this learning occurs amid one's own ever-changing characteristics and under varying environmental and social situations. Noticing relationships, considered by Polanyi[23] to be a largely tacit process, seems to underlie the effective orchestration of resources.

Access to sources of knowledge about the self and world is limited by one's current level of knowledge and control and, of course, biased by it. That is, our perception of the world, and ourselves as agents in that world, is relative to our current capacities. As these capacities change, so do the relevancies of self and environment change and produce unique experiences. (See , for example,

Gibson et al.[11], analysis of the perceptual interests of walkers vs. crawlers.) For example, the achievement of bipedal locomotion, the onset of handedness, the onset of speech, and the change in scale as a function of growth each presents unique experiences and unique constraints that alter the way we view ourselves and the world, alters the way others view us, and alters our problem-solving capacity. And each achievement spurs the (re)organization of supporting resources and reflects itself in the emergence of movement(s) complementary to the new state.

For example, as one achieves bipedal locomotion, surfaces take on new meaning. The individual must now attend to those aspects of surface and object that afford support and pathway. Chairs are no longer "to go under" or "to pull up on," they are "to go around" or "to hold on to." Similarly, when handedness becomes established, the role of the preferred and nonpreferred hand in our actions is redefined and biases what can be considered an effective environmental structure to support our actions. We then perceive the environment from this bias so that it will complement our orientation within it in light of the demands of the task. At the same time, the way in which body parts and internal/external forces are related to each other changes to suit the new state(s). Once any significant achievement is attained (i.e., crawling or walking), old relationships supporting previous behaviors are no longer relevant and quickly disappear. They will only reappear if they again become relevant because of some trauma or change that makes them the preferred relationship—but even then, they will be altered in some way that is suitable to the new state (Thelen and Ulrich[29] offer a detailed treatment of emergent relationships).

The gain in control over the understanding, orchestration, and deployment of resources during infancy and early childhood is apparent in the child's products—her/his movements. And, her/his movements obviously appear very different in infancy than they do in early childhood or adulthood or old age. What remains the same is the *responsiveness* of movement form to currently effective constraints inherent in the morphology, physical and social environment, and field of external forces. Also pervasive is the need to gain control over the factors that influence the organization of movement and over the production of the movement itself. Each gain in control attained by the child is viewed as enhancing her/his competence and redefining her/his field of opportunity—i.e., making accessible that which was previously inaccessible.

We do not feel that infants (or adults for that matter) are gaining control over specific patterns of movement or neural outflow. Rather, we view these patterns the emerge as a function of maturation, experience, and environmental context. Producing a particular pattern of movement is not the likely goal of the infant. Rather, we view infants as eminently interested in their surroundings for the primary purpose of acting within it—calling mom or dad, shaking the crib, grasping the object, getting to the table, clapping hands, and so on. We view infants as gaining control over the orchestration of any available skeletomuscular and neuromotor processes and social or environmental phenomenon to support this endeavor of on-going action amidst ever-changing personal and environmental characteristics. Achieving the goal has primacy.

To achieve the goal, the individual will self-organize to complement (reflect) the demands of the action in the current context.[21,28] This self-organization is reflected in the spatial and temporal organization of the movement. The details of the movement, whether it subserves exploration, communication, object manipulation, body stability, body transport, or (more often) multiple purposes, will emerge as a function of context. And context is defined as the momentarily effective state of the environment and the individual at the time of the action. We view the spatial and temporal characteristics of the movement, and the strategies supporting it, as a reflection of its underlying neuromotor control. The movement itself is a coherent, dynamic structure acquiring its organization by reference to some goal[17] and emerging as an adaptation to the constraints imposed by the infant's morphology, cognitive level, and perceptual skill; the field of external forces; and the nature of physical and social objects and events.[13]

The organization of movement is a total body response to context and purpose. A change in any of these variables will result in a change in the organization of movement. The total body response represents many nested interactive "dialectics" among body parts and processes that serve to mutually restrict and challenge each other.*

---

* As Gordon[12] points out, the act of reaching out for an object is limited by the current ability to stabilize the torso. Yet, the very act of reaching (and over-reaching) incites a compensatory response from the supporting musculature that will indeed serve to strengthen and differentiate itself, in turn laying the groundwork to enhance the extent of reach. Gordon aptly refers to this as an example of a proximal-distal dialectic. But, this idea is equally applicable to all emerging compensatory relationships.

Understanding and controlling these dialectics enhances competence and spurs further change. The organization of movement at any one point in time represents a context-appropriate, compensatory, coordinative relationship among body parts and between body and environment. A large part of motor skill learning is devoted to the progressive understanding and control over the coordinative relationships, however transient.

With reference to walking, we view a particular gait or manner of walking to emerge as a function of needs, potentialities, and limitations (as will be further explored in our subsequent chapter on learning). The idea is to locomote—to develop competence in locomotion. As an early walker, Elizabeth is not learning a walking pattern. Rather, she is learning to manage her body and any objects she carries or manipulates while she locomotes. She will experience any number of gait patterns toward this end. She is learning the ways and means of allocating her available resources in the service of a particular locomotor problem, be it to run, get to her playroom, or go to her parents. The solutions to the particular motor problem will involve different styles and rates of gait, slowing, stopping, starting and restarting; different pathways; and different implications for arm and leg use.

What follows is a discussion of five weeks in Elizabeth's life during which she experiences changes in morphological resources underlying locomotion and, over time, establishes a limited number of locomotor patterns that serve a limited range of solutions. She experiences a repertoire of gaits that serve her unique needs and emerge directly from available resources.

ANALYSIS OF ELIZABETH'S CASE

Before the Injury

Elizabeth is a child who has recently achieved independent locomotion. Implied is that she has the prerequisites or substrates necessary to support this act—i.e., strength of leg extensors, the ability to achieve lateral stability, etc. Her locomotor pattern, as Tomlinson tells us, is a "typical toddler gait pattern." Presumably, her parents, educated in physical therapy, have provided an environment that encourages developmentally appropriate activity—that is, activity which encourages the child to participate in the process of problem solving and exploration without knowingly imposing preconceived notions of how the world should be viewed or how the motor problem should be solved. We also assume that Elizabeth has had

time to explore herself as a moving system in many environmental contexts and has reaped the physical and social rewards of achieving independent locomotion.

Typically, in infancy, walking is studied as a leg action that occurs either during independent locomotion or during induced stepping on a treadmill. We believe this to be a limited view of this act. Walking is not a leg action, but rather a total body response to context and purpose. Campos and Berthenthal[6] argue that the achievement of self-produced locomotion plays a pervasive role in development. It produces unique experiences with regard to maintaining equilibrium and enhancing visual attention to surface of support. Similarly, it makes the infant aware of the constraints and opportunities of her/his own physical structure as she/he becomes cooperatively linked to support this precarious act. This cooperation is not limited to the development of a coordinative relationship among body segments and the environment. It also extends to the corralling of social cooperation (from caregivers, parents, other children) to facilitate this complex action. The onset of walking and the constraints of bipedal locomotion change the relevancies in the physical and social environment. Thus, the attainment of bipedal locomotion induces or corrals a subset of synergies to support the emerging product. All synergies will essentially support a basic, compelling set of substrates that underlie bipedal locomotion: the action of a central pattern generator operating on an upright system with very specific morphological characteristics. The ensuing walk has a form that complements this complicated array of variables.

As argued in a previous paper[17], walking is viewed as a dynamic form that itself can undergo transformation and change and emerges when its supporting substrates are present in an individual/environment. The form of the walk emerges in response to the surrounding conditions that sustain it. Since these surrounding conditions are likely to vary and be subject to perturbation, the walk must be responsive to the environment and tolerate a bandwidth of perturbations so its purpose prevails. If these conditions are exceeded (i.e., over-the-ground speed exceeds that which a walk can tolerate or a morphological change that precludes a walking form), the walk will transform into another form—perhaps a run or a crawl that may or may not be suited to the overall goal of locomotion. The form of locomotion that emerges is a self-organizing and meaningful response to the individual-environment interaction under currently prevailing conditions (see also Reference 7). The details of the form are not specified by inherent principles or purposes, but rather emerge during the course of the action. Gait patterns subserve the mechanical, morphological, and environmental demands of the task, embodying these demands in its spatial and temporal organization.

A Toddler's Gait.   Elizabeth's gait prior to the injury reflects her particular developmental status and physical structure. As can be seen in Figure 4-1, an early walker has a movement form that emerges in response to the morphology that supports it. In this case, the top-heavy toddler remains very erect, waddling from side to side (rather than the characteristic falling forward and regaining of balance with each step that appears in later childhood). The top-heavy toddler is incapable of controlling her/his mass (in the confines of a walk) by propelling it outside of the base of support. Thus, the walking strategy is often one that ensures that the center of gravity is minimally displaced in a forward direction.

At the same time, the leg action is relatively undifferentiated. The leg does not really swing.* The lateral displacement that is characteristic of a top-heavy toddler does not compel a leg swing. Rather, it compels a leg lift with its concomitant hip and knee flexion and relatively rigid ankle. It also compels a sideward shift of weight to the supporting leg—a preparatory extension of the nonsupporting leg and a "plop" (or lateral reshifting of weight) to the newly extended leg with the now nonsupporting leg often acting as a cantilever for balance. The primary action occurs at the hip and knee, with the spine and arms acting in a compensatory manner to complement the side-to-side waddle. When no object is being manipulated, the arms are generally used as cantilevers in the maintenance of balance. Arm swing is not mechanically necessary in a lateral, waddling walk. Arm swing only emerges when leg swing emerges.† Clearly, an infant needs no arm swing. The toddlers arms are not linked to the leg swing, but rather to postural stability and to object manipulation. In a toddler's walk, the entire body has assumed a coordinative relationship that is com-

pensatory and dialectic. The underlying constraints influencing the basic form of the walk similarly apply to the many different derivatives that the walk will assume as it adapts to changing goals and circumstances.

Elizabeth, through preliminary months of exploration and gains in strength and balance, is familiar enough with the affordances of her anatomical linkages to modulate the forces around her joints to produce torques where needed in support of a walk. That is, she has solved the force problems underlying the achievement of upright posture, lateral stability, and translatory motion. She has begun to learn how to selectively apply her strength to the particulars of the walking problem. She is probably thrilled (as are her parents) and focused on her new skill. Her degree of competence is complementary to her morphology and to her ability to control it. Within these limitations, she has probably just begun to or will soon shift from focusing on the act of walking in itself, to focusing on what walking now affords her—to get to Dad, to get the milk, the toy, etc.—and to simply experience the joy of accomplishment and the thrill of speed and freedom inherent in the walk itself. And now, she falls.

After the Injury

In the Cast   Spending 23 days in a long-leg plaster cast is a unique experience. What was a lower limb system with eight degrees of freedom about the hip, knee, and ankle is suddenly reduced to a system of three degrees of freedom about the hip alone. What was a shared responsibility among hip, knee, and ankle musculature for management of this system and the forces it received during weight bearing is now solely borne by the hip musculature. What was a system capable of manipulating moment of inertia around the joints for temporal and force advantages has been reduced to a system incapable of reducing moment of inertia about the hip—a temporal and force disadvantage of a long, rigid lever. What was a leg of a specific weight is now heavier due to the added weight of the cast.

The impact of these changes in the weight, degrees of freedom, and dynamic characteristics of the leg is felt throughout the body. And even though this analysis is focused on walking, the morphological change imposed by the cast will impact on all activities and emergent movement solutions. All previously developed cooperative relationships have to be redefined.

In the case of walking, preeminent are those relationships underlying lateral support (Thelen et al,[28] and Higgins[14-16]) and movement of the

---

* Leg swing emerges in a more mature walk in response to the stretching of the rear leg in a forward/backward stride, the pushoff of the rear foot and the forward displacement of the torso. A leg swing is exhibited by an individual who is capable of incorporating mechanical and reactive phenomena in the organization of movement.[16]

† Some excellent sources for the analysis of infant and mature walking patterns include Bril and Breniere[5]; Craik et al.[8]; Forssberg[10]; Murrary[22]; and Thelen, et al.[29]

FIGURE 4-1 Top-heavy walker. An early walker has a movement form that emerges in response to the morphology. In this case, the top-heavy toddler remains very erect, waddling from side to side. From Wickstrom.[30]

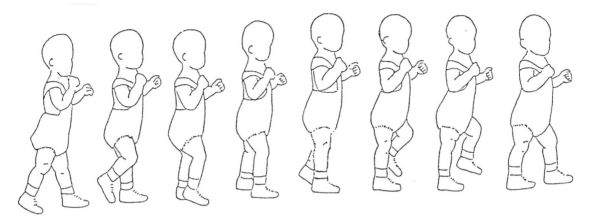

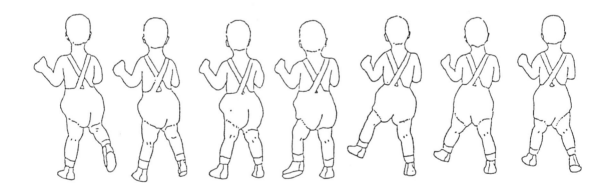

casted leg. The roles and relationships among torso, affected limb, and nonaffected limb will alter. For example, the abdominal and other spinal musculature may assume an increased burden in movement synergies; she can no longer use knee action for bringing the foot off the ground in the "swing" phase or in the propulsive phase. Indeed, the fact that the knee and ankle are restricted by the cast poses a different muscle control problem both for the support and "swing" phases of the movement. In addition, the contralateral hip musculature will play an entirely different role in controlling the walk. So much so that the child may adopt a totally different strategy in the way

that the weight is shifted to the unaffected side. The timing between lower limb segments will be altered to deal with the asymmetrical characteristics between the legs and the neuromotor and biomechanical implications of such asymmetry. The lack of "give" in the "new" leg redefines its set of affordances in the infant's repertoire of actions. Everything changes—except the need to locomote.

On the other hand, the "new" leg is less complicated to control than the "old" leg. There are fewer degrees of freedom to be regulated. The stiffness about the knee and ankle now come "for free" in terms of muscle force. The rigid cast provides instant stability and resistance and produces a new complement of reactive forces that can potentially be transferred to the torso. This "new" leg has different capacities. It is a new tool.

It took Elizabeth 14 days to adopt a pattern of gait that compensated for the additional weight and restrictions imposed by the cast. During this adjustment period, Elizabeth was learning about the new leg, learning how to use her available strength in order to move it to suit her purposes, and learning a new complement between casted leg, noncasted leg, torso, and surround.

Elizabeth's initial week was apparently spent without self-initiated transport. We suspect that she was exploring her new leg in a limited fashion and subsequently developing a newly defined muscle aggregate to move the limb (and concomitantly, the strength needed in the aggregate). Exploration would answer such tacit questions as: How much does this leg weigh? How much force does it take to lift it? Does it hurt? What can it do? I'd like to go to my play area, how can I get there? Simply attempting movement in a supine position will activate muscle synergies, test their efficacy, and begin to develop the strength and tentative coordination underlying use of the new leg. This is not idle time.

Within a week, she was creeping. Elizabeth's resort to creeping was a reversion to a previously experienced (and probably mastered) form of locomotion that poses little danger from falls. She did not yet have adequate control over the new leg in order to incorporate it into an upright locomotor pattern. Her goal was to locomote and she marshalled the synergies she was currently able to control in order to achieve her goal. By using a creep, she became increasingly familiar with the affordances of her new leg and its implications for the rest of her body. The position of her leg in creeping was suited to the constraints of the cast, the capabilities of the remaining joints and musculature, and the demands of the task—it worked.

Tomlinson reports that within two weeks she was able to walk upright for short distances with the right leg abducted and externally rotated. She spent minimal time in stance on the right and had minimal weight shift to the right. This gait pattern is one that seems complementary to the constraints of a stiff right leg and the restrictions underlying a toddler's walk. Actually, a casted leg is more suited to be incorporated into a toddler gait than into a more mature gait pattern (i.e., one demanding a swing). Let's examine how the emergent form may be construed as complementary to the toddler's constraints.

The abducted right leg is quite suitable for a "typical" toddler's gait—that is, it is in a good position to receive the body's weight as it is laterally shifted to that side. We imagine that by externally rotating the leg, it is placed in a position to be lifted by the stronger hip flexors during the "swing" phase. An externally rotated leg also places the foot in a better position to support pivoting in any direction. Nonetheless, the abducted and externally rotated casted leg was seemingly used as a walking stick. It was a stiff receiver of lateral forces which were then transferred back to the body.

The report that she spent minimal time standing on the casted leg and minimal time during weight shift to that side may indicate that the casted leg was primarily used for lateral support and as a rebounding device—a natural use for a stiff leg. Standing on the casted leg in single support would seem counterproductive, a mismatch between form and function. The knee and ankle would not be available to "give" in the maintenance of equilibrium or in assisting in a step in any direction. Thus, time spent in stance on the casted leg may have been appropriately minimized in order to avoid falling. At the same time, the minimized time spent on the right side may have resulted from both the way she used the leg and the inherent (biomechanically derived) temporal demands of incorporating a casted leg into a toddler's walk. Since the leg appeared to be used as a rebounding device, time in stance would indeed be minimized. (It would be interesting to see if a corresponding increase in stance time of the unaffected leg occurred and to more closely examine the shifts in the spatial organization of the movement of the unaffected leg.) The shift in the spatial and temporal organization of the walk is an indication of her solution to the lateral support and propulsive problems so critical to independent locomotion.

During this time, Elizabeth became somewhat used to controlling the casted leg by using newly grouped muscle aggregates. She very likely developed a neuromotor control strategy that exploited the cast and organized its reaction force into the structure of the movement. Similarly, she learned to exploit the affordances of the noncasted leg and torso in this newly fashioned walk.

Out of the Cast Apparently, when the cast was removed, Elizabeth had no (or minimal) changes in range of motion and strength. Her behavior upon seeing and feeling her healed leg is interesting. She takes time to explore it in a number of settings. Again, before she is able to use the leg, she must understand what it affords her. The time she spent in the cast, moving a single-joint leg, left her with no immediately available strategy for simultaneously and cooperatively controlling the hip, knee, and ankle. Recall that the knee and ankle were held in position, thus freeing the musculature from the task of controlling their position. The positive outcome is a simpler system to control. The negative outcome is a loss of (or failure to develop) coordination among successive lower limb segments in support of leg action. This is revealed in Elizabeth's inconsistent use of the ankle and knee and in the failure of her strategies to provide the stiffness needed for support. There also seemed to be no ground-up or peripherally induced coordination from the ankle to the knee and hip. She had no control strategy to apply stiffness about these joints in relation to her weight-bearing tasks. The cast had provided this control, but now she must rally the resources to do so.

Tomlinson does not describe how the child kicked her leg during diaper change—only that both legs seemed capable of exerting the same amount of force. Implied is that the failure of her healed leg to supply the support needed for locomotion was not due to any loss in strength. Rather, it appears to be due to a loss in control over how to apply available strength to this new system.

Again, the need to locomote is pervasive, not the need to produce a "normalized" walk. Elizabeth applies a successful strategy to walk by the afternoon of the day in which the cast was removed. Not surprisingly, she reverts to using the same position that the leg assumed while in the cast (similar to her reversion to creeping when the cast was new). Her right leg is held in a relatively fixed position allowing her the freedom to locomote without the added problem of learning to control and coordinate eight degrees of freedom. Clearly her interest is in mobility. However, maintaining this fixed leg position was at a cost to her energy; it did not come "for free" as with the cast. This pattern was to break down after ten days.

Reverting to her cast gait seems likely for a number of reasons. Elizabeth had not been walking long enough prior to the injury to have established a working relationship among lower limb segments that she could reliably apply after the injury. The cast gait was characterized by the casted leg being used as a rebounding stick. Elizabeth then attempted to use her healed leg in a similar fashion. However, the healed leg is not suited for this purpose. It is not naturally stiff; it

needs to be held stiff, which is an inefficient solution and not complementary to the characteristics of the healed leg. This solution cannot endure. Elizabeth will experience a redefinition of the muscle aggregates supporting the walk (and all other activities). As with the cast-on experience, she will need to make a crucial integrative adjustment in the control of the hip musculature (on both sides) now that the knee and ankle are again free to participate directly in the movement.

The first sign of this adaptation is observed at the ankle. She appears to release it from its held position. That this first release occurred most distally is interesting. The now floppy ankle can begin to exert its ground-up influence on the knee, hip, and spine, allowing a transfer of energy. Tomlinson indicates that the gait pattern was more symmetric, with less weight shift to the right and less time in single support on the right. Elizabeth is now in transition. She occasionally applies her stiff leg control strategy and occasionally allows her ankle and leg to relax. The latter strategy facilitates a transfer of energy through the knee and hip and indicates a neural adaptation of generating torques at selected points in the step cycle rather than throughout. This later pattern is of course the more efficient—especially for a three-joint leg system that is on the verge of a pendular swing. She is beginning to incorporate reactive phenomena in the use of the leg, to exploit the pendular capabilities of the leg, and to apply stiffness only when needed. The spatial and temporal organization of the movement has shifted to complement both the characteristics of her freely movable leg and her ability to control it.

Some Comments on the Adjustment Periods

It is interesting that the periods of transition to cast-on and cast-off locomotor forms are approximately the same. Elizabeth's movement emerged in each condition at about the same rate, which could be a reflection of her movement potentiality at this period of developmental time.* During these transitional periods, new brain-behavior-body-environment relationships are explored and exploited. It is often believed that adjustments made after the removal of a cast are due to a loss of strength in the casted musculature. However, it

---

* Dependent upon the nature and type of injury, these periods of adjustment or adaptation may exhibit a very different time course. It would be interesting to examine the duration and transformations occurring in the transitional periods in older children and adults with comparable injuries.

might be more useful to view the transitional process as one of learning (or relearning) to use the available strength. Considerable evidence now exists to support the notion that the transitional period in developing a new locomotor of any form may not be much a strength development issue as it is a matter of learning how to apply available strength to a new set of conditions—particularly in the lateral hip musculature.[3,9,25,27] As mentioned previously, changes in coordination of the affected leg during the "cast-on" period altered the hip action on both sides. The musculature responsible for the observed adjustments was used in a very different way. Elizabeth's musculature had not lost strength; but rather the net neural drive to the musculature had been applied and expressed in a different way. Neural adjustments in force parameterization, based on exploration and experience, characterize the shift or transition to a new locomotor form—what many current investigators refer to as neural adaptation.[2,4,20,26] The idea that there may be a developmentally-based neural adaptation time would be interesting to pursue.

In Conclusion

It might be suggested that what is being learned or being acquired by Elizabeth during this time—preaccident, "cast-on," and "cast-off"—is the ability to generate and control variations of gaits, each of which serves her needs and goals at a particular moment. As more and more gaits emerge, each in relation to a specific goal and set of constraints, she will have learned a variety of ways or means of allocating resources to solve particular locomotor problems.

It is not at all likely that Elizabeth was thinking about how to use her leg. She was thinking about locomoting. Her complex control strategy prior to the accident was not applicable to the casted leg (i.e., which offered its own stiffness). She quickly exploited the characteristics of the casted leg, incorporating its properties into the organization of the movement. When the cast was removed, the leg had capabilities that she could not currently control. Thus, the time in transition after the removal of the cast accomplished two things: (1) it gave her the opportunity to (re)discover the affordances of a system with eight degrees of freedom using an initial walking style that was familiar, safe, and easy to control; and (2) it allowed the necessary time for neural adaptation.

Throughout it all, Elizabeth achieves her overall goal of locomotion. Despite the parents' concern over what they felt was a lingering "cast" gait, a complementary movement pattern emerged, which Tomlinson refers to as "normal." Our perspective would beg consideration for all the patterns that emerged to be viewed as "normal." Whether they are acceptable to the parent, therapist, or child/adult is another issue.

What is quite nice about this case study is the clear example of continuously evolving gait patterns each demonstrating responsiveness to Elizabeth's evolving states. Given time and freedom to explore in a safe and nurturing environment, Elizabeth achieved her goals utilizing the resources she had to her avail. Her movement solutions were complementary to those resources and approached efficiency for each unique set of conditions. Inappropriate solutions did not prevail when conditions changed. There was no need to teach Elizabeth to walk, but rather, to support her in her goal-directed activity. Elizabeth solved the problem.

We are delighted that there was no attempt to "normalize" her locomotor pattern. We are not so sure that parents, significant others, and/or therapists would play such a passive role with an older child or an adult. Freedom of movement in a safe environment by an active problem solver is a powerful and trustworthy means of supporting the emergence of motor skill.

REFERENCES

1. Arend S: Developing the substrates of skillful movement, *Motor Skills: Theory into Practice* 4(1):1, 1981.
2. Binder-Macleod SA: Force-frequency relation in skeletal muscle. Reported at Conference on Motor Learning, Teachers College, Columbia University, March 1992.
3. Bohannon RW: Significant relationships exist between muscle group strengths following stroke, *Clin Rehab* 4:27, 1990.
4. Bohannon RW: Relevance of muscle strength to gait performance in patients with neurologic disability, *J Neurol Rehab* 3(2):97, 1989.
5. Bril B, Breniere Y: Steady-state velocity and temporal structure of gait during the first six months of autonomous walking, *Hum Movement Science* 8:99, 1989.
6. Campos JJ, Bertenthal BI: Locomotion and psychological development in infancy. In Morrison F, Lord K, Keating D, editors: *Applied developmental psychology,* New York, 1989, Academic Press.
7. Clark JE, Whitall J, Phillips SJ: Human interlimb coordination: the first 6 months of independent walking, *Dev Psychobiol* 21(5):445, 1988.
8. Craik R, Herman R, Finley FR: Human solutions for locomotion: interlimb coordination. In Herman RM et al, editors: *Neural control of locomotion,* New York, 1976, Plenum Press.
9. Enoka RM, Fuglevand AJ: Neuromuscular basis of the maximum voluntary force capacity of muscle.

Reported at Conference on Motor Learning, Teachers College, Columbia University, March 1992.

10. Forssberg H: Ontogeny of human locomotor control: infant stepping, supported locomotion and transition to independent locomotion, *Exp Brain Res* 57:480, 1985.

11. Gibson EJ et al: Detection of the traversability of surfaces by crawling and walking infants, *J Exp Psychol* [Human Percept] 13(4):533, 1987.

12. Gordon J: Personal communication.

13. Higgins JR: *Human movement: an integrated approach,* St. Louis, 1977, Mosby.

14. Higgins JR, Higgins S: Temporal and spatial characteristics of infant walking within the first 10 days of independent locomotion: The effects of arm/hand complex use and locomotor patterns. Reported at Motor Development Academy, AAHPERD, April 1990, New Orleans, Louisiana.

15. Higgins JR et al: The development of motor skill in infancy: A paradigm for study, onset of infant locomotion, posture and reaching and grasping, and risk taking and the development of motor competence. Motor Development Academy, AAHPERD, March 31, 1990, New Orleans, Louisiana.

16. Higgins JR: Observations of infant to toddler transition: Time spent in single leg support. Unpublished research project, Teachers College, Columbia University, 1991.

17. Higgins S: Movement as an emergent form: its structural limits, *Hum Movement Science* 4:119, 1985.

18. Higgins S: Motor skill acquisition. In Rothstein JM, editor: *Movement science,* monograph, American Physical Therapy Association, 1991.

19. *Hum Movement Science,* 1992, Special Issue: The social dynamics of development.

20. Jones DA, Rutherford OM: Human muscle strength training: the effects of three different regimes and the nature of the resultant changes, *J Physiol* 391, 1, 1987.

21. Kelso JAS, Schoner S: Self-organization of coordinative movement patterns, *Hum Movement Science* 7(1):27, 1988.

22. Murray MP: Gait as a total pattern of movement, *Am J Phys Med* 46(1):290, 1967.

23. Polanyi M: *The tacit dimension,* New York, 1966, Doubleday.

24. Reed E: Applying the theory of action systems to the study of motor skills. In Meijer O, Roth K, editors: *Studying complex movement phenomena: the motor action controversy,* Amsterdam, 1988, North-Holland.

25. Rutherford OM, Jones DA: The role of learning and coordination in strength training, *Eur J Appl Physiol* 55:100, 1986.

26. Rutherford OM: Muscular coordination and strength training: Implications for injury rehabilitation, *Sports Med* 5:196, 1988.

27. Sale DG: Neural adaptation to resistance training, *Med Sci Sports Exerc* 20(5):135, 1988.

28. Thelen E, Kelso JAS, Fogel A: Self-organizing systems in infant motor development, *Dev Review* 7:39, 1987.

29. Thelen E, Ulrich BD: Hidden skills: A dynamic systems analysis of treadmill stepping during the first year, *Monographs of the Society for Research in Child Development* 56(1):1991.

30. Wickstrom RW: *Fundamental motor patterns,* Philadelphia, 1983, Lea & Febiger.

CHAPTER 5

Dynamical Systems Perspective

Jane E. Clark

Key Terms

Attractor

Control parameters

Environmental constraints

Intralimb coordination

Interlimb coordination

Organism constraints

Task constraints

From the dynamical systems perspective, the case report on Elizabeth presents a good example of a "dynamical system" in action. A dynamical system is a system that changes. Clearly, Elizabeth (i.e., the dynamical system) has changed. From the newly walking infant to the casted hobbler who finally returns to independent walking, Elizabeth's walking behavior has evolved, dissolved, and reemerged. Why have these changes occurred? How does the dynamical systems approach explain what happened to Elizabeth?

To begin, the dynamical systems approach views any behavior as arising from a multitude of constraints. Elizabeth's behavior at any time in her life emerges from the constraints within herself (organism constraints), those constraints in her environment (environmental constraints), and those constraints inherent in the task at hand (task constraints). All these constraints shape the observed behavior. So when we see Elizabeth taking her first steps at 9 months, we must recognize that the constraints within and surrounding Elizabeth have come together in such a way that when Elizabeth is confronted with the task of getting from here to there, she walks. After her fall, her leg is casted and with it comes major changes in organism constraints. For example, the cast changes the leg's mass and fixes the ankle at 45° of plantarflexion and the knee at 30° of flexion. But again with these new organism constraints, Elizabeth finds a behavioral regimen that permits the achievement of her goal of locomotion.

When one or more constraints are capable of changing the system's behavior, it is presumed that we have found a control parameter(s). Control parameters are those constraints that, when scaled in magnitude, move the system from one state to another. For example, while not necessarily positive in its effect, the cast and its ancillary constraint changes (i.e., leg mass and joint immobilization) became control parameters—changing Elizabeth's ambulatory behavior. Normally, we are seeking control parameters that have positive effects on behavior. Indeed, to distinguish control parameters that seem to restrict or hold back development, we refer to them by a separate term, *rate limiter*. In other words, the cast was a rate limiter to Elizabeth's walking development. Once the rate limiter is eliminated, walking development should resume.

But after the cast was removed, Elizabeth did not immediately return to the walking behavior she evidenced prior to casting. Why? The answer again lies in changing constraints. Casting not only affected the locomotor behavior, but it also may well have affected other organism constraints (e.g., strength, range of motion). While the case report indicates that Elizabeth's range of motion (ROM) and strength appeared normal, neither of these organism constraints was tested in the task context. System behavior, including ROM and strength, depend on the task. According to the case report, anecdotal observations of these characteristics were made. But is it possible that if ROM and strength were examined in upright bipedal gait, they may well have shown deficits? The case report mentions that Elizabeth was frustrated, presumably because her right leg did not provide reliable support. Is it not possible that after twenty-three days in a cast Elizabeth's lower leg muscles were weakened for a task such as walking where, for brief periods, she must completely support her body weight on one leg? Just as the cast had acted as a rate limiter, now one or more organism constraints (e.g., strength, ROM, and/or some other system characteristic) would seem to be holding back Elizabeth's locomotor development.

While concepts such as constraints and control parameters may well resonate metaphorically with those seeking to diagnose and treat gait disorders, it is the analytical tools and concepts of dynamical systems that provide its strongest arguments for serious consideration. Using a dynamical systems approach, Elizabeth's behavior can be captured in a low-dimensional description that we can then study for its stability and loss of stability as control parameters are manipulated. For example, work in our laboratory has shown that both interlimb and intralimb coordination can be modelled as coupled nonlinear limit cycle oscillators[1,2]. This type of model can be mapped as an attractor (i.e., a limit cycle or coupled limit cycles, described as a torus). As illustrated in the chapter by Clark, a low-dimensional description of walking, such as that offered by a limit cycle attractor (or coupled limit cycle systems), captures the behavior of a highly complex system. Thus, if we were to study Elizabeth's behavior prior to her fall, during her casting, and then in the time period immediately after the cast's removal, we should be able to see the effect on the attractor of the changing control parameters. Particularly interesting would be the time from the cast's removal until the reemergence of a normal gait pattern. Systems in transitions, such as Elizabeth's following the removal of the cast, provide a unique window on understanding the operative constraints. By manipulating task constraints, such as providing support, we may well reveal the rate limiter to the return of Elizabeth's normal gait.

In summary, the dynamical systems perspective on the case report sees Elizabeth's ambulation as a function of constraints found in Elizabeth herself, her environment, and the task she seeks to undertake. When one or more of these constraints are changed to some critical level, a new behavior will emerge. While changes in some constraints may well have a positive effect on behavior, clearly others, such as the cast, may have a negative impact. The important point, however, is that to change behavior you must change one or more constraints.

REFERENCES

1. Clark JE, Phillips SJ: A longitudinal study of intra-limb coordination in the first year of independent walking: a dynamical systems analysis, *Child Dev* 64:1143, 1993.
2. Clark JE, Truly TL, Phillips SJ: On the development of walking as a limit cycle system. In Thelen E, Smith L, editors: *Dynamical systems in development: applications,* Cambridge, Mass, MIT Press (in press).

PART II

CONCEPTUAL FRAMEWORKS FOR AMBULATION

♦ The development of the tools for measuring gait has preceded consensus on how the body elaborates this complicated task. This section provides a detailed review of several theories developed to explain how walking is produced. A mathematical model, a neural control model, a motor learning model and a dynamical systems theory model are each presented as a conceptual framework for understanding human locomotion. The chapter on motor learning also provides a link between theory and practice by offering a conceptual framework for the reacquisition of gait.

C H A P T E R   6

MATHEMATICAL MODEL

Joseph Mansour

KEY TERMS

Body segment parameters

Degrees of freedom

Free body diagram

Inverse dynamics

Joint movements

Lagrangian mechanics

Model

Newtonian mechanics

Rigid body

Support moment

This chapter is concerned with and limited to the mathematical modeling of mechanical features of gait. It should be clear from other chapters in this section that understanding the mechanics of gait is not the only area where models could be of use. However, as we will see, a mechanical model of gait has many applications. In addition to being used to investigate purely mechanical characteristics of walking, a mechanical model of gait could also be used in conjunction with other modeling approaches described in this book.

Models are idealized representations of a system or phenomenon. They can be conceptual, experimental, analytical, or a combination of these classifications. A "rigid body" is an example of a *conceptual* description of material behavior. In a rigid body the distance between two arbitrarily chosen points is always fixed. Certainly, this is an idealization since every material deforms when loaded. However, idealizing deformable behavior as rigid has proven to be useful for many applications. *Experimental* models may be used to verify a calculation, discover a new behavior, or in situations where analytical models would be inaccurate or where insufficient information is available to develop a mathematical model. For example, scale models are sometimes used to experimentally evaluate the characteristics of a ship or airplane. Experimental "animal models" are sometimes used to study abnormal biological processes, such as the etiology of osteoarthritis.[38] *Analytical* models are used in engineering and physical science where there is sufficient knowledge to construct a mathematical theory or where experimental measurements cannot be made. There are many aspects of gait analysis where quantities cannot be measured experimentally. For example, joint moments cannot be measured but they can be estimated from a mathematical model. Rigid body dynamics is an example of an analytical model.

Models are usually developed to investigate some specific behavior. Certain significant mechanical characteristics of gait warrant the development of a model. Gait is produced by the interaction of active and passive forces and gravity. Active forces are generated by the contraction of skeletal muscle. Passive forces are generated from the deformation of noncontractile tissues surrounding the joints (for example, ligament and joint capsule). This interplay of forces acting on material bodies and their accompanying movement is clearly described by a mathematical model based on the laws of physics. Using such a model it is possible to determine features of gait, such as

joint moments, that cannot be measured experimentally. Such a model can also be used to investigate the sensitivity of an output to changes in input parameters. For example, the sensitivity of the motion (output) to changes in muscle forces (input) can be evaluated using a mathematical model of gait. A sensitivity analysis is not limited to this muscle-force limb-motion example. Gait is produced by the coordinated action of multiple muscles producing the movement of many limb segments. Limb segment motions are coupled; that is, the movement of one segment affects the movement of other segments. Models may be used to investigate the sensitivity of limb segment dynamic interactions.

A mathematical model that "walks" under the action of joint moments or muscle forces can be used to evaluate theories of locomotion. For example, are the six "determinants of gait"[44] necessary for normal walking or is the idea of a "support moment"[50] generally applicable to gait? While such ideas can be tested using a mathematical model of gait, it is important to recognize that a purely mechanical model would not necessarily provide any insight into the physiological mechanisms by which muscle forces are controlled. Control issues can, however, be investigated using a mathematical model of gait when the control system is well characterized. Functional Electrical Stimulation (FES) systems are being developed to restore upper and lower extremity movement in people with paraplegia and tetraplegia.[11, 33] Systems that provide gait-like movements are being used by persons with paraplegia. In such systems electrical signals are applied to the muscles through either surface or indwelling electrodes. The pulse width and interpulse interval of these signals may be controlled to produce the desired muscle force and accompanying joint movement. The control of these quantities is quite complex owing to the properties of muscle and the need to control multiple joints. Many controllers can and have been designed for use in functional electrical stimulation systems. However, the testing of these controllers on human subjects is costly in terms of both risk to the subject and laboratory time. As an alternative to human tests, testing is done in a model environment by coupling the controller to a mathematical model of gait.

Well-characterized models of gait or other movements can also be used to evaluate experimental surgeries such as tendon transfers or joint arthrodesis. Transferring a tendon causes the point of application of a muscle force to change; it is a well-defined mechanical process describable in mathematical terms in a model. What could be more difficult to describe is the change in passive moment at a joint, which could result from the surgery. Arthrodesis corresponds to a loss of motion, which translates in a model to a reduction in the number of degrees of freedom.

FORMULATION

A mathematical model of gait is simply a set of equations that describe the interaction of applied forces and movement of limb segments. These equations are expressions of the basic laws of physics. In general, two approaches have been used to formulate the equations of motion for gait: one based on Newtonian mechanics or one based on Lagrangian mechanics, also known as analytical mechanics.

For a given system of admissible coordinates, both the Newtonian and Lagrangian approaches lead to the same system of equations. While there is no clear advantage to using one approach or the other, each has some notable advantages and disadvantages. The Newtonian approach may be somewhat easier to envision since it is based on a free body diagram of each part of the system being studied. All forces, both internal and external, are explicitly displayed in the equations developed from a Newtonian approach. In contrast, a Lagrangian approach is developed for the entire system, not from free body diagrams of each part. Constraint forces that do no work do not appear in a Lagrangian formulation. If our goal is to determine the resultant forces at a joint then the Newtonian approach is preferable because these forces do not appear explicitly in a Lagrangian formulation of limb dynamics since they do no work. If our goal is simulation of motion, either approach could be used; however, the Lagrangian may be somewhat simpler due to the explicit absence of workless constraint forces, which would be eliminated mathematically if the Newtonian approach was used.

In the preceding discussion we identified two uses of the equations that describe the rigid body dynamics of gait, calculation of net resultant forces and moments at the joints, and simulation of motion. While these both use the same equations, the desired result is obtained by very different means. These ideas are illustrated with a simple example. For a physical pendulum shown in Figure 6-1 (that is, a pendulum with distributed mass rather than a point mass at the end of a string) the equation of motion is

$$I_0 \ddot{\Theta} + mgr \sin \ddot{\Theta} \text{ ite} + F_H l + M_0 = 0 \qquad (1)$$

FIGURE 6-1 Physical pendulum used to illustrate inverse and direct dynamics. The pendulum has a distributed mass similar to a limb. A moment M_O acts at the support (O) and is analogous to a joint moment in gait. External forces, F_V and F_H, act on the end of the pendulum similar to the foot-floor reaction forces in gait.

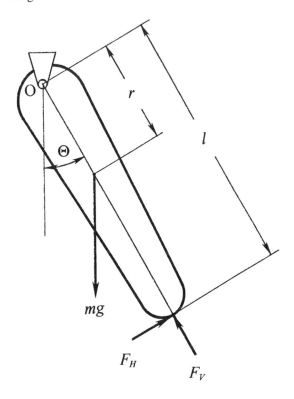

where M_0 is the joint moment, and F_H and F_V are the components of a force applied at the end of the pendulum at a distance l from the support. Since F_V does not have any moment about point 0, it does not appear in Equation 1. I_0 is the moment of inertia of the pendulum with respect to an axis through the support; m is the mass of the pendulum; r is the location of the center of mass of the pendulum; and Θ and $\ddot{\Theta}$ are the angular position and acceleration of the pendulum. Note that a dot over a quantity indicates its time derivative, e.g., $\dot{\Theta}$ is the first derivative of the angular position Θ and therefore represents the angular velocity of the pendulum. Although simplified, with respect to gait this example contains many of the same elements that would be present in a multilink model of walking. In gait, each joint moment is the resultant of the moments of all active muscle forces as well as passive moments. In this example, the joint moment is equivalent to M_O. The

Table 6-1   Degrees of freedom of a hypothetical, three-dimensional model of single limb support

Joint	Degrees of Freedom 3-D Model	Degrees of Freedom 2-D Model
Stance leg ankle	3	1
Stance leg knee	1	1
Stance leg hip	3	1
Swing leg ankle	3	1
Swing leg knee	1	1
Swing leg hip	3	1
Lower trunk	3	1
Upper trunk	3	1

forces F_H and F_V are equivalent to the ground reaction forces in gait. Also, like a limb, this pendulum has a distributed mass rather than having all of its mass concentrated at a single point.

Typically in gait analysis, equations of motion such as Equation 1 are used in either of two ways: to find resultant forces and moments or to simulate motion. The first case is sometimes known as inverse dynamics. Given the kinematics of the pendulum (e.g., Θ, $\dot{\Theta}$, and $\ddot{\Theta}$, or limb segments), which might be obtained experimentally using a video, optoelectronic, or cine film system, and the external force, which in the case of gait is measured with a force plate, the resultant forces and moments at the joints are found by simply adding each of the terms on the left hand side of this equation.

Alternatively, motion can be simulated or predicted based on known joint moments. That is, we determine the angular position of the pendulum (Θ) or a limb segment. In this case the motion is predicted by integrating the differential Equation 1 subject to a set of initial conditions on angular position (Θ) and angular velocity ($\dot{\Theta}$). For example

$$\Theta(t = 0) = \Theta(0) = \Theta_0$$

and

$$\dot{\Theta}(t = 0) = \dot{\Theta}(0) = \dot{\Theta}_0$$

where Θ_0 and $\dot{\Theta}_0$ are known values of the initial position and angular velocity of the pendulum. If we were modeling the swing phase of gait, these conditions might express the position and angular velocities of the thigh, shank, and foot at toe off. The exact form of the solution of Equation 1 will depend on the form of the joint moment, $M_0(t)$, and the ground reaction forces. For a sinusoidal

joint moment, $M_0(t) = M \sin \omega t$, zero external force, and with the requirement that the displacement is small so that $\sin\Theta \approx \Theta$, the displacement $\Theta(t)$ is found by integrating equation 1

$$\Theta = \frac{M_0}{mgr} \frac{\sin \omega t}{\left(1 - \dfrac{\omega}{\omega_n}\right)} \tag{2}$$

where the natural frequency of the pendulum, ω_n is

$$\omega_n = \frac{gr}{r_g^2}$$

and r_g is the radius of gyration of the pendulum. By using a solution such as Equation 2, not only is the motion predicted, but the solution can also be used to investigate the sensitivity of the motion to changes in input parameters such as initial conditions or moments of inertia. Unlike gait, this example has only one degree of freedom; only the angular position, Θ, needs to be specified to fully describe the position of the entire system.

A model of gait requires several degrees of freedom. For example, a model of planar motion of just one swing leg has three degrees of freedom: the flexion-extension angle at the hip, knee, and ankle. Twenty or more degrees of freedom might be needed for a bilateral three-dimensional model of single limb support (Table 6-1) even though this complex model does not include varus-valgus or internal-external rotation at the knee or any head or arm motion. In double limb support, the requirement that both feet be on the ground reduces the number of independent coordinates needed to define the position of the model. For example, a planar model of double limb support including only the lower extremities has four rather than six degrees of freedom. Any four of the six angles describing the position of the limbs are independent coordinates and the remaining two coordinates are dependent on the other four. To see this, imagine that the position of both feet and shanks are specified by four independent angles. These angles and the position of the feet on the ground fixes the position of both knees. Since the lengths of the thighs are fixed and must be joined to the knees, the hip position is determined by the intersection of two circles whose radii are the thigh lengths and whose centers are at the knees. This shows that the thigh positions are not independent of the four given angular coordinates: only four independent angles describe the position of this system.

As the number of degrees of freedom increases, the complexity of the equations of motion also increases. For systems of more than three or four degrees of freedom it becomes impractical to attempt to develop the equations of motion by longhand calculation. Numerous approaches have been developed for generating these equations spurred, at least in part, by developments in robotics where similar issues must be faced.* Automated computer-based algorithms have been developed using both Newtonian and Lagrangian mechanics. Some of these algorithms are primarily numerical in that they compute values of each term in each equation of motion with little regard for algebraic simplification. Other algorithms are based on an algebraic development of the equations of motion in much the same way as one would do longhand, except the algebra is done on a computer. Using this approach, Ju and Mansour[29] showed that the number of calculations could be greatly reduced using Kane's dynamical equations (a variation on Lagranges' equations) implemented and algebraically simplified using the symbolic manipulation package MACSYMA (Symbolics Inc., Cambridge, Mass.).

To simulate motion, joint moments must be specified. It has been common practice to specify the resultant joint moment without regard for the force-generating properties of muscle. In other words, muscle actions are replaced by a pure moment generator without regard for changes in muscle force that would accompany length or velocity changes in the muscle. Nominal values for these moments are sometimes derived from joint moments computed from the inverse dynamics.

Muscle, however, does not produce a constant force. The force in a muscle depends on its activation, length, and velocity. The moment a

muscle produces will then depend on its force as well as the muscle moment arm with respect to the joint. In the past fifteen years, models that simulate a wide range of muscle responses have been under development.[8,19,54,55,56,57] Several applications of muscle-driven mechanical models of movements have been investigated, including gait,[53] kicking,[17] jumping,[43] and manual grasp.[32] If a muscle model is coupled to the mechanical model, some means must be provided to specify muscle activation. In applications with a clear objective, such as kicking a target in the minimum time, methods of optimal control have been used to specify the activation parameters. While one could imagine having activation specified manually for each muscle rather than by a controller, the number of muscles used in gait and the variations of the activation over a gait cycle make this an essentially impossible task.

Body Segment Parameters

The mass, moments and products of inertia, and location of the center of mass of limb segments are essential for describing their dynamical behavior. It should be noted that Equation (1) has no explicit representation of the pendulum, which is instead represented by its mass, moment of inertia, and location of its center of mass.

Body segment parameters for limbs have been determined using a variety of approaches. Dissected cadaver limbs—thigh, shank, foot, etc.— may be weighed to determine mass and location of center of mass.[9] Moments of inertia have been determined by mounting the limbs on a pendulum and measuring its natural period of oscillation.[2] Oscillation of limbs in living individuals has also been used to determine body segment parameters.[4,16] Alternatively, mass of body segments in living individuals have been determined by water immersion to first determine volume; and then, using a density averaged over bone and soft tissue, the mass is determined.[7] Yet other approaches have modeled the shape of a limb—e.g., as a frustum of a cone—and from this assumed shape and average density, body segment parameters are calculated.[15,20] A refinement of an assumed overall shape for a limb is the use of a shape for discrete "slices" of the limb. Jensen obtained "slices" from biplanar photographs of a limb that were digitized to obtain major and minor axes of an assumed elliptical shape of each slice.[26, 27] These shape data and an average density are then used to determine body segment parameters. Since slices are obtained photographically, this approach is suitable for use on live individuals for obtaining products as well as moments of inertia.

---

* References 3, 18, 25, 29, 30, 31, 40, 46, 51, 52.

It is worth noting that it is *always* possible to find a set of axes through any point in a rigid body such that the products of inertia are all zero but the moments of inertia are nonzero. Such axes are known as principal axes. Some of the preceding techniques for determining body segment parameters will yield moments and products of inertia with respect to whatever point and coordinate axes are used. From these data the principal axes can be found. We often seek principal axes of inertia since, if they are used, the equations of dynamics take a much simpler form. However, if principal or nonprincipal axes are used, the same dynamical behavior will be described. In many of the following applications of mathematical modeling of gait, it has been assumed that principal axes of inertia are known.

Applications

Several applications of mathematical models of gait were briefly introduced at the beginning of this chapter. Some of these will now be reviewed in greater detail. Several applications have used mathematical models to evaluate the relative importance of the "six determinants of gait."[44] These descriptors were proposed based on observation of normal and pathological gait. Pelvic rotation (in the horizontal plane), pelvic tilt or list (above or below the horizontal plane), and stance phase knee flexion-extension are three determinants that act to flatten the trajectory of the center of gravity of the body when compared with a stiff-legged, compass gait. The interaction of foot and knee mechanics during stance (two additional determinants) helps to provide a smooth transition of the trajectory of the center of mass from step to step. Finally, lateral displacement of the pelvis provides the lateral movement of the center of mass.

As noted previously, models are often developed to investigate particular aspects of a complex system. The mechanics of the swing phase of gait have been studied by several investigators. Mochon and McMahon developed a ballistic model to investigate the mechanisms that influence the time for the swing leg to move from toe off to heel strike.[36] The model was "ballistic" in that limb motion was determined entirely by initial conditions (position and angular velocity of the limbs at toe off) and gravity—no active moments of muscle forces acted on the limbs in this model. The absence of muscle moments was motivated by electromyographic measurements, which have shown relatively little activity in the muscles of the swing leg. This model also included two of the determinants of gait believed to be most signifi-

FIGURE 6-2 Comparison of the range of swing times measured experimentally (vertical lines) with swing times predicted by the ballistic model (shaded area) and the half-period of a compound pendulum model of the leg. The experimental and pendulum data are from Grieve and Gear (13). Reprinted from Mochon S, McMahon, TA (1980). Ballistic walking. *Journal of Biomechanics* 13:49, with kind permission from Pergamon Press Ltd, Headington Hill Hall, Oxford OX3 OBW, UK.

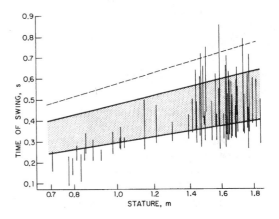

cant: knee flexion and hip flexion.[44] The model included three segments: a stiff-stance leg and a thigh and shank of the swing leg. The foot of the swing leg was rigidly attached to the shank, and all motion was two dimensional. The mass of the upper body was concentrated at the hip. Equations of motion were formulated using a Lagrangian approach and were solved subject to several constraints based on experimentally observed characteristics of gait.

Model simulations predicted swing times based on qualitative evaluation of the data that were in good agreement with experimental measurements (Figure 6-2). The agreement between experimental and predicted swing time was particularly good for people greater than 1 meter tall. These results are consistent with experimental results, which have shown that children probably use different mechanisms to achieve a normal swing phase than do adults.[13] This purely ballistic model gave good predictions of both joint angles and the horizontal component of the foot-floor contact force, but predictions of the vertical component of this force were less accurate.

An improved model of ballistic walking was developed to better predict the vertical component of the foot-floor reaction force.[37] The model was similar to that used above except that now the stance leg was not stiff; it consisted of thigh and shank segments with a hip and knee. This model added two determinants of gait: knee and ankle interaction and pelvic rotation. These additional determinants were found to be insufficient to adequately predict the vertical foot-floor force during gait. The improved model did, however, show that the additional determinants of gait were important for increasing walking speed.

In an independent investigation, Pandy and Berme continued the investigation of the contribution of the six determinants of gait to the predicted foot-floor contact forces.[41,42] They employed two models, one for the phase from toe off to opposite heel off and another from heel off to heel strike. These models did not include pelvic list or transverse pelvic rotation. Simulations gave a good approximation of the vertical and fore-aft components of the foot-floor force in the initial phase of swing. However, they did not fully reproduce the fore-aft component of the horizontal force in the phase from heel off to heel strike (Fig. 6-3).

These results are somewhat different from those found by Mochon and McMahon,[36, 37] who were not able to reproduce the vertical foot-floor force with the foot and ankle interaction determinant of gait. These discrepancies illustrate the need to weigh the assumptions made in any model. In the ballistic walking model the ankle of the stance leg was permitted to plantarflex or come to neutral, but there was no dorsiflexion as was permitted in the model presented by Pandy and Berme. Pandy also points out the limitations of planar models that unnaturally couple the stance and swing legs. Since there is no pelvis in a planar model, the right and left hips are always located at the same point—the influence of pelvic rotation and tilt are absent. All of these studies suggest the need for a pelvic segment that would allow the hips to move independently. Pelvic list would impart an acceleration to the upper trunk. Even a small acceleration of the upper trunk could have a profound effect on the vertical component of the predicted ground reaction forces, although it would have relatively little effect on the horizontal component of this force.

Recognizing the limitations of a two-dimensional model of gait, Pandy and Berme developed a three-dimensional model for single limb support (Figure 6-4).[42] A massless spring damper system crossing the knee of the stance leg is used to produce the flexion-extension behavior of the knee in the phase from toe off to opposite heel off. This model was used to investigate the effect of five of the six determinants of gait on foot-floor reaction forces: stance knee flexion-

Figure 6-3 Comparison of simulated and measured foot-floor contact forces for the period from opposite toe off to heel off. Simulations are derived from a planar model of gait. Reprinted from Pandy MG, Berme N (1988). Synthesis of human walking: planar model for single support. *Journal of Biomechanics* 21:1053, with kind permission from Pergamon Press Ltd, Headington Hill Hall, Oxford OX3 OBW, UK.

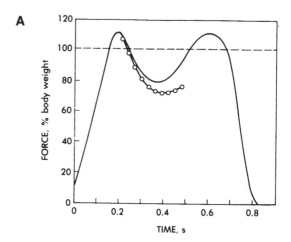

A

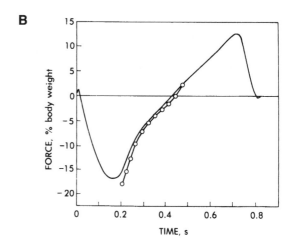

B

extension, foot and knee interaction, pelvic list, and transverse pelvic rotation. Somewhat surprisingly, pelvic list was found to have relatively little effect on the vertical component of the foot floor reaction force. As was found in previous studies with planar models, stance knee flexion-extension and foot-knee interaction were the primary determinants of the vertical force. The presence of transverse pelvic rotation in the three-dimensional model was found to be an important factor in the development of the horizontal ground reaction force (Figure 6-5).

FIGURE 6-4 A three-dimensional model for simulating gait. This is a refinement of the two-dimensional model used to predict the ground reaction forces in Figure 6-3. This model incorporated five of the six determinants of gait. Reprinted from Pandy MG, Berme N (1989). Quantitative assessment of gait determinants during single stance via a three-dimensional model—part 1. Normal gait. *Journal of Biomechanics* 22:717, Copyright 1989, with kind permission from Pergamon Press Ltd, Headington Hill Hall, Oxford OX3 OBW, UK.

FIGURE 6-5 Ground reaction forces predicted by the model shown in Fig. 6-4 (circles) compared with measured experimental data. The more complete three-dimensional model has improved the prediction of the vertical component of the ground reaction but the fore-aft force prediction has lost some fidelity when compared with the results shown in Fig. 6-3. Reprinted from Pandy MG, Berme N (1989). Quantitative assessment of gait determinants during single stance via a three-dimensional model—part 1. Normal gait. *Journal of Biomechanics* 22:717, with kind permission from Pergamon Press Ltd, Headington Hill Hall, Oxford OX3 OBW, UK.

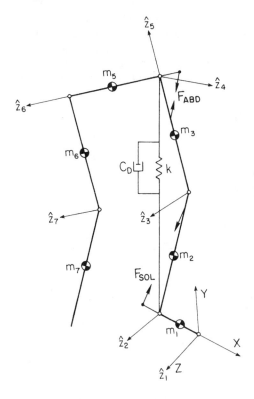

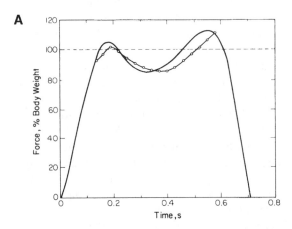

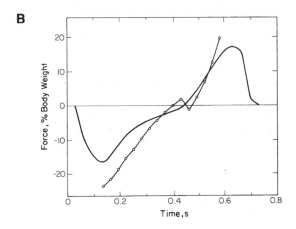

There are, of course, many features of gait not encompassed by the "six determinants." Mena et al. used a model to investigate which one of the many possible factors had the greatest influence on producing a normally appearing swing leg motion.[34] They modeled the dynamics of just the swing leg, that is, the thigh, shank, and foot suspended from a hip that moved in both the horizontal and vertical direction. This study was motivated by observations of gait in children with cerebral palsy where abnormalities in limb movement were particularly evident in the swing leg.

The swing leg was modeled with three independent degrees of freedom, the angles that the thigh, shank, and foot make with the vertical. Alternatively, intersegmental angles could be used, but

using angles relative to a fixed reference simplified the equations of motion. A Lagrangian approach was used to formulate the equations of motion leading to three coupled equations, one for each degree of freedom. The fact that the equations are coupled, just as the thigh, shank, and foot are coupled means that these equations must be integrated simultaneously to obtain limb position. This is true of all of the simulation studies discussed in this chapter. Some information about the swing leg motion can, however, be obtained from these equations without integrating to obtain position as a function of time.

The equation for the thigh or Θ degree of freedom is   (3)

$$K_{11} \dot{V}_{0_y} \cos \Theta + K_{12} V_{0_z} \sin \Theta + K_{13} \ddot{\Theta} + K_{14} \sin \Theta$$
$$+ K_{15} \cos(\Theta - \ddot{\Phi})\Phi + K_{16} \sin(\Theta - \Phi) \dot{\Phi}^2$$
$$+ K_{17} \cos(\Theta - \Psi) \ddot{\Psi} + K_{18} \sin(\Theta - \Psi) \dot{\Psi}^2 = T_t$$

where the K_{ij} are constants that depend on the body segment parameters; Θ, Φ, and ψ are the angles at the thigh, shank, and foot; and T_t is the net joint moment acting on the thigh. Equations for the shank and foot degrees of freedom are similar. The first two terms in this equation expresses the influence of the acceleration of the hip, $\dot{V}_{0_y}$ and $\dot{V}_{0_z}$, on the dynamics of the swing leg. The next two terms look like the pendular dynamics in Equation 1 except that the constants K_{13} and K_{14} include the body segment parameters for all segments, not just the thigh. The next four terms depend on the angular velocity and angular acceleration of the shank and foot and could be thought of as representing the interaction of shank and foot dynamics with thigh dynamics. This equation clearly shows that the dynamics of the thigh depends on the dynamics of the shank and foot as well as the acceleration of the hip. The equations for the shank and foot show similar results in that their dynamics depend on the acceleration of the hip, pendular dynamics, and interactions with the other segments.

To what extent do segment interactions influence the dynamics of any segment? To address this question Mena et al. compared the magnitude of the interaction and pendular terms using a logarithmic magnitude ratio (LMR) defined by

$$\text{LMR} = \log_{10}\left(1 + \frac{NL}{P}\right)$$

where NL represents one of the nonlinear interaction terms and P represents one of the pendular terms in the equations of motion. A logarithm of the ratio was used since there was a large difference in magnitude of the nonlinear and pendular terms. Since the logarithm of zero is not defined, it was necessary to add the constant, 1, to the LMR. If a pendular and nonlinear interaction term are equal, the LMR = $\log(2) = 0.3$. Using data from a normal subject, calculation of the LMR showed that the pendular motion of the thigh and shank was not strongly influenced by the interaction of the other segments (Figures 6-6 and 6-7). In

FIGURE 6-6   Dynamic interaction of the thigh as measured by the log magnitude ratio (LMR). The algebraic terms used in these comparisons appear in the equations of motion for a three-link planar model of the swing leg, e.g., Equation 3. Thigh-shank interactions are measured by terms with coefficients K_{15} and K_{16}, and thigh-foot interactions are measured by terms with coefficients K_{17} and K_{18}. Part A compares pendular gravitational terms with interaction terms and part B compares pendular inertial terms with interaction terms. Reprinted from Mena D, Mansour JM, Simon, SR (1981). Analysis and synthesis of human swing leg motion during gait and its clinical applications. *Journal of Biomechanics* 14:823, with kind permission from Pergamon Press Ltd, Headington Hill Hall, Oxford OX3 OBW, UK.

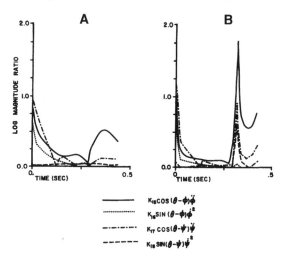

contrast, foot dynamics were strongly influenced by thigh and shank dynamics (Figure 6-8).

Simulations of motion were then performed to gain further insight into the relative importance of initial conditions, body segment parameters, and joint moments on swing leg motion. These parameters were varied about nominal values obtained from a normal gait cycle. The moments on the thigh, shank, and foot were estimated from the inverse dynamics, using normal gait kinematic data. Parameters in the equations of motion were independently varied to determine their influence on limb movement.

Simulations showed that the angular velocity of the limbs at the start of the swing phase have a much greater effect on the swing leg motion than do angular positions. In particular, the initial angular velocity of the thigh was necessary for the leg to execute normal swing leg motion. Using nominal joint moments but varying body segment

FIGURE 6-7 Dynamic interaction of the shank as measured by the logarithmic magnitude ratio (LMR). The algebraic terms used in these comparisons appear in the equations of motion for a three-link planar model of the swing leg, e.g., Equation 3. Shank-thigh interactions are measured by terms with coefficients K_{25} and K_{26}, and shank-foot interactions are measured by terms with coefficients K_{27} and K_{28}. **A** compares pendular gravitational terms with interaction terms, and **B** compares pendular inertial terms with interaction terms. Reprinted from Mena D, Mansour JM, Simon, SR (1981). Analysis and synthesis of human swing leg motion during gait and its clinical applications. *Journal of Biomechanics* 14:823, with kind permission from Pergamon Press Ltd, Headington Hill Hall, Oxford OX3 OBW, UK.

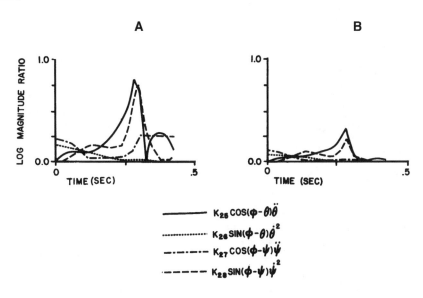

FIGURE 6-8 Dynamic interaction of the foot as measured by the log magnitude ratio (LMR). The algebraic terms used in these comparisons appear in the equations of motion for a three-link planar model of the swing leg, e.g., Equation 3. Foot-thigh interactions are measured by terms with coefficients K_{35} and K_{36}, and shank-foot interactions are measured by terms with coefficients K_{37} and K_{38}. **A** compares pendular gravitational terms with interaction terms, and **B** compares pendular inertial terms with interaction terms. Reprinted from Mena D, Mansour JM, Simon SR (1981). Analysis and synthesis of human swing leg motion during gait and its clinical applications. *Journal of Biomechanics* 14:823, with kind permission from Pergamon Press Ltd, Headington Hill Hall, Oxford OX3 OBW, UK.

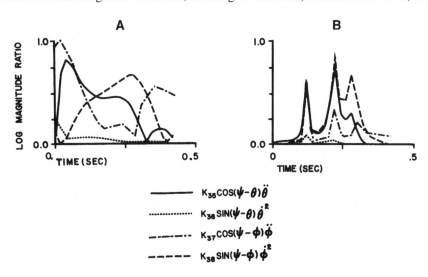

FIGURE 6-9   Free pendular motion of the leg as predicted by a dynamic simulation. All of the joints were modeled as frictionless hinges and no moments were acting at any of the joints. The limb segments started from a normal position at toe off and with normal angular velocities. Reprinted from Mena D, Mansour JM, Simon SR (1981). Analysis and synthesis of human swing leg motion during gait and its clinical applications. *Journal of Biomechanics* 14:823, with kind permission from Pergamon Press Ltd, Headington Hill Hall, Oxford OX3 OBW, UK.

FIGURE 6-10   Constrained pendular motion of the leg as predicted by a simulation model. The joints were frictionless, but each was constrained to an anatomically normal range. The constrained motion of the thigh and shank more closely resembles normal than in the unconstrained case. Reprinted from Mena D, Mansour JM, Simon SR (1981). Analysis and synthesis of human swing leg motion during gait and its clinical applications. *Journal of Biomechanics* 14:823, with kind permission from Pergamon Press Ltd, Headington Hill Hall, Oxford OX3 OBW, UK.

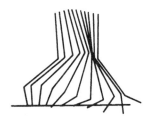

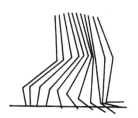

parameters showed that swing leg motion was more sensitive to reductions in mass and moment of inertia of the limb segments than to increases in these parameters. Moments acting on the thigh and shank had relatively little effect on the motion of these segments, but a moment on the foot was necessary to control this segment. The relative lack of importance of the thigh and shank moments and the results of the LMR comparisons suggest that the thigh and shank behave as pendula. However, simulations without thigh and shank moments and with the hip and knee modeled as frictionless hinges led to abnormal motion (Figure 6-9). Although the thigh and shank motion appear to be close to normal for more than half of the swing phase, the knee is severely hyperextended in the last third of swing. If, however, the knee is constrained so that it cannot hyperextend, the thigh and shank motion are close to normal throughout the swing phase (Figure 6-10). The constraint of knee extension was modeled as an elastic collision between the thigh and shank.

The results of these simulations were used to propose a set of minimum conditions needed to produce a normal swing phase (Table 6-2). The only moment that is necessary is on the foot. The thigh and shank behave as constrained pendula to prevent hyperextension of the knee. The results summarized in this table assume a normal hip trajectory. The results summarized in Table 6-2 show that little active control is needed to execute a near normal swing leg motion. Only the foot needs to be controlled to prevent extreme rotation

at the ankle. However, swing leg motion is not exactly like that of a pendulum. Constraints at the knee are needed to prevent hyperextension. These results are consistent with ballistic hypothesis proposed by Mochon and McMahon except that a foot moment is required. In the ballistic models, the foot was rigidly fixed to the shank so that there was no need for a moment to control this segment.

A possible implication of the results summarized in Table 6-2 is that person with an above-knee amputation should be able to execute a normal swing leg motion provided the prosthetic limb has the same body segment parameters as the removed limb. A person with an above-knee amputation should be able to generate an angular velocity of the thigh at toe off. The knee of a prosthetic limb is constrained to prevent hyperextension and the foot is controlled in many applications by simply making the ankle a fixed joint. The implication that near normal swing leg motion could be achieved with an anatomically weighted prosthesis is, however, contrary to current prosthesis design practices: prostheses are commonly made much lighter than the limbs they replace.

The effects of prosthesis mass and mass distribution were evaluated experimentally by Menkveld et al.[35] Subjects walked with their usual lighter-weight prosthesis as well as with their own prosthesis with weight added to bring it to the weight of the removed limb. Results of simple gait analysis showed that increasing the mass of the shank segment improved the subjects' feeling of being able to control their prosthesis. Quantitative

TABLE 6-2   Minimum conditions needed for normal swing leg motion

	Moment	Constraint	Mass, Moment of Inertia
Thigh	Not needed	Not needed at hip	Normal or greater
Shank	Not needed	Needed at knee	Normal or greater
Foot	Required	Not used at ankle, controlled by moment	Normal or greater

gait analysis showed that the collision between the thigh and shank, at the knee hyperextension stop, occurred later in the gait cycle with the heavier prosthesis than with a lighter one. In sharp contrast, increasing the mass of the stump-socket segment of the prosthesis caused considerable discomfort to the subject.

The effects of altering the mass of a prosthesis were also evaluated using a model of the swing phase of a person with an above-knee amputation.[48] The swing leg was suspended from a moving hip as in the model used by Mena et al., however the ankle was fixed and the knee was controlled by passive forces arising from either Coulomb or viscous damping. Simulations were performed for a range of walking speeds from slow to fast. The effects of five combinations of prosthesis body segment parameters were simulated at each walking speed. The simulated gait was compared with the normal gait data used to obtain input parameters.

Simulations showed that a heavier prosthesis generally produced a more normally appearing gait than lighter prostheses. For a given walking speed there was a clear minimum in deviation from normal gait for a particular Coulomb damping at the knee. That is, at one walking speed, simulations using a frictional knee controller more closely matched normal gait than at other speeds. This result, which is consistent with clinical experience, suggests limited utility of a frictional controller with respect to changing walking speed. In contrast, a viscously damped knee showed relatively uniform performance over a range of walking speed. The clear message from these simulations is that a prosthesis with normal body segment parameters outperforms lightweight prostheses has yet to be tested clinically. Other factors such as the general health of the amputee could be important factors in determining the correct body segment parameters for a prosthesis.

The use of functional electrical stimulation (FES) to restore gait in people with paraplegia has been an area of intense research.[11, 33, 53] Using func-

tional electrical stimulation, assisted gait at near normal speed has been obtained. The use of an assistive device such as a walker has, however, been an essential part of FES implementations. The feasibility of unassisted gait with functional electrical stimulation was investigated by Yamaguchi and Zajac using a mathematical model.[53] The body was modeled with eight degrees of freedom as shown in Figure 6-11. The thigh, shank, and foot of each leg were modeled with one degree of freedom, flexion-extension. Two degrees of freedom were assigned to the trunk, flexion-extension and abduction-adduction. The foot of the stance leg rotated about the metatarsal joint, which was assumed to be fixed to the ground. A unique feature of this model was the use of muscle like actuators to drive the motion rather than joint moments or pure force generators acting along a muscles line of action. The muscle consisted of a contractile element with series and parallel elasticity in series with a nonlinear elastic tendon. The details of the muscle model are given in a number of studies.[55, 56, 57] Muscle stimulation patterns were found using a dynamic programming approach coupled with open loop simulation. Including muscle elements made the model more human like at the expense of an increased cost of computation. The model identified phases of the gait cycle where control was particularly difficult due to limited muscle strength or the need for precise positioning of limb segments (Fig. 6-12). Since the model was driven by individual muscles, their functional importance in each phase of the gait cycle could be identified.

The results of this simulation study showed that by using functional electrical stimulation, persons with paraplegia could walk, although their walking speed might be limited. This conclusion was based on muscle strength needed for walking and the requirements for controlling multiple limb segments. For example, it was estimated that plantarflexion moments of approximately 120 Newton meters (Nm) are needed during push off in normal gait (53). This was believed to be twice the typical

FIGURE 6-11 A three-dimensional model with eight degrees of freedom used to study the feasibility of restoring gait in paraplegic people using functional electrical stimulation. From Yamaguchi GT, Zajac FE (1990). Restoring unassisted natural gait to people with paraplegia via functional neuromuscular stimulation: A computer simulation study. *IEEE Trans. Biomed. Engr.* 37:886.

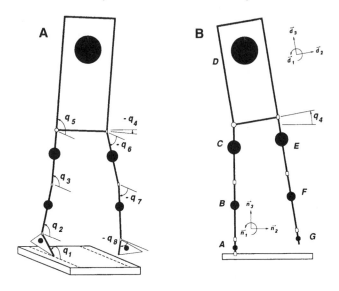

FIGURE 6-12 Stick figures showing the results of simulations of the feasibility of electrically stimulated gait in persons with paraplegia demonstrating a variety of possible outcomes: **A** collapse of the stance leg; **B** foot-ground contact occurring prematurely during swing; **C** a longer-than-normal step due to excessive extension at the knee; and **D** an essentially normal step. From Yamaguchi GT, Zajac FE (1990). Restoring unassisted natural gait to individuals with paraplegia via functional neuromuscular stimulation: A computer simulation study. *IEEE Trans. Biomed. Engr.* 37:886.

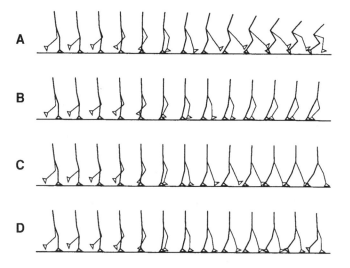

strength of plantarflexors in people using functional electrical stimulation.

It is instructive to assess this conclusion obtained from simulation in comparison with that which might be obtained from inverse dynamics, i.e., computing joint moments from force plate and kinetic data. If joint moments needed for normal gait were compared with those generated by a subject walking with functional electrical stimulation, it would be clear that insufficient strength is being developed. Why then is a simulation of gait valuable in assessing feasibility of electrically stimulated gait when the much simpler inverse dynamics appears to yield similar information? The answer lies in the ability of a simulation to show the movement that would result from attempting to walk with impaired muscle strength or control. Simply comparing joint moments does not give any indication of the functional *potential* for movement using weaker muscles or a different set of muscles than those used in normal gait. Simply arguing that a particular level of joint moment is needed for gait based on data from normal gait could easily lead to an incorrect conclusion, since such an argument does not consider the possibility of compensatory moments at other joints or that the ensuing motion could be functional but not necessarily normal in appearance. In contrast, a simulation does show the potential movement that could be achieved with limited muscle control and strength.

From observation of abnormal gait, it is clear that people can walk in some fashion despite impairments to their neural control system, muscles, and/or joints; some level of compensation is used to produce a functional, but not necessarily normal gait. Winter proposed one type of compensation in what he called the support moment.[50] The support moment is based on the idea that one function of the legs, in gait, is to prevent collapse of the body. To do so requires a net extensional moment at the joints of the leg or legs supporting the body. Winter defined the support moment as the sum of the moments at the hip, knee, and ankle where a sign convention based on flexion-extension was used. From a series of gait analyses (involving 24 normal subjects, 9 patients, and 3 jogging trials), it was observed that the sum of the moments at the hip, knee, and ankle always produced a net extension of the lower extremity. Ankle moment showed little change from walk to walk, while hip and knee moment showed greater variability from walk to walk. From the moment data is appeared that some muscular compensation between the hip and knee was used, possibly to rest some muscles for a few steps and then use these rested muscles while others then produced less effort. Physically, one could imagine a situation in the stance leg where additional hip extension moment is used to enhance knee extension in a phase where knee extensors are in a resting mode. This idea of using muscles at one joint to compensate for a lack of muscle effort at another joint has many potential implications for rehabilitation of abnormal gait. Could weakness in muscles crossing one joint be compensated for by using muscles crossing another joint? Again, this is a question that cannot be answered by observing the joint moments, but it can be answered by simulation.

The extent to which the support moment concept can be used to compensate for weakness at a joint was investigated for the double limb support phase by Chiang[5] using a modification of the planar model developed by Ju.[28] This model included the thigh, shank, and foot of each lower extremity and a two-segment trunk. The feet were modeled with curved plantar surfaces.[45] These curves were chosen to produce near normal foot kinematics during double limb support. The model was driven by joint moments derived from those used in a normal gait but modified to give simulated joint kinematics similar to those used in the normal gait. Two cases will be reviewed here: compensation for a reduced support moment by modifying the moment at an individual joint and a normal support moment with a modified distribution of moment among the joints.

If the support moment was less than normal, the leading (weight acceptance) leg-ankle moment could not be modified to compensate for the deficiency even though knee and especially hip moment could be modified to compensate for the loss. In the trailing leg, a 50% reduction in the support moment could be compensated for by hip and ankle moment, but not by knee moment. If the support moment of the trailing leg was less than 50% of normal, no means of compensating for this loss could be found.

The effects of using a normal support moment abnormally distributed among the joints led to results that were strongly dependent on the leg and joint. Redistributing the leading ankle moment to hip and knee produced little effect on the gait, probably since this moment is relatively small in the phase that was investigated. In contrast, redistributing the trailing ankle moment to hip and knee of that limb caused relatively large changes in kinematics. Redistributing leading knee moment generally led to poor foot kinematics, and attempts at redistributing trailing leg knee moment led to generally poor kinematics for all joints of this limb. In general, a loss of some leading and trailing hip moment could be compensated for at other joints provided not more than half of it is distributed to the respective ankle joints. In summary, the results of these simulations suggest that with a normal support moment the knee moment cannot be lost. Limited amounts of hip or ankle moment can, however, be lost and compensated for at other joints.

In summary, each of the investigations described attempted to answer a question related to mechanical features of gait. The works reviewed here are by no means all inclusive of the field of modeling of gait. In the past 25 years there has been a renewed interest in modeling and simulation of gait,* although the basic mechanics and formulations of such investigations were published at the end of the last century.[12] The development of numerous computer algorithms have made it possible to implement equations of motion for multilink systems with relative ease and accuracy. Using a computer to develop equations of motion has made it possible to develop models with a greater number of degrees of freedom than could be obtained from longhand calculation.

Presumably, increasing the number of degrees of freedom to depict the multiple movements possible at each joint, produces a model more representative of gait. The utility of a model, however, depends on how well it represents features of gait. Simulation models discussed in this chapter "walk" by applying some input, such as joint moments or gravity, for example. The output of these models is limb kinematics (typically displacement, velocity, and acceleration are of interest) and, where applicable, forces between the foot and floor. The ability of the model to produce acceptable output variables for reasonable estimates of the input variables is one measure of the utility of the model.

Simulations of walking have been driven by joints moments, muscle-like forces or, in some cases, gravity as the only forces acting on the limbs. As muscle models are developed and means for estimating their parameters become better established, the use of muscle-like actuators will likely become more common in mathematical models of gait and other activities. Muscle is not a pure force generator; its force depends on activation length and velocity. Using musclelike actuators rather than pure force or moment generators gives a more realistic response of the mechanical model to applied forces. One feature absent in all of the models described in this chapter is a neural control system, although considerable work has been done on the control of bipedal walking and standing from an engineering point of view.[14, 23, 24, 49] As our understanding of the neurophysiology of walking increases, there is no reason why mechanical models of walking cannot be used to test control hypotheses in much the same way that purely mechanical concepts have been investigated.

References 1, 5, 6, 21, 22, 28, 34, 36, 37, 39, 40, 41, 42, 45, 47, 48, 53.

REFERENCES

1. Beckett R, Chang K: An evaluation of the kinematics of gait by minimum energy. *J Biomech* 1:147, 1968.
2. Braune W, Fischer O: Center of gravity of the human body. *Human Mechanics: Four Monographs Abridged* Technical Documentary Report AMRL-TDR-63-123:1, 1963.
3. Cesareo G, Nicolo F: DYMIR: A code for generating dynamical model of robotics. *Proc 1st Int IEEE Conf Robot* March 13–15:115, 1984, Atlanta.
4. Chandler RF, Clauser CE, McConville JT, et al: Investigation of the inertial properties of the human body. *Technical Report DOT, HS-801,* 430, Wright-Patterson Air Force Base, Ohio, 1975.
5. Chiang KH: A dynamic model of human gait with applications to functional neuromuscular stimulation, PhD Thesis, Dept of Mech and Aero Engr, Case Western Reserve University, 1992.
6. Chow CK, Jacobson DH: Studies of human locomotion via optimal programming. *Math and Bioscience* 10:239, 1971.
7. Contini R: Body segment parameters (pathological), Technical Report no. 1584.03, New York University, School of Engineering and Science, University Heights, New York, 1970.
8. Crago PE: Muscle input-output model: The static dependence of force on length, recruitment, and firing period. *IEEE Transactions on Biomedical Engineering* 39(8):871, 1992.
9. Dempster WT: Space requirements of the seated operator, WADC Technical Report 55–159, Wright Patterson Airforce Base, Ohio, 1995.
10. Drillis R, Contini R, Bluestein M: Body segment parameters: A survey of measurement techniques. *Artif Limbs* 8(1):44, 1964.
11. Edwards BG, Marsolais EB: Energy costs of ambulation with reciprocal gait orthosis, electrical stimulation, long leg braces and hybridge: A case study. *Clin Kinesiology* 44(2):43, 1990.
12. Fischer O: Theoretical fundamentals for a mechanics of living bodies. *Human Mechanics: Four Monographs Abridged* Technical Documentary Report AMRL-TDR-63-123:58, 1963.
13. Grieve DW, Gear RJ: The relationship between the length of stride, step frequency, time of swing and speed of walking for children and adults. *Ergonomics* 9:379, 1966.
14. Gubina F, Hemami H, McGhee RB: On the dynamic stability of biped locomotion. *IEEE Transactions on Biomedical Engineering, BME-21,* 102, 1974.
15. Hanavan EP: *A mathematical model of the human body* AMRL-TR-64-102, Behavioral Sciences Laboratory, Aerospace Medical Research Laboratories, Aerospace Medical Division, Air Force Systems Command, Wright-Patterson Air Force Base, Ohio, 1964.
16. Hatze H: A new method for the simultaneous measurement of the moment of inertia, *in situ* the damping coefficient and the location of the centre of mass of a body segment. *European Journal of Applied Physiology and Occupational Physiology* 34:217, 1975.
17. Hatze H: The complete optimization of a human motion. *Math and Bioscience* 28:99, 1977.

18. Hatze H: A complete set of control equations for the human musculo-skeletal system. *J Biomech* 10:799, 1977.

19. Hatze H: A myocybernetic control model of skeletal muscle. *Biol Cybern* 25:103, 1977.

20. Hatze H: A mathematical model for the computational determination of parameter values of anthropometric segments. *J Biomech* 13:833, 1980.

21. Hatze H: Neuromusculoskeletal control systems modeling: A critical survey of recent developments. *IEEE Transactions on Automatic Control, AC-25(3):375, 1980.*

22. Hatze H: Myocybernetics: A new development in neuromuscular control. *Journal of Cybernetics,* 10:341, 1980.

23. Hemami H, Jaswa VC, McGhee RB: Some alternative formulations of manipulator dynamics for computer simulation studies, *Proc 13th Allerton Conf on Circuit Theory* October:124, 1975, University of Illinois.

24. Hemami H, Farnsworth RL: Postural and gait stability of a planar five-link biped by simulation. *IEEE Transactions on Automatic Control, AC-22:452, 1977.*

25. Hollerbach JM: A recursive Lagrangian formulation of manipulator dynamics and a comparative study of dynamics formulation complexity. *Transactions on Systems Management and Cybernetics,* 10(11):730, 1980.

26. Jensen RK: Changes in segment inertia proportions between 4 and 20 years. *J Biomech* 22(6/7):529, 1989.

27. Jensen RK: Estimation of the biomechanical properties of three body types using a photogrammetric method. *J Biomech* 11:349, 1989.

28. Ju M-S, Mansour J: Simulation of the double limb support phase of human gait. *J Biomech Eng* 110:223, 1988.

29. Ju M-S, Mansour J: Comparison of methods for developing the dynamics of rigid body systems, *International Journal of Robotics Research,* 8(6):19, 1989.

30. Kane TR, Levinson DA: Dynamics: theory and application. New York, 1985, McGraw-Hill.

31. Levinson DA: The derivation of equations of motion of multi-rigid-body systems using symbolic manipulation, *AIAA* paper TP76-816, 1976.

32. Mansour JM, Rouvas C, Sarangapani J, et al: Quantitative functional anatomy of finger muscles: Application to controlled grasp, to appear in *NATO Advanced Workshop, Advances in the Biomechanics of the Hand and Wrist,* 1992.

33. Marsolais EB, Kobetic R, Barnicle K, et al: FNS application for restoring function in stroke and head-injury patients. *J Clin Eng* 15(6):489, 1990.

34. Mena D, Mansour JM, Simon SR: Analysis and synthesis of human swing leg motion during gait and its clinical applications. *J Biomech* 14(12): 823, 1981.

35. Menkveld S, Mansour JM, Simon SR: Mass distribution in prosthetics and orthotics: Quantitative analysis of gait using biomechanical model simulation, *Transactions of the 27th Annual Meeting,* Orthopaedic Research Society, 1981.

36. Mochon S, McMahon TA: Ballistic walking. *J Biomech* 13(1):49, 1980.

37. Mochon S, McMahon TA: Ballistic walking: An improved model, *Math and Bioscience* 52:241, 1980.

38. Moskowitz RW: Experimental models of osteoarthritis. In Moskowitz RW, Howell DS, Goldberg VM, et al (Eds): *Osteoarthritis: diagnosis and management.* Philadelphia, 1984, WB Saunders.

39. Onyshko S, Winter DA: A mathematical model for the dynamics of human locomotion. *J Biomech* 13:361, 1980.

40. Pandy MG, Berme N: A numerical method for simulating the dynamics of human walking. *J Biomech* 21(12):1043, 1988.

41. Pandy MG, Berme N: Synthesis of human walking: A planar model for single support. *J Biomech* 21(12):1053, 1988.

42. Pandy MG, Berme N: Quantitative assessment of gait determinants during single stance via a three-dimensional model. Part 1. Normal gait. *J Biomech* 22(6/7):717, 1989.

43. Pandy MG, Zajac FE, Sim E, et al: An optimal control model for maximum-height human jumping. *J Biomech* 23(12):1185, 1990.

44. Saunders JB, Inman VT, Eberhart HD: The major determinants in normal and pathological gait. *J Bone Joint Surg* 35A:543, 1953.

45. Stein JL: Design issues in the stance phase control of above knee prostheses, PhD Thesis, Dept of Mechanical Engineering, MIT, Cambridge, Mass, 1983.

46. Stepanenko Y, Vukobratovic M: Dynamics of articulated open-chain active mechanisms. *Math and Bioscience* 28:137, 1976.

47. Townsend MA, Seireg A: The synthesis of bipedal locomotion. *J Biomech* 5:71, 1972.

48. Tsai C-S, Mansour JM: Swing phase simulation and design of above knee prostheses. *J Biomech Eng* 108:65, 1986.

49. Vukobratovic M, Stokic D: Contribution to the decoupled control of large-scale mechanical systems. *Automatica* 16:9, 1980.

50. Winter DA: Overall principle of lower limb support during stance phase of gait. *J Biomech* 13:923, 1980.

51. Wittenburg J: *Dynamics of systems of rigid bodies.* Stuttgart, 1977, BG Teubner.

52. Wolz U, Wittenburg J: MESA VERDE: A program for the symbolic generation of equations for multibody systems. *ZAMM,* 66(5):399, 1986.

53. Yamaguchi GT, Zajac FE: Restoring unassisted natural gait to paraplegics via functional neuromuscular stimulation: A computer simulation study. *IEEE Transactions on Biomedical Engineering,* 37(9):886, 1990.

54. Zahalak GI: A distribution-moment approximation for kinetic theories of muscular contraction. *Math and Bioscience* 55:89, 1981.

55. Zajac FE, Stevenson PJ, Topp EL: A dimensionless musculotendon actuator model for use in computer simulations of body coordination: Static properties. *Proc N Amer Congress Biomechanics* Montreal, Quebec, Aug. 25-27:245, 1986.

56. Zajac FE, Stevenson PJ, Topp EL: A dimensionless musculotendon model. *Proc 8th Ann Conf IEEE Eng Med Biol Soc* 601, Ft. Worth, TX, 1986.

57. Zajac FE: Muscle and tendon: Properties, models, scaling and application to biomechanics and motor control. *Crit Rev Biomed Eng* 17:359, 1989.

CHAPTER 7

THE NEUROPHYSIOLOGY OF HUMAN LOCOMOTION

Charles T. Leonard

KEY TERMS

Central pattern generator

Convergence

Divergence

Flexor reflex afferents (FRAs)

Golgi tendon organ

H-reflexes

Mesencephalic locomotor region (MLR)

Muscle spindle

Neurochemistry

Ontogenetic development

Positron emission transaxial tomography (PETT)

Subthalamic locomotor region (SLR)

Few human activities generate as much innate human interest as locomotion. Consider the following examples: Learning to walk is the most anxiously awaited developmental milestone by parents and grandparents. Interest in walking is not limited to infants. Therapists and physicians often relate that the first question asked by patients with back and leg injuries is, "Will I be able to walk again?" Similarly, individuals with even a long-standing paraplegia often report that they dream of walking.

Despite our fascination and years of scientific inquiry, we still do not know how we manage to get from point A to point B in an upright position. Controlling bipedal locomotion is not an easy task. The central nervous system (CNS) somehow must generate the locomotor pattern, generate appropriate propulsive forces, modulate changes in center of gravity, coordinate multilimb trajectories, adapt to changing conditions and changing joint positions, coordinate visual, auditory, vestibular and peripheral afferent information, and account for the viscoelastic properties of muscles. It must do all of this within milliseconds and usually in conjunction with coordinating a multitude of other bodily functions and movements. Dissecting each contributing variable and determining relative influences of each in order to develop a model for the control of human locomotion is a daunting scientific task.

Although the examination of human gait has received considerable scientific attention, many questions remain unanswered. This chapter will provide the reader with currently available information regarding the neural control of locomotion but will not, in most cases, provide definitive answers as to the neural control of locomotion. Definitive answers, unfortunately, are not yet available. This will become quite evident in the subsequent discussion of several unresolved theoretical issues. The chapter first attempts to acquaint readers with the questions concerning neural control of locomotion and perhaps assist the readers in formulating their own conceptual framework from which to analyze experimental results. The chapter will then introduce several experimental approaches being used by scientists to resolve these debatable issues, followed by a presentation of the results that have been obtained thus far.

NEURAL CONTROL OF HUMAN LOCOMOTION

This section describes issues currently being investigated by neuroscientists and others. These topics are only a small sampling of the many questions being explored through research, but they represent areas of inquiry that generate considerable debate.

Human Locomotion: Innate or Learned?

Reflexive movements of the human fetus begin at about 8 weeks gestation.[96] Infants with anencephaly also exhibit some ability to move their legs in a coordinated stepping manner.[113] These data would seem to support the idea that the human locomotor pattern is reflexive and therefore innate. According to this view, any change in afferent input brought about by a changing environment or goal-directed behavior merely serves to modulate a preexisting pattern. The machinery necessary to carry out human locomotion is contained within the spinal cord and brainstem centers. Nonhuman animal studies add further support to the innate, hard-wired theory of human locomotion.

For example, cats with totally transected spinal cords still maintain the ability to ambulate and coordinate limb movements.[100] They lose righting and equilibrium responses, but maintain the ability to walk and to appropriately alter limb positions for obstacle avoidance.[39] A collection of neurons contained within the spinal cord termed *central pattern generators* (CPGs) have been identified as being responsible for generating the locomotor rhythm.[46]

The limited human research that is available, however, suggests that spinal cord CPGs may not have the same primacy of control as in other species. The role of higher brain centers, such as the cerebral cortex, may be considerably different in humans than it is with other species. Human data, in fact, suggest that learning plays a critical role in the attainment of an adultlike, bipedal, plantigrade gait pattern. The examination of the development of independent locomotion in children provides some evidence for this conclusion.

Goal-directed ambulation generally begins at about 10 months of age. During the next few months childrens' biomechanical and muscle activity patterns exhibit considerable intra- and inter-subject variability.[69,87] This variability cannot be explained by a hard-wired reflexive model of walking. Rather, this interval of time in a child's life appears to reflect a period of trial and error in the attainment of walking. Learning also occurs in adults. Adults maintain the ability to change their ambulation pattern. For instance, individuals with lower extremity amputations learn to modify ambulation patterns to optimize prosthetic use.[116] Although it remains a debatable point, it is this author's viewpoint that existing data provide more support for learning than for hard-wired reflexive models. This does not, in any way, imply that the learning process does not involve hard-wired pathways such as CPGs or genetically predetermined CNS connectivity. CPGs almost certainly play a role in human locomotion. Differences between humans and other mammalian species with regard to CPG functioning provide additional clues indicating that learning may play a large role in the attainment of human bipedal locomotion.

Existence of CPGs in Humans

There is little doubt that central pattern generators (CPGs) exist in many, if not all, vertebrate species. To date, however, scientists have been unable to provide evidence for an autonomously functioning spinal cord CPG in humans or other mature primates.[30] Some data have been presented that are suggestive of the existence of CPGs in humans,[15] but this work has failed to provide conclusive evidence for autonomous CPG functioning as occurs in lower mammalian species. The CPG, if it does exist in adult humans, appears unable to independently generate coordinated rhythmic locomotion.

From a logical point of view, one would reason that CPGs exist in some form in humans. Entire neural pathways are rarely lost during evolutionary development.[102] It should not, however, be overly surprising that the role of the CPG in generating locomotion has changed with phylogenetic development. Quadrupedal locomotion requires the coordination of 4 independently moving limbs. Human bipedal locomotion has halved this complexity, but it also results in increased equilibrium demands. Equilibrium control is, to a large degree, a supraspinal function. Neuroanatomical data indicate the existence of more descending supraspinal pathways in humans than in any other species. The corticospinal tract makes more monosynaptic and polysynaptic connections in the cervical and lumbar spinal cord of humans than in other species.[6] Because of this difference, it is conceivable that the autonomous nature of spinal cord CPGs is lost in favor of the added influences of descending systems. This conjecture leads to the next question.

Cerebral Cortex Involvement in Locomotion

Many supraspinal centers have obvious roles to play in human locomotion. Cerebellar and vestibulospinal systems are among the best delineated.[18] Known functions of the cerebral cortex with regard to locomotion include cognitive aspects of motor control, visuomotor coordination, and motor planning. The possible role of the cerebral cortex in the generation and coordination of human locomotion remains controversial. The existence of locomotor activity in nonhuman animals following spinal cord transection argues against a role for the cerebral cortex in the generation of locomotion. The neural circuitry required for quadrupedal and other forms of vertebrate locomotion, however, may be entirely different than that required for bipedal locomotion.

Bipedal gait is a uniquely human activity. In addition to increased equilibrium demands, bipedal gait involves increased anticipatory muscle activations, the functional stretch reflex (FSR), and bodily responses to the unweighting of a limb and single leg stance.[19] All of these functions rely on cerebral centers.[27] Sir John Eccles, one of the most noted neuroscientists of all time, states, "The rhythmic movements of human walking are not explicable by spinal mechanisms, and only imperfectly by lower cerebral levels such as the vestibular inputs to the reticulospinal and vestibulospinal pathways.... Undoubtedly a bipedal gait had entailed a drastic reorganization of the central nervous system."[27]

The following findings also seem to indicate an increased role for cerebral involvement in human locomotion: (1) Motor cortical neurons fire tonically and phasically during and preceding movement and in time with stepping movements.[3,31,34] (2) Some automatic reactions involve long-loop cortical reflexes.[75,76] These long-loop reflexes are abolished following damage to the cerebral cortex.[20] (3) Reciprocal inhibition of antagonist muscles required for voluntary movements such as locomotion is lost following perinatal damage to sensorimotor cortical pathways.[71] (4) The cerebral cortex of humans connects monosynaptically and polysynaptically to a multitude of spinal cord neurons including alpha and gamma motoneurons.[6,103] (5) Muscle spindle afferents project to the cerebral cortex and are under the influence of the cerebral cortex.[9,77]

Ontogenetic Development and Locomotion

The locomotor pattern of a human infant differs considerably from that of the mature adult.[35,69,87,112] Obviously many biomechanical and somatic changes contribute to these changes. An intriguing question, however, is whether the neural substrate for locomotion actually changes over time. Nonhuman animal studies have indicated that the neural substrate for certain reflexes and motor behaviors do indeed change over time.[42,66,98] For instance, in the cat a reflex known as low threshold placing is initially controlled at a segmental level but very quickly after birth becomes dependent on an intact sensorimotor cortex.[1,67] Changes in the neural substrates subserving movement during development have considerable clinical relevance with regard to the effects of brain damage. Following perinatal brain damage, the stage of development of surviving pathways as well as pathways that have been damaged are factors that contribute to functional outcome.[42,66]

Although there is no direct evidence that the neural substrate for human locomotion changes with development, experimental evidence suggests human locomotion is first controlled segmentally and then becomes progressively more dependent on supraspinal systems, which is similar to certain motor behaviors of other mammalian species. Human newborns exhibit stepping behaviors immediately after birth even though descending projections are not fully developed or completely myelinated.[35,93] Infants with anencephaly also exhibit similar stepping movements.[113] Apparently, the cerebral cortex is not necessary for early infant stepping.

Years ago it was suggested that "encephalization" was responsible for the transition from the infant stepping pattern to an adult pattern of locomotion.[93] Infant stepping was regarded as a reflex that later became inhibited by descending systems. It was further believed that the original circuits that generated reflexive stepping were not used in the adult. More recently it has been suggested that spinal CPGs generate the basic locomotor rhythm and supraspinal systems serve to initiate and drive the CPGs.[46,36] Experimental evidence suggests that neither explanation adequately addresses the enhanced involvement of supraspinal centers in the generation and control of human locomotion.

The progression to a mature gait pattern involves a transition from a stereotyped synergistic pattern to one in which anticipatory postural changes and precise fractionated movements replace fixed synergistic movements.[35,69,87,112] The corticospinal tract fractionates movement in the upper extremity.[95] Similarly, it may serve to fractionate the locomotor pattern so that a coordinated, energy-efficient gait is obtained. Individuals who have suffered perinatal damage to the cerebral cortex, internal capsule, periventricular white matter, or the pyramids never develop a mature gait pattern.[25,69] Rather, they continue to exhibit many characteristics of early reflexive stepping. This finding provides additional indirect evidence that supraspinal pathways, and specifically corticofugal pathways, are necessary for the attainment of a mature gait pattern. It is unlikely that supraspinal centers supercede CPGs. Rather, it is more probable that descending systems *integrate* with existing spinal cord circuitry in order to fractionate lower extremity movement and provide greater adaptability to changing afferent conditions.

SCIENTIFIC APPROACHES TO THE NEUROBIOLOGY OF LOCOMOTION

Diverse neuroscientific approaches are used to examine questions relating to human locomotion. The following section will describe briefly the type of information that is discerned from each approach.

Invertebrate Studies

"The neurobiology of swimming in the leech."[63] "Interneuronal circuitry underlying cyclical feeding in gastropod moluscs."[7] Not exactly titles you might expect to yield essential information regarding human locomotion. Despite the esoteric titles, studies performed with invertebrates and lower-order vertebrates have done much to increase our knowledge of human locomotion. Our understanding of the action potential, the neuromuscular junction, the role of calcium in muscle contraction, chemical synaptic neurotransmission, membrane conductance changes, and postsynaptic potentiations were all derived from the study of invertebrates. Another example is the current problem facing neuroscientists in determining the mechanisms responsible for the generation of temporally sequenced muscle activity during locomotion. Invertebrate studies are invaluable for researching issues such as these.

Because of the relative simplicity of the invertebrate nervous system, individual neurons can be identified, the total sum of their afferent and efferent connectivity characterized, and their relation to movement of the animal described. The cellular basis of central pattern generators can be examined and manipulated. For instance, different neurotransmitters can be introduced and their effects monitored via intra- and extracellular recordings. These studies can also be performed with some lower-order vertebrates such as the lamprey eel. Elegant studies are being performed with the lamprey eel that permit an analysis of membrane properties and neural network circuitry subserving lamprey locomotion.[50] These principles can then be applied to other vertebrates and eventually to humans.

Nonhuman Vertebrate Studies

All vertebrates have the ability to ambulate. This ability necessitates reciprocal activations of muscles and coordinated multijoint movement in both humans and nonhuman animals. These characteristics are shared with human locomotion. Because no current methods exist that permit the direct analysis of neural connectivity in humans, neuroscientists must rely on nonhuman animal studies. The advantages of using nonhuman animals are many. Behavioral data can be obtained throughout the life span of an animal. Specific lesions to various parts of the CNS can help to identify the relationship between lesioned structures and motor behavior. Behavioral recovery following CNS damage can be observed. Neurophysiological properties of a functioning animal can be determined. Neuroanatomical studies can determine neural circuitry of the developing animal and the fully mature animal as well as the effects of various CNS lesions on neural connectivity. Neurophysiological and neuroanatomical studies can be correlated to behavior and to behavioral changes following therapeutic interventions.

As essential as these studies are for the understanding of human locomotion, the major drawback is that quadrupedal locomotion, or even the quasi-bipedal locomotion of some primates, is not the same as human plantigrade bipedal locomotion. Additionally, the expansion of the human cerebral cortex poses some problems. It is difficult to apply all nonhuman data to humans. For this reason it is imperative that neuroscientists and others continue to examine human gait. Even though many principles derived from nonhuman studies have been shown to apply to humans, it is just as likely that humans have evolved neural and biomechanical strategies that are as unique as their method of locomotion.

Human Gait Analysis

The intricacies of human gait and other movements are being unraveled with the use of clinical neurophysiological techniques. Positron emission transaxial tomography (PETT), H-reflex testing, cortical magnetic stimulation, electromyography (EMG), and computerized three-dimensional motion analysis provide information regarding the neural and biomechanical control of human movement. All of these methods can be used with fully conscious humans. In many cases, the tests can be carried out on a freely moving individual. This is vitally important because neurons and neural pathways respond differently during different tasks.[94,111]

PETT scans monitor the metabolic activity of cortical areas and thus provide insights into what areas of the brain are active during various tasks. One study of considerable relevance indicated that association areas of the brain are used for the acquisition of a task, whereas basal gangliar structures become more involved once the task is learned.[105] H-reflexes indirectly measure the level of excitability of alpha motoneurons. Techniques have been developed that permit detection of alpha motoneuron modulations during various movements including locomotion.[70,111,16] Other H-reflex testing procedures provide information regarding other neural pathways involved in human locomotion.[59,60,71] Cortical magnetic stimulation provides a painless way to determine what areas of the body are controlled by various cortical areas.[80] The technique has been used to demonstrate that the cortical control of movement is different between a nondisabled population and individuals with cerebral palsy.[14] Surface EMG and computerized gait analysis are particularly useful in integrating the examination of neural and biomechanical control of movement.

Figures 7-1 and 7-2 provide graphic depictions of the kinematics and muscle activation patterns of the human step cycle. These data supply information regarding muscle temporal sequencing, muscle amplitudes, duration of contractions, muscular co-contraction, joint kinematics, movement kinetics, changes in interjoint degrees of freedom, and the relationships between each variable. Information from human gait studies have been correlated with data from nonhuman animal studies and have led to insights into the neural control of locomotion.[65,68,69,118] Gait analysis data, either alone or in conjunction with other techniques such as H-reflex testing, provide an uncommon opportunity to interface and synthesize neural and biomechanical analyses. Neuroscientists are increasingly aware that the biomechanics of locomotion not only place constraints on the system, but also serve to modulate neural responses.[10, 28]

Integrating Biomechanical and Neurophysiological Data

Peripheral receptors in joints and muscles detect changes in muscle length and force, joint position, and possibly weight-bearing status of the limb. Conceptually, therefore, the nervous system is aware of at least some biomechanical aspects of movement. How it makes use of this information remains a mystery. A number of studies have now shown that changes in the biomechanics of a movement alter neural responses.*

---

* References 10, 23, 26, 28, 43, 49.

FIGURE 7-1 **A,** EMG recordings from 5 leg muscles of a nondisabled woman during overground locomotion. **B,** Joint angular excursions of both legs of the same subject during overground locomotion. These data are representative of normal temporal EMG sequencing and joint excursions. LG = lateral gastrocnemius; TA = tibialis anterior; HM = biceps femoris; RF = rectus femoris; GM = gluteus maximus; RHS = right heel strike; LTO = left toe off; LHS = left heel strike; RTO = right toe off. Data and graphs for figures 7-1 and 7-2 were generated by a 3-D computerized, 4-camera, 200 Hz, VP-320 Motion Analysis system.

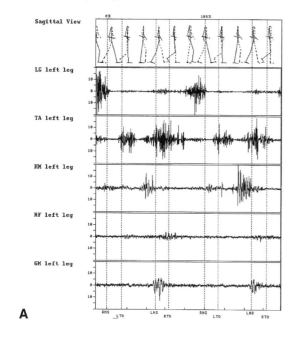
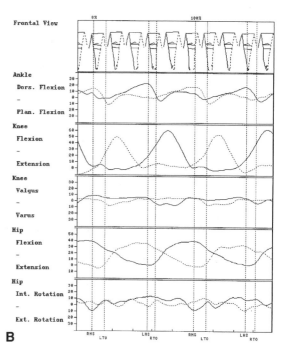

The generation and control of locomotion can be roughly divided into two phases: (1) descending commands from higher brain centers signal subcortical systems to initiate movement; and (2) information relating to the subsequent movement is relayed back to the nervous system. Changes in afferent sensory information will alter motor responses. Through their analyses of feedback and feedforward systems, biomechanists and engineers have much to offer to our understanding of locomotion. They provide information that includes, but is not limited to, forces acting on a limb, torque generation, relationships between torque production and joint angle changes, control of limb trajectories, descriptions of interjoint kinematics, and changes in mechanical relationships over time.[53] The control of these parameters requires feedback mechanisms.

Feedback from peripheral receptors assists in the refinement of on-going movement. For instance, engineers use feedback loops in robotic design. *Servoregulation* is a term they use to describe the process by which a feedback signal (afferent sensory discharge) is compared with the set point (desired motoric output) in order to make necessary corrections for successful completion of the task.[53] The vocabulary may be different, but neuroscientists and engineers have been struggling with similar problems within their respective fields. The human body is governed by the same physical contraints as any other moving object. The CNS must make use of biomechanical information for the final shaping of its motoric output. Similarly, neuroscientists, biomechanists, engineers, and mathmeticians must make use of the knowledge base of various disciplines in order to decipher the intricacies of movement. This interchange will continue to clarify the various mechanisms inherent to human locomotion. Similarly, the study of human pathology also aids our understanding of human locomotion.

Neural Plasticity Studies

Various injuries and diseases of the nervous system impact locomotion. For instance, Huntington's disease involves progressive deterioration of the striatum and cerebral cortex; Parkinson's disease results from depletion of dihydroxyphenylalanine

FIGURE 7-2   **A** and **B,** EMG recordings of leg muscles of an 11-year-old boy with spastic type diplegic cerebral palsy during overground locomotion. Notice the lack of normal temporal sequencing when compared with the nondisabled subject. Also note that although he has diplegic involvement, EMGs reveal different activation patterns and different problems between the two legs. For instance, more paresis is in evidence in the left leg as indicated by decreased EMG amplitudes. **C,** Kinematic analysis reveals multiple problems including a crouched gait, excess hip internal rotation, and an ankle that is maintained in dorsiflexion. It remains a challenge for clinicians and scientists to determine which EMG and kinematic abnormalities are due to neurological impairment and which are compensatory responses to the disability.

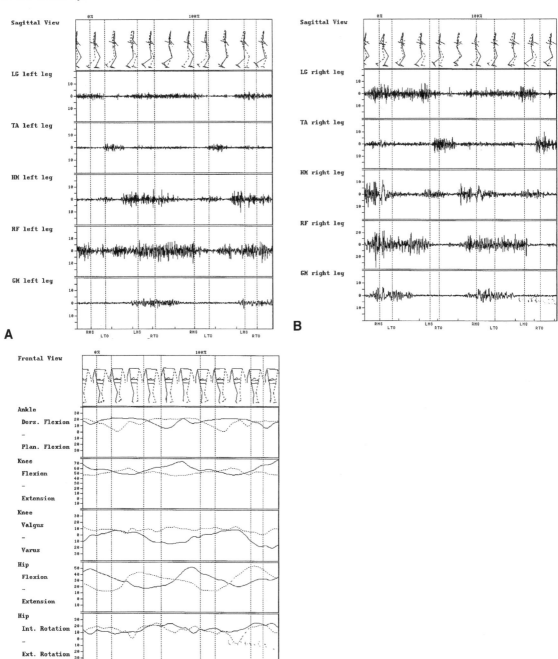

(dopa) secreting cells within the substantia nigra; syringomyelia begins by weakening postural muscles; and spinal cord injuries and cerebral vascular accidents result in varying degrees of motor dysfunction. By studying the effects these diverse processes have on motor performance, neuroscientists gain insights into the functioning of various pathways and neural structures. Examining the differing behavioral effects of CNS lesions occurring during different stages of ontogenetic development yield information pertaining to development and CNS maturation. Processes of neural recovery following damage, termed *plasticity,* also provide important clues, not only to neural responses to injury but also to mechanisms involved in motor learning. Recovery and learning both involve the concept of synaptic plasticity. Investigations into synaptic plasticity also reveal how transmission and structural change of the synapse are affected by use and disuse as well as whether external influences such as physical and pharmacological therapies can change these processes.

NEURAL COMPONENTS INVOLVED IN HUMAN LOCOMOTION

Questions relating to human locomotion and methods of inquiry have been presented thus far. What follows is a synthesis of what has been found to date regarding the contribution of various neural components to human locomotion.

Principles of Neural Convergence

Principles of convergence and divergence greatly enhance the relative activity and influence of any given neuron. Convergence refers to multiple afferent input onto a single neuron or nucleus. Divergence refers to the multiple outputs of a neuron or nucleus. It also greatly increases the realm of influence of a neuron.

Convergence occurs at every level of the CNS. Segmentally, interneurons and motoneurons receive multiple inputs (Figure 7-3).[52] A single alpha motoneuron may receive more than ten thousand contacts.[86] The complexity increases in supraspinal centers. Determining which input has greater relative influence is a difficult task. The difficulty of this task is increased by changes in the relative influences of afferent input within a situational context,[31-33,44] the position of the limbs,[10] weight-bearing status,[92] and anticipatory motor set.[32]

Convergence is an important concept to bear in mind during subsequent paragraphs of this chapter in which inputs and outputs of various neural structures as well as discernment of function based

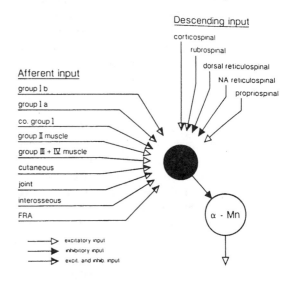

FIGURE 7-3 Convergence of multiple descending systems and multisensorial afferent input onto interneurons mediating nonreciprocal group I inhibition to alpha motoneurons. Ia inhibitory interneurons that mediate reciprocal inhibition receive similar convergent input. The main difference is that Ia inhibitory interneurons do not receive Ib input but receive a rich input from the vestibulospinal tracts. The alpha motoneuron also receives convergent input from multiple sources. co. = contralateral; FRA = flexor reflex afferents; NA = noradrenergic.[52]

on connectivity are discussed. This information is useful for a global understanding of the neural influences on locomotion. Because of the complexity introduced by convergence and divergence, however, descriptions of neural connectivity alone may be insufficient for an accurate determination of what initiates, generates, and maintains locomotion.

Central Pattern Generators (CPGs)

Central pattern generators refer to a grouping of neurons or neural circuits that can generate coordinated movements autonomously. CPGs for locomotion have been identified in the vertebrate spinal cord.[62,73] CPGs can generate coordinated locomotor movements even in the absence of all movement related afferent feedback.[48,51] Since this original discovery, the CPG theory of the control of locomotion has undergone considerable refinement. Although CPGs form an innate neural network that independently can activate coordinated stepping, this capability does not imply that the network or its output is invariant. CPGs have the ability to change output depending on speed requirements,[37,108] and in response to obstacle avoidance.[2,38] Although CPGs can operate without afferent input, CPG activity is constantly modified by available sensory input.[46] This is a crucial distinction and one that has been misinterpreted by those who have questioned the role of CPGs in locomotion.[115] CPG activations are constantly modified by on-going internal and external sensory changes.

At any given moment or stage of a step cycle, the importance and consequences of various afferent inputs change. For instance, during the transition from stance to swing, hip flexor stretch receptors may be the primary sensory input that initiates change in CPG output.[49] During other stages and conditions, other sensory input may be of primary importance. These observations have yielded the concept of command neurons. Command neurons are defined as those neurons that respond to sensory input and initiate CPG activity. Different movements or different conditions may activate different command neurons. Command neurons, in turn, activate specific neural discharge sequencing within the CPG. Thus, different movements are possible depending on which command neurons within the CPG are activated.

Activity within the CPG and the patterns of movement that result from CPG activation appear to be influenced primarily by three factors: (1) supraspinal center input, (2) the type and degree of afferent feedback, and (3) the influences of limb and body position on afferent feedback. Since it is becoming clear that the nervous system processes more information than was previously thought, CPG models of locomotion will continue to be modified as new information becomes available. Change in neural outputs depend on joint angle and interjoint positions.[10,11] Weight-bearing status of a limb also affects neural transmission of some neurons.[92] Perhaps changes in center of gravity are recognized in the CNS by a unique integration of multisensorial afferent input or by peripheral receptors yet to be defined. These additional factors will have to be considered in any future analysis of CPG functioning in human locomotion.

Peripheral Receptors and Afferents

Locomotion results in a wide array of sensory changes. Afferent information derived from the muscles can be considered among the most important of these changes. Control of bipedal locomotion requires constant monitoring of muscle length and tension. This monitoring is provided by spindles, which are sensitive to changes in muscle length, and golgi tendon organs, which are responsive to muscle tension.

Muscle Spindles   Muscle spindles are sensitive to changes in muscle length. Some spindles respond to the rate of change in muscle length whereas others respond to absolute length changes. Although this has long been accepted spindle physiology, recent studies have questioned whether the spindle actually does accurately monitor changes in muscle length during certain movements.[55] Spindles are innervated by gamma motoneurons. The gamma motoneuron determines the sensitivity of the spindle to stretch. The sensitivity of the spindle then changes with the requirements of the movement. Therefore, the spindle not only serves as a feedback receptor but also as a feedforward mechanism. Gamma and alpha motoneurons are controlled in parallel from supraspinal centers.[74] (A number of introductory neuroscience textbooks contain additional information about spindle physiology and anatomy.) Spindle discharge is transmitted via Ia afferents. Because dynamic changes in muscle length occur during the human gait cycle, some discussion of Ia afferents is warranted.

Ia afferents are the largest diameter peripheral nerve fibers and thus have the fastest conduction velocities. Stretch of a muscle activates the spindle and initiates transmission in the Ia afferent. One result of Ia afferent activation is monosynaptic excitation of the stretched muscle and its synergists. It will also synapse on an interneuron—the Ia inhibitory interneuron—which inhibits the muscle that is the antagonist to the stretched muscle. The Ia afferent also gives off collaterals that will ascend in the dorsal columns of the spinal cord to higher brain centers.[6] One hypothesis states that these ascending projections inform higher brain centers (e.g., cerebellum, cerebral cortex) of changing conditions. Higher brain centers can then modify gamma and alpha motoneuron discharge to meet the requirements of the changing condition. Changes in the excitability of motoneurons by higher brain centers is one way that a hard-wired reflex can be modified. Other mechanisms, such as presynaptic inhibition, can also modify reflex output.

Presynaptic inhibition of Ia afferents decreases the amount of transmitter released by Ia afferents and can be accomplished by descending projections, motoneuron collaterals, or by interneurons. Therefore, the same amount of spindle activity may result in varying amounts of excitation and inhibition. Modulation of the interneurons that are interposed between the Ia afferent and other neurons can also modify reflex responses. A tremendous amount of convergence onto interneurons from a variety of sources takes place (Figure 7-3).

Through the integration of all input, including others that have yet to be discovered, segemental reflexes such as the stretch reflex are influenced by activity in other parts of the nervous system.

Golgi Tendon Organs and Ib Afferents Golgi tendon organs (GTOs; tendon organs) are contraction-sensitive mechanoreceptors that are innervated by fast-conducting Ib afferent fibers. Their speed of conduction is only slightly less than the Ia fibers that innervate muscle spindles. Researchers once thought that GTOs responded to excess tension that developed in an overly stretched muscle. They now know that GTOs have a low threshold and are sensitive to any type of muscle contraction, independent of the amount of stretch placed on the muscle. Muscle contraction will always elicit a GTO response whereas a stretch does not always stimulate GTO firing.[58,61] Stimulation of GTOs appears to inhibit homonymous and synergistic motoneurons and excite antagonist motoneurons. The majority of Ib fibers synapse on interneurons within the spinal cord. Ib input converges with a multitude of other afferent and supraspinal input.

GTOs have been hypothesized to play a role in ambulation.[22,92] GTOs are thought to constantly alter the force output of different muscles in order to meet the requirements of on-going movement.[103] The timing of the locomotor rhythm is strongly influenced by Ib afferents.[22] Input from Ib afferents inhibit flexors during the stance phase of gait.[92] It would appear, therefore, that changes in Ib afferent activity may play a role in regulating the stance-to-swing transition in gait. Considering the extensive multisensorial convergence onto Ib interneurons and Ib supraspinal projections, it will not be surprising if future studies indicate a broader role for the Ib afferent system in the control of locomotion.

Flexor Reflex Afferents (FRAs) Flexor reflex afferents refer to a multisensorial and interneuronal reflex system that has been hypothesized to be partially responsible for the generation of locomotion.[77] The afferents included in this reflex pathway include mechanoreceptors, cutaneous afferents, nociceptors, joint afferents, and muscle afferents.[103] The reason these various high threshold afferents are grouped together is that their stimulation causes the same motoric reflex response. FRAs exert either an inhibitory or excitatory effect on the motoneuronal pool of a limb. Activity in one motoneuronal pool generally results in inhibition of antagonist pools. Alternating activity between various motoneuron pools forms

the basis for rhythmic locomotor activity.[103] FRAs, therefore, may play a vital role in human locomotion.

FRAs send projections to higher brain centers and receive input from descending supraspinal centers. During locomotion, stimulation of FRAs may result in differing motoric outputs. For example, a cutaneous stimulation applied during limb extension in the cat will result in limb flexion. Applying the same cutaneous stimulation during limb flexion will result in extension of the limb.[101] This finding and that of other researchers shows that reflex activity can be altered based on the position of the limb.[10] Biomechanists have been suggesting this idea for quite some time. Knowledge of the effects of FRAs on locomotion potentially have some clinical usefulness, such as the use of cutaneous stimulation to enhance the ambulation of individuals who have had a stroke.[40]

Brainstem Electrical stimulation of neural centers located in the nonhuman mammalian midbrain and brainstem causes spontaneous locomotion.[88,90,106] Three such centers are the mesencephalic locomotor region (MLR), the pontine locomotor region (PLR), and the subthalamic locomotor region (SLR). These centers receive and integrate diverse descending and afferent input, then their efferent output goes to spinal CPGs. Although stimulation of any of these centers in nonhuman vertebrates elicits coordinated locomotion, the effects of lesioning the centers or their projections is somewhat different. The primary role of each center in an intact animal, therefore, is likely to be different.

The mesencephalic locomotor region (MLR), located ventral to the inferior colliculus, receives afferent input from the basal ganglia, the limbic system, and the sensorimotor cortex.[13] It connects with spinal circuitry via the reticulospinal tract.[89] The MLR appears to be an important relay station between cortical limbic drives and CPGs. By nature of the sympathetic inputs to the limbic system, the MLR may be the center by which the "flight" component of the "fight or flight" sympathetic response becomes manifest.

The pontine locomotor region (PLR) is located caudal to the MLR and may actually be contiguous with it. It has been suggested that there is a pontomedullary locomotor strip that extends from the MLR to the upper cervical spinal cord.[107] Stimulation of this area changes postural tone and alters firing within the MLR.[82]

Electrical stimulation of the subthalamic locomotor region (SLR), located in close proximity to the subthalamus, also elicits locomotion. If this region is disconnected from cortical centers in the cat, the animal can ambulate spontaneously but loses all obstacle avoidance ability. The SLR, therefore, appears to be necessary for the modulation of the locomotor pattern. A lesion immediately caudal to the SLR in cats will result in the disappearance of all spontaneous locomotion.[45]

Cerebellum The cerebellum is one of the most intriguing neural structures involved in motor control and locomotion. It is one of the biggest enigmas of the central nervous system. Neuroscientists have been able to classify all the cells of the cerebellum, its projections have been mapped, and its afferent input is well defined. We know everything about it, yet we still do not understand how it does what it is hypothesized to do.

The cerebellum is hypothesized to compare motor commands emanating from the cerebral cortex with the resultant afferent consequences of the movement.[12] It is essential for the smooth execution of voluntary movement. Some regions of the cerebellar cortex are active prior to a movement and appear to preset the body for the intended movement. Other regions of the cerebellum are not active prior to a movement. Rather, they become active during the movement and reflect the afferent result of the movement. The cerebellum encodes reaction times of intended movement and the patterns of muscles used.[13] In other words, it contributes to coordination of muscle activity.

The cerebellum is also important for our ability to adapt to a changing environment. Optimal movement solutions are devised at the cerebellar level based on trial and error. By constantly comparing the afferent consequences of a particular movement sequence with the desired outcome, an optimal movement solution is developed. With repetitive trials, adaptation will yield to learning. Motor learning takes place when adaptations provide the desired outcome to a specific stimulus. Many CNS structures are involved in motor learning, but the cerebellum is absolutely essential in developing selective associations.[114] Although the cerebral cortex provides insights into motoric outcome, the cerebellum is necessary for the development of smooth motoric responses resulting from the learning of a motor task. The afferent and efferent connections of the cerebellum provide some insight into how this might be accomplished.

The cerebellum receives somatotopically organized input from the cerebral cortex (motor areas 4 and 6, visual and auditory cortices), the brainstem

nuclei such as vestibular nuclei, and the midbrain.[13] The ventral and dorsal spinocerebellar tracts relay information from the peripheral muscle spindles, GTOs, and joint afferents to the cerebellum during movement. These tracts relay somewhat dissimilar information. Both tract systems are phasically active during locomotion. The dorsal tract conveys information about the activity of individual muscles. The ventral tract receives more diffuse input and appears to be involved in comparing the descending copy of the motor program for locomotion with the resultant changes in the periphery.[4,5] Cerebellar output indirectly affects spinal cord interneurons and motoneurons and the motor cortex. Its affect on spinal cord circuitry is via its initial connections with vestibular nuclei. Its influence over the motor cortex is via its input to the ventrolateral nucleus of the thalamus. It has a direct connection with the red nucleus.[13]

Similar to examination of cerebellar connections, the study of the effects of cerebellar lesions can provide useful information regarding its functioning. Cerebellar lesions result in the decomposition of movement. Muscles that normally act synergistically lose their ability to do so. Errors in direction, muscular force, and velocity are common. Intentional tremors and nystagmus often result. Lesions that affect the vestibular component of cerebellar function result in a wide-based staggering gait and an inability to make correct postural adjustments to movement. Individuals may be able to compensate somewhat for cerebellar dysfunction but the movements are slow, clumsy, and require much concentration. All fluidity and grace of movement are lost following lesions of the cerebellum.

To summarize briefly, the cerebellum coordinates movement, assimilates parameters necessary for motor learning, creates programs and subprograms for specific movements, establishes an internal model of expected afferent consequences of a motor act, preprograms alpha and gamma motoneurons, integrates vestibular reflexes, and provides ongoing comparisons of descending motor commands with changing peripheral and internal conditions.

Basal Ganglia The basal ganglia is composed of the caudate nucleus and the putamen (collectively referred to as the striatum), the globus pallidus, and the subthalamic nucleus. Input is received from the cerebral cortex, thalamus, and substantia nigra. The main output, via the globus pallidus, is to the thalamic nuclei that will, in turn, project to the supplementary motor and motor cortices.[21] The basal ganglia plays an important role in motor control. Although this role cannot be precisely defined, diseases of the basal ganglia provide insights into the tremendous importance of the basal ganglia with regard to movement. Diseases that affect the basal ganglia include Huntington's chorea, athetosis, and Parkinson's disease. These disorders result in disruption of motor control and lead to serious motor control disabilities. Observations of patients with athetosis provide a clinical example of the importance of the basal ganglia for locomotion. Patients with athetosis are unable to control limb movement and have fluctuating muscle tone and poor stabilization of the trunk musculature. Other clinical disorders of the basal ganglia include akinesia, a loss of voluntary movement; extrapyramidal dyskinesia, a difficulty in performing movement accompanied by involuntary, unsuppressible movement; and bradykinesia, a slowness of movement.

The functions of the basal ganglia with regard to movement and locomotion remain a mystery. Based on current understanding it is thought that the basal ganglia process afferent information from the periphery and the cerebral cortex and somehow impact motor planning. They play a role in the initiation and termination of movement. Some basal gangliar neurons fire before movement, whereas others fire after movement and after neurons within the SM cortex have already finished firing.[21] Neurons within the basal ganglia respond to sensory input only if the sensory input is related to movement.

To further complicate our understanding, some neurons that respond to a given sensory stimulus will only be activated in a given situational context.[21] The basal ganglia may alter motor output based on sensory input by integrating sensory stimuli and determining which stimuli will be used by the CNS to impact movement. They not only integrate sensory information, but also appear to attach situational significance to it.

In addition to its as yet undetermined role in motor planning, the basal ganglia is intimately connected to the limbic system.[54] The significance of this has not yet been determined although clinicians have long noted an association between the motor impairments and flat emotional affect of patients with Parkinson's disease.

Cerebral Cortex Depending on your point of view, the cerebral cortex is either the omnipotent ruler who lords over the kingdom or a slave to its constituents' wishes. The study of the role of the cerebral cortex during human movement, including locomotion, is perhaps the most challenging for today's neuroscientist. No other species has undergone such a dramatic expansion of the cerebral cortex. Did the cerebral cortex evolve solely for the development of speech and self-reflection? The dramatic increase in monosynaptic and polysynaptic cortical projections onto spinal motoneurons and interneurons would suggest otherwise. As stated by Wise and Evarts, ". . . the fact that spinal cord in phylogenetically more primitive forms organizes detailed movement sequences does not imply a failure of cerebral cortex to have a parallel function in more advanced forms."[117]

As discussed previously in this chapter, cortical neural activations precede movement and fire phasically during locomotion.[3,31,34] Many neuroscientists now refer to the corticospinal tract as being responsible for fractionating movement. To begin to understand the potential role of the cerebral cortex with regard to locomotion, it is advantageous to understand something of its organization.

The cerebral cortex has both a horizontal laminar and vertical columnar organization. Human cortical neurons differentiate and migrate to their final horizontal laminar location during fetal development.[109] Cell differentiation and horizontal migration patterns appear to be genetically determined.[29,109] At 8 weeks gestation in the human, cortical neurons and thalamic projections interact at the cortical plate before the final migration to the cortex.[97] It is also interesting to note that the first fetal movements are detected at 8 weeks gestation.[96]

Cortical neurons also organize themselves in functionally related vertical columns. Unlike horizontal laminations, vertical columns are extremely plastic and their organization is activity dependent.[109] Damage to peripheral nerves of a monkey results in the expansion of the cortical representation of those areas receiving sensory input from remaining peripheral nerves.[79] Stimulation of a single whisker vibrissae of a rat will increase its cortical representation.[24] Our final movement repertoire and our ability to respond to sensory stimuli is apparently dictated by experience. How cortical neurons contribute to our movement repertoire is a story just beginning to be understood.

Visual system research provided the first clues as to the functioning of cortical neurons during movement. Neurons within the primary visual cortex respond to very specific stimuli. Some neurons only respond to movement occurring in the periphery of the visual field, others during stimulations to the fovea. Some neurons fire in response to vertical lines, others to horizontal or oblique lines.[79] Similarly, it was found that sensorimotor cortical neurons collectively encode very specific movement parameters. Some neurons contribute to the encoding of direction of movement, whereas others encode force or velocity.[8,31,41, 110] It does not appear that single neurons dictate final behavioral outcome. Final movement performance is determined by the collective firing of cortical neurons. The resultant collective activations of groupings of neurons create a vector field. This summation determines final motor outcome.[41] Cortical vector fields thus indirectly prescribe movement characteristics such as force and velocity. Similar organization has been described for subcortical nuclei and the spinal cord.[8]

Neurons within functionally related cortical columns transform afferent sensory stimuli into a generalized motor plan. Direction, amplitude, velocity, and the final desired outcome of the intended movement can be prescribed. Subcortical regions further refine the response taking into account joint positions and interjoint degrees of freedom. It should be emphasized that although experimental evidence supports this computational model, it remains theoretical at this point. A function of the cerebral cortex, that has moved beyond the theoretical and into the realm of a generally accepted premise is the involvement of the cerebral cortex in movement-related reflexes known as long-loop, long-latency, or transcortical reflexes.

Long-loop reflexes refer to the modulation of spinal reflex circuits by supraspinal centers. Long-loop reflexes are identified by their relatively long latencies. Muscular responses to a muscle stretch can be divided into the M1, M2, and M3 phases.[64] In the wrist, the M1 response occurs at about 25 milliseconds, the M2 at 50 to 80 ms, and the M3 at about 85 to 100 ms. In the lower leg, M2 responses occur at approximately 100 ms. The M2 and M3 responses have been shown to be dependent on an intact sensorimotor cortex and have thus been termed transcortical reflexes[20,91] (Figure 7-4). Shaping of segmental reflex activity is vitally important for anticipatory reactions. Locomotion is an example of a motor act that incorporates anticipatory reactions to loading and unloading of the limb (Figure 7-5). Supraspinal centers determine the "motor set" required for a certain movement by altering segmental reflex responses. For instance, the motor set required for walking over uneven terrain in the dark differs from that required for walking on your living room carpet.

Figure 7-4 A and B, Stretch reflex potentiations of the gastrocnemius muscle recorded from nondisabled subjects. A*b,* Recordings from subjects with spinal cord injuries that resulted in spastic paraplegia. B*b,* Recordings from the affected sides of subjects with adult-onset cerebral vascular accidents (CVAs). The M2 phase of the gastrocnemius stretch reflex normally occurs at about 100 ms. The M2 response is absent below the level of the lesion following spinal cord injury and is absent on the affected side of subjects with adult-onset CVA subjects. These findings are consistent with the fact that long-loop responses (M2; M3) are dependent on intact supraspinal connections. Specifically, the responses are dependent on intact connections from the motor cortex.[13]

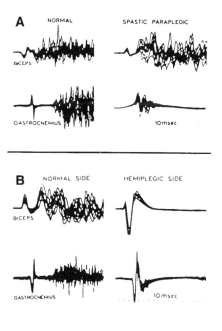

Long-loop reflexes alter segmental reflexes in order to achieve a desired motor output.[33,34,57,81] For instance, they will inhibit segmental reflexes if the segmental reflex response opposes a desired movement. Conversely, they will enhance segmental reflex activity if the reflex assists in a desired movement.[84] Long-loop/transcortical reflexes serve a feedforward function. The set established for running presumedly differs from that required for walking. Muscle torque output, muscle temporal sequencing, and H-reflex changes are considerably different between these two modes of locomotion.[17,47,85] The motor set established via transcortical reflexes is at least partially responsible for these changes. Further evidence is provided by work showing disruption in these modulations and

FIGURE 7-5 Neurophysiological model of human ambulation. Circles within each domino represent neural populations innervating a specific muscle group. Propriospinal projections extend up and down spinal cord segments to coordinate other parts of the body. Commisural fibers to the contralateral side of the spinal cord assist bilateral coordination.

● = Command Neuron: the neuron that is initially depolarized that will trigger Central Pattern Generators (CPGs). Different neurons may act as the command neuron, dependent on current conditions and limb position. Neurons within CPG receive rich convergent input from afferents, brainstem nuclei, and cerebral cortex.

—< = Excitatory Input

—● = Inhibitory Input

<—> = Do not necessarily indicate a direct projection

CST = Corticospinal tract; VST = Vestibulospinal tract; RST = Rubrospinal tract; RetST = Reticulospinal tract.

This model is useful for understanding how on-going afferent information might modulate CPG activity and the mechanisms by which the CST fractionates movement. It is also a useful model for understanding the potential neural mechanisms involved in spasticity and motor control dysfunction following damage to the CST.

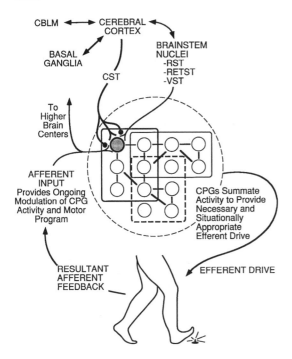

other segmental mechanisms following damage to the sensorimotor cortex or its projections in humans.[13,20,56,71] Considerable evidence points to the important rule that the cerebral cortex plays in the generation of coordinated locomotion in humans.

NEUROCHEMICAL CONSIDERATIONS

Knowledge of the connectivity of various neural systems contributing to the control of locomotion is a necessary step toward understanding the neural basis of human locomotion. Events that occur at a molecular level are equally important. Neurochemical processes underlying synaptic transmission have as much of a role to play in final behavioral outcome as actual physical connectivity between neurons. Transmission changes that occur pre- or postsynaptically can dramatically modulate activity within any given neural pathway. An understanding of some of the neurotransmitters and postsynaptic membrane receptors involved in movement enhances our abilities to understand the mechanisms involved in human locomotion. It is also vital to our understanding and development of drugs that can influence movement and movement-related disorders.

Postsynaptic Receptor Physiology

The postsynaptic membrane contains highly specialized membrane proteins called receptors. These receptors respond in a certain way to specific neurotransmitters. The way in which a receptor responds determines whether the postsynaptic neural membrane will become more permeable to Na^+, K^+, Ca^{++}, or Cl^-. This, in turn, determines whether the neurotransmitter will have an excitatory or inhibitory effect on the postsynaptic neuron. Increased permeability to positively charged ions results in excitation, and permeability to negatively charged ions yields inhibition. Different neurons contain different membrane receptors. A single neuron may have receptors for a variety of neurotransmitters. Therefore, each neuron will respond differently to any given stimulus. For instance, NE may be excitatory at some receptor sites and inhibitory at others. The interaction between neurotransmitters and receptor sites increases the diversity available within any given pathway.

Neurotransmitters

To be classified as a neurotransmitter, a substance must meet certain pharmacological criteria. A simplified definition of a neurotransmitter is any substance that is released synaptically by a neuron and has an effect on another neuron or organ. The tremendous growth in identifying neurotransmitters is evident when reviewing the literature. In 1981, nine substances were identified as neurotransmitters.[104] Today the number of known neurotransmitters is about ninety.* Following is a brief discussion of some transmitters known to be involved in motor control and human locomotion.

Acetycholine   Acetycholine was the first neurotransmitter to be identified.[86] It is the transmitter of the neuromuscular junction. Acetycholine is released by alpha and gamma motoneurons, thereby controlling intrafusal and extrafusal muscle contraction. It is not just found at the neuromuscular junction. The reticular formation and the striatum are rich in acetycholine-containing cells. Interestingly, the physiological action of acetycholine is somewhat different between the peripheral and central nervous systems.[86] In the peripheral nervous system it is excitatory, and its action is very short lived. In the CNS, the action of acetycholine is slow and diffuse.[86] This speaks to the importance of the receptor site in determining excitatory or inhibitory effects of a given neurotransmitter. Cholinergic neuron projections include the hippocampus, thalamus, and cerebral cortex. Considering these projections, it is clear that acetycholine will have effects on locomotion and other neural functions in addition to neuromuscular transmission. As an example, a dramatic decrease in acetycholine occurs in individuals diagnosed with Alzheimer's disease.[86] Alzheimer patients not only exhibit mental deterioration but motoric deterioration as well.

Glutamate and Aspartate   The role of glutamate and aspartate in the CNS is analogous to the role of acetycholine in the peripheral nervous system. These neurotransmitters cause brief point-to-point excitation within the CNS. Glutamate tends to be a bit more potent than aspartate in its ability to cause neural excitation.[78] Excess accumulation of glutamate can be toxic to neurons. This condition is known as excitotoxicity.[86] There are reports in the literature that consumption of large amounts of the artificial sweetener, Aspartame, which is structurally related to aspartate, causes symptoms that could be related to excitotoxicity. Monosodium

glutamate, often used in Chinese cooking, has caused similar effects.[78] Cortical pyramidal cells are rich in glutamate and aspartate. It is one of the transmitters used by the corticospinal tract. There are many glutamate and aspartate receptors within the cerebral cortex, yet no neural pathway has yet been associated with these receptor sites. Glutamate and aspartate are also found in high concentrations in the mammalian hippocampus, amygdala, cerebellum, red nucleus, striatum, and thalamus. Glutamate is also the neurotransmitter used by the endings of primary afferents.[78]

GABA   Gamma-aminobutyric acid (GABA) is the major transmitter for point-to-point *inhibition* in the CNS. Similar to glutamate, it can be found in the cerebral cortex and the spinal cord in addition to other structures concerned with motor control such as the cerebellum and the basal ganglia.[83]

Two types of receptors are receptive to GABA. GABA(A) receptor sites are postsynaptic receptors and are responsible for mediating postsynaptic inhibition. The GABA(B) sites are on presynaptic autonomic and central nerve terminals. GABA(B) receptors reduce the outflow of excitatory neurotransmitters such as glutamate and norepinepherine, serving a modulatory function.[78]

Many clinically administered drugs interact with GABA. Its inhibitory effects, therefore, can be manipulated somewhat. Benzodiazpines, such as diazepam, which are prescribed to decrease anxiety and spasticity, facilitate GABA binding and therefore increase its inhibitory effects. Baclofen, also used to control spasticity, is a GABA(B) agonist.[78] Its administration mimics the inhibitory effects of GABA. Bicuculline is a GABA(A) antagonist. It inhibits the inhibitory effects of GABA and therefore causes excitation. Bicuculline has been used to enhance the ambulation of spinal injured cats.[99]

Glycine   Glycine is an inhibitory neurotransmitter thought to be the transmitter used by spinal cord inhibitory interneurons.[83] It is also found in the cerebral cortex and cerebellum. The actions of glycine at the spinal level are similar to those of GABA. However, the results of these two transmitters are affected quite differently by other substances. Strychnine will block the action of glycine but not GABA. Bicuculline will block GABA but not glycine. This type of drug interaction specificity may one day be used by neuropharmacologists to develop drug therapies for various neurological disorders.

---

* Source: Dr. Craig Johnston, neuropharmacologist; personal communication.

SUMMARY

This chapter is by no means an inclusive review of neurophysiological processes involved in human locomotion. Obvious omissions include the role of the vestibular system in postural control, the visual system for locomotor adaptation, neural and muscular adaptations to muscular fatigue during locomotion, the neuromuscular junction, myotatic reflex influences on locomotion, and processes of neural development that impact on the acquisition of bipedal locomotion. Despite the tremendous strides that have been made, the final chapter on the neural basis of human movement has not been written. The remaining challenges that face scientists and clinicians are considerable.

One challenge will be to determine the neural processes by which the performance of a movement is compared with the intended movement making on-going instantaneous corrections possible. Neural processes underlying task-dependent neural and nonneural modulations add additional complexity to this problem. Determining what factors influence the effects on motor output of any given afferent stimulus during the various phases of the gait cycle will be a critical step toward solving this problem. Perhaps the greatest challenge will be the discovery of therapeutic interventions that will lessen the debilitating effects various neural diseases have on one of the most innate desires of the human animal—the desire to walk upright.

REFERENCES

1. Amassian VE, Ross R: Development in the kitten of control of contact placing by sensorimotor cortex, *Journal of Physiology (Cambridge)* 230:55-56, 1972.
2. Andersson O, Forssberg H, Grillner S: Peripheral feedback mechanisms acting on the central pattern generators for locomotion in fish and cat, *Canadian Journal of Physiology and Pharmacology* 59:713-726, 1981.
3. Armstrong DM, and Drew T: Discharges of pyramidal tract and other motor cortical neurones during locomotion in the cat, *Journal of Physiology (Cambridge)* 346:471-495, 1984.
4. Arshavsky YI, Berkenblit MB, Fukson OI, et al: Recordings of neurons of the dorsal spinocerebellar tract during evoked locomotion, *Brain Research* 43:272-275, 1972.
5. Arshavsky YI, Berkinblit MB, Gelfand IM, et al: Activity of the neurons of the ventral spinocerebellar tract during locomotion, *Biophysics* 17:926-935, 1972.
6. Baldissera F, Hultborn H, Illert M: Integration in spinal neuronal systems. In Brooks VB, editor: *Handbook of physiology: The nervous system II,* Baltimore, 1981, Williams & Wilkens, 509-595.
7. Benjamin PR, Rose RM: Interneuronal circuitry underlying cyclical feeding in gastropod molluscs. In Evarts EV, Wise SP, Bousfield D, editors: *The motor system in neurobiology,* Amsterdam, 1985 Elsevier, 67-73.
8. Bizzi E, Mussa-Ivaldi FA, Giszter S: Computations underlying the execution of movement: a biological perspective, *Science* 253:287-291, 1991.
9. Boyd IA: The isolated mammalian muscle spindle. In Evarts E, Wise S, Bousfield D, editors: *The motor system in neurobiology,* New York, 1985, Elsevier Press, 154-167.
10. Brooke JD, McIlroy WE: Effect of knee joint angle on a heteronymous Ib reflex in the human lower limb, *Canadian Journal of Neurological Sciences* 16:58-62, 1989.
11. Brooke JD, McIlroy WE: Vibration insensitivity of a short latency reflex linking the lower leg and the active knee extensor muscles in humans, *Electroencephalography and Clinical Neurophysiology* 75:401-409, 1990.
12. Brooks VB: The cerebellum and adaptive tuning of movements, *Experimental Brain Research*-(Suppl 7):170-183, 1984.
13. Brooks VB: *The neural basis of motor control,* New York, 1986 Oxford University Press, 1-330.
14. Brouwer B, Ashby P: Corticospinal projections to lower limb motoneurons in man, *Experimental Brain Research* 89:649-654, 1992.
15. Bussel B Roby-Brami A, Yakovleff A, et al: Late flexion reflex in paraplegic patients: Evidence for a spinal stepping generator, *Brain Research Bulletin* 22:53-56, 1989.
16. Capady C, Stein RB: Amplitude modulation of the soleus H-reflex in the human during walking and standing, *Journal of Neurosciences* 6:1308-1313, 1986.
17. Capaday C, Stein RB: Difference in the amplitude of the human soleus H-reflex during walking and running, *Journal of Physiology (Cambridge)* 392:513-522, 1987.
18. Carew TJ: Descending control of spinal circuits. In Kandel ER, Schwartz JH, editors: *Principles of neural science,* New York, 1981, Elsevier, 312-322.
19. Chan CWY, Melvill Jones G, Catchlove RFH: The "late" electromyographic response to limb displacement in man. II. Sensory origin, *Electroencephalography and Clinical Neurophysiology* 46:182-188, 1979.
20. Chan CWY, Melvill Jones G, Kearney RE, et al: The "late" electromyographic response to limb displacement in man. I. Evidence for supraspinal contribution, *Electroencephalography and Clinical Neurophysiology* 46:173-181, 1979.
21. Connor NP, Abbs JH: Sensorimotor contributions of the basal ganglia: Recent advances, *Physical Therapy* 70(12):118-126, 1990.
22. Conway BA, Hultborn H, Kiehn O: Proprioceptive input resets central locomotor rhythm in the spinal cat, *Experimental Brain Research* 68:643-656, 1987.

23. Corcos DM, Gottlieb GL, Agarwal GC: Organizing principles for single-joint movements. 2. A speed-sensitive strategy, *Journal of Neurophysiology* 62:358-368, 1989.

24. Craik RL, Hand PJ, Levin BE: Locus coeruleus affects glucose metabolism in the physiologically activated rat barrel cortex, *Brain Research Bulletin* 19:495-499, 1987.

25. Dubowitz L Finnie N, Hyde SA, et al: Improvement of muscle performance by chronic electrical stimulation in children with cerebral palsy, *Lancet* 1:587-588, 1988.

26. Duysens J, Pearson KG: Inhibition of flexor burst generation by loading ankle extensor muscles in walking cats, *Brain Research* 187:321-332, 1980.

27. Eccles JC: *Evolution of the brain,* London, 1989, Routledge.

28. Edamura M, Yang JF, Stein RB: Factors that determine the magnitude and time course of human H-reflexes in locomotion, *Journal of Neuroscience* 11(2):420-427, 1991.

29. Edelman GM: *Neural Darwinism,* New York, 1987, Basic Books.

30. Eidelberg E, Walden JG, Nguyen LH: Locomotor control in macaque monkeys, *Brain* 104:647-663, 1981.

31. Evarts E: Pyramidal tract activity associated with a conditioned hand movement in monkey, *Journal of Neurophysiology* 29:1011-1027, 1966.

32. Evarts EV, Granit R: Relations of reflexes and intended movements, *Progress in Brain Research* 39:1-14, 1976.

33. Evarts EV, Tanji J: Gating of motor cortex reflexes by prior instruction, *Brain Research* 71:479-494, 1974.

34. Evarts EV, Tanji J: Reflex and intended responses in motor cortex pyramidal tract neurons of monkey, *Journal of Neurophysiology* 1069-1080, 1976.

35. Forssberg H: Ontogeny of human locomotor control I. Infant stepping, supported locomotion and transition to independent locomotion *Experimental Brain Research* 57:480-493, 1985.

36. Forssberg H: Development and integration of human locomotor functions. In Goldberger ME, Gorio A, Murray M, editors: *Development and plasticity of the mammalian spinal cord,* Padova, 1986, Liviana Press, 53–63.

37. Forssberg H, Grillner S, Halbertsma J: The locomotion of the spinal cat. I. Coordination within a hindlimb, *Acta Physiologica Scandinavica* 108:269-281, 1980.

38. Forssberg H, Grillner S, Rossignol S: Phase dependent reflex reversal during walking in chronic spinal cats, *Brain Research* 85:103-107, 1975.

39. Forssberg H, Grillner S, Rossignol S: Phasic gain control of reflexes from the dorsum of the paw during spinal locomotion, *Brain Research* 132:121-139, 1977.

40. Fung J, Barbeau H: Modulatory effects of cutaneomuscular stimulation on the soleus H-reflex in spastic paretic subjects during standing and walking. In Horak F, Woollacott M, editors: *Posture and gait: Control mechanisms,* Portland, 1992, Oregon Press, 27-30.

41. Georgopoulos AP, Schwartz AB, Kettner RE: Neuronal population coding of movement direction, *Science* 233:1416-1419, 1986.

42. Goldman PS, Galkin TW: Prenatal removal of frontal association cortex in the fetal rhesus monkey: Anatomical and functional consequences in postnatal life, *Brain Research* 152:451-485, 1978.

43. Gottlieb GL, Corcos DM, Agarwal GC: Organizing principles for single-joint movements. 1. A speed-insensitive strategy, *Journal of Neurophysiology* 62:342-357, 1989.

44. Grillner S: Interaction between central and peripheral mechanisms in the control of locomotion, *Progression Brain Research* 50:227-235, 1979.

45. Grillner S: Control of locomotion in bipeds, tetrapods, and fish. In Brooks VB, editor: *Handbook of physiology, vol 2: The nervous system II, motor control,* Bethesda, Md., 1981, American Physiological Society, 1179-1236.

46. Grillner S: Neurobiological bases of rhythmic motor acts in vertebrates, *Science* 228:143-149, 1985.

47. Grillner S, Halbertsma J, Nilsson J, Thorstensson A: The adaptation to speed in human locomotion, *Brain Res* 165:177-182, 1979.

48. Grillner S, Perret C, Zangger P: Central generation of locomotion in the spinal dogfish, *Brain Res* 109:255-269, 1976.

49. Grillner S, Rossignol S: On the initiation of the swing phase of locomotion in chronic spinal cats, *Brain Res* 146:269-277, 1978.

50. Grillner S, Wall' n P, Dale N, et al: Transmitters, membrane properties and network circuitry in the control of locomotion in lamprey, *Trends in NeuroSciences* 10:34-41, 1987.

51. Grillner S, Zangger P: How detailed is the central pattern generation for locomotion? *Brain Res* 88:367-371, 1975.

52. Harrison PJ, Jankowska E: Sources of input to interneurons mediating group I nonreciprocal inhibition of motoneurones in the cat, *J Physiol (Lond)* 361:379-401, 1985.

53. Hasen Z, Enoka RM, Stuart DG: The interface between biomechanics and neurophysiology in the study of movement: Some recent approaches. In Buskirk ER, editor: *Exercise and Sport Science,* New York, 1985, American College of Sports Medicine, 169-234.

54. Heimer L, Switzer RD, van Hoesen GW: Ventral striatum and ventral pallidum. In Evarts EV, Wise SP, Bousfield D, editors: *The Motor System in Neurobiology,* Amsterdam: Elsevier, 259-269, 1985.

55. Hoffer JA, Caputi AA, Pose IE: Movement of muscle fibers in cat locomotion: What do muscle proprioceptors sense? In Woollacott M, Horak F, editors: *Posture and Gait: Control Mechanisms,* Portland, 1992, Univ of Oregon Books, 25-27.

56. Horak FB, Esselman P, Anderson ME, Lynch MK: The effects of movement velocity, mass displaced, and task certainty on associated postural adjustments made by normal and hemiplegic individuals, *J Neurol Neurosurg Psychiatry* 47:1020-1028, 1984.

57. Horak FB, Nashner LM: Central programming of postural movements: Adaptation to altered

support-surface configurations, *J Neurophysiol* 55:1369-1381, 1986.

58. Houk JC: Regulation of stiffness by skeletomotor reflexes, *Annu Rev Physiol* 41:99-114, 1979.

59. Hultborn H, Meunier S, Pierrot-Deseilligny E, Shindo M: Changes in presynaptic inhibition of Ia fibres at the onset of voluntary contraction in man, *J Physiol (Lond)* 387:757-772, 1987.

60. Hultborn H, Pierrot-Deseilligny E: Changes in recurrent inhibition during voluntary soleus contractions in man studied by an H-reflex technique, *J Physiol (Lond)* 297:229-251, 1979.

61. Jami L: Golgi tendon organs in mammalian skeletal muscle: Functional properties and central actions, *Physiol Rev* 72(3):623-666, 1992.

62. Jankowska E, Jukes MGM, Lund S, Lundberg A: The effect of DOPA on the spinal cord. 5. Reciprocal organization of pathways transmitting excitatory action to alpha motoneurones of flexor and extensors, *Acta Physiol Scand* 70:369-388, 1967.

63. Kristan WB: The neurobiology of swimming in the leech. In Evarts EV, Wise SP, Bousfield D, editors: *The Motor System in Neurobiology,* Amsterdam, 1985, Elsevier, 58-67.

64. Lee RG, Tatton WG: Motor responses to sudden limb displacement in primates with specific CNS disorders and in human patients with motor system disorders, *Can J Neurol Sci* 2:285-293, 1975.

65. Leonard CT: Neural and neurobehavioral changes associated with perinatal brain damage. In Forssberg H, Hirschfeld H, editors: *Movement Disorders in Children,* Amsterdam, 1992, Karger, 50-56.

66. Leonard CT, Goldberger ME: Consequences of damage to the sensorimotor cortex in neonatal and adult cats. II. Maintenance of exuberant projections, *Devlp Brain Res* 32:15-30, 1987.

67. Leonard CT, Goldberger ME: Consequences of damage to the sensorimotor cortex in neonatal and adult cats. I. Sparing and recovery of function, *Devlp Brain Res* 32:1-14, 1987.

68. Leonard CT, Hirschfeld H, Forssberg H: Gait acquisition & reflex abnormalities in normal children & children with cerebral palsy. In Amblard B, Berthoz A, Clarac F, editors: *Posture and Gait: Development Adaptation and Modulation,* Amsterdam, 1988, Elsevier Press, 33-45.

69. Leonard CT, Hirschfeld H, Forssberg H: The development of independent walking in children with cerebral palsy, *Dev Med Child Neurol* 33:567-577, 1991.

70. Leonard CT, Moritani T: H-reflex testing to determine the neural basis of movement disorders of neurologically impaired individuals, *Electromyogr Clin Neurophysiol* 32:341-349, 1992.

71. Leonard CT, Moritani T, Hirschfeld H, Forssberg H: Deficits in reciprocal inhibition in children with cerebral palsy as revealed by H-reflex testing, *Dev Med Child Neurol* 32:974-984, 1990.

72. Livingstone M, Hubel D: Segregation of form, color, movement, and depth: Anatomy, physiology, and perception, *Science* 240:740-740, 1988.

73. Lundberg A: Reflex control of stepping. In *The Nansen Memorial Lecture, October 10th 1968,* Oslo: Universitetsforlaget, 1-42, 1969.

74. Lundberg A: Control of spinal mechanics from the brain. In Tower DB, editor: *The Nervous System,* New York, 1975, Raven Press, 253-265.

75. Marsden DC, Merton PA, Morton HB: Anticipatory postural responses in the human subject (Proceedings), *J Physiol (Lond)* 275:47P-48P, 1978.

76. Marsden CD, Rothwell JC, Day BL: Long-latency automatic responses to muscle stretch in man: Origin and function. In Desmedt JE, editor: *Motor Control Mechanisms in Health and Disease,* New York, 1983, Raven Press, 509-539.

77. McCrea DA: Spinal cord circuitry and motor reflexes. In Pandolf KB, editor: *Exercise and Sport Science Reviews: Vol 14,* New York,1986 Macmillan, 105-141.

78. McGeer PL, McGeer, EG: Amino acid neurotransmitters. In Siegel G, Agranoff B, Albers RW, Molinoff P, editors: *Basic Neurochemistry* New York, 1989, Raven Press, 311-333.

79. Merzenich MM, Kaas JH, Wall J, et al: Topographic reorganization of somatosensory cortical areas 3B and 1 in adult monkeys following restricted deafferentation, *Neuroscience* 8(1):33-55, 1983.

80. Mills KR: Magnetic brain stimulation: A tool to explore the action of the motor cortex on single human spinal motoneurones, *Trends in Neuro-Sciences* 14(9):401-405, 1991.

81. Moore SP, Rushmer DS, Windus SL, Nashner LM: Human automatic postural responses: Responses to horizontal perturbations of stance in multiple directions, *Exp Brain Res* 73:648-658, 1988.

82. Mori S, Kawahara K, Sakamoto T, et al: Setting and resetting of postural muscle tone in the decerebrate cat by stimulation of the brainstem, *J Neurophysiol* 48:737-748, 1982.

83. Nagai T, McGeer PL, Araki M, McGeer EG: GABA-T intensive neurons in the rat brain. In Bjorklund A, Hokfelt T, Kuhar MJ, editors: *Classical Transmitters and Transmitter Receptors in the CNS, Part II Handbook of Chemical Neuroanatomy,* vol 3, Amsterdam, 1984, Elsevier, 247-272.

84. Nashner LM: Adapting reflexes controlling human posture, *Exp Brain Res* 26:59-72, 1976.

85. Nilsson J, Thorstensson A, Halbertsma J: Changes in leg movements and muscle activity with speed of locomotion and mode of progression in humans, *Acta Physiol Scand* 123:457-475, 1985.

86. Nolte J: *The Human Brain,* St. Louis, 1988, Mosby.

87. Okamoto T, Goto Y: Human infant pre-independent and independent walking. In: Kondo S, editor: *Primate Morphophysiology, Locomotor Analyses and Human Bipedalism,* Tokyo, 1985, University of Tokyo Press, 25-45.

88. Orlovsky GN: Electrical activity in brainstem and descending paths in guided locomotion, *Sechenov Physiol J USSR* 55:437-444, 1969.

89. Orlovsky GN: Connections between reticulospinal neurons and locomotor regions of the brainstem, *Biofizika* 15:171-177, 1970.

90. Orlovsky GN: The effect of different descending systems in flexor and extensor activity during locomotion, *Brain Res* 40:359-372, 1972.

91. Palmer E, Ashby P: Evidence that a long latency stretch reflex on humans is transcortical, *Jrnl of Physiol* 449:429-440, 1992.

92. Pearson KG, Ramirez JM, Jiang W: Entrainment of the locomotor rhythm by group Ib afferents from ankle extensor muscles in spinal cats, *Exp Brain Res* 90(3):557-566, 1992.

93. Peiper A: *Cerebral Function in Infancy and Childhood,* New York, 1963, Consultants Bureau, 1-683.

94. Pierrot-Deseilligny E, Katz R, Hultborn H: Functional organization of recurrent inhibition in man: Changes preceding and accompanying voluntary movements. In Desmedt JE, editor: *Motor Control Mechanisms in Health and Disease,* New York, 1983, Raven Press, 443-457.

95. Porter R: Corticomotoneuronal projections: Synaptic events related to skilled movement, *Proc R Soc Lond [Biol]* 231:147-168, 1987.

96. Prechtl HFR: Ultrasound studies of human fetal behaviour, *Early Hum Dev* 12:91-98, 1985.

97. Rakic P: Specification of cerebral cortical areas, *Science* 241:170-176, 1988.

98. Robinson GA, Goldberger ME: The development and recovery of motor function in spinal cats. I. The infant lesion effect, *Exp Brain Res* 62:373-386, 1986.

99. Robinson GA, Goldberger ME: The development and recovery of motor function in spinal cats. II. Pharmacological enhancement of recovery, *Exp Brain Res* 62:387-400, 1986.

100. Rossignol S, Barbeau H, Julien C: Locomotion of the adult chronic spinal cat and its modification by monoaminergic agonists and antagonists. In Goldberger ME, Gorio A, Murray M, editors: *Development and Plasticity of the Mammalian Spinal Cord,* New York, 1984, Fidia Research Series, 323-345.

101. Rossignol S, Gauthier L: An analysis of mechanisms controlling the reversal of crossed spinal reflexes, *Brain Res* 182:31-45, 1980.

102. Sarnat HB, Netsky MG: *Evolution of the Nervous System,* London, 1974, Oxford Univ Press.

103. Schomburg ED: Spinal sensorimotor systems and their supraspinal control, *Neurosci Res* 7:265-340, 1990.

104. Schwartz JH: Chemical basis of synaptic transmission. In Kandel ER, Schwartz JH, editors: *Principles of Neural Science,* Amsterdam, 1981 Elsevier, 106-120.

105. Seitz RJ, Roland RE, Bohm C: Motor learning in man: A positron emission tomographic study, *NeuroReport* 1:57-66, 1990.

106. Shik ML, Severin FV, Orlovsky GN: Control of walking and running by means of electrical stimulation of the mid-brain, *Biofizika* 11:659-666, 1966.

107. Shik ML, Yagodnitsyn AS: The pontobulbar "locomotion strip," *Neurophysiol USSR* 9:72-74, 1977.

108. Shurrager PS, Dykman RA: Walking spinal carnivores, *J Comp Psychol* 44:252-262, 1951.

109. Sidman RL, Rakic P: Neuronal migration with special reference to developing human brain: A review, *Brain Res* 62:1-35, 1973.

110. Smith AM, Hepp-Reymond MC, Wyss UR: Relation of activity in precentral cortical neurons to force and rate of force change during isometric contractions of finger muscles, *Exp Brain Res* 23:315-332, 1975.

111. Stein RB, Capaday C: The modulation of human reflexes during functional motor tasks, *TINS* 11:328-332, 1988.

112. Sutherland DH, Olshen RA, Cooper L, Woo SY: The development of mature gait, *J Bone Joint Surg [Am]* 62:336-353, 1980.

113. Thomas A, Autgaerden S: Locomotion from pre- to post-natal life. In Thomas A, Autgaerden S, editors: *Locomotion from Pre- to Post-Natal Life,* London, 1966, Medical Books Ltd, 1-88.

114. Thompson RF, Clark GA, Donegan NH, et al: Neuronal substrates of learning and memory: A "multiple trace" view. In Lynch G, McGaugh JL, Weinberger NM, editors: *Neurobiology of Learning and Memory,* New York, 1984, Guilford Press, 137-164.

115. Winter DA: Biomechanics of normal and pathological gait: Implications for understanding human locomotor control, *J Motor Behav* 4:337-355, 1989.

116. Winter DA, Sienko SE: Biomechanics of below-knee amputee gait, *J Biomech* 21:361-367, 1988.

117. Wise SP, Evarts EV: The role of the cerebral cortex in movement. In Evarts EV, Wise SP, Bousfield D, editors: *The Motor System in Neurobiology,* Amsterdam, 1985, Elsevier, 307-315.

118. Yang JF, Stein RB, James KB: Contribution of peripheral afferents to the activation of the soleus muscle during walking in humans, *Exp Brain Res* 87:679-687, 1991.

CHAPTER 8

THE ACQUISITION OF LOCOMOTOR SKILL

Joseph R. Higgins
Susan Higgins

KEY TERMS

Critical feature

Motor skill

Prerequisite

Substate

Task analysis

Taxonomy of motor skills

Total body response

Learning motor skills may be viewed as the progressive gain in understanding and control over the genesis and mastery of the cooperative relationships. These relationships are task-related organizations that serve to unite the individual and the surroundings. This chapter focuses on several ideas concerning this view of motor skill learning and includes how the individual might acquire this skill given a variety of situations and conditions.[*] The frame of reference is upon bringing about a change in movement behavior as it supports the act of locomotion in the variety of situations and conditions from which gait emerges.

Locomotion is viewed as a task or a problem to be solved by the mover. From a perspective of skill learning, understanding the relationship between task and mover serves as a critical starting point for both theoretical and practical considerations. A task analytic approach is suggested as a way of systematically gathering information and establishing the relationship between the mover and the environment for the task at hand.[4] At the same time, this model becomes an essential point of departure for understanding skill and the underlying processes subserving skill.

Finally, we will discuss what constitutes a locomotor problem and why locomotion might be considered a skill involving an infinite variety of solutions, depending upon the task and its context. The mover needs to be viewed as an **active problem solver** who is engaged in understanding the task and the personal resources they have available for solving the problems posed by the task.[†] In the concluding section we discuss several implications for practice that emerge from concepts of motor skill learning. Specific reference to locomotion is made in view of practice.

The Learning of a Motor Skill

Throughout the life span the individual struggles to progressively gain control over the available resources pertinent to their interaction with the external surroundings.[22] **Available resources** are embedded in or emerge from morphological, perceptual/sensory, and physical world assets. These resources are exploited by the mover in attaining a movement goal. Factors, for example, such as body size, muscular strength, degrees of freedom, vision, gravity, etc., are progressively exploited and used as the mover interacts with the environment. These resources are applied to the construction and control of the cooperative relationships that "unite the individual, the task constraints and the surround." (See Chapter 4). The mover comes to understand the utility of her/his available resources in a broad range of tasks and to develop the cognitive and perceptual skill and motor control necessary to exploit these resources toward achieving the mover's own purposes and goals. Ultimately a mover develops a well-coordinated total body response to the problem. This is the essence of learning a motor skill.

The learning of motor skill involves the development of a progressively competent **total body response** to the performance context and purpose of the movement. The total body response is viewed as many nested cooperative relationships between the individual and the surroundings directed towards a particular purpose or goal (the motor problem). For example, cooperative relationships must be developed between limb segments and the torso, between perceptual systems and the limbs and torso, between perceptual systems, limbs, torso and the external world. Furthermore, each of these relationships must be consistently available for the mover to draw upon—that is, the relationships must come under the performer's control both in their construction and their execution. The appropriate and progressive development of these cooperative relationships represents the motor learning process.

Each gain in control represents an increased compliance with the external world and a changing understanding of the task-individual-environment interaction. Motor control ultimately is the selective allocation of muscular tension across the appropriate joint-segment relationships in the body.[‡] The learner discovers how much tension to apply, where the tension is allocated, and how long the tension is applied. A well-controlled motor response will exhibit task-appropriate differential allocation of tension or force that is integrated with

---

[*] When we use the term *acquisition,* it can mean either acquiring a skill for the first time or reacquiring a skill following some physical or neural insult. We also use the term *learner* throughout and should be considered in the broadest sense to include patients, children, adults, athletes, etc.

[†] In terms of practice, it should be noted that the learner *and* the practitioner/teacher are both active problem solvers, and in a teaching/learning setting the interaction between the two should receive attention. The teacher and learner interact not only with each other but with the motor task(s) to be solved at any moment in time. From their unique perspectives, each must analyze the motor problem(s) to be solved and create an appropriate movement solution—the *practitioner as facilitator* and the *learner as mover.*

[‡] Within a learning context, motor control might be considered as the act of *gaining control.*

the external forces.§ What makes a force or level of tension the appropriate amount depends on the particular movement or motor problem being solved at a particular moment in time. Allocation of force/ tension is specific to the problem being solved, the nature of the internal and external forces available to the mover, and the nature of the lever systems to which those forces are applied. Forces are selectively applied to each tentative solution, results are analyzed, and changes are made. In this way, the learner comes to understand both the problem and the resources. For example, when confronting walking with crutches for the first time, the learner comes to understand what underlying resources are available for stability and for mobility, what crutches afford, and how crutch and individual can be cooperatively related to the task at hand.

Gain in control is expressed by the learner in at least two ways: (1) cognitively and perceptually and (2) motorically. The goal or purpose of the movement, the constraints imposed by the individual's morphology, and the environmental context and the field of external forces merge to form the motor problem to be solved. As the learner comes to understand the elements that constitute the motor problem and the relationship between available resources, the movement solutions emerge to complement them. Initially the learner explores different ways or means of organizing the body-environment relationship to achieve the goal—for example, where and how to allocate force for stabilization of the upper body and for mobility using the crutches for alternately providing support and mobility. The insights gleaned from these initial encounters help establish cooperative relationships that can then be mastered and generalized. Understanding is achieved as a function of the time spent exploring the **means-end relationships.**‖ The individual progressively gains control in relation to the management of the body center of mass (COM) and the appropriate trunk and segment relationships. This development of progressive control is seen, for example, in the increased use and regulation of the number of participating segments, increased range of motion (ROM), generally improved flow of the movement, and improved and increasingly effective use of the body-posture system.[34]

Each gain in control (or competence or understanding) supports the next gain. As the first discoveries are made, the learner is challenged to master the appropriate solutions and, at the same time, extend the repertory to apply these solutions to an increasing number of situations and conditions. Exploring previously limiting conditions, for example, or exploring the environment in a different way or under different conditions brings the learner to a new level of understanding and control. This interactive cycle of discovery, mastery, and application occurs continuously as the learner encounters and reencounters each task or situation.[22] These aspects of the process of learning should be viewed in most circumstances as occurring simultaneously; initially, however, it is the discovery aspect that seems to begin the process. Discovery involves the learner's understanding of the goal and task demands and then developing the means of achieving the goal through movement.

Locomotion as a Motor Skill

Understanding locomotion as an emergent movement form that undergoes progressive development of control requires some understanding of skill. Locomotion is a crucial resource for the individual. It is an action, realized through any number of movement forms, that serves to transport the individual through the environment. Locomotor skill is defined as the individual's effectiveness in achieving this transport function under very limited or very diverse conditions. At the same time locomotion as a skill can be employed or empowered in a larger action. Skill as elaborated by Susan Higgins, is an "... aspect of the on-going function of an individual" and is expressed by some level of control over goal-directed movement; it is the acquired ability to consistently solve a movement problem under a variety of conditions.[22]

Locomotor skill might be thought of as expressing the individual's competence in controlling the locomotor act in the service of a goal-directed behavior. In this context, skill is the individual's ability to use locomotion as a problem-solving tool. The individual is limited in skill (the degree to which they are able to accomplish the goal effectively) by their current capacities (including physical or morphological, experiential, and emotional). Furthermore, skill is represented by the individual's ability to apply available resources toward achieving a solution to the motor problem being encountered and is viewed as being relative to the individual's developmental, cognitive, fitness, and competence levels.[22]

Skillful movers are skillful problem solvers. Skill is relative to the individual's state at any

---

§ We use tension and force interchangeably to mean specifically the effective output of muscles across joints that are interacting to produce segmental movement.

‖ For a more in-depth discussion of the means-end relationship in the acquisition of skill, the reader is referred to Higgins S,[22] and Gentile AM.[10,11]

moment in time. The adolescent with cerebral palsy (CP), for example, may be a skillful runner relative to what her/his motoric and developmental state afford. Regardless of the condition of the body, the individual analyzes a variety of situations and acts appropriately given the unique demands of each situation. The adolescent with CP learns from the results of his/her actions, from the failure or success of the chosen motor solution, and from observing the movements/actions of others. The knowledge gained is used to produce alternative solutions or to improve the efficiency and effectiveness of subsequent actions. The adaptations and compensations are a function of what is required of the task—locomotion—and the state of the moving system itself. In several case studies, Winter shows that an adaptation of muscle use, a shift from one joint to another for primary control, compensates for the inadequate control across other joints.[36] For example, lack of control of tibialis anterior may be compensated for by "hyperactive" hip extensor muscles, which compensate for forward propulsion. What is of particular interest in Winter's findings is that the need to locomote and the action of locomotion allow any number of muscle activations to compensate for the inadequately functioning muscles.[35,36] A movement emerges that produces a walk; the system is clearly able to adapt, to compensate for limitations, and to learn to use its available resources constructively.

Skill can be viewed as a product of our genetic potential and our experiential history. The degree of skill achieved can be enhanced by psychological factors such as motivation, perceptual and cognitive abilities; by physiological factors such as fitness level; and by sociocultural factors such as parental and peer influence.[22] Even though genetic and structural potential are important factors underlying skill development, the role of experience is often the critical determinant. We elaborate upon this notion of the importance of experience in the concluding section when we discuss instruction and practice.

Locomotion solves a basic need of the individual: the need to transport the body from one location in space to another. It is this basic need that is pervasive as the individual learns how to locomote from one point to another within a variety of spatial and temporal conditions (see Chapter 32 for more details). Any number of factors limit the type of locomotion resolution; for example, the individual may not have the use of the legs, or may be unable to talk or hear or see, or may have a congenital condition such as talipes, or may be recovering from a stroke. With reference to locomotion, the condition of the individual partially forms the problem. Additionally, each individual will have a different solution to the problem. In one instance the individual may have to learn how to rally social support from others. In other instances support is rallied from within to control a wheelchair or to manage a special orthotic device. In all cases the individual rallies and masters the support necessary to accomplish the locomotor act.

Locomotion is a skill; the need to locomote is a pervasive aspect of being human. The movement form supporting this act differs depending on the morphological, cognitive, and perceptual state of the individual. The form will differ depending upon the goal and the particular motor solution needed to meet that goal.[*] Given a particular individual configuration of morphology the act of locomoting may be narrowed to walking. The walk requires that the individual be able to stand upright and to alternately swing the leg from a position of double support to single support.

Skillful locomotion occurs when the individual is able to modify the means or locomotor pattern so as to be effective given different environmental situations (surfaces, stairs, ramps, objects, and people) and task conditions (distances, speeds, and directions). The skillful mover has control over a variety of locomotor solutions and has learned how to modify the pattern to suit the demands of a particular environment and task. In order to appropriately enlist a crawl rather than a walk, for example, the mover must understand which aspects of the environment to pay attention to and which to ignore. How a surface and surrounding structures and objects can be traversed and the state of the mover will determine what locomotor form is appropriate.

Learning a locomotor skill entails both acquiring control of the movement itself and the knowledge of external conditions that affect the movement. Locomoting, of necessity, will not be the same from one instance or encounter to the next. There may be different surfaces, objects and people over and around which the locomotor action must contend.

Learning to manage and manipulate a wheelchair is illustrative of this point. The different surfaces, objects, and people, and whether they are in motion or stationary will alter the way the locomotor act itself emerges. In any situation, the

---

[*] For example, the situation will determine the type of locomotor action that is appropriate. If the mover's goal is to go into a cave and the opening does not afford upright posture, the obvious solution is then to crawl. The size of the opening affords crawling and not walking.

individual's basic need is to reliably respond to an increased variety of conditions so goal achievement is possible. This is what skill is all about; it involves the consistent and effective achievement of the goal under a variety of task and environmental conditions and with the least amount of expenditure of energy for that person at that time.

Some individuals are unable to be responsive to all possible conditions and are therefore precluded from developing reliable solutions to certain conditions.[22] The solutions are outside their cognitive, perceptual, mechanical, and motoric capabilities or capacity. Experience helps individuals become aware of their limits or limiting conditions and then develop locomotor skill appropriate to various contexts given their capacity.

The principles and ideas expressed so far work across the range of types of locomotion because they are appropriate for all motor skill. The remainder of the discussion will be limited to consideration of those individuals who are capable of generating a walk to solve a motor problem.

WALKING EMBEDDED IN A LARGER ACTION

Locomotion is the act of getting from one place to another, it is an action. **Gait** is the means of achieving this action and is specified by the goal and nature of the task.[†] The goal might be to carry a doll from the bedroom to the kitchen where the child's parents are preparing dinner. Carrying the doll and the urgency of the need to bring the doll to the kitchen constitute the emerging action. The movement solution for carrying out the action includes the incorporation of the individual's permanent or transient anatomical features, assitive devices, etc., along with the turns and changes of rate required to get from bedroom to kitchen. The emotional component or perceived immediacy of the goal interacts with the morphological state and determines the rate of her/his gait, making it a walk or a run, a creep or a crawl.[‡]

Many of our actions involve locomotion as a support function toward achieving a goal: running to catch a ball, carrying a cup and saucer from the sink to the table, or carrying the doll in the previous example. In these tasks gait can be viewed as supporting the functional goal (a walk, a run).

Locomotion is the skill that involves not only functional use of the leg but also of the arm/hand complex. The arm/hand complex[§] is used in support of the locomotor act, or it can be integrated into the action as a process involving the primary aspect of movement goal. For example, pumping the arms to enhance the run vs. carrying a cup of coffee or a glass of milk. Carrying a hot cup of coffee across the room (complicated by the type of vessel that contains the coffee), demands stabilization and management of the object in the hands. The mover attends to that aspect of the task allowing the locomotor processes for walk to emerge in keeping with the problem solution. If the individual is using some form of locomotor assistive device and simultaneously needs to carry an object, a different set of problems is posed for the mover that results in a different action solution. It is the systematic understanding of these functional aspects of the movement and task and of the different factors and how they may effect the emerging movement solution that have been ignored in traditional views of gait. It should also be noted that the mover's attention will be twofold when the function of the arm/hand complex becomes primary, i.e., the goal to not spill the coffee holds one's attention on the cup along with where one is going. When the arm/hand complex is complementary to the locomotor act, the focus is generally singular, i.e., where one is going.

The relationship between the walk and the independent use of the arm/hand complex depends upon the task and environmental constraints. Observations of toddlers in the initial phases of bipedal locomotion clearly reveal that from the beginning walking emerges in concert with the

---

[†] The distinction between locomotion and gait can be clarified: *locomotion* is an action involving the change in position of the body and limbs in space and time; *gait* is the particular manner or style of moving on foot—it can be a walk, a jog, or a run. Walking is a particular form of gait.

[‡] According to S. Higgins,[21] gait is considered a dynamic and biological structure that subserves locomotion and, by definition, has a set pattern of foot falls, affords stability, and "exhibits a periodic relationship among successive states of the supporting limbs." As the tempo is varied from the preferred to very, very slow or upward to very fast, no apparent change in foot fall pattern develops. At extremely slow speeds the alternating periods of double support and single support change to include an

additional double support phase; when the tempo increases beyond a "limit," the walk becomes a jog or run, eliminating the double-support phase and producing alternating periods of contralateral single-leg support.

[§] The term *arm/hand complex* is used to emphasize the notion that the hand is served by the arms and the entire shoulder complex; it can be argued that the trunk and legs also serve the functions required by the hand(s). Morphologically and functionally the *arm/hand complex* is used in manipulatory activity of the hand(s) and should be considered a complex involving the skeletal, articulatory, muscular, and sensory and motor nervous systems as they collectively and integratively interact in the service of the hand. In the past we have referred to the functions involving this complex as limb manipulation.

TABLE 8-1   A Strategy for Task Analysis

1. Identify the task(s) and specify the goal and subgoals.
2. Amass information concerning:
   a. The *action,* including classification of the function of the action and movement.
   b. The *environment,* including the influence of both direct and indirect conditions.
   c. The *mover/patient,* including his/her characteristics, abilities, and whether the minimal prerequisite skills for success are present.
   d. The *prerequisite skills* required of the client.
   e. The *expectations* of outcome and movement outcomes.
3. Develop a strategy to make up for any deficits identified in #2.
4. Plan the intervention strategy based upon the preceding information concerning the individual-task-environment interaction.
   a. With the broader context in mind, systematically plan the action-goal-task encounter and include an observational strategy focusing upon the critical aspects of the action and outcomes that can be used for patient feedback and evaluation of the effectiveness of the strategy.
   b. Structure the environment for appropriate task-action encounter, including attention to the broadest range of conditions possible.
   c. Clarify the goal and subgoals.
5. Effect the strategy.
   a. Observe the performance of the mover.
   b. Record *what happened:* what was the outcome, and what was the approach and effect of the movement solution?
6. Evaluate the observations.
   a. Compare *expectations* and *what happened.*
   b. Provide feedback based on the comparison above and assist the mover/learner in making decisions about the next encounter.
   c. With the mover, plan the next intervention/task-action encounter.

Adapted from Arend and Higgins.[4]

arm/hand complex. The arm/hands either function in support of the walking itself or function independently of the walk as when carrying or manipulating an object.[18,19]

A walk is a category of gait pattern that under certain circumstances subserves the locomotion function. The walk is an emergent property of the individual who is capable of upright posture, single leg support and lateral stability, and alternately generating and resisting self-produced forward momentum. If an individual has the capacity to control these factors and has an intact central pattern generator, walking will emerge when the conditions in the environment supporting it prevail. Once walking emerges as a self-organizing, meaningful response to the individual-environment interaction, the individual brings the response under control, subsequently modifying it in relation to an infinite or increasing variety of task and environmental conditions.

Regardless of her/his state, the mover is engaged in a constant quest to gain control over task, environmental conditions, and production of solutions. A skill like walking is not a leg pattern or a movement pattern that can be imparted, but rather is a total body response generated by the individual who is actively solving a specific motor problem. It is not the control of a particular joint or segment, but rather how the critical features of the movement affect and determine the development of control. Gait solutions emerge which are appropriate for the individual's current condition or state and in relation to the task.[25]

LEARNING AND THE TASK ANALYTIC APPROACH

The importance of a careful and systematic **task analysis** cannot be overemphasized in understanding locomotion. This strategy provides the basic understandings required for learning and subsequently structuring the learning environment. A task analysis is a cyclic process that integrates planning/designing instruction and practice, observation, intervention, and evaluation.[4,17] Table 8-1 provides guidelines for consideration in this process.

The critical factors that affect any learning situation are systematically identified through a task analysis. Factors such as goals and subgoals, perceptual demands and subskills inherent in the task, relationships between the movement and the environment, substrates of control, and related prerequisites are systematically identified. This information is then used as a basis for developing a theoretical understanding of gait. In the interest of brevity we address only three points from this framework: (1) identification of the goal and sub-goals, (2) classification of the skill, and (3) identification of prerequisites. These points are of particular importance and illustrative of the task analytic approach.

Identification of Goals and Subgoals

A critical activity is identification and consideration of the relationship between the goal (and the subgoals) of the action and the functional significance of the use of the limbs (the integration of body/torso, legs and arms). The investigator considers the task conditions and identifies the motor problems the mover must solve. Goals serve as the basis for organizing the movement and are a function of the movers potentialities, the movement needs, and the task constraints. It is not a specific movement pattern that is identified by the mover. Instead, the mover assesses the nature of the goal and the problems needing resolution and then determines how the movement must be organized to meet the goal. There is no single solution for any given task condition. The variety of task conditions and solutions is limited only by the context and the state of the individual.

The movement solutions to movement goals often involve the integration of the locomotor process and arm/hand complex manipulation. The goal and subgoal of the movement are identified with respect to function of both the locomotor and manipulatory systems. (There are tasks that involve manipulation of objects with the feet/legs while at the same time locomoting. These tasks are analyzed in terms of the the functional relationship between the locomotion system and the manipulatory system.)

Identifying subgoals as parts of the movement is helpful in determining which aspects of the movement need special attention, which aspects are most critical, and which are most tractable. Subgoals are identified for each phase of a movement, thus linking movement and goal. For example, a purpose of the swing phase of the walk is to move the nonsupport leg forward to provide a new base of support. In addition, other subgoals of the swing phase include lateral support or balance on a single leg, deceleration of the swing leg, creation of a reactive force for moving the com forward, or control of the foot contact at the end of the swing. Finally, some subgoals need to be identified in relation to arm/hand complex use. The arm/hand complex can be used in producing walk, in the service of the walk, or independently in order to accomplish another aspect of the goal.

Classification of Skills

In order to deal with the complexity of the situations that can arise with this functional approach, an overall organizing system is needed. This system takes into account both the conditions of the environment that constrain or dictate how movement solutions will emerge as well as how the processes for control and regulation of posture, locomotion, and arm/hand complex movement are integrated. A *Taxonomy of Motor Skill* was outlined in the early 1970s by Gentile and Higgins.[12] This taxonomy and its modifications provide an organizing scheme for the classification of motor skills underlying perceptual motor processes and information about critical learning variables affecting a particular skill.[10,11,17] *

To briefly describe the taxonomy, we begin by considering each of the two dimensions along which skill is classified. One dimension considers the types of environmental conditions that directly affect how movements are organized: objects, people, and surfaces are stable or moving, and events or situations remain the same or change from one movement execution to the next. The second dimension considers the nature of movement or function of the action involved in the solution of the task: whether the body remains in one place and is thus stable or whether the body is being transported from one place to another (locomotion). Superimposed on this body stability or locomotion function is the presence or absence of arm/hand complex involvement in a dual task. The use of the arm/hand complex can be integrated into the stable body or a larger locomotor action in order to bring about change in the environment.

Examination of the functional relationship between locomotion and limb use provides, among other things, a way of viewing and considering dual tasks. Walking with an assistive device such

---

* For a more detailed discussion of this model approach and representation of these taxonomic dimensions, with examples of tasks and task characteristics that include perceptual and information processing demands, the reader is referred to the tables presented in Gentile.[10]

as a cane or crutches involves use of the arm/hand complex in the service of the locomotor function. Running to catch a bus while carrying packages, on the other hand, is illustrative of the idea that the arms can be decoupled from the locomotor process and used in the service of another function—in this example, carrying an object. Using the arm/hand complex for other purposes, such as carrying an object, alters both the temporal and spatial organization of the pattern of locomotion.[18,19,20]

This is an example of a dual task condition involving both locomotion and the independent use of the arm-hand complex. By assuming an upright and bipedal posture, the upper limbs are freed from serving postural support functions and locomotion. Humans exploit this ability to locomote with their upper limbs decoupled for serving another purpose. As a result we have a marvelously large repertoire of potential actions in which we can use both upper limbs and lower limbs interactively or independently in order to solve an infinite variety of motor problems. Studying or observing movement under conditions in which the limbs are used for purposes other than in the service of locomotion provides an interesting window to understanding the organization of movement. This approach provides a practical and systematic way of varying task constraints around a primary movement function.

The assumptions underlying the stability/locomotion and independent limb function are based on evidence that specialized neural pathways and cortical and subcortical centers are responsible for regulation and integration of posture, locomotion, and arm/hand use and manipulation.[13,14,15,16] In terms of function, the learner/performer must regulate and maintain postural control for each particular task as well as integrate the required locomotor and arm/limb control processes into the action.

For every task some form of postural support must be exercised. Task analysis provides a means of understanding the condition(s) or state(s) under which the posture must be regulated and controlled, how posture functions in supporting or serving both locomotion and arm/limb use. The task may involve only maintaining a stable position in space, as with sitting or standing, or the preparation for initiating a gait process. On the other hand, the task may demand that the performer walk across the room, or cross the room carrying an object, etc. An infinite variety of conditions can be considered that are illustrative of the interaction of postural support alone, the role of posture while locomoting, or the act of loco-

moting and using the arm/hand complex. From the performer's perspective, larger and larger action sequences may also be integrated or incorporated into the action as experience with the tasks is gained. The end result is a more efficient and functionally successful outcome.

For example, crossing a room in order to bring an object from the table to the chair in the corner poses a significant motor problem for the individual using a walker or crutches. The goal would be to transport an object from its place on the table to another location in the room. Along with this primary goal, several subgoals serve to define the problems to be solved: initiating gait, crossing the room, navigating around furniture, approaching the table, slowing down and stopping, reaching for and grasping the object, turning and initiating the gait in the direction of the chair, locomoting to the chair, slowing down and stopping, and finally placing the object on the chair. In this action, the function of object acquisition, manipulation, and transport is served by the arm/hand process; that part of the goal requiring the transport of the object and the individual is subserved by the locomotor process. The postural support function now supports both the locomotion and the object stability and manipulation functions. The hands are free to manipulate and retrieve the object, transport it, and place it in a new spatial location within the room. The complication here, however, is that the solution for acquiring and then transporting the object must be solved quite differently when using crutches. For example, the mover may work out a solution for carrying the object—say a book—by slipping it between the forearm and the crutch itself. A perfectly satisfactory solution given that the object does not have to be carried too far and that its weight is not too great.

Ultimately, the mover has functionally organized her/his locomotor movements/actions—including the use of the arm/hand complex—to suit the demands of the task and her/his morphological status at that moment in time given her/his experiential and developmental history. The movements were organized in space and time to "fit" the context. Studying the organization of movement, either theoretically or practically, from this functional perspective provides a means of separating interacting variables and identifying their independent and collective effects.

Identification of Prerequisite Skills

In a 1980 article Susan Higgins first introduced the idea of substrates for control and related prerequisites as tools or resources available to the learner

Table **8-2** Substrate Categories for Identification of Prerequisite Skills

1. **Postural control:** appropriate integration of body and limb orientation for stability and transport.
2. **Dynamic equilibrium:** maintaining balance during all forms of movement, including stopping, intitiating, and maintaining locomotion.
3. **Exploratory movements:** informing the mover about the environment and physical world; functionally incorporated into on-going actions(s) in order to support perceptual processes.
4. **Independent arm use:** allows mover to manipulate devices in the service of locomotion or to simultaneously engage in two tasks (dual task condition).
5. **Integration of postural control and limb manipulation:** progressively larger and more efficient and successful action units are incorporated into functionally larger and more appropriate units.
6. **Symmetrical and asymmetrical use of torso and/or limbs:** reciprocal and symmetrical arm swing or asymmetrical arm use when carrying an object during locomotion.
7. **Differential relaxation:** absence or presence of efficient use of muscle tensions in producing the movement required for the realization of the action.
8. **Use of momentum:** incorporating the motion already in effect into the on-going movement or action; the use of existing internal or external force in the service of the on-going action in order to minimize the energy production needs of the muscle.
9. **Generation of force:** identify what force problems are to be solved for any task and what is required by the mover to generate the appropriate force.
10. **Absorbing force:** task constraint requiring absorption of force generated either internally or externally; going down a ramp or stairs as contrasted with ascending same.

Adapted from S. Arend.[4]

for engaging in increasingly complex movement behavior or actions.[2,3] Identifying and determining the level of prerequisite development for the general and the specific case provides the investigator with a means of deciding what aspects of a particular task need to be dealt with before the mover is ready to engage in a particular task. Does the mover have sufficient upper body strength or balance/equilibrium control to manage walking?* Identifying prerequisite skills provides a systematic set of functions to help the investigator understand the mover-task relationship *and* determine the apparent competence and capacity for effectively and efficiently producing an action in response to a goal and motor problem. Actions are the functional integration of the substrates or prerequisite skills that have contributed to the relative level of efficiency of the individual. They are used by the mover in achieving the goal.

Furthermore, these substrates have a close, if not direct, relationship to underlying motor control processes.

In Table 8-2 we identify ten substrates of control that have particular implications and relevance in working with individuals in a variety of locomotor action contexts. The ten substrates identified constitute a noninclusive list from which specific prerequisites can be identified and examined under varying conditions.† We suggest that the substrates be used to identify the particular prerequisite skill necessary for a particular task and individual. Each substrate is the relationship of the individual and the task influenced by the constraints imposed by environment, morphology, and field of external forces. The identified prerequisites form one of the bases for designing and structuring the intervention strategy and subsequent practice.

* On the issue of muscular strength, a significant body of literature indicates that initial gains in strength can be accounted for by variables associated with learning; for example, motor unit recruitment. In some cases sufficient strength may be available, but the individual is unable to apply it for the specific task. Initially this would imply that learning how to recruit motor units in the service of specific task conditions is of critical importance. This view should be considered both theoretically and practically. For further discussion of this idea and considerations for practice, the reader is referred to Bohannon RW,[6,7] Enoka RM and Fuglevand AJ,[9] Jones DA and Rutherford OM,[24] Loeb GE,[23] Rutherford OM and Jones DA,[30] Rutherford OM,[31] and Sale DG.[32]

† According to Arend S[3] the theoretically derived prerequisites can be arbitrarily categorized on four levels: (1) *knowledge base,* which includes both perceptual and cognitive knowledges; (2) *physical control,* which includes ability to modulate forces at joints and properly sequence limb segments; (3) *subskills* possessed, which directly relate to task solution; and (4) *fitness,* which includes appropriate strength, endurance, and flexibility. These categories and the abilities identified under each express the minimum necessary "tools" or resources for successfully participating in a specific task. The practitioner will want to develop her/his own set of categories that emerge from the context and type of setting in which the process of intervention is being carried out.

TABLE 8-3   Practitioner's Role in Instruction and Practice

1. Facilitate the development of motor skill.
2. Provide a nurturing, safe, supportive, and facilitory environment for bringing about change in functional movements.
3. Analyze tasks.
4. Identify prerequisite skills required of task(s) and compensate deficits identified.
5. Clarify the goal of the movement and minimize goal confusion.
6. Establish appropriate conditions for understanding task and task conditions:
   • Observation
   • Demonstration
   • Functional problem solution
   • Clarification of perceptual demands and relevant environmental features
7. Identify the critical features of the movement for both observation and for instruction and practice.
8. Select tasks requiring a variety of locomotion strategies that incorporate dual task and varied environmental conditions.
9. Capitalize on learner's successes and failures.
10. Provide feedback appropriate to task and skill level of learner.
11. Employ appropriate motivational strategies.

Prerequisites are the minimal necessary conditions needed to successfully participate in a task to produce the successful action.[2] These conditions involve the mover's knowledge base, perceptual skill, motor control, training or fitness, and emotional security. The prerequisites are the necessary "tools" that allow the mover to engage in complex behavior. These tools are generally acquired as a function of experience with a wide variety of action-task situations or contexts. The mover must meet the minimal prerequisites in order to succeed in the task. Once identified, prerequisite skills are evaluated by observing performance in a series of less complex tasks that demand the same or similar knowledge.

INSTRUCTION AND PRACTICE

Ideas and concepts emerging from and about motor learning should be considered with respect to how they influence practice. The notions gleaned from experiments and from practice merge so as to inform the practitioner about motor skills and how they are acquired.[11] The practitioner brings a broad knowledge base for problem solving in a specific context, while the learner is usually focused upon a specific goal within that context.[11] For the learner the solution for the locomotor problem is emergent and inherent in the interaction between self and task.[*] Facilitating

the acquisition of skill begins with identifying the substrates and prerequisites of skill that the learner has available at a particular moment in time.[3,17] As a model for designing strategies for facilitating skill (providing instruction and structuring practice), special emphasis is given to how the practitioner systematically analyzes the task-individual-environment interaction as described above.

Changing the functional use of locomotion takes place through instruction and the establishment of practice routines and strategies. Two aspects of the learning setting over which the practitioner has direct control are instruction and practice. The teacher designs instruction and practice so that the learner develops appropriate and effective movement strategies under a broad range of contexts. Instruction and practice are designed so that the learner develops appropriate and effective movement strategies. Table 8-3 outlines 11 primary roles for the practitioner to consider in facilitating the acquisition of skill. The list is not complete; for more details, see both Gentile[10,11] and S. Higgins[22] for more detail.

We view the practitioner as being a facilitator of skill.[†] In this instance the practitioner facilitates gait by applying concepts that emerge from "motor learning." The role of the practitioner in the general context of facilitating skill involves: (1) enhancing the problem-solving capacity of the

---

[*]   For a more detailed discussion of the idea of movement as an emergent property see chapter 4 and reference 17.

[†]   By practitioner we mean the principal agent for facilitating change in motor behavior: the teacher, coach, therapist, and parent, to name a few.

individual; (2) enhancing the morphological resources available to the individual; (3) facilitating the development of the cognitive and perceptual bases for skill; and (4) providing and structuring contexts appropriate for instruction and practice. The effectiveness of the practitioner in bringing about change is largely contingent on involving the learner as an active problem solver.[1]

During instructional and practice periods, the learners must be actively engaged in finding task solutions with functional significance to them. Practice should not be restricted to the teaching session, but designed to extend outside to the broader and functional settings.

This is an important consideration for the practitioner who has relatively little contact time with the client. What the client does outside the instructional/practice setting has considerable impact upon the progress of learning. The practitioner, therefore, must plan for and incorporate this analysis into the instructional period so that the learner can practice independently while away from formal instruction and supervision. Here again the learner needs to understand how to incorporate not only the physical practice requirements but also how to rally the social support systems described earlier.

The learner must become immersed in the learning process and invested, as an intelligent participant, in (re)securing his/her competence in solving motor problems. Strategies for securing active learner participation are critical to the achievement of both teaching and personal goals. In the past several years much has been written about the "active learner."[1] The active involvement of learners in their own learning within a safe and nurturing environment is both motivational and instructive. From this perspective, solutions to the movement problems confronting the learner must be dealt with so that she/he actively moves or attempts the movement with little assistance from the practitioner, other than minimal body support. Passively moving the limb(s) does not appear to contribute to learning a skill or the solution of a task. Consider the following discussion regarding observation of the task as a more critical way of providing understanding about the movement itself. The teacher's role is to develop ways of encouraging and facilitating the learner's ability to analyze the task in order to "derive" her/his own solution to the problems posed.

We conclude our discussion of instruction and practice with an expanded discussion of demonstration and observation and the use of critical features of the movement in instruction and practice.

Observation and Demonstration

The topological characteristics or the form of the movement seem to convey to the learner more useful information than does descriptive information about the absolute motions involved.[33] In facilitating the (re)acquisition of walking, for example, observation and demonstration are the primary source of information about the form and structure of the movement.

Observation of others in the process of learning a skill and subsequently receiving feedback about the observed movement appears to promote motor skill learning.[26,27,28] This is an especially important idea that can be readily incorporated into instructional setting. In essence, these authors and others have suggested the following: (1) guided observation and demonstration is a potent form of instruction, and (2) providing feedback about another's movement conveys useful and accessible information for the learner.

Using other movers as models for various movement solutions—noting that there is no *ideal* form or movement suggested—and specific comments or feedback from a teacher about the movement observed will enhance performance. The mover learns from the observation of others, especially when the teacher comments on the critical aspects of the observed movement. Apparently the observer gains insight and information about the movement that can be incorporated into her/his own movement solutions. In the initial process of motor skill learning, the learner benefits more from the guided visual information than from information derived proprioceptively or kinesthetically.

This approach can be expanded to include observation of video-taped movements by other learners in a variety of contexts. It is a way of expanding the movement problem repertory beyond the formal teaching/learning setting; the video may show an individual or individuals struggling during the initial learning process while on a busy street, or navigating through a home, or climbing onto a public bus. In addition, video can be used for the active self-observation of the mover's performance. In all cases the objective is to help the learner actively solve the movement problem at hand, to help in arriving at alternative solutions, and to develop their own strategies for solving an increasing variety of movement problems.

Critical Features of the Movement

In our strategy for analysis and intervention (developed first in 1976) we noted that for understanding, observing, and providing feedback about

TABLE 8-4 Biomechanical Derivatives and the Critical Features of the Walk

1. Displacement of the body center of mass in a forward direction:
   • COM or pelvic girdle in front of pushoff foot
2. Regaining of control during the resistive phase:
   • Heel contact occurs with foot in front of COM
3. Lose and reestablish successive bases of support:
   • Alternating periods of single and double support

the movement, it was essential to identify the critical features of the movement. **Critical features** are those aspects of the observable movement that are essential for success and thus are least modifiable.[4] Carr and Shephard later refer to these as "essential components" of the movement.[8] One of the principal outcomes of the task analysis is identification of those critical features of the movement that have a direct relationship to the task.

For a given individual and task conditions, certain features of the observable movement must be present for a successful walk. These features are least modifiable. Though specific task conditions and a particular individual will alter the specific details, we have identified three general biomechanical derivatives in Table 8-4 from which critical features for the walk are described. The movement form must incorporate these features in order to produce what is considered a walk.

These three critical features can be expanded to include more detailed consideration of the walk such as:

1. Control of COM in relation to base of support
2. Foot use in relation to COM during pushoff, swing, and landing
3. Timing of placement of handhold or placement of assistive device
4. Use of arm/hand complex, critical in use of assistive device or engaging in dual task
5. Head torso involvement, not as crucial as above, in service of arm/hand complex and transport function of legs

Disturbances in walking resulting from some motor dysfunction might be considered in terms of an inability to solve one or more subgoals of the task.

Knowing what features to look for serves not only in providing instruction and feedback, but also helps the learner focus upon specific aspects of the movement, especially when observing others. Subgoals and critical features are often closely related. For example, walking with an assistive walker, 4 subgoals can be identified, each having a counterpart prerequisite and critical feature: (1) prevention of lower limb collapse; (2) maintenance of postural support of upper body; (3) maintenance of equilibrium during double and single support; and (4) control of foot trajectory for safe ground clearance and gentle foot/heel contact. Appropriate subgoals or critical features become part of the substance of instruction.

During both instruction and practice the learner should be allowed to fail—all within the basic safety net. Practitioner and learner both benefit from observing or experiencing a movement breakdown or a nonfunctional or unsuccessful solution to the motor problem. Allowing the opportunity for failure or "misses" promotes novel movement solutions. In the end these responses serve as a means of understanding the movement-problem-action relationship. Often in the initial stages of learning more is learned from failures or near misses than from the specification of the movement pattern or specifying a particular solution.[28]

Some Remarks about Practice

Bernstein first brought to our attention the idea that practice must involve the learner in the search for optimal solutions to the current motor problem.[5] The practice of solutions to the motor problem seems to promote learning, not the repetition of a particular movement, pattern, or solution.[5,10,22,29] Practice is the time-consuming aspect of the learning process. Instructional time usually does not provide sufficient time for adequate practice. The practitioner needs to develop meaningful and self-motivating practice routines for the learner. Working out or designing practice is as important as is the instructional design for each teaching/learning session. Preparing the learner for practice with a purpose must be designed into the instructional session. Knowing what to practice and how to practice is as important as knowing how much to practice. As learners gain competence and move out of the initial stage of the learning process, they can become increasingly more involved with the design of the practice routine; they understand what they should be considering and looking for as they practice.

Practice should be both appropriate for the task and for the level of skill and experience of the individual. For example, climbing stairs might be done under a variety of conditions: stairs with hand rails on only one side, stairs with other people on them, flights of stairs that change direction, etc. Individuals learning to walk with a cane, walker, or crutches need practice going up and down curbs and edges of varying heights, over terrain that is variable with respect to its compliance and/or condition of the surface.

Finally, providing the appropriate motivational atmosphere cannot be emphasized enough as a critical aspect of promoting the process of learning. The practitioner creates a specific learning problem for the mover, one that is solvable and at the same time challenging, based on a thorough understanding of the task and the learner. On the other hand, the learner must recognize that her/his role in the process is to accomplish a goal defined in concert with the practitioner through movements organized so that they match the demands of the environment.

CONCLUSION

Concepts gleaned from "motor learning" suggest that practitioners be familiar with and operate out of some frame of reference that will guide their thinking, observation, and ability to structure instruction and practice. In addition, the primary role of the practitioner is to support, nurture, and facilitate an atmosphere and setting in which the mover can develop and (re)learn strategies for locomotion under a variety of task conditions and constraints. This setting should include an opportunity for encountering a wide variety of movement-related problems while at the same time providing the learner with freedom to explore her/his own solutions. Solutions should not be imposed by the teacher; instead a careful task analysis including evaluation of the learner will help the practitioner clarify the goal, the environmental constraints, and the task conditions most directly affecting the learner.

The teacher can only clarify what the goal is, identify crucial and relevant aspects of the environment, and structure the task; she/he cannot specify the detail of the movement or movement solutions. All patterns of movement that emerge should be considered appropriate relative to the individual and the task conditions at that particular moment in time. Through structured and careful practice, the patterns will change as new understandings and different strategies are applied by the learner. Engagement of the learner as the active discoverer of relationships regarding self,

movement, environment, task problem to be solved is a laudable teaching and therapeutic goal.

REFERENCES

1. Ada L, Canning C, Westwood P: The patient as an active learner. In L, Ada Canning C, editors: *Key Issues in Neurological Physiotherapy,* Oxford, 1990, Butterworth-Heinemann, Ltd.
2. Arend S: Developing the substrates of skillful movement, *Motor Skills: Theory into Practice* 4:3-10, 1980a.
3. Arend S: Developing perceptual skills prior to motor performance, *Motor Skills: Theory into Practice* 4:13-20, 1980b.
4. Arend S, Higgins JR: A strategy for the classification, subjective analysis and observation of human movement, *Journal of Human Movement Studies* 2:36-52, 1976.
5. Bernstein NA: *The Coordination and Regulation of Movements,* Oxford, 1967, Pergamon Press Ltd.
6. Bohannon RW: Significant relationships exist between muscle group strengths following stroke, *Clinical Rehabilitation* 4:27-31, 1990.
7. Bohannon RW: Relevance of muscle strength to gait performance in patients with neurologic disability, *Journal of Neurological Rehabilitation* 3(2):97-100, 1989.
8. Carr J, Shepherd R: A motor learning model for rehabilitation of the movement-disabled. In Ada L, Canning C, editors: *Key Issues in Neurological Physiotherapy* Oxford, 1990, Butterworth-Heinemann Ltd, 1–24.
9. Enoka RM, Fuglevand AJ: Neuromuscular basis of the maximum voluntary force capacity of muscle (publication pending), reported at Conference on Motor Learning, Teachers College, Columbia University, New York, March 1992.
10. Gentile AM: Skill acquisition: Action, movement and neuromotor processes. In Carr J, Shepherd RB, Gordon J, Gentile AM, Held JM, editors: *Movement Science: Foundations for Physical Therapy in Rehabilitation,* Rockville, Md., 1987, Aspen Publishers, Inc.
11. Gentile AM: The nature of skill acquisition: Therapeutic implications for children with movement disorders. In Forssberg H, Hirschfeld H, editors: *Movement Disorders in Children, Med Sport Sci* Basel, 1992, Karger, 31–40.
12. Gentile AM, Higgins JR, Miller EA, Rosen BM: Structure of motor tasks. In *Mouvement, Actes du 7 Symposium in Apprentissage Psycho-motor du Sport.* Quebec, Ont., Canada, Professionalle de L'Activité Physique du Quebec, 11–28.
13. Ghez C: The control of movement. In Kandel ER, Schwartz JH, Jessell TM, editors: *Principles of Neural Science,* New York, 1991a, Elsevier, 533-547.
14. Ghez C: Posture. In Kandel ER, Schwartz JH, Jessell TM, editors: *Principles of Neural Science,* New York, 1991b, Elsevier, 596–608.
15. Ghez C: Voluntary movement. In Kandel ER, Schwartz JH, Jessell TM, editors: *Principles of Neural Science,* New York, 1991c, Elsevier, 609–625.

16. Gordon J: Spinal mechanisms of motor coordination. In Kandel ER, Schwartz JH, Jessell TM, editors: *Principles of Neural Science,* New York, 1991, Elsevier, 581–595.

17. Higgins JR: *Human Movement: An Integrated Approach,* St. Louis, 1977, Mosby.

18. Higgins JR, Higgins S: Temporal and spatial characteristics of infant walking during the first 10 days of independent locomotion: The effects of arm/hand complex use and locomotor patterns. Reported at Motor Development Academy, AAHPERD, New Orleans, April 1990.

19. Higgins JR: Observations of infant to toddler transition: Time spent in single leg support. (Unpublished research project), Department of Movement Sciences and Center for Infants and Parents, Teachers College, Columbia University, New York, 1991.

20. Higgins JR, Doyle J, Hopkins D, Horton S: The effect of object manipulation on the movement organization of preschool age children's jumping pattern: a temporal and kinematic analysis (manuscript in preparation), 1993.

21. Higgins S: Movement as an emergent form: Its structural limits, *Human Movement Science* 4:119-148, 1985.

22. Higgins S: Motor skill acquisition, *Journal of the American Physical Therapy Association* 71:48-64, 1991.

23. Loeb GE: The functional organization of muscles, motor units, and tasks. In Binder MD, Mendell LM, editors: *The Segmented Motor System* Oxford, 1990, Oxford University Press.

24. Jones DA, Rutherford OM: Human muscle strength training: The effects of three different regimes and the nature of the resultant changes, *Journal of Physiology* 391:1-11, 1987.

25. Marshall RN, Jennings LS: Performance objectives in the stance phase of human pathological walking, *Human Movement Science* 9:599-611, 1990.

26. McCullagh P, Caird JK: Correct and learning models and the use of model knowledge of results in the acquisition and retention of a motor skill, *Journal of Human Movement Studies* 18:107-116, 1990.

27. McCullagh P, Stiehl J, Weiss MR: Developmental modeling effects on the quantitative and qualitative aspects of motor performance, *Research Quarterly for Exercise and Sport* 61:344-350, 1990.

28. McCullagh P, Weiss MR, Ross D: Modeling considerations in motor skill acquisition and performance: An integrated approach. In Pandolf KB, editor: *Exercise and Sport Sciences Reviews* 17:475-513, Baltimore, 1989, Williams & Wilkins.

29. Newell KM: Motor skill acquisition, *Annual Review of Psychology* 42:213-237, 1991.

30. Rutherford OM, Jones DA: The role of learning and coordination in strength training, *European Journal of Applied Physiology* 55:100-105, 1986.

31. Rutherford OM: Muscular coordination and strength training: Implications for injury rehabilitation, *Sports Medicine* 5:196-202, 1988.

32. Sale DG: Neural adaptation to resistance training, *Medicine and Science in Sports and Exercise* 20(5):135-145, 1988.

33. Scully DM, Newell KM: Observational learning and the acquisition of motor skills: Toward a visual perception perspective, *Journal of Human Movement Studies* 11:169-186, 1985.

34. Seefeldt V, Haubenstricker J: Patterns, phases, or stages: An analytical model for the study of developmental movement. In Kelso JAS, Clark JE, editors: *The Development of Movement Control and Coordination*, New York, 1982, John Wiley and Sons, 309-317.

35. Winter DA: Biomechanics of normal and pathological gait: Implications for understanding human motor control, *Journal of Motor Behavior* 21:337-356, 1989.

36. Winter DA: *The Biomechanics and Motor Control of Human Gait: Normal, Elderly and Pathological* Waterloo, Ont., 1991, University of Waterloo Press.

CHAPTER 9

DYNAMICAL SYSTEMS PERSPECTIVE ON GAIT

Jane E. Clark

KEY TERMS

Attractor

Collective variables

Context-conditioned variability

Control parameters

Degrees of freedom

Emergent behavior

Environmental constraints

Organism constraints

Self-organization

Stability

State space

Systems approach

Task constraints

For the normal adult, the task of walking from here to there requires little effort and even less attention. A careful examination of the constituents involved in walking, however, reveals that this seemingly simple act arises from a nervous system comprised of billions of neurons and a musculo-skeletal system of over a thousand muscles and more than 200 bones and 100 moveable joints. How, out of such neuromusculoskeletal complexity, can a person walk across a crowded room or in a moving bus without falling? The Russian physiologist Nikolai Bernstein recognized this dilemma over a half century ago.[1] That is, any theory of motor control must solve two problems if it is to be tenable; these problems are (1) the degrees-of-freedom problem and (2) the problem of context-conditioned variability.

The degrees-of-freedom problem refers to the control problem inherent in a system with many individual components (i.e., neuronal, muscular, skeletal, and sensory). Context-conditioned variability, on the other hand, is a function of the indeterminacy between the brain and the effectors. The brain does not play the muscles like a keyboard; i.e., the same command does not always result in the same movement. Rather, the neuro-muscular system must be coordinated within ever varying anatomical, mechanical, and physiological contexts. Bernstein identified the challenge of finding a theory of motor control and coordination that adequately explained how skilled movement could occur in the face of these two problems.

DYNAMICAL SYSTEMS PERSPECTIVE

Over the last decade or so, a theoretical perspective has emerged that may answer Bernstein's challenge. This perspective is called dynamical systems theory and is about systems that change over time.[3,9] While the origins of dynamical systems are in the mathematical and physical sciences dating back almost a century, its more recent formulations have been extended to a variety of complex systems from the weather to mother-child interactions. The dynamical systems perspective also has emerged in the movement sciences. Over a decade ago, Kugler, Kelso, and Turvey[7] were the first to see the possibilities that such a perspective would offer to the understanding of movement control and coordination. Since that seminal paper, many have extended and elaborated upon the approach. Some have sought to use the approach in the most analytically rigorous manner; others have used the concepts in a more metaphorical manner. But while there are many differences among those seeking to develop this new perspective on motor control and coordination, there are some general principles that appear to be common.

A Systems Approach

One of the revelations of twentieth century science is the realization that reducing a complex system to a *simple* system or studying parts of the system in isolation does not always help us understand the system itself. This is particularly true in the study of biological systems. Indeed the behavior of humans is incredibly complex because of the interaction of many subsystems comprised of many constituents. Walking to the kitchen, for example, involves multiple interacting subsystems (e.g., neural, muscular, skeletal, motivational, perceptual, etc.), each of which is a complex system itself. Clearly, one's success in walking to the kitchen can be dramatically affected by the state of any one of these systems.

The dynamical systems approach recognizes the importance of studying systems. Causality is multidimensional and multilevel. To understand why someone walks a certain way we must look at multiple subsystems and their processes. We also must appreciate the nature of the interaction between the various constituents. The state of one element of the system may well affect or be dependent upon the state of another element(s).

Behavior as Emergent from a Multitude of Constraints

The dynamical systems approach to motor behavior and specifically to ambulation views behavior as *emergent*. Behavior is not directed by the brain (i.e., by some omniscient executive), but emerges from the external and internal *constraints* that surround the goal-directed action. Constraints set the boundaries or the limits for behavior. These constraints arise from three sources: the organism, the environment, and the task.[8] *Organism constraints* are those constraints that are embodied in the individual mover. The multiple subsystems and their processes represent organism constraints. Organism constraints include the physical attributes of the mover (such as height, weight, strength, and neuromaturation) as well as the psychological characteristics (e.g., cognitive development and motivation). *Environmental constraints* refer to the environment that surrounds the mover. For example, on earth our movements are continuously constrained by gravity. A slippery surface or rough terrain would also be considered environmental constraints. The environment also includes the sociocultural milieu. Although perhaps subtle in effect, our culture shapes our movements. Take for example, the different manner in which eating is accomplished in different cultures. The manipulation of knives and forks in Europe is different from the actions employed in the United States, and both are very different from the use of chopsticks by Asians. The *task* comprises the third category of constraints. What does the task demand of the mover? How fast must we make the movement? How accurate must the movement be? When must the movement be initiated? Task requirements constrain the movement. Indeed, while the organism and environmental constraints sit ever-present as a surrounding web, the task demands marshall the neuromuscular system into the pattern of coordination we observe.

To look at ambulation from a dynamical systems perspective is to see locomotor behavior emerge from the constraints embodied in the individual (i.e., organism), surrounding the action (i.e., the environment), and manifested in the task. Clearly, a broken leg, weakened ankle muscles, or diminished vision are organism constraints that affect locomotion. It is important, however, to realize that *all* the structural and functional capabilities of the human body constrain our movements. The knee's structure, for example, constrains the type of locomotion humans are capable of achieving as does the shape of the foot. The global environment and the specific task required also shape the movements we see. Walking across a frozen, icy pond changes the way we walk. Walking upstairs or down, on a balance beam or under it all result in changes to our movement.

The view that movement is an emergent property of the system's constraints differs dramatically from views such as motor programming or schema theories in which movements are commanded by motor programs stored in the central nervous system (CNS). From a dynamical systems perspective, movements emerge from constraints, not from detail-specific motor commands issued by a centrally stored program. The dynamical systems perspective realizes the importance of the CNS, but treats the CNS as a source of constraint not as an omniscient executive commanding individual muscle fibers. Constraints also address the degrees-of-freedom problem since constraints act to reduce the degrees of freedom within a system.

Self-Organization

The concept of constraints alone cannot explain movement. To understand the emergence of movement, another theoretical construct must be intro-

duced, namely, self-organization. *Self-organization* is that property of a system in which system components organize themselves into spatial and temporal patterns. No prior instructions are inherent in the system. For example, if you put ice cubes in a saucepan and heat the pan, the ice cubes will melt leaving you with a pan of water. If you continue to heat the water, it will eventually condense to steam. The instructions for this transformation are not within the ice cube or the water. Rather as an environmental constraint (temperature) is scaled to a critical level, the molecules move from one state (the ice cube) to another qualitatively different state (water) and finally to yet to another state (steam). No individual molecule is being instructed to move to a specific space at a specific time. The molecules are moving solely as a result of the system's dynamics—the cooperative action of many constrained molecules.

Biological motion such as human walking gives rise to spatial and temporal organization. From a dynamical systems perspective, this order arises from the self-organization of the many subsystems involved in this movement. For example, the neural substrate plays an important role in walking; but in many theoretical formulations about gait, it would seem that the CNS was the only system involved. Clearly, central pattern generating networks of neurons, spinal reflexes, and supraspinal influences all contribute to the unfolding action. But at issue is the nature of their role. Within dynamical systems theory, the neural substrate is one source of constraint for the behavioral outcome of locomotion. Indeed at another level of analysis, it is possible to examine the neural network itself for self-organizing properties.

Movement Behavior as Pattern Formation

Understanding the nature and principles underlying pattern formation is a fundamental issue in dynamical systems theory. In the movement sciences, this approach recognizes that the motor skill behavior of humans gives rise to dynamic patterns. The precise spatiotemporal organization observed between the trunk, thigh, and shank during a walking cycle, for example, represents a *pattern* of order and regularity. For motor skills, we seek to identify patterns that correspond to particular tasks or functions. Hence walking, running, and galloping may be seen as different locomotor patterns. By focusing on patterns and variables that capture these patterns, referred to as *collective variables,* our high dimensional complex system can be compressed into a lower dimensional description. For example, in locomotion the pattern of foot falls may be used to distinguish between symmetric and asymmetric gait forms (e.g., between running and galloping). These interlimb patterns arise from the interaction of hundreds of muscles, bones, and neurons. But in one variable, the phasing relationship between foot falls, we can describe the lower extremities' interlimb coordination. This collective variable compresses the complexity of the neuromusculoskeletal system into a description that captures the essence of the system. The movement has a pattern and the dynamical systems approach seeks to understand the nature of that pattern and how it is formed.

Stability and Instability

An important concept of dynamical systems theory is the notion of *stability*. Stable behaviors are ones that resist small perturbations. If you are walking along the street and you trip on a rough patch of sidewalk (i.e., you experience a small perturbation), you are likely to regain your walking pattern. For you, walking is a stable pattern of coordination. But imagine the newly walking infant attempting to walk through the clutter of toys in the living room. Even the smallest perturbation can send the infant back to crawling. For the newly walking infant, walking is not a stable behavior, however, crawling is.

The stability and instability of movement patterns come from the surrounding constraints. Some constraint configurations result in stable, preferred patterns, while others make stability difficult. For example, the strength of the leg extensor muscles of a newly walking infant may be insufficient to provide a stable walking pattern. Once the strength constraint achieves a specific level of function, the walking pattern may stabilize. Of course it may not, since the instability may have multiple causes. However, if we can identify a variable that when scaled (up or down) to a critical level causes the pattern to change, we have found a *control parameter*. In the example of the ice-to-water-to-steam transition, temperature acts as a control parameter. If changing strength were to result in a stable walking pattern, it too would be considered a control parameter. Clearly the identification of control parameters is an important goal in seeking to change one pattern of behavior into another or to stabilize unstable patterns.

ANALYTICAL TOOLS AND CONCEPTS

One of the major strengths of the dynamical systems approach is the powerful analytical tools and concepts that it offers for examining movement. Certainly, Newton as well as Lagrange,

Euler, and Laplace, among others, have provided a rich reservoir of analytical techniques for those who study locomotion. However, each approach is not without its limitations. An analysis of gait using Newtonian mechanics generates an incredible number of kinematic and kinetic variables.[10] But once having collected and analyzed all these variables, how does one decide which ones are important? Biomechanical analysis of adult hemiplegic gait, for example, may result in more than 50 variables that differ from normal gait (stride length, swing/stance ratio, knee range of motion, etc.). If we want to change the gait of a person with hemiplegia, how do we use the information obtained from the biomechanical analysis? What variables are important for changing the pattern of locomotion? Biomechanics is mute on these questions.

The dynamical systems perspective, on the other hand, seeks to address these questions. In the late nineteenth century, the French mathematician Poincaré was, it has been said, the first to recognize the limitations of Newtonian physics and to emphasize the importance of the global, qualitative character of the system's dynamics. Complex, high dimensional dynamical behavior, according to Poincaré, may be described in low dimensional qualitative dynamics. In other words, systems with many degrees of freedom (high dimensional) can be captured in a description of far fewer variables. This approach requires that we capture the behavior we are studying at an instant (referred to as the *state* of the system) and then continue to map the system as it evolves in time (referred to as the system's *trajectory*). The state of the system and its trajectory are mapped in state space. *State space* is defined as the map of all possible states of the system. If the system is a stable dynamical system, then we should find that all the trajectories will be attracted to a specific region of the state space. When this occurs, we have found an attractor. An *attractor* is the low dimensional subset of state space to which all the nearby trajectories converge. There are three fundamental types of attractors: point, periodic (sometimes referred to as limit cycle), and chaotic.[11] Point attractors are attractors whereby all trajectories come to a point. The periodic or limit cycle attractors form closed orbit trajectories. The chaotic attractor is neither a limit cycle nor point, but it is not easily described since its trajectories tend to approach a region and then diverge.

Characterizing a system's behavior by attractor descriptions has important implications for understanding the system. First, each attractor has specific properties that lead to predictable dynamical behavior. Knowing whether a system can be described by a limit cycle or a point attractor leads to very different qualitative predictions about the system's behavior. Second, it may be possible to identify equations that describe the attractor's motion. The latter, of course, would offer important precision to the predictive power of those seeking to explain the system's behavior. Finally, in the future, identifying general classes of behavior based on similarities in attractor dynamics may be possible.

WALKING FROM A DYNAMICAL SYSTEMS PERSPECTIVE

To help us work through all this terminology and perhaps provide a more compelling story about the power of the dynamical systems approach, we take two specific examples. The first example comes from a normal adult and the second comes from an infant who has just begun to walk.

To begin, let us consider the normal adult walking cycle (Figure 9-1). Humans locomote on two legs comprised of three segments each (thigh, shank, and foot). Atop the two legs is the trunk-head-arm unit. While the trunk-head-arm complex is important, for our purposes in this example, we will consider only the lower extremities (specifically, the largest segments, the thigh and shank). In Figure 9-1, look closely at the shank and thigh motions. Beginning with the left-most figure, the thigh starts near the vertical, swings forward and then back. The shank (again starting with the left-most figure) begins back, swings forward then rotates back. Both segments seem to show the cyclic motion of a pendulum, one fixed at the hip, the other at the knee.

In viewing walking from a dynamical systems perspective, our first task is to capture the system's behavior (i.e., walking) with a low dimensional

FIGURE 9-2 An exemplar phase portrait of the shank motion of a normal adult for one complete walking cycle (AD501).

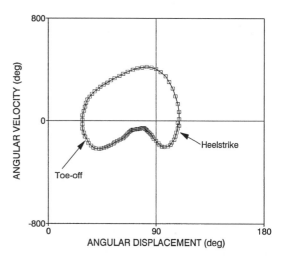

description (i.e., an attractor). We start by trying to identify an attractor, because once we have done so, we can then explore the dynamics of that attractor—observing how it changes with various changes in the organism, environment, and/or task.

Thus beginning very simply, let us follow the behavior of the lower leg (the shank) during walking. To do this, we must find a variable(s) that captures the state of the system at any one time and then measure the system's state over time. It just so happens that for the motion of the shank only two variables are needed to capture the shank's behavior. These two variables are the shank's angular displacement (its inclination to the horizon) and its velocity (Figure 9-2). Of course we could select other variables (kinetic and potential energy, electromyographic signals from selected muscles, etc.). The selection of variables depends in part on the questions you are interested in answering. But not all variables will give you a complete description of the system, nor will they reveal an attractor. Indeed a good deal of time may be spent finding appropriate variables to capture the behavior of interest.

In Figure 9-2, angular velocity of the shank is plotted on the *y*-axis and the angular displacement is plotted on the *x*-axis. This graph represents the state space for the shank's behavior in one normal adult walking cycle. Any one *instant* in the shank's motion is represented by the □. For example, at the moment of toe off, the shank is approximately at a 30-degree inclination and −150 degrees per second angular velocity. The trajectory then moves clockwise through the shank's swing phase until heel strike (110 and 50 degrees per second).

FIGURE 9-1 The walking cycle of a normal adult.

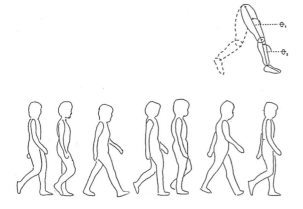

FIGURE 9-3 **A,** The phase portrait of the shank motion for four walking cycles of a normal adult (AD501). **B,** The phase portrait of the shank motion for four walking cycles with 17.5% of the subject's body weight affixed to the ankle. (Same subject as portrayed in Figure 9-3, *A*.)

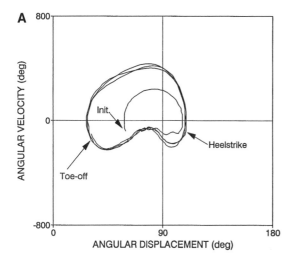

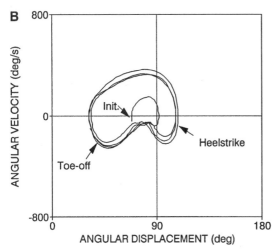

Figure 9-3, *A* reveals why the term *attractor* is used to describe the state space representation of the shank's behavior. In this figure, four continuous walking cycles are plotted in state space. Notice how all but the first cycle tend toward the same region of the state space. As the system starts into its motion (i.e., initiation or "Init."), there is a *transient,* representing the time it takes for the system to stabilize into its behavioral regimen. For the normal adult walker, this transition takes place within less than a cycle as the shank's motion is quickly drawn into the attractive region of state space.

The phase portrait (the term used to describe the state space representation of the shank) that emerges of the shank is one of a limit cycle attractor. Recall that a limit cycle attractor is one in which the trajectories form a closed periodic orbit. We now have a low dimensional description of the behavior emanating from an incredibly high degree-of-freedom system (namely, the neuromusculoskeletal system). But we have more than just a description of the shank's behavior. Once we have found an attractor to capture our system, we also can explore its properties. When will it change? What control parameters will destabilize the system? Under what conditions is it stable? For example, what happens if there is a significant change in an individual's strength or posture? How does the attractor change? Also, knowing what kind of attractor models the system can give us predictive capabilities.

If, for example, our system can be modeled as a limit cycle attractor, then we know much more about the system. For example, a limit cycle system is attracted to specific regions of state space and if slightly perturbed will return to these attractive regions. If we perturb the adult walker with an ankle weight of 17.5% of body weight attached to one leg, what might we expect to happen to the shank's motion? If Figure 9-3, *B* we see the same adult's phase portrait for the weighted shank. Clearly there is little effect on the attractor.

In the case of a newly walking infant, the problem might be viewed as one in which the system is seeking the attractive region of state space. In the months prior to walking, infants demonstrate stable crawling behavior. But adopting the upright bipedal position and attempting to locomote is an unsteady proposition. Does our dynamical description allow us to see that instability in the attractor? Figure 9-4, *A* is a phase portrait of an infant who is within a day or two of taking her first steps. Indeed at the time of testing she never takes more than three to five independent steps. Many of her walking attempts result in falling. Figure 9-4, *A*, however, is the shank's motion during a successful three-step walk. Compared to the phase portrait of the adult (Figure 9-3, *A*), the infant's shank motion while in a particular region of state space, is not consistently drawn to the same region cycle after cycle as is the adult's. However when we examine this same infant's walking two months later (Figure 9-4, *B*), we see quite clearly that the infant's system has stabilized onto the attractor. What has changed? Probably a number of things. In our longitudinal study of infant walking, we have argued that at least two control parameters might be responsible for the changes: leg strength and balance.[2]

FIGURE 9-4 **A,** The phase portrait of the shank motion for four walking cycles of a newly walking infant (KN-T1).
B, The phase portrait of the shank motion for four walking cycles of the same infant 2 months later (KN-T16).

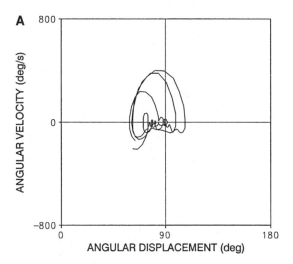

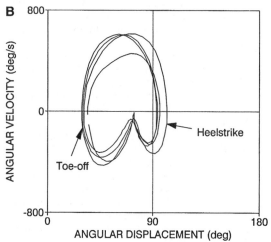

DIAGNOSIS AND TREATMENT OF GAIT DISORDERS

A few years ago, Kelso and Schöner[6] suggested a research strategy that might offer a good starting point for using the dynamical systems approach in the diagnosis and treatment of gait disorders. They identified five steps that they called the synergetic strategy: (1) identifying a collective variable, (2) mapping the collective variable onto an attractor, (3) identifying a control parameter(s) that affects the attractor, (4) studying the attractor's stability and loss of stability as control parameter(s) change, (5) establishing the relationship(s) among various levels of analysis.

Finding an Attractor

For gait analysis then the first step as we discussed earlier is finding the collective variable that can be mapped as an attractor (Steps 1 and 2). If we are interested in segmental motion, then segmental angles of inclination as illustrated in our earlier examples may be sufficient. If the coordination between the segments is of interest, then intersegmental angles (e.g., the knee and ankle) and their velocities may be used.[4] Signals from muscle activation may also prove to be useful, although little has been done with this type of data. This is in contrast with both EEG signals from brain activity and ECG signals from the heart, both of which have been used to map the behavior of these dynamic systems.[5] In fact, phase plane portraits have been extensively used in identifying the potential for heart attacks.

Manipulating Control Parameters

Once an attractor has been identified, then it is possible to study the effects of manipulating control parameters (Step 3). Control parameters represent the treatment. The patient's behavior is a function of all the surrounding constraints. It is the art and science of therapeutics in which the critical constraints that shift the system to a new behavior (i.e., the control parameters) are identified. With the attractor identified, a control parameter or more than one control parameter can be manipulated and the behavior of the system through its phase plane portrait can be observed. Relevant control parameters can be found in the patient, his/her environment, and/or in the task. An orthosis, strength training, canes, and similar interventions are all potential control parameters that can assist the patient and may help stabilize behavior.

Another way to view constraints other than ones that are manipulated to change behavior is to see that some constraints may act as *rate limiters,* which hold back the change. Here again these constraints may be identified and then the same principles applied, namely, to find the critical constraint and change it.

Stability and Instability

As control parameters are manipulated, what effect is there on the attractor? Is it stabilized? Destabilized? By analyzing the attractor's stability, we can begin to understand the effect of the control parameter on the system. Some movement patterns may be more stable than others, while some may be inherently unstable, requiring considerable constrarinment to maintain the pattern. Various handicapping conditions bring with them different organism constraints. How do the constraints change the pattern? Is one pattern more stable than another? Why? In addition, some pathologies result in rigid behavior. Stability in these systems may well be maladaptive, restricting any change in behavior. But here again these issues may be explored through the use of attractor dynamics.

Summary

A brief overview of the dynamical systems approach to gait has been presented. This approach has been contrasted with other perspectives, and arguments are offered for why this approach may be a useful one for the study of movement control and coordination. A very brief description of the tools and concepts of dynamical systems was offered. For those readers interested in a more in-depth study of the approach, a listing of selected readings is included after the references. Finally, adult and infant gaits were examined from this perspective, and a strategy for employing the approach to gait was outlined.

References

1. Bernstein N: Biodynamics of locomotion, In Whiting HTA, editor: *Human motor actions: Bernstein reassessed.* Amsterdam, 1984, Elsevier (Original work published in 1940).
2. Clark JE, Phillips SJ: A longitudinal study of intralimb coordination in the first year of independent walking: A dynamical systems analysis, *Child Development* 64:1143-1157, 1993.
3. Crutchfield JP, Farmer JD, Packard NH, Shaw RS: Chaos, *Scientific American* 254(12): 46-57, 1987.
4. Forrester LF, Phillips SJ, Clark JE: Locomotor coordination in infancy: the transition from walking to running. In Savelsbergh GJP, editor: *The development of coordination in infancy.* Amsterdam, 1993, Advances in Psychology Series, North Holland.
5. Glass L, Mackey MC: *From clocks to chaos.* Princeton, NJ, 1988, Princeton University Press.
6. Kelso JAS, Schöner G: Self-organization of coordinative movement patterns, *Human Movement Science* 7:27-46, 1988.
7. Kugler PN, Kelso JAS, Turvey MT: On the concept of coordinative structures as dissipative structures. I. Theoretical lines of convergence. In Stelmach GE, Requin J, editors: *Tutorials in motor behavior,* New York, 1980, North Holland, 3-47.
8. Newell KM: Constraints on the development of coordination. In Wade MG, Whiting HTA, editors: *Motor development in children: Aspects of coordination and control,* Boston, 1986, Martinus Nijhoff, 341-360.
9. Rosen R: *Dynamical system theory in biology, vol I: Stability theory and its application.* New York, 1990, Wiley, John.
10. Sutherland DH, Olshen RA, Biden EN, Wyatt MP: *The development of mature walking.* Oxford, 1988, Blackwell Scientific Publications, MacKeith Press.
11. Thompson JMT, Stewart HB: *Nonlinear dynamics and chaos,* New York, 1986, John Wiley.

Suggested Readings

Abraham RH, Shaw CD: *Dynamics: The geometry of behavior. Part I: Periodic behavior.* Santa Cruz, Calif, 1982, Aerial Press.

Clark JE, Truly TL, Phillips SJ: On the development of walking as a limit cycle system. In Thelen E, Smith L, editors: *Dynamical systems in development: applications.* Cambridge, Mass, 1993, MIT Press, 71-93.

Clark JE, Whitall J: Changing patterns of locomotion: From walking to skipping. In Woollacott M, Shumway-Cook A, editors: *Development of posture and gait across the lifespan,* Columbia, S.C., 1980, University of South Carolina Press, 128-151.

Forrester LF, Phillips SJ, Clark JE: Locomotor coordination in infancy: the transition from walking to running. In Savelsbergh GJP, editor: *The development of coordination in infancy,* Amsterdam, 1993, Advances in Psychology Series, North Holland.

Garfinkel A: A mathematics for physiology, *American Journal of Physiology (Regulatory Integrative Comp. Physiology)* 245:R455-R466, 1983.

Glass L, Mackey MC: *From clocks to chaos,* Princeton, NJ, 1988, Princeton University Press.

Kelso JAS, Mandell AJ, Schlesinger MS: *Dynamic patterns in complex systems,* Singapore, 1988, World Scientific.

Kugler PN, Turvey MT: *Information, natural law, and the self-assembly of rhythmic movement,* Hillsdale, N.J., 1987, Lawrence Erlbaum Associates.

Nicholis G, Prigogine I: *Exploring complexity: An introduction,* New York, 1989, W.H. Freeman.

Scholz JP, Kelso JAS: A quantitative approach to understanding the formation and change of coordinated movement patterns, *Journal of Motor Behavior* 21:122-144, 1989.

Schöner G, Kelso JAS: Dynamic pattern generation in behavioral and neural systems, *Science* 239:1513-1520, 1988.

Stewart I: *Does God play dice?* Cambridge, Mass., 1988, Basil Blackwell.

Thelen E: Development of coordinated movement: Implications for early human development. In Wade MG, Whiting HTA, editors: *Motor development in children: Aspects of coordination and control,* Boston, 1986, Martinus Nijhoff.

Thelen E, Ulrich BD: Hidden skills: A dynamic systems analysis of treadmill stepping during the first year, *Monographs of the Society for Research in Child Development* 56(1), (Whole Serial No. 223).

PART III

THEORY, TECHNOLOGY, AND NORMATIVE DATA

♦ This section addresses theory associated with measuring certain parameters, measurement technology and any normative data available. The first chapter bridges the terminology gap in measurement theory between engineering and clinical professionals. The theory associated with the measurement or reliability is discussed, differences in the terminology are presented and methods to determine the acceptability of a measurement tool are presented. The rest of this section reviews variables used commonly to measure some aspect of the walking pattern. Current "standard" clinical methods used to describe patterns of gait using visual analysis without instrumentation are presented. Subsequent chapters address the theory, technology and normative data associated with footfall measures, joint kinematics, kinetics, and EMG, respectively.

CHAPTER 10

RELIABILITY
AND MEASUREMENT THEORY

Michael J. Strube
Anthony Delitto

KEY TERMS

Accuracy	Ratios
Agreement	Reliability
Change scores	Sensitivity
Error	Specificity
Generalizability theory	Standard error of measure
Precision	Validity

RELIABILITY

Everyone has an implicit understanding of *reliability*. We all know what it means to have a reliable friend or a reliable toaster. Indeed, we tend to take reliability for granted and not give it much thought, until the relied upon friend fails our expectations or the toaster fails to offer up the expected morsel. Reliability is no less important in science. It underlies one of the central and defining features of research: systematic observation. Through careful and reliable assignment of numbers to represent the properties of observable phenomena, scientists can communicate in a common language, providing the basis for inferential advances that are the cornerstones of theory.[14,75,99]

Given the crucial position of measurement in all branches of science, it is not surprising that much attention has been given to reliability and its implications for scientific inference. In this chapter we will provide an overview of measurement and reliability. We will clarify commonly used and confused terms, describe the major measurement models, demonstrate the calculation and interpretation of the most common reliability estimates, and comment on the numerous caveats and problems that confront the applied researcher. Recognizing that the technical literature on measurement is inaccessible without modest training in mathematics, our focus will be on translating important principles and ideas so that they can be used by researchers with average exposure to design and statistics.* Although our examples will come from the measurement of gait, the underlying principles are general and apply with equal force to other measurable phenomena.

Measurement and Error

The intent of any measurement is to capture the true nature of an observable phenomenon. The hope is that the assigned number can "stand for" the observed event or characteristic, that is, the assigned number is a trustworthy or reliable proxy. Yet, as all researchers know, the success of this translation from fact to number is often fraught with difficulties. For example, measurement of range of motion (ROM) can be influenced by placement of the goniometer, training of the ob-

server, and motivation of the subject. Each may produce a discrepancy between the true ROM and the observed ROM. The measurement of skeletal kinematics can likewise be hampered by soft tissue movement that displaces skin markers over the putative centers of rotation.[112] Surface motion artifacts can likewise introduce errors in the measurement of joint forces when accelerometers are attached to the skin.[63] In all these cases, there is the potential for important discrepancies between the underlying characteristic being measured and the assignment of numbers to that characteristic. The simple fact that observations are subject to error is the starting point for definitions and theories about reliability.

To state matters more formally, any observed score, *x,* can be thought of as containing two major components: a true score component (t) and an error component (e). The true score component represents the characteristic (e.g., ROM, ground reaction force, walking velocity, stance time) that is expected to remain constant over repeated measurements in the absence of intervention. The error component represents the positive or negative score increments arising in a particular measurement occasion that are unrelated to the characteristic of interest (e.g., momentary lapse of concentration by an observer; poorly controlled ambient lighting during videotaping). This independence of true score and error allows a simple definition of observed score: $x = t + e$. The variability of observed scores can then be represented as the sum of true score variability and error variability:†‡

$$\sigma_x^2 = \sigma_t^2 + \sigma_e^2. \tag{1}$$

In other words, the relative rank order of individuals based on observed scores is in part due to underlying differences in their true scores and in part due to random variability. This additive nature of true score variability and error variability allows a convenient and traditional definition of reliability. Reliability (r_{xx}) represents the ratio of true score variance to observed score variance:

$$r_{xx} = \frac{\sigma_t^2}{\sigma_t^2 + \sigma_e^2}. \tag{2}$$

---

* A comprehensive coverage of measurement theory is beyond the scope of this chapter. Interested readers are encouraged to pursue additional sources that provide elaboration of the points made here (References 2,17,18,32,47,49,67,69,76). In addition, many measurement topics are related to design and statistical issues that cannot be covered here. These are also discussed elsewhere (References 25,29,57,58,72,74,100,101,110).

---

† For this part of the discussion, measurement errors are assumed to be normally distributed random variables with a mean influence of zero, to be uncorrelated with true scores, and to be uncorrelated with true scores and error scores on subsequent measurement occasions. Errors may also be systematic; we discuss this point again later.

‡ To avoid unnecessary clutter, most statistical equations in this chapter will be given in terms of population parameters. It will be assumed that sample estimates are used in particular applications.

This ratio is also generically known as an *intraclass correlation*. From this definition it is clear that as measures approach the status of being error-free (i.e., $\sigma_e^2 \to 0$), reliability coefficients approach a value of 1.0, and the actual relative standing of individuals on the characteristic of interest is reproduced by the measure. Similarly, as error variability increases ($\sigma_e^2 \to \infty$), reliability approaches 0, and the actual relative standing of individuals on the characteristic of interest is lost at the level of measurement. It is also possible to interpret the reliability coefficient in correlational terms; the square root of the reliability coefficient, sometimes called the *index of reliability,* is equal to the correlation between true scores and observed scores:

$$r_{tx} = \sqrt{r_{xx}}. \qquad (3)$$

Thus, from a statistical standpoint, the reliability coefficient provides a meaningful index of how dependably a measure maps onto or is correlated with the underlying characteristic being assessed.

The variance-ratio definition of reliability is convenient, but it also hides an important truth about measurement and reliability. Specifically, it treats error as though it arises from one source. In fact, there can be numerous sources of error for any measurement occasion, and the consequences of multiple error sources are important to recognize. One might assume that because error is random, multiple error sources will cancel each other out. It is true that over repeated measurement occasions the impact of all random error sources will be an average increment of 0 to the true score. But, because separate error sources are also assumed to be independent, their separate variances are additive and inflate the variance of the observed score relative to the contribution of the true score. It is better to think of the error variability in Equations 1 and 2 as having multiple additive components:

$$\sigma_e^2 = \sigma_{e_1}^2 + \sigma_{e_2}^2 + \sigma_{e_3}^2 + \ldots + \sigma_{e_k}^2. \qquad (4)$$

An important implication is that reliability assessment requires attention to many possible sources of error. We discuss this issue in more detail in later sections. Until then it is easiest to pretend that error is a unitary phenomenon.

Error "Terms"

Given this traditional, statistical definition of reliability, it is possible to compare alternative labels that have been used synonymously. Most common have been the terms *repeatability, dependability, homogeneity, generalizability,* and *consistency.*

The use of these terms is understandable given the foregoing discussion. A reliable measure can be expected to repeat the same score on two different occasions, provided the characteristic of interest does not change. Likewise, a reliable measure can be depended on to give a close approximation to the true score. Several reliable measures of the same characteristic should converge on the same true score and thus indicate homogeneity. And, based on one measurement with a reliable instrument one can generalize to what would occur on future similar measurement occasions.* One common theme that runs through these terms is that scores obtained on different measurement occasions should be consistent if there is little error.

Other terms have been used as well, but these are more often confused with other measurement concepts. For example, the terms *precision* and *accuracy* are often used in place of *reliability.* These terms are used appropriately when, for example, a researcher is interested in the expected variability of one person's score over measurement occasions. For example, to what degree will repeated measurements of an individual's free-walking gait velocity vary? That is, how accurate or precise is any one measure as an estimate of that person's true or typical gait velocity? This is clearly a matter of reliability because observed scores will vary in random ways over measurement occasions to the extent that error is present. In fact, the standard error of measure, σ_{meas}, used in the calculation of probability intervals around individual scores, is directly related to reliability:

$$\sigma_{meas} = \sigma_x \sqrt{1 - r_{xx}}. \qquad (5)$$

The σ_{meas} represents the standard deviation of error scores and is sometimes preferred as a measure of reliability because it gives an indication of error magnitude scaled in the original score units.[35] Thus, as reliability increases, the standard deviation of error scores decreases, and estimates of true scores based on observed scores become more precise or accurate.†

---

*   One potential problem with the casual use of the term *generalizability* is that it is also associated with a well-formulated theory of reliability that will be discussed later.[32]

†   One technical point is important here. The σ_{meas} as defined by Equation 5 may not be the best estimate of error score variability for every respondent. Recent advances have been made in the estimation of error variability for different score levels.[6,36,70] Those sources should be consulted if probability intervals around individual scores are to be calculated. The general point remains true, however: Reliability increases the precision of estimating true scores from observed scores.

The terms *precision* and *accuracy* have also been used to mean *correct* or *valid* measurement, typically in terms of prediction. For example, when the average person refers to an unreliable weather prediction or an unreliable stock market prediction, the implication is that later facts contradict the prediction (i.e., the prediction was inaccurate). Yet, the measurements of weather-related factors (e.g., temperature or barometric pressure) or economic factors (e.g., short-term interest rates or GDP) might still be very reliable in the sense that they contain little error; they just may not mean what the forecasters think they mean and thus have little *validity* for predicting other events (e.g., the likelihood of rain or a bull market).* Similarly, gait measures (e.g., cadence, velocity, muscle activation, power) may demonstrate high reliability but be disappointing in their ability to predict important outcomes (e.g., recovery of mobility for adequate daily functioning following a stroke). Correct prediction relies on the gait characteristics being valid measures of outcome-related processes. Validity is a separate issue that we will treat briefly later.

Precision is also defined frequently as the degree of exactness or discrimination with which a quantity is stated, and accuracy is defined frequently as "the quality of freedom of mistake or error."[9] Used in this way, both precision and accuracy require a standard against which the measure can be compared, and thus are better used with reference to bench testing of equipment that will be used in gait assessment. For example, the precision and accuracy of a force platform would relate to how well the transducers in the platform translated known loads applied in appropriate planes. The distinction between validity and reliability is important here. The force platform could be biased in a systematic but repeatable way, always producing results that deviate by a predictable amount from the known standard. The rank ordering of individuals measured on the same force platform would be repeatable, but the labeling of an individual's score (a validity issue) would be in error because the obtained score would systematically underestimate or overestimate the actual ground reaction force. Of course, calibration of equipment removes this bias problem.

Two additional terms that are often used in relation to reliability are *sensitivity* and *specificity*. These terms have a meaning particular to classification and prediction and should best be reserved for that purpose; they should be used very cautiously in other contexts. *Sensitivity* is the proportion of times that a measure correctly identifies a disorder or condition when the disorder or condition is, in fact, present. *Specificity* is the proportion of times that a measure correctly identifies a disorder or condition as being absent when the disorder or condition is, in fact, absent. These characteristics are related to reliability because correct classification relies on a reliable measure, but the terms should not be confused with the definition of reliability described earlier.

The term *sensitivity* has an additional use in measurement that we should also mention. Sensitivity of measurement sometimes refers to the resolving power of the instrument. An insensitive measure cannot discriminate underlying differences of interest. Consequently, obtained score differences will not reflect the actual rank ordering of individuals on the characteristic of interest. Sensitivity is application specific, however. A measure may be adequately sensitive for one purpose but not for another.

To be complete, it is also useful to contrast the present use of the term *reliability* with its use in engineering. According to Dummer and Winton, the generally accepted definition of reliability is ". . . the characteristic of an item expressed by the probability that it will perform a required function under stated conditions for a stated period of time."[34,33,114] This failure-analysis conception of reliability is closer to the lay person's understanding of the term, but it is not fundamentally different from the measurement use. In both cases, there is a central concern with error.

The Central Role of Reliability in Inference

If the uses of measurement were confined to simple description, then reliability might be a relatively minor concern. Measurement, however, is typically the first step toward more important inferences and decisions. Often, as mentioned earlier, researchers want to use their measures to predict, diagnose, and infer important things about their respondents. For example, suppose that a clinician wished to use a measure of ankle dorsiflexion ROM (x) to predict the peak ankle power during gait (y). If such prediction were possible, a relatively easy-to-collect static measure could be used to forecast an important characteristic of gait dynamics. The correlation between the two variables (r_{xy}) gauges the direction and strength of their relation and serves as the basis for generating a prediction equation. The ability to detect any relation, however, depends on the reliability of the individual measures. Intuitively, it should be clear

---

* A similar example is given by Feldt and Brennan.[35]

that if one measure is composed largely of random error, then it shouldn't be able to predict anything. That intuition is correct and can be stated more formally:

$$r_{xy} = \rho_{xy} \sqrt{r_{xx}r_{yy}} \qquad (6)$$

where ρ_{xy} is the error-free correlation between x and y (a hypothetical value), and r_{xx} and r_{yy} are the reliabilities of x and y respectively. This formula makes clear that the ability to detect a true underlying correlation is limited by unreliability in either measure. Accordingly, the ability to predict, diagnose, and classify is dependent on the reliability of measures. This point cannot be stated too forcefully. All effort in constructing elegant theories and conceptual models will be wasted if the measures used in validating those models are unreliable. Thus, for example, attempts to verify mathematical and biomechanical models of gait (see chapters 6 and 19) rest on the use of reliable measures of model components. Without reliable measures, model invalidity is indistinguishable from poor measurement. Reliability is thus a necessary condition for validity.[76]*

Reliability does not guarantee validity, however, and great care must be taken to ensure that measures are meaningful in addition to being reliable. Indeed, the challenge in gait analysis may not be the precision of instrumentation or the reliability of assessment techniques as much as it is the attempt to find meaningful measures of ambulation that are related to and predictive of the functional limitations and disabilities of people. Demonstrating validity for a measure may be more difficult than demonstrating reliability.

Validity essentially refers to the interpretation of scores, and those interpretations may be several steps removed from a simple description of the measurement operation. This is most clear, of course, in scientific disciplines where the characteristics of interest are hypothetical constructs like personality traits, attitudes, or intelligence. In these cases, scores on paper and pencil questionnaires are interpreted as indicators of underlying characteristics, which is a fairly long leap of inference that requires considerable evidence to justify. Nonetheless, arguments about interpretation of scores can arise in any science if only because there are as many validities for a measure as there are applications.[73] Thus, for example, the

use of gait measures (e.g., stride length, cadence, velocity, stance, etc.) to evaluate normal gait (e.g., in recovery) requires an agreed upon definition of normal gait and the establishment of criterion scores for the labeling of patients. These choices move the measure beyond simple demonstrations of replicable observation and are often open to debate. These debates and their solutions make up the bulk of scientific progress. They can only be settled, however, after reliable measures have been developed.†

Reliability Estimates

Measurement Models.   Thus far we have discussed reliability as though it were a unitary construct. At a general level that is true. But at the level of estimation where reliability coefficients are calculated and interpreted, the issues become more complex. Reliability estimates rest on sets of assumptions about measurement, or *measurement models*. Over the years numerous measurement models have been proposed, each producing reliability estimation procedures that are appropriate when the accompanying set of assumptions are valid. We cannot cover all of the numerous measurement models adequately here.‡§ Nonetheless,

---

† Further information on validity can be found elsewhere (References 29,47,73,76,96).

‡ These developments are described adequately elsewhere under several titles including classical theory, theory of true scores and error scores, the model of parallel tests, domain sampling theory, and generalizability theory.[32,35,47,76] The identification of the model that best fits the data can be informed in part by covariance structure modeling approaches such as LISREL,[56] EQS,[3] and EzPATH.[97] Description of these procedures is beyond the scope of this chapter, but they provide a potentially powerful way to explore measurement model assumptions.[7,77] Researchers should not mindlessly apply a reliability formula without first carefully examining their data and measurement assumptions.[98] Indeed, development of a well-articulated measurement model should precede a reliability study.[7,8]

§ Recent advances in the development of item response theory (IRT) should also be considered by researchers. Item response theory was developed in part in reaction to important practical limitations in traditional measurement theories.[50,51] Item response theory is an item level approach that attempts to model the functional relation between an underlying latent trait or factor (e.g., walking ability) and an observed response to a particular test item (e.g., rated ability to walk without noticeable stagger). Provided that an IRT model is appropriate, the advantages of IRT measures over measures developed via classical measurement theory are substantial. The most important characteristic is invariance. Invariance means that the item characteristics (e.g., difficulty, discrimination) do not depend on the ability distribution of the sample that is measured. Likewise, ability estimates for a given respondent do not depend on the particular set of items that are completed. This allows different sets of items (all measuring the same underlying characteristic) to be used in different samples without sacrificing the ability to compare the samples. A second desirable feature of IRT-based

---

* Stated differently, increasing the reliability of measures increases the statistical power of significance tests involving those measures.[53,59,109,115] For additional discussion of the impact of reliability on statistical relations, see Bollen[7] and Fleiss and Shrout.[44]

researchers must be attentive to the measurement assumptions that underlie reliability estimation. If those assumptions do not appear to be valid, alternative estimates must be sought. In the discussion that follows, we will focus our attention on two general approaches to reliability that have wide applicability. They correspond to reliability estimations for interval level data and for ordinal and nominal level data.

Generalizability Theory.   When the data that are collected are at least interval in nature, a flexible approach to reliability is provided by generalizability theory.[11,32,90,91]* Generalizability theory explicitly recognizes and attempts to model the multidimensional and systematic nature of error that we referred to previously. Underlying generalizability theory is the assumption that many error sources exert a systematic influence that can be estimated and separated from the random error component. For example, different observers might provide consistently different ratings (i.e., some are harsher or more lenient in their detection of a gait characteristic) or a certain time of day produces systematic differences in measurements. The identification of systematic error sources, or biases, thus places limits on the generalizability of measures from one measurement occasion to another. Because an ignored systematic error source biases the interpretation of true scores, generalizability theory has been correctly described as blending the concepts of reliability and validity.[32]

Generalizability theory distinguishes between two primary types of reliability studies: generalizability (or *G*) studies and decision (or *D*) studies. G studies provide the raw information about reliability on which application decisions, or D studies, are based. The importance of the distinction

will become apparent as we proceed; for the moment it is sufficient to know that many different D studies or reliability inferences can be made using the information provided by the same G study.

A G study begins with the definition of the *universe of admissible observations,* defined explicitly by the conditions of measurement. These conditions are called *facets* in generalizability theory. They can be thought of as attempts to identify the measurement conditions that could threaten the interchangeability of observations. Consider, for example, the task of quantifying the gait of patients with anterior cruciate ligament insufficiency. The gait variable of knee position at heel strike may be of some importance because it captures the "bent-knee gait" commonly seen in patients with knee disorders (whether such a variable actually best represents gait is a validity issue and not the focus of our discussion). The first step is to identify potential error sources (facets) that could threaten the interchangeability or generalizability of scores across measurement occasions. We might wish to consider the following two facets: (1) therapists who examine the patients and (2) walking velocity. By specifying these conditions of measurement, we allow a specific examination of whether measurement of bent-knee gait depends on differences between examiners or the velocity at which patients walk when measured. Different therapists might exhibit systematic biases in reading the strip chart from the potentiometer and different results might be obtained if patients are induced to walk at different speeds. Of course, our reliability interpretation would be open to question if we were to leave out any other important sources of error. Thus, in the design of the reliability study, the identified facets must be exhaustive of important error sources.

In the language of generalizability theory, the universe of admissible observations then has two facets: therapists and walking velocity. By specifying these conditions or facets of measurement, we argue that all important sources of systematic variation in observed scores have been identified. Using the results of a G study, we can then test whether an observed score obtained under any combination of these facets can be considered interchangeable with an observed score obtained under any other combination.

The conduct of a typical G study follows the logic of a random effects analysis of variance. All facets of the design, including the units of observation (i.e., subjects or patients), are considered random samples from their respective populations. Strictly speaking, random sampling should be

---

measures is that they can be constructed to have known discrimination for a specified ability range. Because the individual items are the fundamental units of IRT, a test can be constructed that has the desired item characteristics for a particular problem (e.g., distinguishing those with marginal walking ability from more severely impaired walkers). Third, the potential for test bias is lessened because the items that do not demonstrate invariant parameters across different samples can be eliminated. Finally, and with particular importance to the topic of this chapter, the reliability of each item in IRT can be assessed without reference to any other item, unlike traditional measurement theories in which interitem relations define reliability.

* Interval level data have scale differences that are equivalent across the range of the scale. For example, the difference between 30° and 40° on the Fahrenheit temperature scale is the same as the difference between 50° and 60°. Ratio scales (e.g., ROM) have this equal interval characteristic as well as a true zero point defined by the absence of the characteristic being measured.

TABLE 10-1 Sources of variance and expected mean squares for a two-facet G study

Source	Expected Mean Square
Patient (p)	$\sigma^2_{ptv,error} + n_v\sigma^2_{pt} + n_t\sigma^2_{pv} + n_tn_v\sigma^2_p$
Therapist (t)	$\sigma^2_{ptv,error} + n_v\sigma^2_{pt} + n_p\sigma^2_{tv} + n_pn_v\sigma^2_t$
Velocity (v)	$\sigma^2_{ptv,error} + n_t\sigma^2_{pv} + n_p\sigma^2_{tv} + n_pn_t\sigma^2_v$
$p \times t$	$\sigma^2_{ptv,error} + n_v\sigma^2_{pt}$
$p \times v$	$\sigma^2_{ptv,error} + n_t\sigma^2_{pv}$
$t \times v$	$\sigma^2_{ptv,error} + n_p\sigma^2_{tv}$
$p \times t \times v$, error	$\sigma^2_{ptv,error}$

carried out by first explicitly defining the population and then by randomly sampling from that population. In practice, the levels of each facet are more likely to be convenience samples. Provided that the levels are considered exchangeable with any other potential level of the facet, the analysis can proceed under the random effects model. Once the facets are identified, levels of each facet are sampled and observations are obtained. In the previous example, we might have three therapists measure knee position readings from strip chart recordings of patients walking at two different velocities. The design would be a Patient × Therapist × Velocity completely crossed factorial.

An analysis of variance (ANOVA) of the G study provides the raw material for estimating different sources of variance and for estimating reliability. Recall that reliability is defined as the ratio of true score variance to obtained score variance.* What we seek from the ANOVA are estimates of these variance sources, and in particular, a means of separately estimating the numerous error sources. In an ANOVA, the total variation in scores is partitioned into separate components corresponding to the factors or variables in the design. This variation is estimated by the *mean squares*. The mean squares are, in turn, combinations of the *variance components* needed by generalizability theory.

In the previous example, the ANOVA would produce seven mean squares corresponding to the different sources of variation in observed scores. These are listed in Table 10-1 and represent the familiar ANOVA main effects and interactions.

The only novel feature of this analysis is that patients are treated as though they were levels of a factor, which is always true but hidden in most traditional treatments of ANOVA. The expected mean squares are also listed in Table 10-1.†

In generalizability theory, we need estimates of each variance component. For example, the estimated variance of universe (or true) scores is σ^2_p. This can be estimated from the mean squares in Table 10-1 by the following calculation:

$$\sigma^2_p = \frac{MS_p - MS_{pt} - MS_{pv} + MS_{ptv,error}}{n_tn_v}. \quad (7)$$

Other variance components can also be estimated through manipulation of the mean squares. Once estimated, the variance components can be examined to determine the most important sources of variation in scores. Ideally, the universe score variation is quite high, suggesting that obtained score differences are due largely to differences in the patients' underlying universe scores.‡ But, other sources may contribute as well, and these sources can be separately estimated. One convenient way to assess the relative contribution of each source is to express each as a proportion of the total variability. Thus, for example, the proportion of total variability due to universe scores could be calculated as follows:

$$\frac{\sigma^2_p}{\sigma^2_p + \sigma^2_t + \sigma^2_v + \sigma^2_{pt} + \sigma^2_{pv} + \sigma^2_{tv} + \sigma^2_{ptv,error}}. \quad (8)$$

Examination of the relative proportions of variance can identify potentially large sources of error that would threaten the generalizability of scores across particular facets. For example, a particularly large Patient × Therapist component would indicate that the relative rank ordering of patients varied across therapists, and thus different therapists' measurements may not be interchangeable. This situation would indicate the need for better training to achieve standardized measurement across therapists.

The G study illustrated in Table 10-1 represents just one of many possible designs. It is also possible that some facets are best considered fixed

---

* In generalizability theory, the concept of *true score* is replaced by the concept of *universe score,* the average score an individual would obtain over all observations in the universe of admissible observations. The notion of universe score is explicitly constrained to the measurement conditions defined by the facets of measurement.

† Expected mean squares for many common designs can be found in Cronbach et al.[32] and Shavelson and Webb.[90] Rules for generating expected mean squares are given by Myers and Well.[74]

‡ Our description of generalizability theory assumes that respondents are the object of measurement; that is, inferences are to be made about differentiation of respondents. Generalizability theory, however, is symmetrical and can be used to assess differentiation for other facets.[15,16]

rather than random. A facet would be considered fixed if the levels of the facet were the only ones of interest or if they exhausted the population.[64,92] Another design alternative is to include nested factors. This design feature arises most often from necessity or logistical convenience. For example, it might be decided that time of day (morning and afternoon) is a potentially important source of error, but it is not feasible to have the same therapists examine all patients at both time periods. Instead, different therapists could conduct the tests in the morning and afternoon. In this type of design, therapists are nested within time periods and patients are crossed with time periods.

The important implication for the G study is that the sources of variance and their respective mean squares will be different for a nested design or fixed effects design than for a completely crossed random effects design. Some of the sources estimated separately in a crossed design are confounded in a nested design. In the nested design just described, it is not possible to separately estimate the Therapist main effect and the Therapist × Time of Day interaction; their effects are confounded. Similarly, the Patient × Therapist interaction is confounded with the combination of the Patient × Therapist × Time of Day interaction and random error. Nested designs represent a trade-off between informativeness and logistical or economical necessity. Calculations necessary for fixed effects and nested effects models are described more thoroughly by Cronbach et al. and Shavelson and Webb.[32,90]

Once the G study is conducted, the variance components can be used to estimate the generalizability of observations in different potential applications. These decision, or D, studies allow a researcher to determine the consequences of different measurement conditions. For example, one can ask what the generalizability (reliability) would be if more or fewer levels of a facet (e.g., therapists, walking velocities) were used in a future application. Similarly, the effects of different nested designs can be explored to determine the most economical way to achieve a desired level of generalizability. Each D study defines a different *universe of generalizability*. To aid in the comparison of different designs, generalizability coefficients can be estimated. *Generalizability coefficients* are the generalizability theory equivalents of reliability coefficients in traditional measurement theory. They are defined in similar ways as the proportion of obtained score variance that is due to true score variance. But, generalizability theory defines true score (i.e., a universe score) as the average score across the universe of admissible observations, a somewhat different

definition than used in traditional measurement theory.[90] For that reason, the resulting reliability estimates are called *generalizability coefficients* to indicate the different definition.

Generalizability theory also makes a distinction between *relative* and *absolute decisions.* For example, if we were to develop a treatment regimen for the bent-knee gait described previously, we would not ordinarily include all patients with anterior cruciate ligament insufficiency. Instead, we could establish a criterion by which we recruit into the study those patients with the 10 worst bent-knee gaits (as measured by knee flexion at heel strike). This would represent a relative decision because patients are admitted to the study depending on where they rank relative to other potential patients. Alternatively, we may wish to establish an absolute criterion for bent-knee gait (e.g., at least 5 degrees); only patients exceeding the criterion would be recruited for the study. In this case, each patient is judged according to an absolute cut-score rather than relative to other potential patients.

The sources of error for these two decisions are different. For relative decisions, the only sources of error are those that influence the relative rank ordering of patients: all interactions between patients and other facets. A Patient × Velocity interaction, for example, would indicate the rank ordering of patients and their eligibility for treatment depend on the particular velocity at which they are tested. Other sources, for example a Therapist main effect, affect all patient scores a similar amount and do not influence relative rank ordering. For absolute decisions, on the other hand, *all* sources of variance other than the universe score variance are sources of error. For example, if a substantial proportion of variance is due to the Therapist facet, then the impairment scores for patients could be spuriously high or low because they were examined by a particularly "harsh" or "lenient" therapist. This variance source would affect the absolute value of scores and subsequent treatment eligibility according to a standard cut-score criterion.

The two different kinds of decisions give rise to two different coefficients. For relative decisions, the estimate $(E\rho^2)$ is known as the *generalizability coefficient,* and is defined as follows using the notation from Table 10-1:

$$E\rho^2 = \frac{\sigma_p^2}{E\sigma_x^2} = \frac{\sigma_p^2}{\sigma_p^2 + \sigma_{rel}^2} \quad (9)$$

where σ_{rel}^2 is the error variance for a relative decision. The estimate represents the expected

TABLE 10-2   Knee position at heel strike recorded by three therapists

	Summary Statistics			
	Mean	**Standard Deviation**		
Therapist 1	12.800	6.157		
Therapist 2	12.500	6.091		
Therapist 3	13.200	6.937		

	ANOVA Summary			
Source	**MS**	**Estimated Variance Component**	**Proportion of Variance**	
Patients (p)	95.667	27.312	.665	
Therapist (t)	2.467	.000	.000	
$p \times t$, error	13.730	13.730	.335	

squared correlation between observed scores and universe scores.* A similar estimate can be derived for absolute decisions. This estimate is called an *index of dependability*[12]:

$$\Phi = \frac{\sigma_p^2}{E\sigma_x^2} = \frac{\sigma_p^2}{\sigma_p^2 + \sigma_{abs}^2} \qquad (10)$$

where σ_{abs}^2 is the error for an absolute decision.

A closer look at the error variance components for these two estimates reveals the power of D studies to anticipate the generalizability of a particular application. The relative error term for the design in Table 10-1, σ_{rel}^2, is defined as follows:

$$\sigma_{rel}^2 = \frac{\sigma_{pt}^2}{n_t} + \frac{\sigma_{pv}^2}{n_v} + \frac{\sigma_{ptv,error}^2}{n_t n_v}. \qquad (11)$$

The absolute error term, σ_{abs}^2, is defined as:

$$\sigma_{abs}^2 = \frac{\sigma_t^2}{n_t} + \frac{\sigma_v^2}{n_v} + \frac{\sigma_{pt}^2}{n_t} + \frac{\sigma_{pv}^2}{n_v} + \frac{\sigma_{tv}^2}{n_t n_v} + \frac{\sigma_{ptv,error}^2}{n_t n_v}. \qquad (12)$$

In both equations, different values for the different n can be substituted to estimate the generalizability of a design with, for example, a single therapist ($n_t = 1$) measuring patients at three different velocities ($n_v = 3$). Alternatively, we can decide which lengthening of the measure, more therapists or more velocities, will produce the most efficient

way to achieve a desired level of generalizability. One potential limitation to such D studies, however, is that they are constrained by the characteristics of the original G study. Only facets defined in the G study can be examined in a D study. Also, a nested G study will not allow separate estimates of all the variance components needed for a completely crossed D study due to the inherent confounding of effects. Accordingly, G studies should be defined with some anticipation of application, or designed to allow the broadest range of D studies by using a completely crossed random effects design with as many plausible error sources as can be included.

Two numerical examples will now be given to illustrate calculation of generalizability coefficients. The first example is based on a simple one-facet design. We begin with this simpler design because it allows clear reference to other common procedures cited in the literature and because it allows easy demonstration of potential interpretation problems. As a first example, suppose that the knee positions at heel strike of 20 patients were measured independently by three examiners from strip chart recordings.* The data can be framed as a one-way repeated measures ANOVA. Hypothetical data are displayed in Table 10-2. The coeffi-

---

*   As noted previously, sample estimates would be used to calculate the generalizability coefficient. The resulting estimate is a biased but consistent estimate.

*   There are other variations on this design. For example, each individual could be examined by a different set of observers. This and other less common designs are described elsewhere.[32,64,90,92]

cients for this design can be calculated from the following equations:

$$E\rho^2 = \frac{\sigma_p^2}{\sigma_p^2 + \dfrac{\sigma_{pt,error}^2}{n_t}}, \tag{13}$$

and

$$\Phi = \frac{\sigma_p^2}{\sigma_p^2 + \dfrac{\sigma_t^2}{n_t} + \dfrac{\sigma_{pt,error}^2}{n_t}}. \tag{14}$$

If we planned to use the average of three therapists in future research and were only interested in relative rank ordering, then we would use Equation 13 with $n_t = 3$. The generalizability would be .856. If, on the other hand, we planned to use just one therapist's ratings in future research (i.e., $n_t = 1$), the expected generalizability would be .665. The corresponding estimates for absolute decisions (Equation 14) are also .856 and .665 because there is no variance for the therapist component. When therapist differences are present, the absolute decision model produces lower estimates than the relative decision model because observer mean differences are not considered a relevant source of error in the relative decision model. Of course, the difference between the model estimates will depend on the size of the observer mean differences. When observer differences are indistinguishable from random error, the two models are equivalent (as is the case in this example). Note also that the k-observer relative decision estimate is equivalent to coefficient alpha, a reliability estimate commonly referred to in the measurement literature. In fact, all common reliability estimates can be framed in the generalizability model.[35]

The single observer estimates provide lower estimates than the k-observer estimates; a composite would naturally be expected to be more reliable than any one component. These estimates may diverge considerably when more than two observers are used and single-observer reliability is only modest. In both the relative and absolute decision models, the k-observer estimates are equivalent to the Spearman-Brown prophesy formula applied to the single-observer estimates for a measure of length k:

$$r_{kk} = \frac{kr_{11}}{1 + (k-1)r_{11}} \tag{15}$$

where r_{kk} is the reliability of a k-part measure and r_{11} is the reliability of a single part.

The single-facet design provides a useful vehicle for demonstrating important interpretive issues. As Lahey et al. point out, low reliability values may not reflect a large degree of random error or unreliability in the traditional sense; other potential problems must first be ruled out.[64] A series of examples highlights these problems. First, consider the hypothetical data in Figure 10-1, the raw data for the example in Table 10-2. These data exhibit a high degree of variability in knee positions across patients. In order for reliability to be established there must be sufficient variability for differences to be detected. Figure 10-2, by contrast, contains data with far less variability. Such data might arise, for example, if walking velocity were imposed on subjects (e.g., on a treadmill) or the sample was very homogeneous. In this case, the estimates based on the average of three therapists are much lower: .526 and .520. It might be inappropriate to conclude in this case that the measure is unreliable. Instead, there is insufficient variability to assess reliability. It would be better to suspend judgment until a fairer test is conducted. It could also be concluded that the measure *is* unreliable when used under these measurement conditions.

Figure 10-3 indicates a different problem. In this case, Therapist C has used a fundamentally different measurement technique, such as calculating the knee position from a baseline that is 90 degrees different from the other two raters. The result is a strong Therapist × Patient interaction that is pooled along with random error into the residual term. As a consequence, the reliability estimates are deflated. In fact, the variance component estimate for the universe score (σ_p^2) is negative and thus the generalizability coefficients are zero. Sizeable negative variance components are a cue that something is seriously amiss in the data.* One way to detect such problems is to examine the pairwise correlations among raters (a more formal procedure is described by Lahey et al.).[64] In this example, the correlations quickly reveal that one therapist is using a rating rule opposite to that used by the other therapists: $r_{ab} = .828$; $r_{ac} = -.577$; and $r_{bc} = -.622$. It would be inappropriate to conclude that these data are unreliable because the relations among therapists are quite strong. Instead, a simple rescaling of the data removes the systematic problem. When rescaling cannot be used with confidence, the reliability study should be reconducted with better training designed to eliminate systematic rule variation.

---

* Some negative variance components would be expected due to sampling variability. These are treated as though they were zero.

FIGURE 10-1   Hypothetical knee flexion measurements from three therapists.

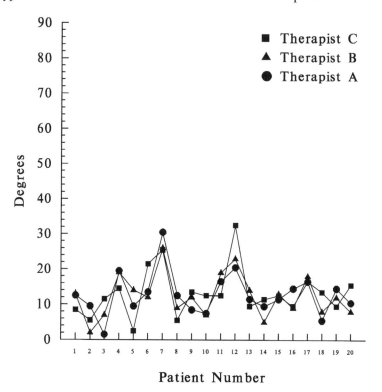

FIGURE 10-2   Hypothetical knee flexion measurements containing insufficient variability.

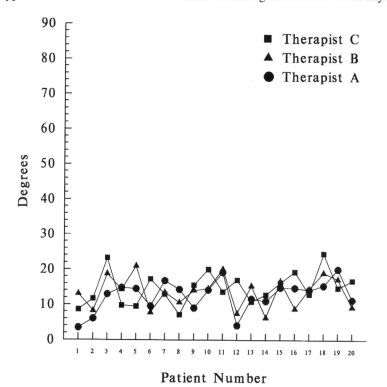

FIGURE 10-3   Hypothetical knee flexion measurements containing a therapist × patient interaction.

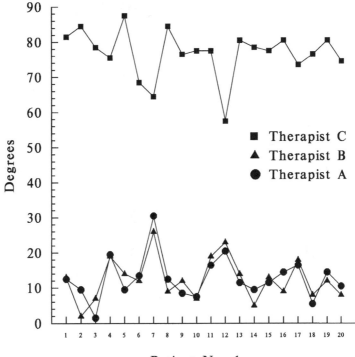

This example highlights an additional point about generalizability theory coefficients: they are averages of individual rater reliabilities that might be quite heterogenous.[81] It is good practice to examine the data closely to ensure that generalizations are defensible statements about the typical judge or observer (or other measurement facet).

A final problem is indicated in Figure 10-4 and highlights the basic difference between relative and absolute decision models. In this figure, the data from Figure 10-1 have been transformed so that all ratings for Therapist B have been increased by 10 degrees. These systematic differences are reflected in the absolute decision model estimate (for the average of three observers) of .655, but not the relative decision model estimate of .856.*

The previous example can be expanded to demonstrate the calculation of estimates from generalizability theory when there is more than one facet. We can return to the original example and assume that the three observers independently assess the same patients at two different walking velocities. The G study design is thus a completely crossed Patient × Therapist × Velocity factorial. A random effects ANOVA can be used to estimate the mean squares for all effects in the model; these are listed in Table 10-3.

The components of variance and the proportions of variance in Table 10-3 indicate that universe scores (the Patient source of variance) are a substantial source of variance in obtained scores. Also sizable, however, is the component for the Patient × Therapist interaction. This term indicates that the relative rank ordering of patients is not consistent across the three therapists; each therapist provides somewhat different rank orderings of the patients. There is also a small effect for occasions; knee position at heel strike is systematically different for the two walking velocities.

The results of the G study can in turn be used to estimate the generalizability for numerous possible applications. For example, we can estimate the reliability of a measure taken at one

---

*   The frequently cited intraclass correlation approach to reliability (e.g., Lahey et al.[64]; Shrout & Fleiss[92]) is a special case of generalizability theory in which a single facet is specified. In that case, the distinction between relative and absolute decisions and the distinction between random and fixed effects cannot be made separately because generalizability theory does not recognize a single fixed facet design.[90] The fixed effects and random effects intraclass correlation estimates reduce to generalizability estimates for relative and absolute decisions respectively.

FIGURE 10-4 Hypothetical knee flexion measurements containing baseline differences.

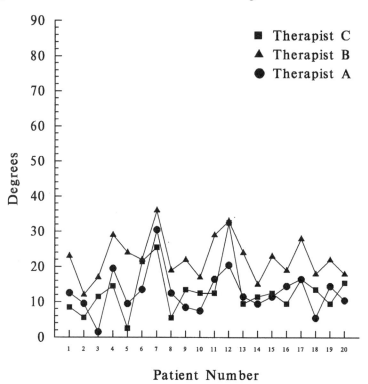

velocity ($n_v = 1$) by one therapist ($n_t = 1$) by substitution in Equations 9 through 12:

$$E\rho^2 = \frac{\sigma_p^2}{\sigma_p^2 + \dfrac{\sigma_{pt}^2}{n_t} + \dfrac{\sigma_{pv}^2}{n_v} + \dfrac{\sigma_{ptv,error}^2}{n_t n_v}}, \qquad (16)$$

and

$$\Phi = \frac{\sigma_p^2}{\sigma_p^2 + \dfrac{\sigma_t^2}{n_t} + \dfrac{\sigma_v^2}{n_v} + \dfrac{\sigma_{pt}^2}{n_t} + \dfrac{\sigma_{pv}^2}{n_v} + \dfrac{\sigma_{tv}^2}{n_t n_v} + \dfrac{\sigma_{ptv,error}^2}{n_t n_v}}. \qquad (17)$$

For relative and absolute decisions, the estimates are .768 and .720 respectively. If three measures will be collected in a future application, the relative consequences of increasing the number of therapists and the number of measurement velocities can easily be compared. For one therapist and three randomly selected velocities (i.e., $n_t = 1$ and $n_v = 3$), the relative and absolute estimates are .777 and .758. On the other hand, for three therapists and one velocity ($n_t = 3$ and $n_v = 1$), the estimates are .908 and .846. Clearly, a decrease in measurement error is best achieved by increasing the number of therapists rather than the number of velocities at which patients are examined.

The relative imprecision due to velocities versus therapists can be estimated in a different way using Equations 16 and 17. We can ask the question, "If I have only one therapist available for measurement, what is the upper bound for generalizability as I increase the number of measurement velocities?" Substituting $n_t = 1$ into Equations 16 and 17 and letting n_v increase to infinity, which effectively eliminates the terms with n_v in the denominator, it can be shown that the upper limits for generalizability for a single therapist are .782 and .779. On the other hand, if only one velocity can be used ($n_v = 1$) but the number of therapists is potentially unlimited ($n_t \to \infty$), then the upper limits for generalizability are 1.000 and .926. These conclusions are no surprise. The information from the G study clearly indicated that the relative rankings of patients varied more across therapists than across velocities.

In summary, generalizability theory provides a powerful way to investigate the influence of different potential error sources and a flexible means for planning future measurement problems. Generalizability theory, however, requires measurement on at least an interval scale. This assumption will be reasonable for many gait variables (e.g., velocity, stride length, stance time, power, etc.).

TABLE 10-3   Knee position at heel strike measured by three therapists at two velocities

<table>
<tr><td colspan="4" align="center">**Summary Statistics**</td></tr>
<tr><td></td><td></td><td align="center">**Mean**</td><td align="center">**Standard Deviation**</td></tr>
<tr><td>Therapist 1</td><td>Velocity 1</td><td>14.543</td><td>7.755</td></tr>
<tr><td></td><td>Velocity 2</td><td>17.141</td><td>8.400</td></tr>
<tr><td>Therapist 2</td><td>Velocity 1</td><td>14.381</td><td>6.929</td></tr>
<tr><td></td><td>Velocity 2</td><td>17.992</td><td>7.390</td></tr>
<tr><td>Therapist 3</td><td>Velocity 1</td><td>14.526</td><td>8.034</td></tr>
<tr><td></td><td>Velocity 2</td><td>16.519</td><td>7.661</td></tr>
</table>

ANOVA Summary

Source	*MS*	Estimated Variance Component	Proportion of Variance
Patients (*p*)	300.504	45.722	.720
Therapist (*t*)	4.406	0.000	.000
Velocity (*v*)	224.232	3.632	.057
p × *t*	26.547	12.716	.200
p × *v*	.737	0.000	.000
t × *v*	6.682	.278	.004
p × *t* × *v, error*	1.115	1.115	.018

On the other hand, many gait variables are best thought of as nominal or ordinal categories. For example, ratings of presence or absence of gait abnormality or ratings of degree of abnormality on a simple three- or four-category scale are common in observational gait analysis systems (see Chapter 11). Classification decisions (e.g., diagnoses) also commonly require placement of patients into discrete categories. These kinds of measures are best examined using an agreement model of reliability.

Agreement.   The measurement of agreement in classification might seem simple and easily assessed by calculating the proportion of agreement in categorization by judges. This approach, however, has a fundamental flaw that is easily demonstrated. Imagine two raters asked to classify 100 patients into one of two categories: normal gait and abnormal gait. Furthermore, presume that instead of actually observing the gait of each patient, the two raters each independently draw successive classifications out of hats, with each hat containing 90 pieces of paper with "normal gait" written on them and 10 pieces of paper with "abnormal gait" written on them. The classification process can easily be seen to be random. Yet

this process will yield an expected proportion of agreement between the two judges of .82. The probability of two independent events (e.g., both judges classifying a patient as having normal gait) is equal to the product of their individual probabilities (e.g., .9 × .9). When those individual probabilities are high, the likelihood of agreement by chance alone is also quite high. To provide an appropriate measure of agreement, the proportion of agreement must be corrected for agreement expected by chance. The most popular chance-corrected measure is Cohen's kappa:

$$\kappa = \frac{p_o - p_e}{1 - p_c} \tag{18}$$

where p_o is the observed proportion of agreement, and p_c is the proportion of agreement expected by chance.[23] Kappa is an intuitively appealing agreement statistic because it is readily interpreted as chance-corrected agreement. Numbers greater than zero indicate agreement above chance levels and numbers below zero indicate agreement below chance levels (e.g., one judge using a classification rule that is the inverse of that used by another judge).

Table 10-4   Calculation of kappa for two judges and two rating categories

		Cross-Classification Table		
		Judge 1		
		Stagger Absent	**Stagger Present**	**Marginal**
	Stagger Absent	32 (.64)	5 (.10)	37 (.74)
Judge 2	**Stagger Present**	6 (.12)	7 (.14)	13 (.26)
	Marginal	38 (.76)	12 (.24)	

Kappa Calculations

$p_o = .640 + .140 = .780$

$p_c = (.740 \times .760) + (.260 \times .240) = .625$

$\kappa = (.780 - .625)/(1 - .625) = .414$

Although numerous other agreement statistics have been proposed,[41,102,116] kappa remains the most useful because the basic formula has been modified and extended to apply to other variations on the categorical judgment theme. For example, kappa has been extended to allow more than two raters,[27,40,105] different raters for each subject,[40,89] missing data,[105] nonexclusive categories,[45,60] time-based nominal scales,[28] and weighting for partial agreement.[24] This latter extension is particularly noteworthy because it allows the use of kappa for ordered categories. In addition, the sampling theory for kappa is well understood, at least for large samples[40,43,52]; robust small sample standard errors appear to be adequately estimated by jackknife techniques.[60,89]

Kappa is not without its problems, however.[95,106,107] Its maximum value is dependent on the base rate, sensitivity, and specificity, indicating that it is best thought of as a family of reliabilities specific to different response rates in the population.[48,108] Practically, this means that comparison of kappas across samples is appropriate only if their response rates are reasonably similar. Suggested alternatives (e.g., Yule's Y[95]) also have interpretive problems,[20,93,107] thus kappa remains the most flexible agreement statistic and should be used routinely when categorical or ordinal reliability estimates are desired. In addition, however, the patterns of agreement and disagreement should be examined carefully because the overall kappa statistic often hides important information at the level of particular categories or combinations of judges—a problem similar to that demonstrated with generalizability theory. For example, some pairs of judges may agree more than other pairs, and some categories may achieve higher agreement than others.*

To demonstrate the calculation of kappa, two examples will be provided. In the first, two judges classify subjects into two categories. In this case, suppose that a clinician wished to construct a simple checklist of gait characteristics, each rated dichotomously as normal versus abnormal or present versus absent. Such a checklist, if reliable, could allow a quick assessment of normal gait. Each item on the checklist could be examined for reliability by having two raters independently assess a sample of individuals. Assume, for example, that the variable *stagger* was rated as present versus absent for a sample of 50 patients. The independent observations of the two raters would allow classification of patients into a two-fold table. (See hypothetical data in Table 10-4.) The main diagonal of this table allows calculation of observed proportion of agreement; in this case, p_o = .780, seemingly high agreement. But, because so many of the subjects exhibit no stagger, this simple proportion of agreement is inflated by chance agreement. In fact, the judges would be expected to agree 62.5% of the time if they were drawing classifications out of hats and the hats contained classifications in the same proportions

---

* Further discussions of this topic can be found in the following sources: 20,27,40,66,103,104.

Table 10-5 Calculation of weighted kappa for two judges and four ordered categories

		Judge 1				
		0	**1**	**2**	**3**	**Marginal**
	0	12 (.06)	94 (.47)	10 (.05)	6 (.03)	122 (.61)
	1	4 (.02)	4 (.02)	16 (.08)	0 (.00)	24 (.12)
Judge 2	2	2 (.01)	8 (.04)	0 (.00)	22 (.11)	32 (.16)
	3	0 (.00)	0 (.00)	2 (.01)	20 (.10)	22 (.11)
Marginal		18 (.09)	106 (.53)	28 (.14)	48 (.24)	

	Weight Matrix 1				Weight Matrix 2				Weight Matrix 3			
	0	**1**	**2**	**3**	**0**	**1**	**2**	**3**	**0**	**1**	**2**	**3**
0	1	0	0	0	1	1	0	0	1	1	1	0
1	0	1	0	0	1	1	1	0	1	1	1	0
2	0	0	1	0	0	1	1	1	1	1	1	0
3	0	0	0	1	0	0	1	1	0	0	0	1

as those given by the marginal distributions in Table 10-4. When this level of chance agreement is taken into account, the true agreement (κ) is only .414.

As noted previously, the appeal of kappa arises from its extensions to other important agreement problems. One of the more useful extensions is for data that are ordinal in nature, but do not possess the interval characteristics that justify use of generalizability theory. For example, suppose two judges independently rated a geriatric sample ($N = 200$) using the Gait Abnormality Rating Scale.[111] Each item on the GARS requires an ordered judgment on a four-point scale; each scale measures a different feature of gait (e.g., guardedness, staggering, weaving, shoulder extension). The hypothetical data in Table 10-5 refer to the classifications of two independent judges each rating subjects using the GARS item that measures pathological forward projection of the head relative to the trunk (0 = earlobe vertically aligned with shoulder tip, 1 = earlobe vertical projection falls 1″ anterior to shoulder tip, 2 = earlobe vertical projection falls 2″ anterior to shoulder tip, and 3 = earlobe vertical projection falls 3″ or more anterior to shoulder tip).

Calculation of the simple kappa coefficient yields .015, indicating little agreement. But, simple kappa ignores the ordinal nature of the categories; disagreement between adjacent categories is penalized as harshly as disagreement between more dis-

tantly separated categories. Weighted kappa, on the other hand, allows for different degrees of disagreement. Moreover, the precise nature of the allowable levels of disagreement is defined by the researcher in the form of weight matrices. Three such matrices are listed in Table 10-5. For simplicity, weights have been limited to values of 0 and 1, with 1 indicating that the two categories in question are considered identical (i.e., no disagreement is counted) and 0 indicating that the categories are considered distinct (more finite levels can be used). Each matrix defines disagreement a little differently. The first matrix, in fact, defines disagreement in the same way as simple kappa; each category is distinct and all disagreements are treated similarly. Weight matrix 2 defines disagreement more liberally. In this case, if judges classify a subject in adjacent categories, no disagreement is counted. This might be a reasonable model if one judge appears to exhibit a systematic shift in classifications (e.g., a relatively harsh judge).* The third matrix reflects an interest in distinguishing severe

---

* Another approach to these data is to calculate the Spearman rank-order correlation. For these data, $r_s = .639$. Clearly, the judges are consistent in the rank order sense if not in the absolute sense (i.e., simple kappa). The disadvantage to the rank-order correlation approach is that it defines disagreement in only one way. Consequently, the method is less flexible than weighted kappa.

projection from all other categories. If a diagnostic decision will hinge on such a cutoff, the decision rule can be incorporated into reliability calculations using an appropriate weight matrix. The three different weight matrices yield quite different results: .015, .738, and .495. The different results that are produced by different weights underscores an important point; reliabilities are application specific; they are bound by the conditions of measurement and interpretation. In this sense, the use of weight matrices resembles D studies in generalizability theory.*

Common Problems and Pitfalls in Reliability Assessment

In this section we describe some common problems that threaten the appropriate use and interpretation of reliability estimates. One major theme underlies many of the problems we will discuss and may help readers to identify other potential problems in their own research: the conditions under which reliability are assessed must mimic the proposed specific uses of the measure. In this sense, there are as many reliabilities for a measure as there are applications for the measure. This view of reliability is explicit in the distinction between G studies and D studies in generalizability theory, but it underlies proper interpretation of other models as well. There are two related implications that deserve emphasis. First, clear specification of the intended uses of a measure necessarily identifies the expected error sources—anything that can be expected to change from measurement occasion to measurement occasion. Second, specification of error sources, along with obtained scores, fully determines the nature of true scores—anything that remains constant from measurement occasion to measurement occasion. Thus, each application defines true score and error somewhat differently. The important point is that improper

specification of error sources will confuse true score and error components and render reliability estimates uninterpretable. Common error sources include random variabilities arising within individuals (e.g., fatigue, motivation), situational factors (e.g., distracting or unpleasant measurement environments), evaluator factors (e.g., carefulness, subjectivity), and idiosyncratic match between measurement and respondent (e.g., catching some respondents at their best or having a measure that just happens to favor the skills of some respondents more than others).[35] More specific error sources can arise for any application and pose a particular challenge for all reliability studies.

Violation of Measurement Model Assumptions. All reliability estimates are based on measurement models that make certain assumptions about the data. Reliability estimates can only be trusted if the assumptions hold. Unfortunately, model assumptions are most often taken as a matter of faith rather than verified. In many instances, measurement models are robust to violations of assumptions but that state of affairs cannot be trusted to hold universally.[35,76] Indeed, troubling consequences of assumption violation are appearing with greater frequency in the literature.[94] Good sense and good research practice demand examination of the plausibility of the assumptions that underlie reliability estimation and determination of the consequences of assumption violation.

Inappropriate Sampling of Respondents. One of the most common problems in reliability assessment is the use of a sample for reliability estimation that is not representative of the population from which application samples will be drawn. A common practice, for example, is to conduct reliability studies on easily obtained normal samples when the measure will be used for special, impaired populations. Unfortunately, the sources of error variance may be different in kind and number for the reliability sample, and estimated reliability may not apply to future application samples. Furthermore, the variability of true scores may not be representative. When the samples are different, the estimated reliability can either underestimate or overestimate the reliability in the application sample. If the reliability sample is more homogeneous than the intended application sample, there may be little variability in true scores relative to error variability. Reliability estimates will be artificially low. On the other hand, if the reliability sample is unrepresentatively heterogeneous, the true scores may vary more than would be expected in the application sample. In this case, reliability estimates may be artificially high. On

---

* Despite this parallel, generalizability theory estimates are association measures; they primarily gauge the consistency of rank order between judges, time periods, or other measurement facets. By contrast, agreement measures such as kappa impose a harsher standard by penalizing any disagreement (unless appropriate modifications are made, such as weighted kappa). Consequently, different reliability estimates calculated on different types of data ordinarily are not comparable. Indeed, different reliability estimates calculated on the same data set may differ greatly. There are, however, fundamental similarities between the two general classes of estimates we have described. As numerous authors have discussed, the kappa coefficient is an intraclass correlation and the estimates calculated from the two models can agree under certain circumstances.[41,42,84] It is only when the models define error similarly that this correspondence holds, however. In this sense, it is perhaps best to think of agreement models as a special restrictive case of association.[5,40]

the other hand, a heterogeneous sample may also contain more sources of error that could reduce the reliability estimate.

Improper Specification of Error Components. Another common problem is the failure to correctly specify important sources of error. One clear example is the use of a time period in a test-retest study that contains more or fewer error sources than will exist in the application of the measure. If a researcher intends to examine improvement in patient function due to an intervention, the time period that separates the preintervention measure and the postintervention measure defines the appropriate time frame for the reliability assessment of the outcome measure. If instead the reliability assessment time period is too short, important sources of error may not have sufficient opportunity to emerge; they are constants and are counted incorrectly in the true score part of the obtained score. If the time period is too long, more sources of error than expected will affect the reliability estimate; these additional error sources would not ordinarily affect obtained scores in an intervention study using a shorter time frame. In this sense, identification of true score and error may seem somewhat arbitrary because one researcher's true score could be another researcher's error. The important point is to be clear about the specification of true score and error for a particular application and then duplicate those specifications in the reliability study.* This problem can be quite challenging. For example, demonstrating the reliability of a motion analysis system requires replication of complex movements in three planes under carefully controlled conditions, a task not easily accomplished with human targets. Scholz describes a very creative robotic simulation that mimics very closely the intended application with humans.[88] The robotics repeated movements very precisely so that measurement differences were not attributable to changes in the target but to characteristics of the measurement device.

Lack of Standardization.   The sine qua non of testing is standardization of assessment. It ensures

that many potential sources of error are rendered inoperable. Yet this aspect of testing can often be overlooked. We would like to believe that characteristics of the examining room, dress or style of the examiner, time of day, and other apparently mundane features have little impact on measurement. That may be the case, but in the absence of sound evidence for their irrelevance, the safest option is to hold them constant. Indeed, many potential sources of error cannot be anticipated, but they can be ruled inoperable through careful standardization. But, error sources should be held constant only if that level of standardization will be carried over to the application of the measure. Otherwise, reliability estimates derived from a strictly standardized assessment may not reflect the reliability obtained in less standardized applications.

Standardized assessment is particularly crucial for measurement by observers or raters. For example, observational gait evaluation (see Chapter 11) places complex attentional and decision-making demands on raters. Unless raters are trained carefully with thoroughly defined operational definitions, mediocre reliability can be expected. Furthermore it is imperative to verify that observers follow the rating protocol consistently throughout the study. Despite careful initial training, raters may deviate from the protocol over time (a problem akin to measurement drift). The goal is to have raters operate as consistently as a piece of equipment.

The Effect of Measurement on the Respondents.   Measures vary considerably along an active versus passive dimension. Some, such as radiographs or simple observation of stance or walking pattern, have little noticeable impact on respondents. Others, such as muscle strength measures, can influence the characteristic being measured. Repeated muscle strength testing can induce fatigue and introduce both bias and error into the measurement. Two potential problems should be noted here. First, the act of measurement may fundamentally change the nature of the characteristic being assessed. In this case, repeated measures are tapping different true scores because the patient has changed over time. Second, the act of measurement may alter the relative impact of error sources. The combined effect produces reliability estimates of dubious worth; the relative amounts of true score and error shift over time and so provide no stable basis for inference.

Composites, Profiles, and Multidimensional Measures.   Another troublesome source of problems is confusion regarding the level at which reliability should be assessed. This issue is important

---

* The identification of appropriate time periods can be further complicated by any "memory" component to the task. Ideally, the time period is chosen to allow important sources of error to operate and to assume that the true score component remains constant, but to also assume that respondents' memory for previous performance does not bias the results. In practice, this may be difficult to arrange. On physical performance tests, in particular, individuals may be motivated to improve on their previous performances.

when several measures are combined into a composite or profile. For example, ROM of the hip, knee, and ankle provide a useful battery of measures that might be combined to predict stride length. Ambulation profiles (see Chapter 11) likewise consist of multiple tests, in this case to assess walking ability. How should reliability be calculated in such cases? The issue again reduces to how the battery of measures will be used. If individual measures are the most sensible unit of analysis, then reliability should be assessed and interpreted for each measure separately. If, on the other hand, a composite score is to be used, then a reliability estimate based on the composite should be calculated and interpreted.

In general, there is no great difficulty in deriving reliability estimates for composites. A composite (C) is nothing more than a weighted sum of p individual elements: $C = w_1X_1 + w_2X_2 + w_3X_3 + \ldots + w_pX_p$. These weights may be empirically derived (e.g., multiple regression, discriminant analysis) or based on practical or theoretical considerations. From well-known algebraic properties of linear combinations, the variance of a composite can be stated as:

$$\sigma_C^2 = \sum_{i=1}^{p} w_i^2 \sigma_{x_i}^2 + \sum_{i=1}^{p} \sum_{j=1}^{p} w_i w_j \sigma_{x_i x_j (i \neq j)} \quad (19)$$

where $\sigma_{x_i}^2$ is the variance of subpart x_i and $\sigma_{x_i x_j}$ is the covariance between subparts x_i and x_j.[76] Because error components for each subpart are assumed to be independent, the error variance for a composite is simply the weighted sum of the individual error variances:

$$\sigma_{e_c}^2 = \sum_{i=1}^{p} w_i^2 \sigma_{e_i}^2 = \sum_{i=1}^{p} w_i^2 \sigma_{x_i}^2 (1 - r_{x_i x_i}). \quad (20)$$

Finally, the variance-ratio definition for reliability (Equation 2) can be restated in the following form with particular reference to composites:

$$r_{CC} = 1 - \frac{\sigma_{e_c}^2}{\sigma_C^2}. \quad (21)$$

Under different assumptions about the distributions of the subparts, Equation 21 will provide an appropriate reliability estimate.[35,76,87]

To calculate composite reliabilities, researchers must choose the weights carefully. Most often, and often with little thought, the separate components are simply summed. The assumption of equal weights may not be empirically or theoretically justified.[82,83] For example, only under the assumption of equivalent measurement (i.e., parallel forms) and equal conceptual merit does the use of equal weights make sense. Furthermore, if the separate subtests are measured on different scales, their simple summation does not translate into an equally weighted composite. If the separate subtests measure fundamentally different constructs, then their combination into a single score is inadvisable because the empirical weights for the subtests may vary in different measurement contexts. Finally, multiple measures may predict important outcome variables in ways that are more complex than a simple additive model (e.g., interactions or nonlinear relations). The important point is that a combination of measures into a composite rests on assumptions about weights that should be carefully considered and empirically verified.

If it makes little sense to compute a composite score, it may still make sense to calculate a reliability estimate for the battery or profile of tests. Generalizability theory can also be used to estimate reliability of a battery of tests and in particular has a multivariate extension that allows estimation for collections of measures that are quite diverse. In each of these cases, it is perhaps best to think of the estimated reliability as providing information about the global dependability of the profile or measurement protocol.[113] In this sense, if decisions are based on the pattern of individual scale scores, then the reliability of the profile provides information about how much decisions may vary due to random fluctuations in the individual elements of the profile.

Change Scores and Ratios.   Two types of measures closely related to composite scores deserve separate discussion: change scores and ratio scores. Change scores are a common but much debated measure.[31,46,68,85,86] The appeal of a change score is that it provides a direct measure of how much an individual has changed, possibly from before a treatment to after a treatment. For example, improvement in walking ability by hemiplegic patients following implementation of functional electrical stimulation (see Chapter 26) is easily gauged by simple change in performance. Change scores are much maligned, however. The most common complaint stems from their demonstrated low reliability under conditions that might seem quite common. Because a change score is simply a linear combination with weights (w_i) equal to 1 and −1 (i.e., $C = X_1 − X_2$), Equations 19 through 21 can be used to derive an estimate of reliability.* Typically, the simplifying assumption is made that the variances of X_1 and X_2 are equal. Under that restriction, the reliability of a change score can be expressed in the following way:

$$r_{CC} = \frac{\bar{r}_{xx} - r_{x_1 x_2}}{1 - r_{x_1 x_2}} \qquad (22)$$

where $\bar{r}_{xx}$ is the average of the reliabilities for the pretest and posttest measures. Equation 22 indicates that as the correlation between the two measures approaches their average reliability, the reliability of the difference score approaches zero. Even for modest pre/post correlations that differ moderately from the average of the pretest and posttest reliabilities, the difference score reliability can be disappointing. For example, if the pretest and posttest have an average reliability of .800 and their intercorrelation is .650, the difference score reliability is .429. Furthermore, this reliability may be an overestimate because the pretest and posttest reliabilities are likely to be based on a single measurement period and not include time-based error, whereas the pre/post correlation will be attenuated by time-based error.

The aforementioned reliability problem hinges on the assumption of equivalent pretest and posttest variances. But, as many have convincingly argued, that assumption is not likely to be true.[46,62,85] In fact, experimental treatments commonly increase or decrease the variability of measurements. For example, a relatively homogeneous group of poor walkers may respond differently to treatment, producing greater variability in walking ability at posttest compared to pretest. Thus, the conditions under which low change score reliability is often argued to be common, may not be so common at all. Nonetheless correlations involving change scores can be challenging to interpret. As Gardner and Neufeld demonstrate, correlations of pretest with change, correlations of other variables with change, and correlations of two different change scores are influenced by many factors that allow the same correlation value to be produced in many different ways.[46] This is not an inherent limitation to change scores; it simply means that the inherent complexity of change scores must be recognized when they are used.

The problems with the reliability of change scores have led some to dismiss their use in experimental work. The argument is that unreliable outcome measures will lower the power of a between-groups test. That dismissal is not justified, however. As Feldt and Brennan point out, an unreliable difference score will prevent a dependable ranking of individuals *within* an experimental group, but a constant treatment effect that increases or decreases the scores of all subjects in one of the groups may still be detectable.[35] The problem is with confusing within-group reliability with between-group differences in means. Low reliability within groups does not preclude obtaining between-groups differences. Indeed, an effective treatment increases the variability of change scores across groups, in effect increasing the reliability of between-groups change scores. Rogosa et al. make a similar point[85] (see also Humphries and Drasgow[53,54] and Overall[79,80]). They also note that the reliability of a change score depends on the variability of individual growth rates (i.e., change). When those growth rates have little variability within groups, the ability to rank order individuals within a group according to change is low and thus the reliability of the change score is low within treatment groups. But that doesn't mean that the overall level of change cannot be estimated precisely and that differences in change between groups cannot be detected. In fact, average change for a group is estimated most precisely when individuals within the group exhibit little variability in their growth rates.

Nonetheless, there may be conceptual difficulties in the interpretation of change scores that may recommend against their use regardless of their psychometric qualities. For example, if the pretest and posttest are not highly correlated, then the concept of change may be complex and be difficult to define.[4] The use of change scores requires a careful consideration of their reliability as well as their conceptual merit.

Similar interpretive issues surround the use of ratio scores (e.g., percent maximum volitional contraction of a muscle), although there are some important differences. First, a ratio of two measures only makes sense if the individual measures are themselves ratio-level assessments (i.e., possess a true zero point and equal interval scaling). Second, there are potential interpretative difficulties when ratios are correlated with other scales.[25] The resulting correlations may represent primarily a relation with the numerator variable or the denominator variable or both. This ambiguity may be dissatisfying from an inference standpoint no

---

* We discuss only the simple change score. Other versions have been suggested (e.g., weighted reliability measure, residual change) and are discussed at length elsewhere.[26,85] Our general discussion applies to these other measures as well. The reliability of the change score may or may not be a serious problem, depending on the application of the measure.

matter how theoretically sensible the ratio may seem. Third, despite the apparent sensibility of a ratio measure, spurious correlations between ratios and other variables can arise if important assumptions are not met.[38,71] Likewise, statistical problems (e.g., heteroscedasticity) may be created when ratio variables are used.[38] Fourth, one feature of ratios makes them different from other composites: they represent product variables that carry information about the interactive effects of two variables.[10] If the theoretical question that guides the research clearly specifies interactions, then a complete analysis may require including the separate components of the ratio in addition to the ratio.[25,55] Finally, and most important for purposes of this chapter, our previous comments about reliability apply with equal force to ratios. If either component of a ratio is unreliable, the ratio will be unreliable and of no utility. These potential problems with ratios have been discussed at length elsewhere and will not be repeated here.[10,38,39,61] It is sufficient for us to remind potential users of ratios that there are numerous pitfalls that can be avoided through careful attention to available resources.

When Is Reliability High Enough?   If tradition and current practices are any indication, judgments of "good" and "poor" reliability are inevitable. But, reliability coefficients are continuous whereas particular cutoffs tend to place undue importance on particular discrete values. Consequently, some measures are accorded great respect because they successfully leap the artificial hurdle, whereas others are dismissed for just missing the cutoff. The difference between the reliabilities of the measures might be quite trivial, but the conclusions reached about them are not. Nonetheless, reliability cutoffs are a popular shorthand. Numerous favorite benchmarks for acceptable lower limits have been proposed.[13,22,35,65,76] The more important consideration in deciding on a cutoff is how the measure will be used. If the measure will be used in research on modest to large numbers of subjects, then reliabilities in the .70 to .80 range may be tolerable. Correlations are attenuated very little by measurement error in these cases, so detectable effect sizes do not suffer appreciably. Moreover, the power to detect important effects can be enhanced by increasing sample sizes, which may be easier than the efforts usually required to boost a measure's reliability from .80 to .90.[101] On the other hand, when a measure is to be used for *individual* decision-making (e.g., diagnosis or classification), then much higher reliability is required.

In this case, an error has very real individual consequences and great efforts should be made to keep errors at a low level. If an acceptable amount of error around an individual's true score can be specified in advance, Equation 5 can be transformed to give the reliability that will be required:

$$r_{xx} = 1 - \frac{\sigma_{meas}^2}{\sigma_x^2}. \qquad (23)$$

As noted previously, the σ_{meas} may not be constant for all individuals. The level of reliability required depends in part on the score levels at which one intends to make decisions.

Another way to address the issue of whether a reliability coefficient is large enough is to construct confidence intervals around reliability estimates and test the difference between reliability estimates for significance.* Either may be useful when precise statements about a reliability estimate are desired. Moreover, calculation of confidence intervals reminds researchers that sampling error may be substantial and places important limits on the confidence that can be placed in reliability estimates.

Summary and Recommendations

Testing conceptual hypotheses, assigning patients to diagnostic groups, and making decisions about appropriate treatment should not be conducted by lottery. Yet that is the consequence if decisions are based on unreliable measures. As a way of summarizing the contents of this chapter, we offer a short list of recommendations and reminders.

1. Be aware of and examine the plausibility of assumptions underlying reliability estimation. Measurements should be derived based on sound theory, and the measurement model should guide the choice of a reliability estimate.

2. Use large samples when estimating reliability. Reliability theories are large sample models that assume negligible sampling error for subjects. Failure to recognize this could produce disappointing correspondence between reliability estimates achieved in assessment and application samples.

3. A reliability estimate provides a useful summary, but more detailed information should also be examined. For interval level data, variance components and patterns of inter-

---

* For further discussion of significance testing and reliability coefficients, see these sources: 1,19,21,32,35,37.

observer correlation should be examined. For discrete data, patterns of agreement and disagreement should be examined.

4. Think carefully in advance about the sources of error in a potential application. Those sources of error must be represented in the reliability study. When in doubt, include an error source in the reliability study. Error sources are more convincingly ruled out on empirical grounds than through divine revelation. Reliability inferences are limited to the conditions defined by the reliability study. Applications that deviate from those conditions may achieve different reliability.

References

1. Alsawalmeh YM, Feldt LS: Test of the hypothesis that the intraclass reliability coefficient is the same for two measurement procedures, *Applied Psychological Measurement* 16:195-205, 1992.
2. Anastasi A: *Psychological testing,* 4th ed, New York, 1976, Macmillan.
3. Bentler P: *EQS structural equations program manual,* Los Angeles, 1989, BMDP Statistical Software.
4. Bereiter C: Some persisting dilemmas in the measurement of change. In Harris CW, editor: *Problems in measuring change,* Madison, Wis, 1963, University of Wisconsin Press.
5. Berry KJ, Mielke PW Jr: A generalization of Cohen's kappa agreement measure to interval measurement and multiple raters, *Educational and Psychological Measurement* 48:921-933, 1988.
6. Blixt SL, Shama DB: An empirical investigation of the standard error of measurement at different ability levels, *Educational and Psychological Measurement* 46:545-550, 1986.
7. Bollen KA: *Structural equations with latent variables,* New York, 1989, Wiley.
8. Bollen K, Lennox R: Conventional wisdom on measurement: a structural equation perspective, *Psychological Bulletin* 110:305-314, 1991.
9. Booth CJ, editor: *The new IEEE standard dictionary of electrical and electronic terms,* 5th ed, New York, 1993, Institute of Electrical and Electronic Engineers.
10. Bradshaw Y, Radbill L: Method and substance in the use of ratio variables, *American Sociological Review* 52:132-135, 1987.
11. Brennan RL: *Elements of generalizability theory,* Iowa City, Iowa, 1993, American College Testing Program.
12. Brennan RL, Kane MT: An index of dependability for mastery tests, *Journal of Educational Measurement* 14:277-289, 1977.
13. Burdock EI, Fleiss JL, Hardesty AS: A new view of interobserver agreement, *Personnel Psychology* 16:373-384, 1963.
14. Campbell NR: *Foundations of science: the philosophy of theory,* New York, 1957, Dover.
15. Cardinet J, Tourneur Y, Allal L: The symmetry of generalizability theory: Applications to educational measurement, *Journal of Educational Measurement* 13:119-135, 1976.
16. Cardinet J, Tourneur Y, Allal L: Extension of generalizability theory and its applications in educational measurement, *Journal of Educational Measurement* 18:183-204, 1981.
17. Carmines EG, Zeller RA: Reliability and validity assessment. In Sullivan JL, editor: *Quantitative applications in the social sciences,* Beverly Hills, Calif, 1979, Sage.
18. Carnap R: *Philosophical foundations of physics: An introduction to the philosophy of science,* New York, 1966, Basic Books.
19. Cicchetti DV: Testing the normal approximation and minimal sample size requirements of weighted kappa when the number of categories is large, *Applied Psychological Measurement* 5: 101-104, 1981.
20. Cicchetti DV: When diagnostic agreement is high, but reliability is low: some paradoxes occurring in joint independent neuropsychology assessments, *Journal of Clinical and Experimental Neuropsychology* 10:605-622, 1988.
21. Cicchetti DV, Fleiss JL: Comparison of the null distribution of weighted kappa and the *C* ordinal statistic, *Applied Psychological Measurement* 1:195-201, 1977.
22. Cicchetti DV, Sparrow SS: Developing criteria for establishing the interrater reliability of specific items in a given inventory: applications to assessment of adaptive behavior, *American Journal of Mental Deficiency* 86:127-137, 1981.
23. Cohen J: A coefficient of agreement for nominal scales, *Educational and Psychological Measurement* 20:37-46, 1960.
24. Cohen J: Weighted kappa: Nominal scale agreement with provision for scaled disagreement or partial credit, *Psychological Bulletin* 70:213-220, 1968.
25. Cohen J, Cohen P: *Applied multiple regression/correlation analysis for the behavioral sciences,* 2d ed, Hillsdale, N.J., 1983, Erlbaum.
26. Collins LM, Horn JL, editors: *Best methods for the analysis of change: recent advances, unanswered questions, future directions.* Washington, D.C., 1991, American Psychological Association.
27. Conger AJ: Integration and generalization of kappa for multiple raters, *Psychological Bulletin* 88:322-328, 1980.
28. Conger AJ: Kappa reliabilities for continuous behaviors and events, *Educational and Psychological Measurement* 45:861-868, 1985.
29. Cook TD, Campbell DT: *Quasi-experimentation: design and analysis issues for field settings,* Chicago, 1979, Rand McNally.
30. Cronbach LJ: Coefficient alpha and the internal structure of tests. *Psychometrika* 16:297-334, 1951.
31. Cronbach LJ, Furby L: How we should measure "change"—or should we? *Psychological Bulletin* 74:68-80, 1970.
32. Cronbach LJ, et al: *The dependability of behavioral measurements,* New York, 1971, Wiley.
33. Crowder MJ, et al: *Statistical analysis of reliability data,* New York, 1991, Chapman & Hall.

34. Dummer GWA, Winton RC: *An elementary guide to reliability,* 4th ed, New York, 1990, Pergamon Press.

35. Feldt LS, Brennan RL: Reliability. In Linn RL, editor: *Educational measurement,* 3d ed, New York, 1989, Macmillan.

36. Feldt LS, Steffen M, Gupta NC: A comparison of five methods for estimating the standard error of measurement at specific score levels, *Applied Psychological Measurement* 9:351-361, 1985.

37. Feldt LS, Woodruff DJ, Salih FA: Statistical inference for coefficient alpha, *Applied Psychological Measurement* 11:93-103, 1987.

38. Firebaugh G, Gibbs JP: User's guide to ratio variables, *American Sociological Review* 50:713-722, 1985.

39. Firebaugh G, Gibbs JP: Defensible and indefensible commentaries, *American Sociological Review* 52:136-141, 1987.

40. Fleiss JL: Measuring nominal scale agreement among many raters, *Psychological Bulletin* 76:378-382, 1971.

41. Fleiss JL: Measuring agreement between two judges on the presence or absence of a trait *Biometrics* 31:651-659, 1975.

42. Fleiss JL, Cohen J: The equivalence of weighted kappa and the intraclass correlation coefficient as measures of reliability, *Educational and Psychological Measurement* 33:613-619, 1973.

43. Fleiss JL, Cohen J, Everitt BS: Large sample standard errors of kappa and weighted kappa, *Psychological Bulletin* 72:323-327, 1969.

44. Fleiss JL, Shrout PE: The effect of measurement error on some multivariate procedures, *American Journal of Public Health* 67:1184-1189, 1977.

45. Fleiss JL, et al: Quantification of agreement in multiple psychiatric diagnoses, *Archives of General Psychiatry* 26:168-171, 1972.

46. Gardner RC, Neufeld WJ: Use of the simple change score in correlational analyses, *Educational and Psychological Measurement* 47:849-864, 1987.

47. Ghiselli EE, Campbell JP, Zedeck S: *Measurement theory for the behavioral sciences,* New York, 1981, Freeman.

48. Grove WM, et al: Reliability studies of psychiatric diagnosis: theory and practice, *Archives of General Psychiatry* 38:408-411, 1981.

49. Guilford JP: *Psychometric methods,* New York, 1950, McGraw-Hill.

50. Hambleton RK, Swaminathan H: *Item response theory: Principles and applications,* Boston, 1985, Kluwer-Nijhoff Publishing.

51. Hambleton RK, Swaminathan H, Rogers HJ: *Fundamentals of item response theory,* Newbury Park, Calif, 1991, Sage.

52. Hanley JA: Standard error of the kappa statistic, *Psychological Bulletin* 102:315-321, 1987.

53. Humphreys LG, Drasgow F: Some comments on the relation between reliability and statistical power, *Applied Psychological Measurement* 13:419-425, 1989a.

54. Humphreys LG, Drasgow F: Paradoxes, contradictions, and illusions, *Applied Psychological Measurement* 13:429-431, 1989b.

55. Jaccard J, Turrisi R, Wan CK: *Interaction effects in multiple regression,* Newbury Park, Calif, 1990, Sage.

56. Jöreskog KG, Sörbom D: *LISREL 8 user's reference guide,* Chicago, 1993, Scientific Software, Inc.

57. Keppel G, Zedeck S: *Data analysis for research designs,* New York, 1989, Freeman.

58. Kleinbaum DG, Kupper LL, Muller KE: *Applied regression analysis and other multivariable methods,* 2d ed, Boston, 1988, PWS-Kent.

59. Kopriva RJ, Shaw DG: Power estimates: The effect of dependent variable reliability on the power of one-factor ANOVAs, *Educational and Psychological Measurement* 51:585-595, 1991.

60. Kraemer HC: Extension of the kappa coefficient, *Biometrics* 36:207-216, 1980.

61. Kraft M: On "user's guide to ratio variables," *American Sociological Review* 52:135-136, 1987.

62. Labouvie EW: The concept of change and regression toward the mean, *Psychological Bulletin* 92:251-257, 1982.

63. Ladin Z, Wu G: Combining position and acceleration measurements for joint force estimation, *Journal of Biomechanics* 24:1173-1187, 1991.

64. Lahey MA, Downey RG, Saal FE: Intraclass correlations: There's more there than meets the eye, *Psychological Bulletin* 93:586-595, 1983.

65. Landis RJ, Koch GG: The measurement of observer agreement for categorical data, *Biometrics* 33:159-174, 1977.

66. Light RJ: Measures of response agreement for qualitative data: Some generalizations and alternatives, *Psychological Bulletin* 76:365-377, 1971.

67. Linn RL, editor: *Educational measurement,* 3d ed, New York, 1989 Macmillan.

68. Linn RL, Slinde JA: The determination of the significance of change between pre- and posttesting periods, *Review of Educational Research* 47:121-150, 1977.

69. Loevinger J: Objective tests as instruments of psychological theory, *Psychological Reports* 3(Supp. 9):635-694, 1957.

70. Lord FM: Standard errors of measurement at different score levels, *Journal of Educational Measurement* 21:239-243, 1984.

71. Lynn M, Bond CF Jr: Conceptual meaning and spuriousness in ratio correlations: The case of restaurant tipping, *Journal of Applied Social Psychology* 22:327-341, 1992.

72. Maxwell SE, Delaney HD: *Designing experiments and analyzing data: A model comparison perspective,* Belmont, Calif, 1990, Wadsworth.

73. Messick S: Validity. In Linn RL, editor: *Educational measurement,* 3d ed, New York, 1989, Macmillan.

74. Myers JE, Well AD: *Research design & statistical analysis,* New York, 1991, HarperCollins.

75. Narens L, Luce RD: Measurement: The theory of numerical assignments, *Psychological Bulletin* 99:166-180, 1986.

76. Nunnally JC: *Psychometric theory,* New York, 1978, McGraw-Hill.

77. O'Grady KE, Medoff DR: Rater reliability: A maximum likelihood confirmatory factor-analytic

approach, *Multivariate Behavioral Research* 26:363-387, 1991.

78. Olney SJ, et al.: An ambulation profile for clinical gait evaluation, *Physiotherapy Canada* 31:85-90, 1979.

79. Overall JE: Contradictions can never a paradox make, *Applied Psychological Measurement* 13:426-428, 1989a.

80. Overall JE: Distinguishing between measurements and dependent variables, *Applied Psychological Measurement* 13:432-433, 1989b.

81. Overall JE, Magee KN: Estimating individual rater reliabilities, *Applied Psychological Measurement* 16:77-85, 1992.

82. Paunonen SV, Gardner RC: Biases resulting from the use of aggregated variables in psychology, *Psychological Bulletin* 109:520-523, 1991.

83. Perloff JM, Persons JB: Biases resulting from the use of indexes: An application to attributional style and depression, *Psychological Bulletin* 103:95-104, 1988.

84. Rae G: The equivalence of multiple rater kappa statistics and intraclass correlation coefficients, *Educational and Psychological Measurement* 48:367-374, 1988.

85. Rogosa DR, Brandt D, Zimowski M: A growth curve approach to the measurement of change, *Psychological Bulletin* 92:726-748, 1982.

86. Rogosa DR, Willett JB: Demonstrating the reliability of the difference score in the measurement of change, *Journal of Educational Measurement* 20:335-343, 1983.

87. Rozeboom WW: The reliability of a linear composite of nonequivalent subtests, *Applied Psychological Measurement* 13:277-283, 1989.

88. Scholz JP: Reliability and validity of the WATSMART three-dimensional optoelectric motion analysis system, *Physical Therapy* 69:679-689, 1989.

89. Schouten HJA: Nominal scale agreement among observers, *Psychometrika* 51:453-466, 1986.

90. Shavelson RJ, Webb NM: *Generalizability theory: a primer,* Newbury Park, Calif, 1991, Sage.

91. Shavelson RJ, Webb NM, Rowley GL: Generalizability theory, *American Psychologist* 44:922-932, 1989.

92. Shrout PE, Fleiss JL: Intraclass correlations: Uses in assessing rater reliability, *Psychological Bulletin* 86:420-428, 1979.

93. Shrout PE, Spitzer RL, Fleiss JL: Quantification of agreement in psychiatric diagnosis revisted, *Archives of General Psychiatry* 44:172-177, 1987.

94. Smith PL, Luecht RM: Correlated effects in generalizability studies, *Applied Psychological Measurement* 16:229-235, 1992.

95. Spitznagel EL, Helzer JE: A proposed solution to the base rate problem in the kappa statistic, *Archives of General Psychiatry* 42:725-728, 1985.

96. *Standards for educational and psychological testing,* Washington, D.C., 1985, American Psychological Association.

97. Steiger JH: *EzPATH: A supplementary module for SYSTAT and SYGRAPH,* Evanston, Ill, 1989, SYSTAT, Inc.

98. Stine WW: Interobserver relational agreement, *Psychological Bulletin* 106:341-347, 1989a.

99. Stine WW: Meaningful inference: The role of measurement in statistics, *Psychological Bulletin* 105:147-155, 1989b.

100. Strube MJ: Assessing subjects' construal of the laboratory situation. In Schneiderman N, Weiss SM, Kaufmann P, editors: *Handbook of research methods in cardiovascular behavioral medicine,* New York, 1989, Plenum.

101. Strube MJ: Psychometric principles: From physiological data to psychological constructs. In Cacioppo JT, Tassinary LG, editors: *Principles of psychophysiology: physical, social, and inferential elements,* New York, 1990, Cambridge University Press.

102. Suen HK, Ary D, Ary D: A note on the relationship among eight indices of interobserver agreement, *Behavioral Assessment* 8:301-303, 1986.

103. Tanner MA, Young MA: Modeling agreement among raters, *Journal of the American Statistical Association* 80:175-180, 1985a.

104. Tanner MA, Young MA: Modeling ordinal scale disagreement, *Psychological Bulletin* 98:408-415, 1985b.

105. Uebersax JS: A generalized kappa coefficient, *Educational and Psychological Measurement* 42:181-183, 1982.

106. Uebersax JS: Diversity of decision-making models and the measurement of interrater agreement, *Psychological Bulletin* 101:140-146, 1987.

107. Uebersax JS: Validity inferences from interobserver agreement, *Psychological Bulletin* 104:405-416, 1988.

108. Umesh UN, Peterson RA, Sauber MH: Interjudge agreement and the maximum value of kappa, *Educational and Psychological Measurement* 49:835-850, 1989.

109. Williams RH, Zimmerman DW: Statistical power analysis and reliability of measurement, *Journal of General Psychology* 116:359-369, 1989.

110. Winer BJ: *Statistical Principles in experimental design,* New York, 1971, McGraw-Hill.

111. Wolfson L, et al: Gait assessment in the elderly: A gait abnormality rating scale and its relation to falls, *Journal.*

112. Woltring HJ: Data acquisition and processing systems in functional movement analysis, *Minerva Ortopedica e Traumatologica* 38:703-716, 1987.

113. Yarnold PR: The reliability of a profile, *Educational and Psychological Measurement* 44:49-59, 1984.

114. Zacks S: *Introduction to reliability analysis: probability models and statistical methods,* New York, 1992, Springer-Verlag.

115. Zimmerman DW, Williams RH: Note on the reliability of experimental measures and the power of significance tests, *Psychological Bulletin* 100:123-124, 1986.

116. Zwick R: Another look at interrater agreement, *Psychological Bulletin* 103:374-378, 1988.

CHAPTER 11

OBSERVATIONAL GAIT ANALYSIS

Francine Malouin

KEY TERMS

Ambulation profiles

Criterion-related validity

Gait deviation

Inter-rater reliability

Intra-rater reliability

Observational gait analysis systems

Single limb support

Weight acceptance

Observational gait analysis (OGA) describes the qualitative approach of gait analysis used by clinicians. This approach identifies gait deviations in patients from visual observations.[20,23,31] In OGA both the identification and the grading of gait deviations depend on the observer's judgments.[12,31] Although visual assessment of gait is practiced almost on a daily basis by many clinicians, no standardized observational gait analysis system is in universal use.[12,31] While specific and systematic gait evaluation forms and scoring systems have been described,* clinicians in general use a more individualistic approach.[21] Visual gait assessment is appealing for clinicians given the ease, rapidity, simplicity, and low cost of its use in comparison to instrumental gait analysis systems. On the other hand, the subjective nature of what has been referred to by Little[13] as "eyeball assessment" raises many questions concerning the validity and reliability of the measurement derived from this method, and until the reliability of visual assessment is demonstrated, OGA will remain a subjective clinical assessment tool. This chapter will first give an overview of clinical gait evaluation systems that have been developed and review research reports dealing with the reliability and validity of OGA. The indications and limitations of clinical gait assessment systems for clinical practice will be discussed and further research directions will be suggested.

DESCRIPTION OF CLINICAL GAIT EVALUATION SYSTEMS

Clinical gait evaluation systems can be divided into two categories: those known as **ambulation profiles** including, in addition to time-distance parameters, information about walking skills, and others referred to as **OGA systems** that incorporate the evaluation of kinematics—joint-angles and time-distance variables.[23,31]

Ambulation Profiles

Ambulation profiles have been defined either as methods for assessing a patient's ability to ambulate,[24,34] as clinical tests of locomotor skill,[18] or as quantitative methods of assessing ambulatory function.[19,34] In fact, the main reason for developing ambulation profiles is the need to document more objectively the ambulatory status of patients. Ambulation profiles were designed for use in specific patient groups such as children with cere-

bral palsy,[24] persons with severely or mildly disabling neurological conditions,[18] persons with amputation,[19] or for more general use.[34] Items to be evaluated and the scoring methods also vary. Some profiles provide a global score summing the subject's performance for a series of tests, each graded on an ordinal scale,[24,34] whereas others use variables such as time and distance that provide a measure of the subject's performance on an interval scale.[18,19]

Reimers has designed an ambulation profile for children with cerebral palsy, which gives a global score that sums up the performance of the child during sitting, standing, walking, and stair-climbing activities.[24] Points are allotted for the degree of independence achieved for each of the four items assessed. The scoring system is based on demerit points, which are related to the amount of support needed. The more support the child uses, the higher the score (maximum = 100). For instance, a score of 30 is given to a child who cannot walk, while a score of 2 is given if the child walks with a cane. Walking skills are also graded according to the amount of help required to walk, the distance traveled, and the presence of deviations during gait. The maximum value for each item is as follows: sitting, standing, and walking are allotted a maximum of 30 points each; the maximum value for stairs is 10 points. The weighting of the items was determined from experience during a trial period during which the point values were changed to meet the practical needs. When Reimers described this system, it had been in use for assessing the results of surgical treatments in cerebral palsied children for about one year.[24] No data on the validity or reliability of this ambulatory profile are reported.

Another ambulatory evaluation system described by Wolf gives a functional score corresponding to the time needed to walk over different surfaces, taking into consideration the amount of assistance required.[34] The evaluation form consists of a list of eight ambulation situations, which describe the amount of assistance needed by the patient to ambulate. These ambulation situations are ranked from least assistive (no assistance = 1) to most assistive (short leg brace and hemi walker = 8). The patient is required to walk over five different surfaces (floor, asphalt, carpet, obstacles, and stairs) for specified distances. These surfaces are rank-ordered from the easiest (floor = 0.1) to the most difficult (stairs = 0.5). The time required for the patient to complete each activity is recorded with the ambulatory situation (no assistance, or short leg brace, etc.). Then, the time is

---

* See endnotes 1, 2, 5, 14, 20, 24, 30.

multiplied by the appropriate decimal for each of the five tasks. These numbers are added, and the sum is multiplied by the number associated with the ambulatory situation. The total gives a functional score. If a gait deviation is also present it can be taken into consideration by adding a given percentage to the functional score to produce the total score. The lower the total score, the less time required by the patient to complete one or more walking tasks. This evaluation seems particularly interesting to document quantitatively the progress of a patient while providing information on changes in the use of assistive walking devices. It also provides counselors in vocational rehabilitation with relevant information pertaining to job training and work environment.[34] Neither the validity or reliability of this scoring system has been reported.

The reliability of the ambulation profiles developed by Nelson and Olney and colleagues has been studied.[18,19] Nelson's Functional Ambulation Profile (FAP) assesses skills from standing balance to independent ambulation; it can be completed within 10 to 15 minutes and provides a record of time to complete the tasks.[18] It requires only a stopwatch and parallel bars and consists of three phases. In the first or static phase, three tests are arranged in serial order: from bilateral stance, to stance on the non-disabled, to stance on the disabled limb (maximum = 60 seconds). The second phase, or dynamic weight transfer phase, involves rapid shifting of weight from one limb to the other. The third phase, also known as basic ambulation efficiency phase, involves walking through the parallel bars (6m), walking with an assistive device, and walking independently (when possible) over 6m. The intrarater and interrater reliability of the FAP measurements was studied in 31 subjects with neurological deficits. Intrarater reliability was studied by having one rater testing the patients at a 1 hour interval on day 1 (within-day reliability, n = 31) and 2 weeks later (between-day reliability, n = 26). The interrater reliability was determined by having a second rater testing the patients (n = 22). The level of reliability was determined using Pearson correlation coefficients. All correlation coefficients (r) were found to be larger than 0.89, with the highest coefficients for the within day reliability (r = 0.91 to 0.99.) Limb stance (static and dynamic) measurements gave generally larger correlation coefficients. Thus, Nelson's FAP is highly reproducible over time even when the tests are administered by different raters.

Olney and colleagues developed an ambulation profile (14 items) for persons with amputation, that gives information about: (1) fundamental walking skills (7 items); (2) characteristics of free cadence walking (3 items); (3) effort of walking (3 items); and (4) walking endurance (1 item).[19] The fundamental skills consist of the six items assessed in the Nelson's FAP plus an additional item: stair ascent. Speed, cadence, and stride length are measured at free cadence walking. Walking effort is estimated by measuring the pulse rate at rest and after completing the gait evaluation; it is also converted to a percentage of maximum heart rate expected for age. Walking endurance is determined by calculating the distance covered until the patient feels "uncomfortable" or until a maximum of 15 minutes has elapsed. The interrater reliability for this ambulation profile was studied by having two therapists testing concurrently 26 nondisabled subjects. Pearson correlation coefficients were all above 0.90 (range: 0.90 to 0.99) except for one item: speeded ambulation with a walking aid (r = 0.79). A complete test requires 20 to 30 minutes depending upon the duration of the endurance item. Repeated application of this ambulation profile in 59 persons with amputation has proven most valuable to assess progress either by comparing the results of a patient with previous trials or with a known standard.[19]

The reliability of these ambulation profiles exemplify how locomotor skills can be objectively evaluated; they also demonstrate that well-standardized procedures can give reproducible measurements. Among the ambulation profiles described, those developed by Nelson and Olney seem more appropriate for assessment of change on a long-term basis for two main reasons. First, the use of a ratio scale rather than an ordinal scale of measurement suggests that these two ambulatory profiles would be more sensitive to detect progress all along the recovery process. Such an assumption is based on previous reports indicating that locomotor items from functional scales such as the Barthel Index and the Fugl-Meyer sensorimotor tests are less sensitive in detecting improvement for performance approaching a maximum value in comparison to continuous variables such as gait velocity.[25,26] Secondly, because variables such as time, speed, or pulse rate are used as outcome measures, each variable can be analyzed individually and comparisons made with a known standard. A further interesting aspect of Olney's ambulation profile is that factors contributing to improved performance can be singled out. For instance, it is possible to determine if the increased gait speed is associated with a concomitant increase of cadence and/or stride length; Olney's ambulation profile can also help in determining which walking aid can lead to an increase in walking speed without increasing the effort, based on the pulse rate.[19] On the other hand, the ambulation profiles developed by Reimers and Wolf give functional scores that may be considered screening tools to rate the level of performance and the level of functional independence accordingly.[24,34]

Observational Gait Analysis (OGA) Systems

The first OGA system that will be presented was developed by the Professional Staff Association from the Physical Therapy Department and the Pathokinesiology Service at Rancho Los Amigos Medical Center in California. This is perhaps the most comprehensive OGA system known worldwide and for this reason, it will be described in detail. The Rancho Los Amigos OGA system is described in the *Observational Gait Analysis Handbook* that is regularly reedited.[20] This system has been refined during the last 20 years by scores of professionals under the close supervision of Jacquelin Perry. Because the users of OGA systems must develop mental images of normal gait patterns and joint positions, the Handbook first provides information on normal human gait. The information on normal gait consists of the description for the ankle, knee, hip joints, and pelvis of the following variables: range-of-motion (sagittal plane only), muscle actions, torque demands, and functional significance. These variables are described in the text and illustrated for each segment and for each of the eight subphases of the gait cycle (initial contact: IC; loading response: LR; mid stance: MS; terminal stance: TS; pre swing: PS; initial swing: ISw; mid swing: MSw; terminal swing: TSw). Finally, a figure summing the range of motion at each segment (from the toes up to the trunk) during each subphase of the gait cycle provides a reminder of the normal sagittal gait pattern image. Observational gait analysis involves the learning of a new skill that requires much practice and patience before mastering it. Because an organized awareness of normal function must be developed, much emphasis is put on the observational portion of this skill. From this model, pathology is recognized as a deviation from normal function.[23]

After this comprehensive description of normal kinematics, the Handbook presents a pathological gait analysis guide. This guide consists of a series of graphs and accompanying text that illustrate the principal gait deviations, indicate when they can be detected—during one of three basic locomotor tasks: at weight acceptance (WA), single limb support (SLS), and swing limb advancement (SLA)—and their most likely causes and significance. The observer is invited to complete the Gait Analysis: Full Body Form (Figure 11-1), which presents a checklist of gait deviations. On this form, rows represent the gait deviations and the columns the gait phases. To make the evaluation easier the form gives only phases where major (blank boxes) or minor (gray boxes) deviations are expected. The phases where gait deviations are not applicable are represented by black boxes. The process of observational analysis as described by Perry is best performed in two stages.[23] First, a gross review is proposed to sense the flow of action, followed by the analysis in an anatomical sequence starting at the foot and progressing upward. This sequencing helps sort out the multiple events happening at different joints. At each segment the patient's performance is compared to normal and deviations noted. Perry suggested that the evaluator place more emphasis on learning to observe the ankle, knee, and hip since most significant motions occur at these joints.[23] It is recommended that the observer move horizontally across the gait analysis form within each anatomical area. The findings are interpreted as total limb function by summing the gait deviations that occur in each gait phase. The Rancho Los Amigos OGA system follows a problem-solving approach that is also useful for therapy planning.[31] Although in use for many years, however, the reliability and validity of the Rancho Los Amigos OGA system has not been reported. It should be quite interesting to study the reliability of measurements made by raters familiar with this OGA system.

Other gait deviation analysis systems have been developed specifically for the assessment of gait abnormalities common to individuals with rheumatoid arthritis,[5] hemiplegia,[1] or lower limb amputation,[14] or for more general use, such as the Ljubljana Rehabilitation Centre clinical gait analysis described by Stanic.[31] Others have been adapted from existing evaluation forms,[10,30] developed to assess gait deviations in children with cerebral palsy,[4] or evolved from forms used in the Children's Hospital Gait Laboratory in Boston to study the effects of an orthosis on the gait of children with myelomeningocele.[2] Among these, the gait analysis system developed for persons with rheumatoid arthritis (RA) is particularly interesting as it lists gait deviations of individuals with RA according to five main foot deformities.[5] Moreover, in the latter evaluation form, the physical examination findings and treatment goals that

Figure 11-1 Full Body Observational Gait Analysis Form (Rancho Los Amigos System). The rows represent gait deviations and the columns the eight gait subphases. Walking dysfunctions are tabulated by checking the pertinent boxes. The white boxes represent major dysfunctions, the gray boxes, minor dysfunctions, and the black boxes indicate not applicable dysfunctions. (Pathokinesiology Department, reprinted with the permission of the editor, LAREI.)

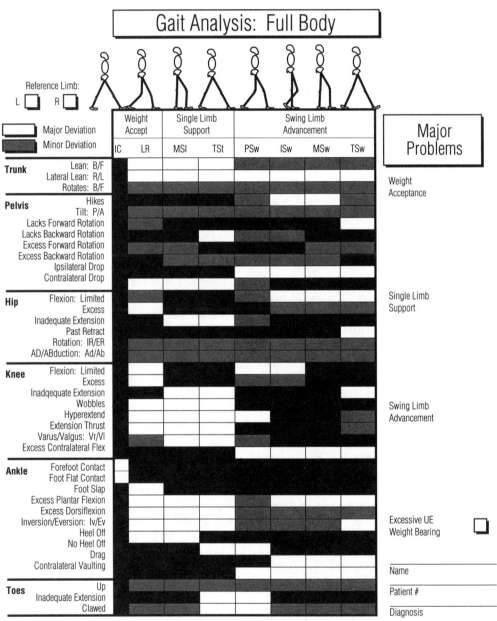

© 1991 LAREI, Rancho Los Amigos Medical Center, Downey, CA 90242

accompany each gait deviation make this system most helpful for the management of gait problems and treatment planning.[11] These clinical gait analysis forms either simply require the observer to check for the presence a gait deviation[1,2,22] or to grade it on a three- or four-point scoring scale.[4,9,10,12,17] In the following section, the OGA systems that were used in reliability and validation studies will be reviewed. As will be shown, in most of these studies,[9,12,17,22,30] only a selected number of gait variables were analyzed.

Studies on the Reliability and Validity of OGA Systems

Fewer than ten studies have looked into the reliability and validity of OGA systems (Table 11-1). Although different methodological approaches have been used in each of these studies, the results are unanimous in pointing out only a moderate level of reliability for intra- and interrater assessments. Because of the many pitfalls associated with these studies, it is perhaps too soon to discard visual analysis of gait as a potentially reliable clinical evaluation tool. For instance, the variables studied, the raters' training, the scoring methods, as well as the data collection and statistical analysis raise many questions. In the following section, attempts will be made to show how the reproduc-

ibility of OGA measurements could be improved. For this purpose the reliability studies as well as the design and results from three validity studies will be reviewed in detail.

Selection of Variables

The few studies that examined the reliability of OGA systems differ markedly in the type and the number of variables chosen as well as the justifications for their selection. For instance, Goodkin and Diller simply adapted a work sheet from the New York Medical School Orthotic Gait Analysis for assessing the gait of 10 patients with hemiplegia.[10] It included a list of 17 gait deviations; among these were three trunk deviations (such as lateral, posterior, and anterior trunk bending), two knee deviations (excessive knee bending, hyperextended knee), five hip deviations (hip abduction adduction, rotation, hiking, and circumduction), and others (insufficient push off, excessive lateral or medial foot contact, toe drag, uneven step length, vaulting, arm swing, and head control). In contrast, Eastlack studied the interrater reliability of videotaped OGA in three subjects with RA and concentrated on five knee deviations (knee flexion at initial contact, at mid-stance, at heel off and at toe off, and genu valgum) and five spatiotemporal variables (stride and step length, stance time, cadence, and step width).[9] The choice of gait

TABLE 11-1   Characteristics of studies on visual gait assessment

Study	Pathology	Raters	Rating Scale	Data Collection	Statistical Analysis	Type of Study[i]
Goodkin and Diller (1973)	Hemiplegia $n = 10$	PT $n = 3$	Ordinal 3 points	Live	Percentage agreement	R
de Bruin et al. (1982)	Cerebral Palsy (children) $n = 18$	Orth. Res.[c] $n = 6$	Ordinal 3 points	Video	None	R
Miyazaki and Kubota (1984)	Hemiplegia $n = 48$	Mixed $n = 5$	Ordinal 4 points	Live	Pearson[e]	R V
Saleh and Murdoch (1985)	Amputation $n = 5$	Mixed $n = 4$	Nominal	Live	Percentage agreement	V
Krebs et al. (1985)	Bilateral KAFO[a] (children) $n = 15$	PT $n = 3$	Ordinal 3 points	Video	Percentage agreement SEM ICCs[f]	R V
Patla and Clouse (1988)	Heterogeneous $n = 8$	Kin. Stud.[d] $n = 5$	Nominal	Video	Occurrence/ nonoccurrence[g]	R
Eastlack et al. (1991)	RA[b] $n = 3$	PT $n = 54$	Ordinal 3 points	Video	Kappa[h] ICCs	R

[a]KAFO: knee ankle foot orthosis; [b]rheumatoid arthritis; [c]orthopaedic residents; [d]kinesiology students; [e]Pearson correlation coefficients; [f]ICCs: intraclass correlation coefficients; [g]Occurrence/nonoccurrence reliability coefficients; [h]Kappa coefficients; [i]R: reliability, V: validation.

variables is also dependent on the type of subjects studied. For instance, Saleh and Murdoch looked specifically at the knee and the ankle-foot during subphases of the stance and swing phase, in addition to step length and step time on the prosthetic leg of persons with an amputation.[30] In contrast, de Bruin and colleagues examined only a few variables such as lumbar lordosis, Trendelenburg gait, knee motion, foot contact, and alternate limb motion during locomotion of children with cerebral palsy.[4]

In only two studies were the gait deviations examined from the foot up to the hip and across subphases of the gait cycle, either during the stance phase only[12] or for the whole stride.[22] Reasons given for limiting the examination of gait deviations to the stance phase included the importance of the stance phase for locomotion and the poor reliability when raters were required to analyze both swing and stance gait deviations.[12,22] Lastly, Miyazaki and Kubota[17] examined a unique combination of variables: fluctuation, symmetry, supportability, variation, shock, push off, cane dependence, and foot contact.[17] These eight variables were chosen for the purpose of comparison with eight waveform indices measured simultaneously with a device detecting vertical forces exerted by the forefoot and the heel. Most frequently scored variables were deviations from the foot to the hip taking place in more than one plane,[10,12,22] as well as trunk deviations.[4,12,17,22] In some studies one or more spatiotemporal variables were also rated: the step length and symmetry being the most frequently examined.[9,17,22] Finally, estimation of push off[10,17,22] has been rated, as well as the use of external support[22] and cane dependence.[17]

As reported above, the selection of gait variables in each of these studies was often based on methodological concerns or the type of patients studied. Consequently, the selection of variables is one of the many aspects that needs to be addressed for the standardization of an OGA system of universal use. For instance, which variables are the most representative of gait capacity and which outcome measures are most relevant to assess effects of therapy on gait disorder are important issues since variables forming the basis of gait assessment must have clinical significance, whether observational or instrumental techniques are used.[3,32,33] The relevance of gait variables for assessment purposes may be dependent on factors in the population studied such as age, pathology, stage of the pathology, and the resulting level of disability. For instance, the nature of gait devia-

tions expected in lower-limb amputees is different from that of adults with hemiplegia or spastic children. The ease with which the gait deviations can be detected depends on the degree of impairment and resulting level of disability. Gait deviations may be more obvious and easier to detect and to grade in a spastic child with a scissors-like gait pattern than in a patient with medial arthroscopic meniscectomy.[8] Moreover, the number of expected abnormal gait variables in each of the subphases, at each of the segments (foot to head), and for all three planes of movement may vary accordingly. In other words, the use of specific evaluation forms—as inspired by the Rancho Los Amigos check form, which includes the gait deviations to be expected at each of the subphases of the gait cycle—should help focus the evaluator on relevant variables.

Study Designs and Populations Studied

Three validity studies compare the results from the OGA assessment to measurements obtained with instrumental gait analysis techniques. For instance, Patla and Clouse compare deviations recognized by OGA assessments to results of measures of angular displacements (sagittal plane) made with protractors on video records advanced frame by frame.[22] Two randomly selected strides were analyzed and joint angles obtained with the protractors were judged to represent normal values if the angle fell within ±2SD of normal reference values. The use of protractors on video records is an interesting way to quantify visual assessments, especially when gait deviation is slight but does not appear the best criterion for validity purposes.[28] In fact, a measurement error is likely associated with this type of measurement (protractors) as with goniometry.[15] Moreover, the measurement of joint angles was made on only two strides while raters based their visual assessment on more strides (five or more).

The second study that attempted to compare the ability of raters to detect gait deviations in individuals with amputations to results from instrumental gait assessment was conducted by Saleh and Murdoch.[30] Their paradigm consisted of inducing predicted gait deviations (from a biomechanical analysis) by changing the prosthesis alignment in five persons with below-knee amputation. In the latter case the raters' judgments were compared to the predicted deviations from the biomechanical analysis and also to those resulting from an instrumental gait analysis system (stick-figures). The main problem with this study is that no criteria were set to define gait deviations such as done by Patla and Clouse.[22] Therefore, failure to detect a given deviation may not necessarily reflect the observer's inability to identify a real abnormality. The level of detection expected from the observers should be set carefully in a concurrent validity study to determine not only if raters are as good as a sophisticated instrument to detect gait abnormalities, but also to estimate the level of detection that can be reliably attained in visual assessment.

The third validation study contrasts with the others since visual rating served as the criterion to validate the clinical use of an objective measuring device.[17] In fact, the authors studied the relationships between visual ratings (mean of four raters) and quantitative indices obtained from a device measuring the vertical ground-reaction force in view of validating the use of their device for clinical gait evaluation. One of the problems with these concurrent validity designs is that the investigators are more inclined to demonstrate the higher accuracy of instrumental gait analysis techniques—which nobody would question—rather than of measuring a reliable level of detection of visual assessment. Thus, no clear demonstration of criterion-related validity of OGA systems has been made.

The level of agreement between raters (interrater reliability) has been examined in most studies, but only two studies[4,12] reported results on the intrarater reliability of OGA systems and three studies addressed validity issues.[17,22,30] In the intrarater reliability studies, raters repeated the rating of the same videotaped gait records at a 1 week[4] or a 1 month interval.[12] The time interval between sessions is an important factor. In fact, it needs to be long enough so that the raters forget the scores they attributed at the first session. A week's interval is probably enough if the raters have many subjects to analyze in the same session. Another way of reducing the carryover and memory bias is to randomize the order in which each of the subjects is assessed.[12]

The sample size is another important concern in reliability studies. There was a wide range (n = 3 to 48) in the sample size across studies (Table 11-1). The sample generally consisted of an homogeneous group of patients such as persons with hemiplegia,[10,17] children with cerebral palsy,[4] children with lower-limb disability requiring bilateral knee-ankle-foot orthoses (KAFOs)[12] and individuals with RA.[9] Only one study included an heterogeneous group of disabled subjects presenting a pathology such as: amputation, cerebral palsy, hip or knee arthroplasty etc.[22] In most studies, the number of raters ranged from three to six, except in one case where 54 raters were recruited.[9] In the latter case, 54 raters assessed the gait of three persons with RA; this design had some drawbacks, however, because of the large number of raters and the small sample of patients.

Assessment Procedures

It is well known that in any reliability study, standardization of the assessment procedures is most critical.[28] Such standardization requires that decision-making criteria are the same among raters or for raters in a test and retest situation. For the evaluation of gait deviations, such a standardization is very demanding because it requires raters to have an internal tridimensional representation of the normal movements from head to feet over the whole gait cycle for comparison purposes. Such an ability develops with time and training.[23] With continued practice and application this observational method becomes an art.[27] Therefore, the training of the raters prior to the onset of the study should be uniform, and background experience should also be considered. The second aspect is the scoring method, which is crucial. The observer may be required to either simply identify the presence of a deviation (nominal measurement) or to grade the magnitude of the deviation (ordinal measure). Lastly, the duration of the observation and the methods used to help focus the gait evaluation of the patients, either in real life or on a videotape, will influence the raters' decisions and should also be standardized.

Rater Training. If we examine the different OGA reliability studies, no consistent training procedures were followed, and the background among raters also differed within each study. The raters were most often health professionals such as physical therapists, physicians, orthopedic residents, physical therapy students, prosthesists, and physiatrists. They all had a clinical background with the exception of one study, where the raters were kinesiology students who, however, had some knowledge of biomechanics and had followed courses on movement assessment.[22] In the majority of the studies, no mention of any rater training was made.[4,10,17,30] The only reference to the raters' background is sometimes an adjective such as "experienced observers"[30] or "senior therapists"[10] or none at all.[17] In the more recent studies, however, some attention has been given to rater preparation. Interestingly, the most elaborate training consisted of a two-hour training session that was provided to kinesiology students.[22] During this training session, the raters were shown videotapes of normal gait patterns, the gait phases were highlighted, normal range (±2SD) of joint movement were identified, and each gait variable was defined. Once they felt comfortable with normal gait, raters were shown a videotape of a patient. The raters were guided by the experimenter in identifying the abnormalities, and they were able to view the tape as many times as they needed during training. In another study, three physical therapists, with more than 5 years experience in gait assessment, were trained in the use of a new OGA form.[12] For this, prior to the study, they viewed the videotapes of three children who were not included in the study but who walked with orthoses as did the children in the study. Training continued until all three raters agreed on the assessments of the gaits displayed during the training session. Lastly, in the study including 54 raters, all were physical therapists with or without previous experience in gait assessment; in the latter case, training consisted simply of informing the observers on how to use the evaluation form without any review of normal gait kinematics.[9] In summary, in all of the studies the OGA evaluation form was unfamiliar to the observers and training consisted mainly of an information on how to use the evaluation form and on the definition of terms.

Scoring Methods.   In two of the studies,[22,30] the raters were asked to identify the gait deviations using a nominal scale, whereas, in all others, they had to grade the gait deviations using a three-point ordinal scale[4,9,10,12] or a four-point scale.[17] The wording was also quite varied; the raters had to score each gait variable as acceptable, needs to be minimized, needs to be maximized,[10] or as inadequate, normal, excessive,[9] or as normal, just noticeably abnormal or very noticeably abnormal.[12] In fact, grading the gait deviation is very demanding and perhaps, before moving to an ordinal scale, it would be wise to demonstrate the reliability of a binary scale as was suggested by Patla and Clouse.[22]

Data Collection and Data Analysis.   Incomplete information was generally available about data collection for the live gait evaluation sessions.[10,17,30] The recording of gait on videotapes was, however, more standardized.[9,12,22] The distance covered, the number of strides, the number of laps and views (lateral and/or frontal), and even the distance between the video camera and the patients were standardized.[9,22] Such standardiza-

tion in the evaluation procedures is a prerequisite if one wants to use a standardized method of analysis. When gait was videotaped, the visual rating was made while the raters viewed the videotape either individually,[22] in small groups,[9] or all together.[12] When the gait was not recorded on videotape, the raters observed the patients independently for an equivalent period of time.[10] In other studies where gait was assessed live, it is not mentioned how the rating sessions were conducted.[17,30] While it is clear that each patient should be assessed by all raters simultaneously for studying interrater reliability, it is not always easily amenable even in a live situation, especially if more than two raters are involved. The use of a video recording certainly decreases the chance for rating disagreement to be related to time or to the patient's performance rather than to the raters' judgments.

Generally, gait videotapes were analyzed individually and raters were free to review the tapes up to five times[12,22] or only twice.[9] The raters were sometimes required to view the tapes of a patient's gait at normal speed to simulate real time visual assessment.[12,22] In a more recent study, slow motion and stop action techniques were used.[9] In the latter case, the speed of the tapes was controlled by the investigator since viewing took place at different facilities where some of the 54 raters met in small groups. Whether the patient is evaluated in a live situation or on videotape, it is important that the parameters used in the analysis be standardized from rater to rater. The information provided to raters prior to the analysis is also very important. For instance, how many strides are representative of a patient's gait pattern? How many times will the rater be allowed to review gait videotapes? Will they do it individually? Will they use real time or slow motion? Will they use markers on the ground[6,7,27] and count the number of frames for measuring gait spatiotemporal variables.[6,7] These are the many aspects that have to be decided and the evaluation protocol standardized accordingly. Instructions to raters must be very clear as well as the methodology, particularly when gait deviations vary from stride to stride as in pathological gait.

Statistical Analysis.   Interestingly, different statistical approaches (Table 11-1) were used among the OGA reliability studies. The choice of statistical tests goes from simple percentage of agreement to kappa coefficients and Intraclass Correlation Coefficients (ICCs). Multiple statistical tests have also been applied on the same data;

this is the case of the study carried out by Krebs, who computed in addition to the percentage of agreement, the SEM, Pearson correlation coefficients and ICCs.[12] Kappa coefficients and two models of ICCs were also compared.[9] Lastly, Patla and Clouse[22] have presented a new method of analysis they identified as occurrence/nonoccurrence interrater reliability coefficient.[22] This method avoids the inflation of reliability scores that takes place when raters agree on a large number of variables that are normal even though they may disagree on variables that are abnormal.[29] The method is similar to the traditional point-to-point reliability but instead of using all the data, the analysis concentrates on either the occurrence or nonoccurrence of abnormality in a measure. Then, the occurrence/nonoccurrence interrater reliability is compared to that of the chance occurrence reliability. The number of combinations of raters showing above-chance reliability is then computed and compared to a maximum possible score. The latter approach and the kappa coefficients are appropriate statistical approaches for nominal and ordinal measures (see chapter 10).

Reliability and Criterion-Related Validity of OGA Systems

Interrater Reliability. If we consider all the reliability studies, visual assessment of gait is at best moderately reliable. Whatever the population studied, the raters involved, the scoring system selected, or the statistical tests applied, no approach seems to yield better results. Observations from one of the first reports dealing with reliability of OGA system indicated percentages of agreement ranging from 60% to 93% (mean: 82.3%, SD: 9.5%) between three physical therapists who evaluated 17 gait deviations in 10 persons with hemiplegia.[10] In a more recent study,[12] in which three physical therapists evaluated the gait of 15 children walking with bilateral KAFO, the level of agreement was not higher despite the fact that raters used videotaped gait sequences rather than the live situations as Goodkin and Diller did.[10] In fact, full agreement was obtained in 67.5% of cases, whereas, disagreement by one point was found in 30% of the observations. The respective ICCs for the total of 18 gait variables (six gait deviations over three subphases of stance) ranged from 0.40 to 0.94 for a mean of 0.73. These ICC values are above the mean ($r = 0.48$) Pearson correlation coefficients (range: $r = 0.43$ to 0.60) reported by Miyazaki and Kubota for the visual assessment of 48 individuals with hemiplegia.[17] In the latter study, however, the following factors

likely contributed to the low reliability level. Raters had received no specific training; they evaluated the subjects live using a four-point scale and were confused about the definition and the interpretation of some of the gait variables. Despite some methodological weaknesses of the latter study, it is worth mentioning that the investigators converted the visual grade, a discrete variable, to a continuous variable prior to the computation of the Pearson correlation coefficients.

In a carefully planned study in which much attention was given to the standardization of the gait videotaping and analysis procedures, the results indicated only a slight to moderate reliability of OGA assessment.[9] More precisely, the level of reliability calculated using kappa coefficients showed a mean value of 0.27 (range: kappa = 0.11 to 0.52) resulting in the lowest reliability levels ever reported. Many factors could explain this low level of reliability. First, kappa coefficients seem to give lower reliability coefficients than ICCs. For instance, when ICCs and kappa coefficients were computed for the same data, higher ICCs values (mean: 0.34) were obtained as compared to kappa coefficients (mean: 0.27) value, suggesting that ICCs overestimate the reliability level and conversely, that the kappa coefficients yield a lower reliability level.[9] Secondly, the lack of training of the 54 raters in normal kinematics in addition to the bias resulting from the nonrandomization of the videotaped gait sequences from the three individuals with RA likely influenced the raters' agreement.

In the only study with a heterogeneous sample (persons with different diseases or disorders), the results also indicate OGA assessments to have a moderate reliability level.[22] Using occurrence/nonoccurrence reliability coefficients, they showed an agreement of 4 to 5 on a maximum possible score of 10. Although raters used a nominal scoring system and received 2 hours of training (including normal kinematics), the raters, who were kinesiology students without previous clinical experience, had never assessed pathological gait. This lack of clinical expertise and also the fact that the raters had to assess patients each with a different disease or condition likely contributed to the low level of raters' agreement. Finally, the results from de Bruin's study are difficult to interpret since the only information provided is that a considerable interrater variation was found.[4]

Among the multiple gait variables studied, some were more reliable than others. This is the case for variables in the stance versus the swing phase.[12,22] On a maximum of 10, variables in the swing phase get as little as 1.7 to 2.2 as compared to 4 to 5 in the stance phase. Gait variables in the sagittal plane also led to higher reliability levels than those in the frontal plane.[9,10,12] A variable such as timing, which involves the integration of time and distance information, has been evaluated very inconsistently (2.2 out of 10) as compared to joint angular displacement (4 to 5 out of 10).[22] On the other hand, the spatiotemporal variables could be assessed by quantitative methods simply by having the subject walk on a walkway with horizontal markers. With a proper video recording system, the evaluator can measure time-distance variables (stance duration, step length, cadence, etc.) by combining frame-by-frame analysis (time) and ground markers (distance).[6,7] This method described as VGT (videographic gait test) has proved highly reliable within (ICC = 0.98 to 0.99) and between raters (ICC = 0.97 to 0.99) for the evaluation of 30 children with cerebral palsy. Comparison of the measurements obtained in 11 nondisabled adults with the VGT to values measured with an instrumental[25,26] technique yielded Pearson correlation coefficients ranging from 0.99 to 0.99 for spatiotemporal variables indicating a high concurrent validity[7] of the VGT.

Intrarater Reliability.   Only one study dealing with intrarater reliability included a statistical analysis.[12] The mean percentage of total within rater agreement (intrarater reliability) reported was slightly higher than that computed for interrater (69% versus 67.5%). The average Pearson correlation coefficient for between rater reliability was 0.60. The main difference between intra- and interrater reliability was a lower level of agreement for gait variables in the horizontal and frontal planes between raters. In the only other study dealing with intrarater agreement, intrarater variations up to 30% were reported.[4]

Criterion-Related Validity.   Results from the validity studies can be perceived as encouraging. In fact, comparison of OGA assessments to angular displacement made by protractors on video records indicated that the capacity of detecting a gait deviation can be quite high (4.2 out of a maximum of 5) for variables such as foot placement.[22] For hip and knee angles, the capacity of detection was lower (1 to 2 out of a maximum of 5). Possible reason for this latter finding is that raters were biased by the patient pathology. For instance, in a patient with hip arthroplasty, the high reliability score contrasted with the low va-

lidity score; raters biased by the patient's pathology judged the variables to be abnormal but quantitative measurements proved them wrong.

If we consider the capacity of a rater to detect gait abnormalities in comparison to predicted deviations from biomechanical analysis or instrumental gait evaluation methods, the pick-up rate can be as low as 22.2%.[30] But if we eliminate the variables associated with time and distance, this detection capacity increases up to 66.4%. Perhaps, the most positive aspect is that when the visual raters detect a gait deviation, in 92.5% of the cases they are right as to the presence of a deviation, suggesting that above a certain threshold the visual assessment can be quite reliable. The question is perhaps more of determining the sensitivity threshold of visual observation since this method has few false positives. Lastly, Pearson correlation coefficients computed between visual scores and waveform indices obtained from a device measuring vertical ground reaction force also indicated that time-distance variables were less accurately scored.[17] The mean Pearson correlation coefficient value was slightly higher ($r = 0.52$ versus 0.42) for variables that did not include a temporal factor.

Summary and Conclusions

Two categories of clinical gait evaluation systems have been described: ambulation profiles and OGA methods. The ambulation profiles assess skills from standing balance to independent ambulation using either a functional score or quantitative methods for measuring time and distance parameters. The OGA methods consist mainly of the evaluation of gait deviations from the visual assessment of joint angles and time-distance variables. While the time and distance variables have been shown to be highly reproducible when measurements were made with objective means (ambulation profiles), they became very inconsistent when raters used visual observation. These findings strongly suggest that raters should use a more quantitative approach for the assessment of spatiotemporal variables.

Among the OGA systems for clinical use, the Rancho Los Amigos system was described in more detail because it is a most comprehensive system. Before using the Rancho OGA form (Figure 11-1), however, it is critical that clinicians read the Handbook explaining how to use the form as well as the principles underlying the Rancho OGA system. Using the Rancho OGA form without the information would be a mistake. Most importantly, clinicians must be aware that there is a discrepancy between their self-assessment of gait analysis capabilities and their real ability. For instance, although data showed only fair reliability among the judgments of 52 raters, only seven did not feel comfortable with their ability to visually assess gait. In a questionnaire study, the majority (18 of 22) of therapists were confident (score > 5 out of 7 points) in the results of their OGA assessments.

The results from the reliability studies clearly indicate that to be recognized as an objective method of evaluation, the reliability level of OGA assessments must be improved. Among the many factors with the potential of improving the reproducibility of visual assessments are the standardization of rater training, a better knowledge of normality, well-developed operational definitions, and a simple scoring system. The standardization of data collection and analysis should also improve the reliability of the observational process. The results from the validity studies are not, however, as clear cut. Validity studies designed to determine reasonable threshold of visual detection of gait deviations are needed in order to be able to develop more appropriate OGA systems and scoring methods. In fact, the human observer can be quite reliable if the task is reasonable.[16] Thus, it should be possible to develop OGA systems with high reliability levels so that the observational gait assessments can be recognized as an objective clinical gait evaluation tool.

REFERENCES

1. Brunnstrom S: Recording gait patterns of adult hemiplegic patients. *Phys Ther* 44: 11-18, 1964.
2. Carroll NC, Jones D, Maschuich W et al: Evaluation pertinent to the gait of children with myelomeningocele. *Prosthet Orthot Int* 6:27-34, 1982.
3. Craik RL, Oatis CA: Gait assessment in the clinic: Issues and approaches. In Rothstein JM, editor: *Measurement in physical therapy.* New York, 1985, Churchill Livingstone Inc.
4. de Bruin H, Russell DJ, Latter JE et al: Angle-angle diagrams in monitoring and quantification of gait patterns for children with cerebral palsy. *Am J Phys Med* 61: 176-192, 1982.
5. Dimonte P, Light H: Pathomechanics, gait deviations and treatment of the rheumatoid foot. *Phys Ther* 62:1148-1156, 1982.
6. Drouin L, Malouin F, Richards CL, et al: Correlations of the gross motor function measure to gait spatiotemporal measurements in disabled children. *Dev Med Child Neurol,* (submitted).
7. Drouin L, Malouin F, Richards CL, et al: Validity and reliability of a new clinical videographic gait test (VGT). *Posture and Gait,* (submitted).
8. Durand A, Richards CL, Malouin F et al: Motor recovery after arthroscopic partial meniscectomy. *J Bone Joint Surg* 75A: 202-214, 1993.

9. Eastlack ME, Arvidson J, Snyder-Mackler L et al: Interrater reliability of videotaped observational gait analysis assessments. *Physical Therapy,* 71:465-472, 1991.
10. Goodkin R, Diller L: Reliability among physical therapists in diagnosis and treatment of gait deviations in hemiplegics. *Perceptual and Motor Skills,* 37:727-734, 1973.
11. Guccione AA: Rheumatoid arthritis. In O'Sullivan SB, Schmitz TJ, editors: *Rehabilitation: assessment and treatment.* Philadelphia, 1988, FA Davis Co.
12. Krebs DE, Edelstein JE, Fishman S: Reliability of observational kinematic gait analysis. *Phys Ther* 65:1027-1033, 1985.
13. Little H: Gait analysis for physiotherapy departments. *Physiotherapy,* 87:334-337, 1981.
14. Lower-Limb Orthotics: New York University Postgraduate Medical School, Prosthetics and Orthotics, New York, 1981.
15. Miller PJ: Assessment of joint motion. In Rothstein JM, editor: *Measurement in physical therapy.* New York, 1985, Churchill Livingstone Inc.
16. Mitchell SK: Interobserver agreement, reliability, and generalizability of data collected in observational studies. *Psychol Bull* 86: 376-385, 1979.
17. Miyazaki S, Kubota T: Quantification of gait abnormalities on the basis of continuous foot-force measurement: correlation between quantitative indices and visual rating. *Med Biol Eng Comput* 22:70-76, 1984.
18. Nelson AJ: Functional ambulation profile, *Phys Ther* 54:1059-1065, 1974.
19. Olney SJ, Elkin ND, Lowe PJ et al: An ambulation profile for clinical gait evaluation. *Physiotherapy Canada,* 31:85-90, 1979.
20. Pathokinesiology Department, Physical Therapy Department: *Observational gait analysis handbook.* Downey, Calif, 1989, Professional staff association of Rancho Los Amigos Medical Center.
21. Patla AE, Proctor J, Morson B: Observations on aspects of visual gait assessment: a questionnaire study. *Physiotherapy Canada,* 39:311-316, 1987.
22. Patla AE, Clouse SD: Visual assessment of human gait: Reliability and validity. *Rehabil Res,* 1:87-96, 1988.
23. Perry J: *Gait analysis: normal and pathological function.* New York, 1992, McGraw Hill.
24. Reimers J: A scoring system for the evaluation of ambulation in cerebral palsy patients. *Dev Med Child Neurol* 14: 332-335, 1972.
25. Richards CL, Malouin F, Dumas F et al: The relationship of gait speed to clinical measures of function and muscle activations during recovery post-stroke. *Proceed 2nd North American Congress on Biomechanics* 299-302, 1992.
26. Richards CL, Malouin F, Wood-Dauphinee S et al: Task-specific physical therapy for optimization of gait recovery in acute stroke patients. *Archives of Physical Medicine and Rehabilitation* 74:612-620, 1993.
27. Robinson JL, Smidt GL: Quantitative gait evaluation in the clinic. *Phys Ther* 61:351-353, 1981.
28. Rothstein JM: Measurement and clinical practice. In Rothstein JM, editor: *Measurement in physical therapy.* New York, 1985, Churchill Livingstone Inc.

29. Roy E, Todd S, Square P et al: Interrater consistency in judging errors in categories. Presented at the North American Conference, International Neuropsychology Society, San Diego, 1985.

30. Saleh M, Murdoch G: In defense of gait analysis. *J Bone Joint Surg* 67B:237-241, 1985.

31. Stanic U, Bajd T, Valencic V et al: Standardization of kinematic gait measurements and automatic pathological gait patterns diagnosis. *Scand J Rehabil Med* 9:95-105, 1977.

32. Winter DA: Concerning the scientific basis for the diagnosis of pathological gait and for rehabilitation protocols. *Physiotherapy Canada,* 37:245-251, 1985.

33. Winter DA: *The Biomechanics and motor control of human gait.* Waterloo, Ont., 1987, University of Waterloo Press.

34. Wolf, SL: A method for quantifying ambulatories activities. *Phys Ther* 59:767-768, 1979.

CHAPTER 12

FOOT FALL MEASUREMENT TECHNOLOGY

James P. Walsh

KEY TERMS

Inferred parameters

Reliability

Resolution

Spatial foot contact patterns
Base of support
Step length
Stride length

Temporal foot contact patterns
Double support time
Single support time

Validity

The task of foot fall technology is to measure one or more of the foot fall parameters described in Chapter 13. The parameters to be measured fall into three categories: spatial parameters, temporal parameters, and combined spatial/temporal parameters. The spatial parameters are stride length, step length, and base of support. The temporal parameters are swing time, stance time, single support time, double support time, and gait cycle time. The combined parameters are average walking velocity and cadence. Similarly, the various methods of measuring gait parameters can be grouped into categories based upon the gait parameter categories. Some researchers have developed methods that focus on the temporal parameters. Others focus on the spatial parameters. Some methods measure both. Most methods determine average walking velocity.

ISSUES INFLUENCING DATA COLLECTION SYSTEMS

The selection of a method for a particular study cannot be based solely on whether the method measures the quantity of interest. Specific experimental aspects of each method can significantly affect the appropriateness of a method for a particular study. The most important of these aspects will be discussed here before going into a detailed discussion of each method.

Resolution

Resolution refers to the precision of the measurement. It is the smallest amount of time or distance by which two measurements may differ. If the measurement technique measures space or time in fixed units, the resolution is limited by the size of the fixed units. The resolution needed for a particular study depends on the magnitude of the effect being tested. For example, if an orthotic device is expected to reduce the left/right asymmetry in stance time by 100 msec or more, the resolution of the stance time measurement must be much smaller than 100 msec. (See chapter 10 for additional discussion of resolution and related topics as they affect the reliability of experimental measurements.)

Inferred versus Measured Parameters

An inferred parameter is not directly measured. Rather, it is derived from direct measurements of other variables. Inferred parameters inherit the combined errors of the actual measurements and sometimes suffer from assumptions that are not strictly true. Averaged gait parameters are by their very nature inferred. For example, average step length might be calculated by dividing the total distance traversed by the number of steps taken. If there is a significant asymmetry between right and left steps, the average step length is not likely to be a good representation of either a right or left step length.

Encumbrance

Theoretically, all measurements affect, to some extent, the quantity being measured. In many cases, these effects are small. However, some methods may modify gait so much as to endanger the applicability of the results. Methods requiring the subject to carry a significant weight, or drag a cable, or walk with a minimum base width, for example, might significantly affect the gait parameters being measured.

Equipment Limitations

A method may use a certain equipment that limits its applicability in some way. For example, a method may depend on bulky equipment that prevents the method from being portable. Or, a method might require special footwear that works well with normal young adults, but cannot be used with children or the elderly. Or, a method might prohibit the use of walking aids, such as canes and walkers.

Degree of Automation

Gait studies require data collection, storage, analysis, and presentation of results. Frequently studies require large numbers of subjects with multiple trials with each subject. The amount of data accumulated in such a study can be enormous. Methods that automate some or all of these steps greatly reduce the time and cost of a study and can affect whether a study is feasible at all.

Compatibility with Other Methods

Measurement of footfall parameters is frequently one aspect of a larger study. Some methods, however, may not be compatible with simultaneous data collection by other measurement techniques, such as (EMG), goniometry, or video recording. For example, a measurement method that depends on the subject breaking a light beam to start data collection, might not work with bright lights required for a slow motion video recording.

Various methods for measuring footfall parameters will be described in the following section. The methods will be grouped together based on the kinds of parameters measured: methods that obtain only inferred parameters; methods that measure either spatial or temporal parameters, but not both; and finally, methods that measure both types of parameters. In each description, the techniques involved in that method are described, and then secondary aspects that will affect whether the method would be appropriate for a particular study are discussed. The list of methods included here is not intended to be exhaustive. Rather, it illustrates the range of approaches that have been presented in the literature.

METHODS OBTAINING ONLY INFERRED PARAMETERS

The simplest method of gait analysis is to ask a subject to walk a measured distance (d) and measure the elapsed time (t_d) with a stop watch. From these simple measurements, one can determine the average velocity (v) as

$$v = \frac{d}{t_d}. \tag{1}$$

If during this walk, we count the number of complete steps (n), and measure the time from the beginning of the first step to the beginning of the last step (t_n), then the cadence (c) is given by

$$c = \frac{n}{t_n}. \tag{2}$$

The average step length (l) may be estimated from

$$l = \frac{d}{n}. \tag{3}$$

Since a complete gait cycle consists of two complete steps, the average gait cycle time (t_{gc}) may be estimated by

$$t_{gc} = \frac{2t_n}{n}. \tag{4}$$

The advantage of this method is its simplicity; it requires little in terms of equipment or experimental technique. It does not encumber the subject at all. It is entirely portable and has general applicability to all subjects. It is not an automated method, but it doesn't need automation since there is so little data involved. Because of these factors, it is especially appropriate for studies of large subject populations.

Clearly this method has many shortcomings. It yields neither spatial nor temporal information about individual step characteristics. It tells us nothing about the degree of symmetry between the right and left sides during the gait cycle. Therefore, the estimate of step length calculated in

Equation 3 might be very different than the average step length on either the right or left side. Furthermore, this estimate of step length and that of gait cycle time (Equation 4) are inaccurate to the extent that the distance d ends with a partial step or partial gait cycle.

METHODS MEASURING ONLY SPATIAL PARAMETERS

In order to obtain more detailed spatial information about individual steps, various methods have been developed to record the position of the individual foot-floor contacts during gait. There are two basic strategies: (1) have the foot physically mark the walkway during floor contact, and (2) cover the walkway with electrical switches, whose positions are known, and that generate an electrical signal in response to foot contact.

Walkway Marking Methods

A commonly used clinical method to obtain spatial data involves recording an imprint of some part of the subject's foot. Such measurement techniques have included inked moleskin on the bottom of the shoe and paper,[1,12] chalked shoes and a black rubber mat, oiled shoes and absorbent paper,[4,14] and walking over thin metal foil that retains the impressions of the feet.[1,3,4,12,14]

In these methods, detailed spatial measurements are made for each step using a ruler or tape measure. This method correctly yields stride length, step length, and base of support. Averages of the gait parameters may also be correctly calculated. Note, however, that the accuracy of the measurements is dependent on accurately imaging the foot on the paper. When the print is made without using moleskin, the technique may not yield well-formed and consistent images of the feet. The moleskin allows for a more precise image, but introduces new sources of measurement uncertainty. The position of the moleskin strips relative to the boundaries of the foot must be included in the measurements. There is a potential increase in the variability in spatial measurements due to trial variability in positioning the moleskin strips on the feet.

Simple time measurements can increase the useful information obtained from this method. A stopwatch can be used to determine the elapsed time for a sequence of complete gait cycles. Using this time, a count of the number of steps, and spatial measurements, the average velocity can be calculated from Equation 1, cadence from Equation 2, average right and left step lengths from

Equation 3, and average gait cycle time from Equation 4, where **d** now is the total distance covered by the sequence of complete gait cycles.

The walkway marking methods are simple and inexpensive to implement. However, these methods may be considered ones that encumber gait. Paper is an unusual surface for walking and might modify a subject's normal gait. Data processing is time consuming due to the detailed manual measurements that must be made on the paper. Storage of the raw data (large sheets of marked paper) can be a problem if the study includes a large number of subjects and/or trials. The method is applicable to all subject populations, although the use of a marker on the bottom of the foot may be unpleasant for some subjects.

Walkways Incorporating Electrical Switches

Walkways incorporating electrical switches have been described by several investigators. These walkways frequently provide both spatial and temporal gait parameter measurements. However, some systems measure only spatial parameters. Representative of these latter systems is one described by Durie and Farley.[5] The measurement setup is illustrated schematically in Figure 12-1. In this system, the walkway consists of several large printed circuit boards laid end to end. Each board consists of a series of long copper strips arranged parallel to each other and perpendicular to the path of progression down the walkway. The strips have small spaces between them to provide electrical isolation from each other. Every other strip is connected together and grounded. The remaining alternate strips are spaced 2 cm from each other and are individually wired into a control box.

Thin (1/8 mm thick) strips of brass shim stock are taped to the bottom of the shoes of the subject to be tested. When the subject's foot makes walkway contact, the strips on the soles of the shoes create an electrical bridge between one of the ungrounded walkway strips and an adjacent grounded strip. Since each of the ungrounded strips is individually wired into the control box, a detection circuit in the box can automatically identify which of the ungrounded strips has been contacted.

The control box is designed to calculate step length automatically. It does this by first temporarily storing the number of the strip that has been contacted. Then, when the next foot contact occurs, the control box identifies the number of the new strip contacted, subtracts the stored number of the previous strip contact, and displays the result on a digital display. It then stores the number of

FIGURE 12-1 A walkway used for measuring spatial gait parameters. The walkway is constructed of a series of identical printed circuit boards. Each board contains a series of interdigitated metal fingers. A metal strip on a subject's shoe provides a bridge between two fingers, allowing a current to flow in the measurement circuit.

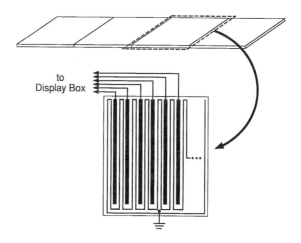

the most recent strip contacted. This process repeats until the subject walks off the walkway.

This method directly measures step length. Stride length can be inferred by adding consecutive step lengths. It gives no information about base of support. If a stopwatch is used to record the elapsed time for a sequence of complete gait cycles, the average walking velocity and average gait cycle time can be calculated. The spatial resolution of this system is limited by the width of the electrical strips and the fact that the identifiable strips alternate with the grounded strips. The resulting resolution is 2 cm.

This method has several advantages. It is inexpensive to implement, doesn't encumber the subject, automates the measurement of step length, is applicable to practically all subjects, and is portable. With some additional circuitry in the control box, this method could easily be extended to gather timing information as well.

The major disadvantages of this method are that it provides no information about the temporal parameters or base of support, and does not distinguish between left and right foot contacts. In addition, it lacks the ability to process the data automatically after the step length has been calculated and displayed. It requires the investigator to manually record successive step lengths as they appear on the digital display, since they are not stored. Further data processing is done outside of the system.

METHODS MEASURING
ONLY TEMPORAL PARAMETERS

Several methods that directly measure only temporal gait parameters have also been reported. These methods are divided into two major groups: (1) those using on electrically conducting walkway with electrical conductors attached to the bottom of the foot/shoe, and (2) those using pressure-sensitive switches attached to the bottom of the foot/shoe.

Using an Electrically Conducting Walkway

These methods are based on the electrical switch formed by the electrically conducting surface of the walkway and an electrically conducting material placed on the bottom of the foot or shoe. When the foot/shoe is in contact with the walkway surface, the switch is closed, and an electrical current can begin to flow in an external circuit. Onset of current flow indicates the beginning of a stance phase, while the termination of current flow indicates the end of a stance phase. This basic approach has been implemented in different ways to obtain different timing information. Two examples will be described below.

The method of Rosenrot et al. is illustrated in Figure 12-2.[13] The walkway is completely covered with a conducting material, which is connected to a low-voltage DC source. Each shoe has a conducting strip attached to its sole. Wires run separately from each conducting strip to a junction box attached to the subject's waist. A cable connects the junction box to a strip chart recorder in the laboratory. The voltage from each shoe strip is plotted using a separate pen on the chart recorder. Figure 12-3 illustrates the kind of plots that would appear on the chart recorder for a normal subject. The traces clearly indicate stance and swing phases for each foot. The investigator can read swing time, stance time, single support time, double support time, and gait cycle time directly from the chart.

This method alone, however, provides no information about the spatial gait parameters. Rosenrot et al. supplemented the method with light beams and photocells at each end of a measured portion of the walkway for the purpose of determining average walking velocity.

The temporal resolution of this method is very good. It is limited by the recording device, i.e. the frequency response of the pen mechanisms and the speed of chart movement. This limitation could be overcome by feeding the signals to a digital computer for more accurate measurements. The

FIGURE 12-2 A walkway system used to measure temporal gait parameters. A low voltage source maintains a constant voltage on the surface of a walkway covered with a conducting material. Metal strips attached to a subject's shoes are connected to a strip chart recorder. As the subject walks, the chart recorder shows the time course of foot-floor contact during successive gait cycles.

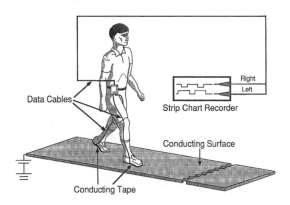

method is fairly inexpensive to implement and maintain and is applicable to all subject populations.

The major disadvantage of this method is the use of a tether cable to convey the foot/floor contact signals to the chart recorder. Dragging a tether cable during walking could modify the subject's normal gait.

The method of Cheung et al. is illustrated in Figure 12-4.[2] The walkway is covered with two wide, longitudinal conducting strips. A small space between the strips prevents electrical current from flowing between the strips. On one side of the walkway, the conducting surface is connected to a 5v DC source. The other side of the walkway surface is connected to a Schmitt trigger circuit. With no input to the Schmitt trigger, the output of the Schmitt trigger is 5v. With an input of 5v to the Schmitt trigger, its output drops to 0v. The output of the Schmitt trigger is led to the input of an analog-to-digital converter installed in a microcomputer. A strip chart recorder may also be placed in parallel with the input to the microcomputer.

Conducting tape strips are applied to the soles of the subject's shoes. A thin wire runs from the subject's waist to the conducting strips on each shoe, connecting them electrically. When both feet are in contact with the walkway, one on each side, a circuit is completed through the foot switches so that 5v is applied to the Schmitt trigger, whose output to the computer then drops to 0v. When either foot breaks contact with the walkway surface, the Schmitt trigger output returns to 5v.

FIGURE 12-3 Sample recording expected from the apparatus shown in Figure 12-2 during normal gait.

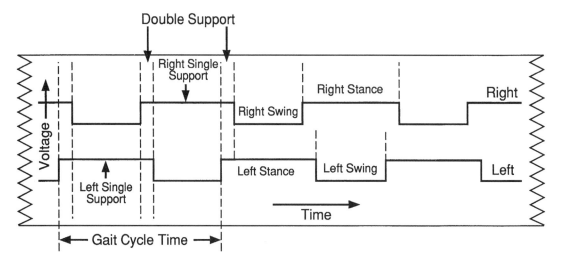

FIGURE 12-4 A walkway system used to measure temporal gait parameters. Right and left sides of the conducting surface are electrically isolated from each other. A wire provides a conducting path between metal strips on the subject's shoes. During stance phase, the metal strips and connecting wire close the circuit allowing current to flow to external measurement instruments. At other times of the gait cycle, no external current flows.

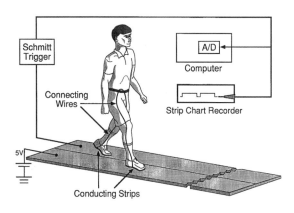

Typical output voltage plots generated during normal walking are illustrated in Figure 12-5. The output voltage is 0v during the double support phases, and 5v at all other times in the gait cycle. All of the temporal gait parameters can be dissected out of this output voltage plot, although automatic processing requires that the investigator tell the computer which foot first made contact with the walkway.

This method can also use light beams and photocells over a measured distance to determine average walking velocity.

This method has several advantages. Its simplicity makes it inexpensive to set up and maintain. No tether runs from the subject to the recording instrumentation that would interfere with the subject's normal gait. The temporal resolution, a function of the sampling rate of the microcomputer, is very good. The authors estimate a resolution of 4 msec. The method is applicable to all subject populations. The use of the computer allows for automatic storage and processing of data, and presentation of results.

Besides the fact that this method yields no information about the spatial gait parameters, its main disadvantage is that it requires the subject to walk with one foot on each side of the walkway. Such a requirement has the potential to interfere with a subject's normal gait and may make measurements of unusual gait involving foot crossovers impossible. In addition, the use of tape applied to the soles of the foot or shoe and wires running along the legs also have the potential for modifying normal gait. This method does not measure activity of each foot independently of the other. The investigator must infer which foot is producing the signal based on knowledge of which foot started the sequence. This aspect has potential for confusion during unusual gait patterns.

Using Pressure-Sensitive Switches Attached to Subject's Foot

An example of a method using pressure-sensitive switches attached to the foot is the commercially

FIGURE 12-5   Sample recording expected from the apparatus show in Fig 12-4 during normal gait.

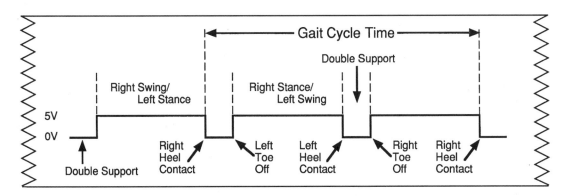

available *Stride Analyzer.** This instrument was used in studies recently reported from the Rancho Los Amigos Hospital in Downey, California.[9,15] It uses special insoles that are inserted in shoes or taped to the bottom of the feet. The insoles contain four pressure sensitive switches that are placed under the heel, at the heads of the first and fifth metatarsal bones, and at the great toe. Wires connect the foot switches to a control box attached to the subject's waist. A light sensor on the control box detects when the subject passes through light beams aimed perpendicular to the line of progression at each end of the walkway. This sensor is used to start and stop data collection automatically. The control box detects openings and closures of the foot switches and records the times of these events. This information is then transmitted to a laboratory microcomputer using either a cable or an FM transmitter. The computer analyzes the data and presents the results both as a graphic display of switch activity and as a numerical table of calculated results. Sample output from the most recent version of the *Stride Analyzer* is illustrated in Figures 12–6 and 12–7.

The graphic display shows both closed and opened periods for all switches on both feet for every gait cycle. The user can quickly identify the various phases of each gait cycle.

The tabular display shows calculated averages of all of the standard temporal gait parameters along with average walking velocity and cadence. Times are presented both in seconds and as a percent of the measured gait cycle.

The *Stride Analyzer* takes advantage of the increased capabilities possible with modern micro-computers. Besides doing detailed analysis and display, the computer allows the user to store the data in a computer file so that the data may be included in a local database or read into other analysis programs. The system also has a built-in database of normals based on data collected from "hundreds of subjects over many years at Rancho Los Amigos Hospital" (B&L private communication). The tabulated results report velocity, cadence, stride length, and gait cycle time as percent of normal using this internal database.

Methods like the *Stride Analyzer* that use foot switches applied to the sole of the shoe or foot have several advantages. By measuring timing information from both feet independently, there is no need to infer which foot is producing the observed signal based on the operator's observation of which foot started the gait sequence. Furthermore, since the switches are placed on several different parts of the sole, the user is able to identify individual events within the stance phase, for example foot flat and heel off. Foot switch sensors also make this method very portable since there is no heavy walkway to be carried around. The use of an FM transmitter to transfer the data from the subject to the computer, while not an essential and exclusive element of the foot switch technology, minimizes encumbrance of the subject's gait.

The use of foot switches embedded in insoles, as they are with the *Stride Analyzer,* has disadvantages as well. A complete set of insoles must be acquired to fit all the subjects of the study. In addition, the insoles may not work correctly if the subject needs an orthotic device within his or her shoe. Furthermore, the presence of the insoles and associated cabling running to the waist-mounted control box has some slight possibility of modifying the normal gait of the subject.

---

* B&L Engineering, P.O. Box 3905, 12309 E. Florence Ave., Sante Fe Springs, CA 90670.

Figure 12-6   Sample graphical output from the *Stride Analyzer* system.

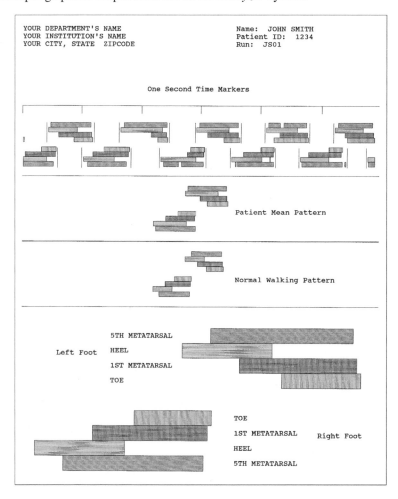

Methods Measuring Both Spatial and Temporal Parameters

Two kinds of methods for measuring both spatial and temporal parameters have been described. One kind uses electrical switches made of electrical elements in the walkway coming into contact with electrical strips on the subject's feet. The other kind uses pressure sensitive stitches embedded in the walkway. In both cases, computers are employed to automate the measurement and data reduction processes.

Using Electrical Switch Elements Attached to Subject's Shoes

Gabell and Nayak report a method superficially similar to the one used by Durie and Farley described above.[7,11] In Gabell and Nayak's version of the method, a walkway surface is constructed using several identical mats containing electrical circuits. One such circuit is illustrated in Figure 12-8. The circuit consists of a constant 4.5v DC source connected in series with a reference resistor and two resistor strings, one string on each side of the mat. From each resistor string, thin brass rods extend parallel to each other from a point between each pair of resistors across to the other side of the mat without touching the rods extending from the opposite side. The set of parallel rods from each side of the mat interdigitate with the rods from the opposite side so that each rod from one side is located between two rods from the other side. Since none of the rods touch each other, the electrical circuit is not closed and no current flows in the reference resistor.

The subject to be tested has thin metal strips attached to the bottom of the heel and sole of each shoe. When the subject steps on a mat, a metal strip provides an electrical bridge between adjacent brass rods from opposite sides of the mat.

FIGURE 12-7   Sample tabulated output from the *Stride Analyzer* system.

```
                        YOUR DEPARTMENT'S NAME
                        YOUR INSTITUTION'S NAME
                    STRIDE ANALYZER REPORT -- WALKING


NAME:          JOHN SMITH              RUN:               JS01
I.D. NUMBER:   1234                    STRIDES:           4
DATE:          05/13/93                DISTANCE (M):      6.00
AGE:           29                      TEST CONDITIONS:
SEX:           M                       WALK
DIAGNOSIS:     Sprained Right Ankle


STRIDE CHARACTERISTICS
                        ACTUAL    %NORMAL
VELOCITY (M/MIN):        60.3      74.0
CADENCE (STEP/MIN):     100.4      92.7
STRIDE LENGTH (M):      1.201      79.8
GAIT CYCLE (SEC):        1.20     106.8


                         -R-       -L-
SINGLE LIMB SUPPORT
    (SEC):               0.429     0.418
    (%NORMAL):           86.4      84.2
    (%GC):               35.9      35.0

SWING (%GC):             33.5      34.5
STANCE (%GC):            66.5      65.5

DOUBLE SUPPORT
    INITIAL (%GC):       15.2      15.4
    TERMINAL (%GC):      15.4      15.2
    TOTAL (%GC):         30.6      30.6


LEFT FOOT (stance = 65.5% GC)
    HEEL            -- Normal contact at 0.0% GC (0.0% Stance)
                       Delayed cessation at 50.6% GC (77.2% Stance)
    5TH METATARSAL -- Premature contact at 3.8% GC (5.7% Stance)
                       Delayed cessation at 63.3% GC (96.6% Stance)
    1ST METATARSAL -- Normal contact at 22.4% GC (34.2% Stance)
                       Delayed cessation at 63.9% GC (97.5% Stance)
    TOE            -- Normal contact at 33.7% GC (51.4% Stance)
                       Delayed cessation at 65.5% GC (100.0% Stance)

RIGHT FOOT (stance = 66.5% GC)
    HEEL            -- Normal contact at 0.0% GC (0.0% Stance)
                       Delayed cessation at 50.8% GC (76.4% Stance)
    5TH METATARSAL -- Premature contact at 4.0% GC (6.0% Stance)
                       Delayed cessation at 64.8% GC (97.5% Stance)
    1ST METATARSAL -- Normal contact at 19.6% GC (29.4% Stance)
                       Delayed cessation at 63.8% GC (96.0% Stance)
    TOE            -- Normal contact at 38.1% GC (57.3% Stance)
                       Delayed cessation at 65.2% GC (98.1% Stance)
```

Figure 12-8 Detection circuit used by the walkway of Nayak et al. to measure spatial and temporal gait parameters. Metal strips on soles of subject's shoes form an electrical bridge between brass rods embedded in the walkway. Current through the test resistor, R_f depends on the location in the walkway of the bridge.

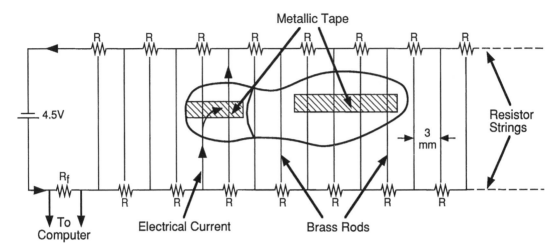

When the bridge forms, the electrical circuit is closed, and current flows through the reference resistor. The amount of current that flows depends on the number of resistors in the circuit. The number of resistors in the circuit depends on the position on the walkway where the contact is made. Therefore the voltage across the reference resistor is an indicator of the position on the mat where the foot contact occurred.

Walkways are constructed using several of these mats placed next to each other. The voltage across the reference resistor from each mat is led to a separate channel of an analog-to-digital converter in an attached computer. The computer samples the reference voltage from each mat at regular intervals. It can tell if a foot has made contact with the mat and, if so, where on the mat the contact was made. In this way, the computer can obtain both spatial and temporal information about the gait cycle.

Nayak et al. and Gabell and Nayak report studies using two walkways based on such mats.[7,11] One walkway was constructed by arranging pairs of mats into two columns about 6 m long. The brass rods in each mat were oriented perpendicular to the line of progression. This walkway was used to measure step length and stride length. The use of separate left and right columns of mats allowed separate left and right measurements. A second walkway of comparable size was constructed with the mats oriented so that the brass rods lay parallel to the line of progression. This walkway was used to measure stride width, although the authors do not indicate which stride width definition was used. (See chapter 13 for a discussion of the various stride width definitions that have been reported in the literature.) Both walkways were used to measure step time, stride time (gait cycle time), and double support time. In these walkways, the rods were spaced 3 mm from each other. The output voltage from each mat was sampled at 50 msec intervals.

This method has several major advantages. A single measurement run yields both spatial and temporal gait parameters. Furthermore, by placing almost all of the measurement apparatus in the walkway, this method leaves the subject relatively unencumbered. Left and right parameters are obtained independently. Excellent spatial and temporal resolution is possible. The use of faster computers now available could easily increase the sampling rate by a factor of 10. By using computer automation of the data collection and analysis, this method can be applied to large population and a local data base can be constructed.

There are several disadvantages of this walkway method. Using metal strip contact to infer foot contact contains the potential for misinterpretation by the computer program. Care must be taken to insure that the length measurement is consistently using signals from the same spot on the foot for every foot contact. Separate left and right measurement systems tend to encumber gait because the subject's normal gait may be modified by trying to avoid crossing over the midline of the walkway. Separate walkways for determining step length and stride width mean that these measurements cannot be obtained simultaneously. Therefore, interactions between these parameters cannot be investigated reliably. Implementation of this method is relatively expensive and requires a considerable amount of electronic and computer expertise.

Using Pressure-Sensitive Switches Embedded in the Walkway

The methods in this group all use a large number of pressure-sensitive switches arranged in transverse rows along the length of a walkway. Each switch is as close as possible to its immediate neighbors. Thus, the entire walkway is covered by the switches. The status of every switch, open or closed, is monitored continuously by an online computer. When a subject walks down the walkway, the computer notes the time that each switch closed and when it reopened. With these data the computer calculates both the spatial and temporal gait parameters.

Three variations of this method have been described, based on the number of switches in each transverse row.

One Switch Per Transverse Row. Gabel et al. describe a system in which each transverse row in the walkway contains one very wide switch.[6] The walkway is connected to a dedicated computer with a gait analysis program in read only memory. The computer monitors the mat for one complete gait cycle, i.e. three foot contacts. At the end of the cycle, the operator enters into the computer the identity of the foot that began the gait cycle. The computer then calculates and tabulates the spatial and temporal parameters for that gait cycle. Since the walkway is only one switch wide, the program is unable to detect a foot contact on a switch that is already closed due to contact by the contralateral foot. Therefore, the system requires that successive foot contacts do not spatially overlap each other. This means that each step length must be greater than the contralateral foot size.

This method has several advantages. There is minimal interference with normal gait since no measurement equipment is attached to the subject. It is applicable to the entire subject population except as noted below. It automates the measurement and analysis process and prints the results. Both spatial and temporal resolution are good. Spatial resolution is determined by the width of each switch, and their separation in the mat. The authors report 15 mm between the active contact

FIGURE 12-9 *GAITMAT* recording system for measuring spatial and temporal gait parameters. Walkway has two longitudinal rows of 256 pressure activated switches. A data collection computer continuously monitors the state of all switches, recording closing and opening times of each switch. Data are transferred to a second computer for analysis and display.

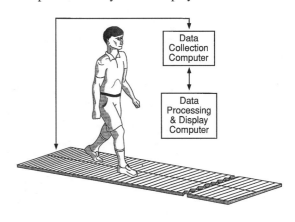

elements of each switch. The temporal resolution is controlled by the interval between each computer scan of each switch. The authors do not report this value.

The main disadvantage of this method is due to having only one switch on each transverse row. As a result, the computer can only distinguish one footprint from the next by having them longitudinally separated. This works well with normal gait, but for subjects with abnormal gait, this requirement may not be satisfied.

Two Switches Per Transverse Row. Taylor describes a system using a walkway containing 512 pressure-sensitive switches arranged in two longitudinal columns of 256 switches with two wide switches in each transverse row.[16] Leiper and Craik describe a more recent version of this system, called *GAITMAT,* having the same switch arrangement, but utilizing more versatile computer support.[10] The setup of this latter system is illustrated in Figure 12-9 and will be described here.

The walkway is 3.8 m long, with an active width of approximately 0.6 m. Each transverse switch is 1.5 cm wide by 30.5 cm long. The mat is connected by a cable to a dedicated microprocessor (Rockwell AIM 65). The microprocessor scans the entire mat at 30 msec intervals. When a switch closes, the microprocessor records the time of closure and the time the switch reopens. Data collection can proceed for up to 80 sec. When data

Figure 12-10 Sample display of the *GAITMAT* gait analysis system. Lower panel shows the pattern of switch closures on the mat. Upper panel shows measured gait parameters for each gait cycle.

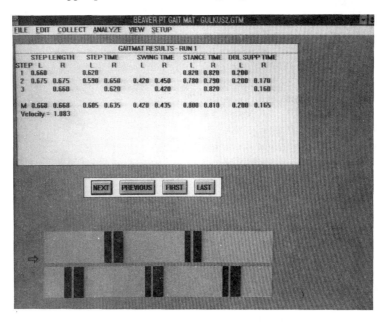

collection is completed, the raw data are downloaded under program control to an IBM compatible computer running the *GAITMAT* analysis and display program.

The *GAITMAT* program display is shown in Figure 12-10. The lower half of the screen depicts the switch array, indicating which switches closed during the current scan. The upper half of the display contains the measured gait parameters for each gait cycle, and the averages of these parameters calculated for the current run.

The program automatically determines the direction of progression, identifies the footprints, and distinguishes between the right and left sides before proceeding with the calculations. The footprint identification algorithm allows for a footprint to have open switches within a footprint, as occurs between the heel and sole of a shoe with a raised heel.

To properly perform a gait analysis, the program requires that right and left feet make contact on opposite sides of the mat. If the subject inadvertently steps on the midline (a partial crossover), or completely crosses over the midline during the gait cycle, the operator can edit the display to indicate which switch closures should actually be located on the other side. The program also allows for the data to be saved into a data file and/or transferred into another program for further data analysis.

The advantages of this system stem from its use of two switches in each transverse row and the incorporation of an inexpensive online personal computer. By using two switches on each transverse row, the system independently measures left and right gait components. It determines all of the usual spatial and temporal gait parameters (except for base of support) in a highly automated fashion. Temporal resolution is 30 msec; spatial resolution is 15 mm. On-line editing of the data allows measurement runs to be used that might otherwise have to be discarded. Facilities for permanent storage of the data and transfer to other programs support development of databases and statistical analyses.

The main disadvantage of this system is that it uses only two switches in each transverse row. Although it is able to distinguish left from right, it is not able to determine the exact lateral location of the feet and therefore not able to calculate base of support. Furthermore, the general requirement for the subject to walk with one foot on each side of the center line might interfere with normal gait.

Multiple Switches Per Transverse Row. Two systems will be described in this category. First, Hirokawa and Matsumara describe a walkway that uses a two-dimensional array of switches based on a lattice of intersecting wires.[8] The lattice consists of a layer of parallel wires running in the longitudinal direction separated by a 3 mm thick foam layer from another layer of parallel wires running in the transverse direction. A small circular hole is cut through the foam layer at the intersection of each longitudinal wire with each transverse wire. The presence of the foam layer around the edges of the hole prevents the wires from touching. When pressure is applied at an intersection the foam compresses, allowing the wires to make contact and provide a current path in an attached electrical detection circuit. The attached electrical circuit is capable of independently scanning the longitudinal and transverse wires to search for closed switches. The output of this electrical circuit is sent to an online microcomputer for analysis. The analysis software reports step length, step width, duration of single and double support phases, foot angle, and velocity.

The operation of the switch lattice in response to applied foot contacts is illustrated in Figure 12-11. The figure shows sample left and right footprints not necessarily collected at the same time. The filled circles represent switches that appear to the detection circuit to be closed when only one foot is in contact with the mat. The open circles represent additional switches that appear to the detection circuit to be closed when both feet are in contact with the mat. The set of switches actually closed by a footstep roughly follows the shape of the footprint, but the external detection circuit is not able to detect this pattern. Rather, it detects a rectangle formed by the group of switches that fall along the extremity of the footprint. This results from an overlap in the current paths of open switches and those of nearby closed switches when the open switches are being tested by the detection circuit. Although the switch at a particular intersection may be open, current can flow from one test wire of the open switch to one or more nearby closed switches until it reaches the other test wire of the open switch, thereby producing a positive detection signal in the external circuit. For example, consider the right footprint in Fig. 12-11. The switch formed by wires X_m and Y_j is open. However, there is a current path from X_m through the closed switch formed with wire Y_k, along wire Y_k to the closed switch formed with wire X_n, along wire X_n to the closed switch formed with wire Y_j, and along wire Y_j to the external circuit. The external circuit is unable to distinguish this circuitous current path from the one going directly through switch (X_m, Y_j). Therefore, the detection circuit erroneously indicates that switch (X_m, Y_j) is closed. For most purposes, this "boundary" rectangle is not a problem because it still can be used to identify step length and step width.

A significant problem does occur, however, during the double support phase of the gait cycle.

FIGURE 12-11 Pattern of detected switch closures in response to foot contact using the instrumented mat of Hirokawa and Matsumara. Filled circles are detected closures with only one foot contacting the mat. Open circles are additional detected closures with both feet contacting the mat. (Modified with permission from Hirokawa and Matsumara.)

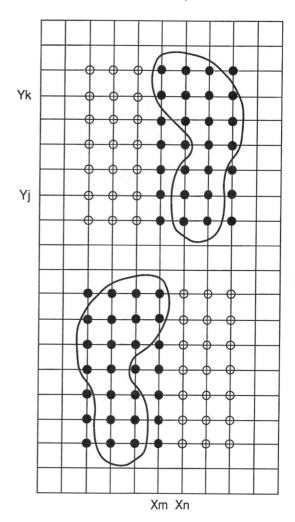

Whenever both feet are in contact with the mat, current flow through nearby closed switches causes the external circuit to detect rectangular patterns whose widths are the combined widths of both footprints. This is indicated by the addition of the open circles in Figure 12-11. An additional complication occurs when the footprints overlap in the longitudinal direction. In that case, the detection circuit identifies a single rectangle whose boundaries are the external boundaries of the two footprints. Hirokawa and Matsumara describe an algorithm based on an idealized footprint shape

FIGURE 12-12 Sample display from the *GAITMAT II* gait analysis system. Lower panel shows the pattern of switch closures on the mat. Upper panel shows measured gait parameters for each gait cycle.

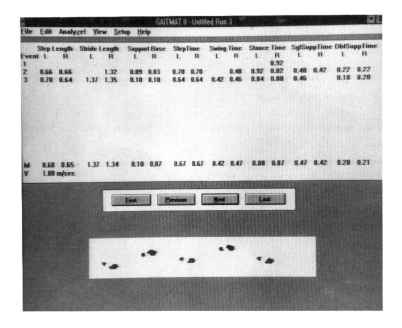

that enables their online computer to distinguish the double support phase from the single support phase and determine the correct single support and double support durations.

This method has all the advantages of the other automated methods that embed the measurement apparatus in the walkway. In addition, the use of multiple switches in the transverse direction removes the encumbrance due to the requirement that the subject walk with one foot on either side of the midline of the walkway.

The primary disadvantage of this method stems from the interaction between open switches and nearby closed switches. This interaction prevents the system from detecting the actual footprint pattern of the subject. In addition, it forces the analysis to rely on a detection algorithm that is based on the shape of an idealized footprint. The authors tested the reliability of this strategy by comparing its spatial parameter measurements with those obtained from one subject walking with painted soles on the walkway covered with paper. They report good agreement. However, much more extensive testing using a large population of subjects with a variety of gait patterns is required to prove the reliability of this algorithm.

Recently, Taylor and Walsh have demonstrated a new version of the *GAITMAT,** the commercially available *GAITMAT II*. This version has several major changes. The surface of the walkway is still covered with pressure sensitive switches, but they are now 15 mm square switches arranged in a matrix of 256 transverse rows with 40 switches in each row. A propriety circuit prevents the appearance of false closures due to interactions between open switches and nearby closed switches. The intermediate, dedicated microprocessor of the original *GAITMAT* has been removed. The GAIT-MAT II walkway is connected directly to an IBM compatible computer. The time required to scan the entire array of switches has been reduced to 10 msec. Temporal resolution is 10 msec, and spatial resolution is 15 mm in both the longitudinal and transverse directions. Total duration of data collection is no longer limited.

Figure 12-12 illustrates the display from *GAIT-MAT II*. The lower half of the display presents a schematic image showing switches that closed during the current run. The upper half of the display tabulates both the resulting measurements for each gait cycle and the averages of these parameters for the entire run. This tabulation now includes the base of support measurement.

Because *GAITMAT II* uses small square switches, the display shows recognizable footprints. The program automatically determines the direction of progression, identifies individual footprints, and distinguishes left and right. It colors the left and right footprints different colors to allow

---

* EQ, Inc, 600 Galahad Road, Plymouth Meeting, PA.

the operator to confirm that the automatic footprint determinations have been performed correctly. The program allows for manual operator intervention to remove spurious switch closures or to correct errors in the automatic detections process.

The automatic footprint detection and identification process works well enough that it is able to correctly distinguish left from right even when some of the left footprints appear to the right of the right footprints. Thus, the subject is free to walk, unencumbered, anywhere on the mat.

The ability to save the data to a file and/or transfer it to other programs for further analysis has been continued from the original *GAITMAT* system.

The use of multiple switches in each horizontal row provides two advantages. First, the system is able to determine base of support directly. Second, the subject is not constrained to walk with one foot on each side of the mat. Thus, there is minimum interference with normal gait. Furthermore, as with other systems of this class, no equipment that might encumber normal gait is attached to the subject. This system is applicable to the general subject population, including those with very abnormal gait patterns.

The major disadvantage of this system is its expense. It would not be appropriate for only a few studies of limited extent. But it could be justified for a clinical or research laboratory doing large numbers of gait analyses on a regular basis.

VALIDITY AND RELIABILITY

In the process of measuring a gait parameter, an observer usually does not measure the gait parameter itself. Rather, he or she measures some object or event with the expectation that the object or event is an indicator of the underlying gait parameter. Such measurements are subject to many sources of error. Two aspects of measurement error, validity and reliability, can influence the methods previously described. The concepts of validity and reliability can be thought to overlap, but for the purposes of this discussion, they will be treated as separate topics. Validity means the aspects of a measurement that depend primarily on the correctness of the assumptions that link the measured object or event to the underlying gait parameter. Validity is not just a yes/no decision but can extend across a range from a high to a low degree of validity. Reliability refers to the aspects of a measurement that depend on the accuracy and precision of the measurement apparatus. For a more general discussion of reliability of experimental measurements see chapter 10.

Spatial Measurements

Three basic strategies for obtaining the spatial gait parameters have been described: walkway marking, walkways covered with transverse electrically conducting strips that form electrical switches with conductive strips on the soles of a subject's feet or shoes, and walkways whose surfaces contain pressure-sensitive switches. The spatial gait parameters of interest are step length, stride length, and base of support.

Walkway Marking.   With the walkway marking methods, the object that is measured is a footprint created as the subject walks across a surface. The validity of the method depends on whether the footprints correctly identify the foot structure of interest. For step length and stride length the marking methods are generally valid. However, since one definition of base of support is the closest transverse distance between right and left feet during a gait cycle, a marking method would not be valid for a base of support measurement unless it could correctly identify the medial edges of each foot. The validity of marking methods is also limited to the extent that walking with something on the sole of the foot encumbers gait.

The location of the footprints on the recording surface can be determined very accurately. This would tend to make such measurements reliable. However, errors will be introduced into the measurement by variability in forming images of the feet on the surface. For methods that apply ink directly to the sole of the foot or shoe, the quality of the image will vary from step to step. Similarly, although moleskin produces more reliable images on paper, variability in positioning the moleskin on the soles of subjects from trial to trial introduces an additional source of error to this method.

Walkways with Conductive Surfaces and Conductive Strips on the Subject's Soles.   The object that is measured is the location of a closed switch formed by a longitudinally oriented strip on the sole of a subject's foot or shoe making contact with a transversely oriented strip on the surface of the walkway. When this method gives no information about the transverse location of the contact it is not valid for base of support measurements. The implementation by Nayak and Gabell includes a second mat whose orientation enables them to measure base of support, but not simultaneously with their step length measurement.[7,11] While the addition of the base of support measure is very important, care must be taken when making inferences about the total gait cycle from two separate measurements. The assumption must be made and tested that the person will walk in the same manner during the separate walking trials.

Measurements of step length (and by derivation stride length) is based on measuring the distance between the same point on the foot on two successive foot contracts. The assumption behind this method, then, is that the observed closures come from the same location on the foot. Efforts must be made to verify this assumption. One possibility is to limit the size of the strips applied to the soles, so that when contract is made, it will be in approximately the same location on the foot. The validity of this method also may be compromised to the extent that the conductive strips attached to the soles of the feet or shoes might modify normal gait.

The reliability of this measurement is a combination of its resolution and inherent variability. The resolution of the measurement is limited by the fixed spacing between successive strips on the walkway. The variability of the measurement includes step-to-step differences in what portion of the strip on the sole forms the switch with the walkway.

Walkways with Pressure-Sensitive Switches.

The distance between closed switches is used to infer spatial gait parameters. Methods in this group that lack a large number of switches in the transverse direction are not valid for base of support measurements. The validity of the step length and stride length inferences depend on using the same location of the foot on successive foot steps. The software that interprets the switch closures and does the calculations must be programmed to use the same portion of the footprint, for example the rearmost closure. This is still not a guarantee of validity since step-to-step variability occurs in which parts of the foot contact the floor. The absence of any measurement apparatus attached to the subject that might encumber normal gait adds to the validity of these techniques.

The reliability of these methods is primarily limited by the spatial resolution of the measurement, which is limited to the spacing of the switches.

Temporal Measurements

Three basic strategies for obtaining the temporal gait parameters have been described: electrically conducting walkways that interact with electrical contacts on the soles of a subject's feet or shoes, walkways with surfaces that contain pressure-sensitive switches, and pressure-sensitive switches attached to the bottom of a subject's feet. The temporal gait parameters of interest are step time and single and double support time.

Walkways with Conductive Surfaces and Conductive Strips on Subject's Feet or Shoes.

The event that is measured is the start and stop of current flow in an external circuit when a switch formed by the conducting surface of the walkway and a conducting strip on the sole of the subject's foot or shoe closes and opens. These are valid indicators of foot contact and foot off and correctly imply the temporal gait parameters. The primary limit of validity for these measurements is the possibility that the metal strips attached to the soles of the feet or shoes and their accompanying wires may encumber normal gait.

The reliability of these measurements is limited by the accuracy and temporal resolution of the instrument used to measure time. In particular, this includes the frequency response of a strip chart recorder or the sampling rate of a computer used to make the time measurements.

Walkways with Pressure-Sensitive Switches.

The event measured is the closing and opening of switches in the walkway beneath a footstep. The validity of the methods depends on the ability of the computer program to correctly identify the switches belonging to each footprint and then use the earliest closure and latest opening to identify foot contact and foot off. This is such a critical item that the program must allow the observer to manually identify these points to the program if it cannot do it correctly. The validity of these methods is enhanced by the absence of attachments to the subject that might encumber normal gait.

The reliability of these measurements is primarily dependent on the resolution of the time measurement instrument. Since this usually is a digital computer, the resolution is the sampling rate of the analog-to-digital converter of the computer.

Pressure-Sensitive Switches Attached to Subject's Feet.

The events measured by these methods are the closings and openings of a small number of switches attached to the bottom of a subject's feet. While one advantage of using such switches is to provide temporal information of events related to specific foot locations, the inference of earliest foot floor contact and latest foot off is not strictly guaranteed. The fact that a switch closes does indicate that the foot is contacting the floor. However, it does not indicate that the closure was the first contact the foot made with the floor, a requirement for both the step time and stance time measurements. Another part of the foot may have made first contact, but no switch was located there. Similarly, the fact that no switch is closed does not indicate that the foot has completed contact with the floor. The validity of this method is also limited by the possibility that the attached switches and accompanying wiring may encumber normal gait.

The reliability of this measurement is limited by a combination of the resolution of the time measurement (the sampling rate of the analog-to-digital converter) and the time measurement errors due to the differences in time between when the foot first contacts the floor and when the first switch closes, and between when the last switch opens and the foot leaves the floor.

CONCLUSIONS

The investigator has many available options when selecting a method for the study of foot fall patterns. The process of selecting an appropriate method for a particular study might utilize the following criteria:

1. *Parameters to be Measured.* The selection must start with what information about foot fall patterns is needed. The less information that is required, the less complex and less expensive is the system needed. In addition, some of the simpler methods are more portable.

2. *Subject Population.* Some measurement techniques will not work well with some groups of subjects, e.g., young children or the elderly. Furthermore, the type of gait patterns expected from the population will affect the selection of the method. Some abnormal gait patterns cannot be studied by certain methods.

3. *Portability.* If the study will collect data from subjects at many different sites (for example, a study of nursing home residents), then the ease with which a system can be transported and set up must be considered.

4. *Size of the Study.* If the number of subjects and the amount of data to be collected from each subject is large, then a method that automates as much of the data collection and analysis as possible is important.

5. *Additional Data Processing.* If the investigator intends to accumulate the data into a database or to do an appreciable amount of statistics on the results, he or she should consider a method that automatically stores

the data in a computer-readable form or that has some other method to make the data available for further processing.

6. *Availability of Engineering Help.* If the investigator is a qualified engineer or has the assistance of such an engineer, then he or she might consider constructing the gait analysis instrumentation in-house, as many of the investigators mentioned earlier have done. However, powerful commercially available footfall analysis systems, like the *Stride Analyzer* and the *GAITMAT II* might be better alternatives.

As with other areas of medical technology, foot fall measurement technology continues to evolve. Modern personal computers show dramatic increases in computing power while at the same time decreasing in cost. The peripheral circuit boards that allow personal computers to interface with sensors for measuring gait-related variables are also increasing in power and decreasing in cost. Developments in computer software are providing better realtime access to sensors and integration with other measurement, analysis, and database systems. This evolution will result in a decline in the prices of commercially available systems and an increase in their capabilities. Future foot fall measurement systems will have the ability to link to statistical and database packages, allowing the development of normal and abnormal gait databases. Powerful notebook computers will allow computer-based measurement systems to be portable. Evolution in sensor technology and increases in the speed of personal computers will allow foot fall measurement systems to give more information about events occurring during the gait cycle, such as the spatial and temporal distribution of pressure on the bottom of the feet. Systems will become available that can be integrated with EMG, goniometry, and full three-dimensional motion analysis systems. Such integration will allow a better understanding of the biomechanical events leading to observed foot fall patterns. As foot fall measurement technology evolves, clinicians and researchers will have a variety of choices that will allow them to increase the information obtained during gait analysis and/or reduce the cost of such studies.

REFERENCES

1. Boening D: Evaluation of a clinical method of gait analysis. *Phys Ther* 57:795-798, 1977.
2. Cheung C, Wall JC, Zelin S: A microcomputer-based system for measuring temporal asymmetry in amputee gait. *J of Prosthet Ortho Int* 7:131-140, 1983.

3. Chodera JD: Analysis of gait from foot prints. *Physiotherapy* 60:179, 1974.

4. Clarkson BH: Absorbent paper method for recording foot placement. *Phys Ther* 63: 345-346, 1983.

5. Durie ND, Farley RL: An apparatus for step length measurement. *J Biomed Eng* 2:38-40, 1980.

6. Gabel RH, Johnston RC, Crowninshield RD: A gait analyzer/trainer instrumentation system. *J Biomech* 12:543-549, 1979.

7. Gabell A, Nayak USL: The effect of age on variability in gait. *J Gerontol* 39: 662-666, 1984.

8. Hirokawa S, Matsumara K: Gait analysis using a measuring walkway for temporal and distance factors. *Med Biol Eng Comput* 25:577-582, 1987.

9. Keenan MA et al: Valgus deformities of the feet and characteristics of gait in patients who have rheumatoid arthritis. *J Bone Joint Surg* 73:237-247, 1991.

10. Leiper CI, Craik, RL: Relationships between physical activity and temporal-distance characteristics of walking in elderly women. *Phys Ther* 71:791-803, 1991.

11. Nayak USL et al: Measurement of gait and balance in the elderly. *J Am Geriatr Soc* 30:516-520, 1982.

12. Ogg HL: Measuring and evaluation of gait patterns of children. *Phys Ther* 43:717-720, 1963.

13. Rosenrot P, Wall JC, Charteris J: The relationship between velocity, stride time, support time and swing time during normal walking. *J Hum Move Stud* 6:323-335, 1980.

14. Shirley MM: Development of walking. In Shirley MM. *The first two years: Study of twenty-five babies.* Connecticut, 1931, Greenwood Press.

15. Skinner HB, Barrack RL: Ankle weighting effect on gait in able-bodied adults. *Arch Phys Med Rehabil* 71:112-115, 1990.

16. Taylor DR: An instrumented gait mat. In *Proceedings of the International Conference on Rehabilitation Engineering*, Toronto, Canada, 278, 1980.

CHAPTER 13

SPATIAL AND TEMPORAL CHARACTERISTICS OF FOOT FALL PATTERNS

Rebecca L. Craik
Lisa Dutterer

KEY TERMS

Base of support

Cadence

Double support phase

Gait cycle

Stance phase

Step time

Stride length

Swing phase

Walking velocity

Ambulation occurs when the center of gravity is efficiently translated through space; it requires the coordinated control of nearly every segment of the neuromusculoskeletal system.[29] Other chapters within the book focus on the use of various kinematic, kinetic, and EMG variables in describing upright walking. The purpose of this chapter is to review the use of foot fall variables to describe walking performance.

Ambulation can be viewed as two different subtasks: progression and "dynamic" postural control. A measure of progression is walking velocity, the result of all factors working to promote walking.[33] Foot contact patterns are the final outcome of the collective motions of all the major segments contributing to ambulation. Since walking velocity is the product of stride (step) length and cadence, the three variables can be treated together to describe performance. The length and timing of each step indicate lower extremity disability when patient data are compared to nonpatient data.[28] Thus, foot placement and temporal factors may be used as outcome measures to reflect the integrity of the neuromusculoskeletal system.

DEFINITIONS

The numerous parameters associated with footfall patterns require definition. This section will provide commonly used operational definitions.[1,10,16] **Walking velocity** is the measurement of distance per unit time. Typically, average walking velocity is expressed in meters per second (m/s) or miles per hour (mph). An individual has a wide range of walking velocities available to meet specific needs. As walking velocity changes, the foot fall patterns change. Therefore, the foot contact patterns are considered velocity dependent.

The **gait cycle** is the fundamental unit of locomotion and has both a temporal and a distance dimension. The gait cycle is defined as the sequence of events that begins with one extremity and continues until that event is repeated with the same extremity. Typically, a gait cycle is the interval between successive ipsilateral foot contacts such as heel strike. Technically, however, it can be considered as the interval between any recurring event that sequentially delineates two steps, e.g., left toe off to subsequent left toe off, right peak knee flexion to right peak knee flexion, etc.

During a gait cycle, **stride length** results in the major displacement of the body along the path of progression. Stride length is the distance from a contact event of one foot to the subsequent contact event of that same foot. Commonly the contact event used is initial contact. Therefore, one stride equals one complete gait cycle. Stride lengths for one individual are symmetrical.

Step length is the linear distance between two consecutive contralateral contacts of the lower extremities. Thus, there are two step lengths, a right and a left, within one stride. When defining step length, the reference is to the advancing limb. Therefore, the distance from initial contact of the left foot to initial contact of the right foot is a right step length.

A temporal variable associated with step length is **step time.** The time for either a right or left step length is the step time. The two steps within one gait cycle have both a distance and temporal component. Thus, if gait is symmetrical the left and right steps are even, and with asymmetrical gait the left and right steps are uneven. **Cadence,** the rhythm of the walking pattern, is defined as the number of steps or strides taken per unit of time. Cadence can be measured directly or derived by taking the inverse of the cycle or the step time.

During one gait cycle the lower extremity spends part of the time in contact with the walking surface and the remainder of the time in the air in preparation for contact with the walking surface. These two portions of a person's step length—the support phase and nonsupport phase—are described as stance and swing. The **stance phase** is the time that the limb is in contact with the walking surface. A gait cycle has two stance phases, a right and a left. Right stance phase begins with initial contact of the right limb and ends with the "take-off" of the right limb. The elapsed time that a limb is in contact with the walking surface is known as **stance time.** The remainder of the gait cycle when the lower extremity is in the air is known as the **swing phase.** The swing phase begins as the limb ends contact with the walking surface, and it ends the moment the same limb makes contact with the surface again. The temporal component of the swing phase is **swing time.** This is simply the elapsed time that one limb spends in the air.

In the ordinary gait cycle the two periods of stance and swing are arranged so that they overlap with one another. The stance phase of one limb overlaps the stance phase of the contralateral limb creating a period in which both limbs are in contact with the ground. The overlapping period of time is known as **double support.** Double and single support phases, rather than stance and swing of one limb, characterize the coordination between the two lower extremities during the gait cycle. Within one gait cycle there are two periods of double support. These two events may be reported separately by designating the trail limb–lead limb. For example, double support time right-left and double support time left-right. Conversely, the elapsed time when one limb is the only point of contact with the walking surface is known as **single support.** One gait cycle has two single support times, one for each lower extremity. Therefore, one lower limb is in single support while the contralateral limb is in swing. The time spent in single limb support for one limb and contralateral swing time are equal.

Base of support or **stride width** is another variable used to characterize the spatial dimensions of the foot fall patterns. A single definition for base of support has not been standardized in the literature. Some investigators report the base of support as the lateral distance between the heels and the angle of the foot placement in relation to the line of progression.[40] Base of support has also been defined as the perpendicular distance separating the midpoints of consecutive heel contacts.[45] If the heel locations have lateral space separating them, then the distance is positive. However, if the consecutive heel locations cross over the line of progression, then the distance is denoted as negative. Still other investigators define the base of support as the mediolateral distance between either the medial or lateral malleoli during the period of double support. The reader is cautioned to read the methods carefully when trying to compare base of support measurements across studies.

The rest of the chapter will examine the use of these parameters to describe the walking patterns of nondisabled and disabled individuals.

NONDISABLED STANDARDS

A common clinical use of gait analysis is, first, to compare a patient's performance with standards or criteria that have been derived from "normal" subjects and then to classify the walking pattern of patients based on the "gait deviation."

If the purpose of the gait evaluation is to describe how a patient's performance differs from "normal," an accurate assessment requires that all differences between the patient's performance and the standard result from the patient's disability. Anthropometric factors, such as stature, leg length, body mass, and body mass index, alter the walking performance of healthy subjects.[38,42-44]

Ideally, a normative data base should include subjects with varying proportions. In this way, the walking pattern of a tall, heavy individual would be compared to a larger sample of individuals with similar physical dimensions. Differences in the gait pattern of the individual could, therefore, be attributed to disease, motivation, or some other feature not included in the data base. At this time, however, no existing data bases adequately account for anthropometric features.

Normalization

Some investigators have attempted to address this lack of a data base, which includes a range of physical dimensions of the subjects, by normalizing the gait variables. One way to control for features that differ between individuals is to normalize them. Another reason variables associated with foot fall patterns are normalized is that control for a particular variable allows researchers to examine relationships among the remaining variables.

Height or, more appropriately, leg length influences step or stride length. A taller subject with long extremities is expected to use longer strides or step lengths than a shorter subject. Therefore, step length and stride length have been normalized to the person's standing height or leg length. The derived variable is a ratio of step length to lower extremity length. The derived variable can then be used to examine the effect of walking velocity, for example, on step length regardless of the person's stature. No standard method for the measurement of leg length has been reported. The reader is cautioned to examine carefully the methodology of a study before using the results as a normal reference.

Other variables that have been normalized include body weight and body mass index (BMI). The BMI is a derived variable of body weight divided by standing height that attempts to control for both weight and height.

The subphases of the gait cycle have also been normalized by dividing the actual time spent in each phase—stance, swing, single and double support—by the total time taken to complete the gait cycle. Cycle times may range from less than 1 second for fast speed walking to as long as 3 seconds for very slow walking velocities. By normalizing the phases of the gait cycle, attention can be focused on how different walking velocities alter the components of the cycle regardless of the actual time. During free speed walking, the stance phase of one limb consumes 60% of one cycle and the swing phase 40%.[29,34,45,47] Single support for both limbs, therefore, occupies 80% of the gait cycle with the two periods of double support accounting for the remaining 20% of the gait cycle.

It is important, therefore, to determine if and how data have been normalized in order to make an accurate comparison of results across studies.

Collection Schemes

The conditions under which footfall data are collected may influence the walking pattern. In the laboratory, the subjects may demonstrate a walking pattern that does not reflect the walking pattern used under "normal" circumstances. Collecting walking data from persons unaware that they are being observed may yield more natural walking patterns; however, the person's motivation for walking at a particular speed still remains unknown in this setting.

We will focus attention on three pedestrian studies to highlight the advantages of collecting foot fall data from large samples of subjects outside of laboratory conditions. In three different studies foot fall variables were studied in naive pedestrians, that is, persons unaware that they were being observed.[15,18,38] In this approach large samples were examined without the constraint of the laboratory and accompanying instrumentation. Drillis observed 752 pedestrians walking on the sidewalk in New York City.[15] Cadence and velocity were determined using a marked distance on the sidewalk. Step length was derived from the cadence and velocity variables. (Refer to Chapter 12 for a description of the methods.) After the observation was made, each pedestrian was asked to report age, height, and weight. The whole sample of pedestrians walked an average of 1.46 m/s (3.26 mph) with a mean cadence or step rate of 1.9 steps/s (112.5 steps/min) and a mean step length of 76.3 cm (30.05 in). Similar results were obtained through the observation of 533 pedestrians in Amsterdam and from 1,106 pedestrians in Philadelphia.[18,38] Molen reported mean walking velocity for the men as 1.39 m/s with a mean cadence of 1.79 steps/s and a derived step length (stride length divided by a factor of 2) of 77.4 cm.[38] The women walked an average of 1.27 m/s with a cadence of 1.88 steps/s and a step length of 67.1 cm. Finley et al reported an average velocity for men as 1.37 m/s with a mean cadence of 1.84 steps/s and a derived step length of 74.1 cm.[18] The women in the study walked with an average velocity of 1.24 m/s with a cadence of 1.94 steps/s and a step length of 63.4 cm. Finley et al observed

walking in a variety of settings including a suburban shopping center, a residential area, and a center city business area.[18] Pedestrians observed at the downtown location walked at a higher mean velocity with longer step length than those at other locations.

The advantage of this investigative approach is that walking is examined in the natural milieu without investigator intervention. The data from the pedestrians are within the range of results reported from studies conducted under laboratory conditions, which suggests that there is face validity to the approach of observing walking behavior under nonlaboratory conditions. Although validity or reliability of the foot fall variables was not addressed in these investigations, it is remarkable to see how similar the results are across the three studies. On the other hand, constraints associated with these studies include the following: (1) the "healthfulness" of the subjects was not determined; (2) the age range of the samples was limited from 20 to 70 years of age; (3) the goal for walking was not examined—for example, walking to work compared to walking for window shopping may require different modes of progression; (4) stride length was derived from cadence and velocity rather than measured directly; (5) stride length was divided by a factor of 2 to determine step length, which assumes symmetry; and (6) the dynamic postural control of the walking behavior was not assessed.

As described in Chapter 12 on foot fall technology, a number of investigators have used a variety of other techniques to describe foot fall patterns in a laboratory condition. In general, the results using these laboratory techniques are consistent with the results reported from the studies of the naive pedestrians. It is important, however, to view results in relation to the laboratory conditions under which the information is collected.

Hageman and Blanke, for example, examined the effect of aging on walking patterns and concluded that women walk faster today than their counterparts 15 to 20 years ago, based on data reported in previous studies.[26] Data collected, however, on small samples under unique laboratory conditions may be different from data collected from another laboratory. The actual values derived from investigations at various laboratories cannot be compared unless validity and reliability of gait variables is established among the laboratories. Hageman and Blanke compared walking from three laboratories. Their own laboratory used high-speed cinematography under optimal lighting conditions. One of the other studies used interrupted light photography, which required the subjects to walk in darkness while a strobe light flashed.[42] The third study required that subjects wear a bilateral electrogoniometric assembly that was attached to the pelvis with a wide band with linked potentiometer centered at each of the lower extremity joints.[19] Differences in age, stature, leg length, or weight among women did not account for the 0.7 to 1.5 m/s range of free speed walking velocities recorded from the three studies. While Hageman and Blanke may be correct in assuming that women walk faster today, the validity of the statement is questioned in view of the diverse laboratory conditions.

Therefore, while it is appropriate to compare *relative* change in walking performance across individuals from different laboratories, the validity of comparing actual data collected under different conditions must be established.

Normative Data

Although Tables 13-1 to 13-5 are not inclusive of all of the literature on foot fall parameters, the tables represent a majority of studies presented in recent years. Tables 13-1 to 13-3 cite the most commonly reported variables: velocity, cadence, and step length. The utility of collecting these three variables has already been addressed. Note that some authors report actual step length and others normalize step length using a variety of methods. Tables 13-4 and 13-5 list studies that selected cycle time and the percentage of stance phase, respectively. It is not clear why these two variables are more commonly reported than other temporal variables such as single support time, swing time, and double support time. The sample sizes have not been included in the tables because all sample sizes are inadequate to reflect the general population. No study has collected data from an adequate number of subjects to serve as a "normative" data base.

"Optimal" performance at free speed for an individual has been commonly described as symmetrical foot placement pattern within a velocity range of 1.2 to 1.5 m/s and with a cadence of 1.6 to 2.0 steps/s (100 to 120 steps/min). Women demonstrate a higher cadence and shorter step length than anthropometrically similar men walking at the same speed.[19,38,42] Such a gender-related difference in walking performance is reported consistently in gait-related research.

Reports that describe the spatial and temporal variables separately for the left and right lower limbs are rare in the literature. In addition, there is a lack of adequate data on actual step length

measurements. Much of the literature has derived step lengths and step time from stride measurements. At this time there is no criterion to determine when the performance between limbs is asymmetrical.

Base of support was not summarized in the tables because there is no consensus regarding an operational definition. Gabell and Nayak, for example, reported a median of 9.6 cm for base of support when measured as the distance between heels at initial contact.[22] Murray, on the other hand, reported a mean of 7.7 cm for base of support, measured as the transverse distance between points approximating the center of the ankle joint.[40] It is not possible to offer consensus regarding the base of support in a normative population.

The precision of the instrumentation used to collect foot fall patterns is often reported, but there are very few attempts to describe the reliability of the walking performance of the subjects over trials or over days. Test-retest reliability for selected foot contact measures has been reported as high in nondisabled women (range, $r = 0.69$ to 0.97), but the sample size was small and the brown paper and inked moleskin method was used.[7] Similar data are not available for nondisabled men. If reliability or consistency of the walking pattern is better defined in the nondisabled population it may serve as a sensitive indicator of disabled performance. For example, a hallmark of the patient with lower limb ataxia may be the inconsistency of the foot contact variables from step to step. Without data that describe the normal variability of performance from step to step, the inconsistency in the patient's pattern cannot be graded as mild, moderate, or severe.

A brief review of the tables, therefore, indicates that we do not possess an adequate normative data base to describe completely the spatial and temporal aspects of the foot fall patterns. In many cases, sample sizes are small; the age ranges are limited; the anthropometric features of the samples are incomplete; a range of walking velocities is not included; and instrumentation differs across studies. Moreover, the majority of the studies that have examined foot fall patterns have been limited to detailing the mean and the standard deviation of each of the variables. The dependence among the variables has not been identified well enough to make it possible for one of the variables to be adequate in describing the walking pattern. A multifactorial analysis may yield a single parameter that effectively describes outcome and simplifies the data collection process. Finally, the variables have not been examined in relation to a

TABLE 13-1 Summary of data from a variety of studies that have examined average walking velocity in younger or older subjects. Many studies report walking in response to a variety of speed commands. Note the range of walking velocities in the younger compared to the older subjects.

Author	Gender	Younger Age (yrs)	Younger Velocity (m/s)	Older Age (yrs)	Older Velocity (m/s)
Blanke & Hageman (1989)	M	20-33	1.31	60-74	1.38
Chao et al (1983)	M	19-32	1.20	32-85	1.27
	F	19-49	1.02	32-85	1.12
Cunningham et al (1982)	M	19-49	1.39	55-66	1.33
	M	19-49	1.08**	55-66	1.04**
	M	19-49	1.71***	55-66	1.60***
	M	19-49	2.25****	55-66	1.93****
Ferrandez et al (1990)	M/F			60-69	1.00
	M/F			60-69	1.31****
	M/F			70-79	0.82
	M/F			70-79	1.08****
	M/F			80-92	0.60
	M/F			80-92	0.84****
Finley et al (1969)	F	18-38	0.82	64-84	0.70
Finley & Cody (1970)	M	?	1.24		
	F	?	1.37		
Gabell & Nayak (1984)	?	21-47	1.37	66-84	1.19
Gifford & Hughes (1983)	?	20-59?	1.30	69-79?	1.18
Hageman & Blanke (1986)	F	20-35	1.60	60-80	1.32
Himann et al (1987)	M	19-39	1.37	63+	1.21
	M	19-39	1.09**	63+	0.95**
	M	19-39	1.71****	63+	1.47****
	M	40-62	1.34		
	M	40-62	1.06**		
	M	40-62	1.62****		
	F	19-39	1.26	63+	0.89
	F	19-39	0.92**	63+	0.67**
	F	19-39	1.59****	63+	1.14***
	F	40-62	1.27		
	F	40-62	0.90**		
	F	40-62	1.58****		
Jansen et al (1982)	M,F	20-29	1.10	60-69	1.10
Larish et al (1988)	M,F	26	1.19	71	1,21
Leiper & Craik (1991)	F			Comm. Act. 65.5-94.5	0.99
					0.47*
					0.73**
					1.17***
					1.57****
					1.03
	F			Exercisers 64.0-81.5	0.43*
					0.74**
					1.24***
					1.57****
					0.89
					0.38*
	F			Sedentary 72.0-90.5	0.62**
					1.07***
					1.29****
Murray et al (1964)	M	20-55	1.52	60-65	1.47
Murray et al (1969)	M	20-55	1.52	60-87	1.26
	M	20-55	2.15****	60-87	1.75****
Waters et al (1988)	M	20-59	1.36	60-80	1.28
	M	20-59	0.79**	60-80	0.83**
	M	20-59	1.84****	60-80	1.61****
	F	20-59	1.29	60-80	1.20
	F	20-59	0.62**	60-80	0.80**
	F	20-59	1.66****	60-80	1.42****

*Very slow speed   **Slow speed   ***Moderately fast speed   ****Very fast speed

TABLE 13-2   The range of cadences exhibited by younger and older individuals when walking at different velocities is summarized here. Refer to Table 13-1 for the different velocity commands.

Author	Gender	Younger Age (yrs)	Cadence (steps/min)	Older Age (yrs)	Cadence (steps/min)
Chao et al (1983)	M	19-32	100	32-85	104
	F	19-49	102	32-85	112
Cunningham et al (1982)	M	19-49	108	55-66	109
	M	19-49	95**	55-66	95**
	M	19-49	119***	55-66	120***
	M	19-49	144****	55-66	135****
Finley et al (1969)	F	18-38	105	64-84	109
Finley & Cody (1970)	M	?	110		
	F	?	116		
Gabell & Nayak (1984)	?	21-47	108	66-84	112
Gifford & Hughes (1983)	?	20-59?	109	60-79?	110
Hageman et al (1986)	F	20-35	119	60-80	120
Himann et al (1987)	M	19-39	108	63+	105
	M	19-39	98.1**	63+	93.2**
	M	19-39	119****	63+	115****
	M	40-62	107		
	M	40-62	94.9**		
	M	40-62	118****		
			115		
			96.3**		
	F	19-39	1.32****		
	F	19-39	114	63+	100
	F	19-39	93.3**	63+	85.0**
	F	40-62	131****	63+	116****
	F	40-62			
	F	40-62			
Jansen et al (1982)	M,F	20-29	131	60-69	135
Leiper & Craik (1991)	F			Comm. Act. 65.5-94.5	109
					72.7*
					91.5**
					123.7***
					140.5****
					105.8
	F			Exercisers 64.0-81.5	63.9*
					87.8**
					119.5***
					141.6****
					106.8
					67.0*
	F				86.5**
				Sedentary 72.0-90.5	120.0***
					136.4****
Murray et al (1964)	M	20-55	117	60-65	115
Murray et al (1969)	M	20-55	111	60-87	111
	M	20-55	132****	60-87	132****
Waters et al (1988)	M	20-59	108	60-80	105
	M	20-59	76**	60-80	78**
	M	20-59	125****	60-80	118****
	F	20-59	117	60-80	112
	F	20-59	67**	60-80	84**
	F	20-59	137****	60-80	124****

*Very slow speed
**Slow speed
***Moderately fast speed
****Very fast speed

TABLE 13-3 The studies included here compare step length in younger and older subjects. Note that several studies report step length normalized to some anthropometric feature.

Author	Gender	Younger Age (yrs)	Younger Step Length	Older Age (yrs)	Older Step Length
Blanke & Hagemen (1989)	M	20-33	0.87 m	60-74	0.94 m
Chao et al (1983)	M	19-32	1.46[a]	32-85	1.56[a]
	F	19-32	1.38[a]	32-85	1.40[a]
Cunningham et al (1982)	M	19-49	0.87[b]	55-66	0.84[b]
	M	19-49	0.76[b]	55-66	0.76[b]
		19-49	0.99[b]	55-66	0.92[b]
		19-49	1.06[b]	55-66	0.99[b]
Finley & Cody (1970)	M	?	0.11		
	F	?	0.98		
Gabell & Nayak (1984)	M,F	21-47	0.75 m	66-84	0.64 m
Gifford & Hughes (1983)	?	20-59	0.83[b]	60-79	0.76[b]
Hageman & Blanke (1986)	F	20-35	1.87[a]	60-80	1.55[a]
Himann et al (1987)	M	19-39	0.76	63+	1.21
	M	19-39	0.67**	63+	0.61**
	M	19-39	0.86****	63+	0.75****
	M	40-62	0.74		
	M	40-62	0.67**		
	M	40-62	0.82****	63+	0.52
	F	19-39	0.65	63+	0.46**
	F	19-39	0.57**	63+	0.58****
	F	19-39	0.75****		
	F	40-62	0.66		
	F	40-62	0.57**		
	F	40-62	0.72****		
Jansen et al (1982)	M,F	20-29	0.59[b]	60-69	0.59[b]
Leiper & Craik (1991)	F			Comm. Act. 65.5-94.5	0.70[c]
					0.50[c]*
					0.62[c]**
					0.74[c]***
					0.78[c]****
					0.74[c]
	F			Exercisers 64.0-81.5	0.51[c]*
					0.64[c]**
					0.80[c]***
					0.85[c]****
					0.64[c]
					0.54[c]*
	F			Sedentary 72.0-90.5	0.44[c]**
					0.69[c]***
					0.73[c]****
Murray et al (1964)	M	20-55	0.90[b]	60-65	0.87[b]
Murray et al (1969)	M	20-55	0.90[b]	60-87	0.82[b]
		20-55	1.08[b]	60-87	0.94[b]

[a]SL/LEL, stride length divided by lower extremity length
[b]SL/Ht, stride length divided by standing height
[c]SL/LEL × 100, step length divided by lower extremity length
*Very slow speed
**Slow speed
***Moderately fast speed
****Very fast speed

TABLE 13-4   The percentage of the gait cycle spent in the stance phase is summarized across studies in young and older individuals.

Author	Gender	Younger Age (yrs)	Younger Stance Phase (% cycle)	Older Age (yrs)	Older Stance Phase (% cycle)
Chao et al (1983)	M	19-32	60	32-85	59
	F	19-32	59	32-85	60
Finley et al (1969)	F	18-38	63	64-84	67
Gifford & Hughes (1983)	?	20-59	55	60-79	57
Jansen et al (1982)	M,F	20-29	69	60-69	69
Murray et al (1964)	M	20-55	61	60-65	61
Murray et al (1969)	M	20-55	61	60-87	60
	M	20-55	57****	60-87	59****

****Very fast speed

TABLE 13-5   Cycle time compared between younger and older individuals.

Author	Gender	Younger Age (yrs)	Cycle Time (sec)	Older Age (yrs)	Cycle Time (sec)
Chao et al (1983)	M	19-32	1.20	32-85	1.15
	F	19-49	1.18	32-85	1.07
Cunningham et al (1982)	M	19-49	1.11	55-66	1.10
	M	19-49	1.27**	55-66	1.27**
	M	19-49	1.01***	55-66	1.00***
	M	19-49	0.83****	55-66	0.89****
Ferrandez et al (1990)	M/F			60-69	1.13
	M/F			60-69	0.98****
	M/F			70-79	1.19
	M/F			70-79	1.04****
	M/F			80-92	1.20
	M/F			80-92	1.03****
Finley et al (1969)	F	18-38	1.14	64-84	1.10
Gabell et al (1984)	?	21-47	1.10	66-84	1.08
Gifford & Hughes (1983)	?	20-59?	1.11	60-79?	1.10
Hageman & Blanke (1986)	F	20-35	1.01	60-80	1.00
Murray et al (1964)	M	20-55	1.03	60-65	1.04
Murray et al (1969)	M	20-55	1.04	60-87	1.13
		20-55	0.88****	60-87	0.94****

**Slow speed
***Moderately fast speed
****Very fast speed

theoretical model of locomotion. Is the system organized, for example, to control for walking velocity, and does cadence or step length vary in a systematic manner to meet the need to change walking velocity? Why does stance time change exponentially over a range of walking velocities when swing time remains relatively constant? The development of a theoretical model for locomotion using foot fall variables may shed light on why the foot fall patterns are altered in light of pathology or aging.

A myriad of variables influence performance in the nondisabled population in addition to anthropometric characteristics and gender. Included are the purpose of walking (e.g., window shopping, reaching the bus before it leaves the curb), environmental constraints, ethnicity, experience, physical activity level, age, level of maturation, and walking velocity. In the next section we will consider effects from three of these factors: age, level of maturation, and walking velocity.

Factors Influencing Gait

Age   Attempts to unravel the relationship between aging and walking date back to at least 1940 and continue today. A number of so-called gait disorders ascribed to age alone are reported in the older clinical literature.[3,4,11,50] Spielberg is apparently the first investigator to systematically observe changes in gait resulting from aging.[48] Three age-related stages in the decline of walking performance were described based on observations of footfall patterns. The first stage (60 to 72 years of age) included a slower walking velocity, shortened steps, lower cadence, less vertical excursion of the center of gravity, and disturbed coordination between the upper and lower extremities. In the second stage (72 to 86 years of age), the normal arm-leg synergy was lost and an overproduction of unwanted movements appeared. The final stage of performance decline (86 to 104 years of age) was typified by a rapid disintegration of the gait pattern with arrhythmical stepping patterns.

The hypothesis that the gait disorders just described are due to age alone is a tentative one. The authors did not provide detailed health screen information for subjects, so changes in walking behavior may reflect both the aging and disease processes. While Speilberg's stages II and III are reminiscent of other clinical walking disorders, the walking patterns are not consistent with descriptions from recent quantitative investigations of "healthy" older subjects.[48]

Drillis states that the age-related velocity decline observed in his results did not follow a natural exponential decay.[15] Comparison between an exponential decay line and actual velocities selected by subjects over 45 years of age reveals that the walking velocities of older individuals are higher than that predicted by exponential decay. Drillis speculates that the higher-than-predicted velocities selected by the older subjects represent their "fight against aging."

An image that emerges from the data listed in the tables is that aging is accompanied by a slower free speed walking velocity, shorter step lengths, and a slower cadence. These features of the older subjects' walking pattern are consistent with Stage I of Spielberg's classification of walking in aging

individuals.[48] The gender-related differences in walking continue with aging; compared to the older men, the older women demonstrate a slower velocity, higher cadence, and shorter step length. Older subjects also appear to demonstrate a greater out-toeing than the younger subjects. This finding was described by Murray with base of support defined as the distances between the heels and the toes.[40] Aging seems to be accompanied by a longer time in the stance phase and a shorter time in the swing phase of the walking cycle. Because swing time for one limb is equivalent to single support time in stance for the contralateral limb, the longer stance time comes from spending a longer time in the two double support phases of the stance period. A hypothesis to be tested is that the longer periods of double support reflect an attempt by the older individual to preserve stability.

Leiper and Craik have examined factors that predict walking speed in the older individual.[35] The contribution of physical activity, age, and body mass index (BMI) to the actual walking velocity was examined using a multiple regression analysis under five different walking conditions—very slow, slow, free speed, fast, and very fast. Across the five conditions, 30% to 45% of the variability was accounted for by age. BMI contributed only a maximum of 3% of the variability. The criterion variables—physical activity, age, and BMI—accounted for only 5% of the variability in the very slow walking condition, which suggests that there is something distinctly different about the very slow walking condition. The women who were active exercisers were able to walk significantly more slowly than the women in the other physical activity groups. The results of this study emphasize the importance of relating variables such as physical activity and age to walking performance. Future studies need to examine the predictive nature of the impairments reported to accompany aging such as muscle weakness, limited range of motion in lower extremity joints, and problems in standing balance.

The normative data on older individuals is incomplete. Many studies consider the upper range of old as 70 years of age, while 70 years of age is defined by some other authors as the younger elder. Results, therefore, may not reflect accurately the effect of aging on the foot fall patterns. Because it is still common practice to collect data in a laboratory and this process selects for an individual who is willing and able to come to the laboratory, the data may not reflect the general population. A study by Gabell and Nayak emphasizes this potential source of error.[22] Only 32 of

1,187 individuals over the age of 64 met the strict selection criteria to be included in the study. Using this elite sample, the investigators reported that healthy older individuals (66 to 84 years of age) walked the same as younger individuals (21 to 47 years of age) when comparing variability in step length, cadence, double support time, and base of support. It is possible, therefore, that the conclusions from this study only apply to "elite" older individuals. Future studies that address the effect of aging on walking performance should strive to include a broad range of older persons who reflect the general rather than the elite older person.

The use of foot fall parameters not only seems to help identify the effects of age but also appears helpful in discerning the functional implications of these changes. Studies need to be conducted to describe what is necessary to function in the society. For example, a study was performed to determine if 79-year-olds could function as pedestrians.[36] Functional capacity of the lower extremities was assessed in 112 women and 93 men. Subjects were asked to walk at free speed and as fast as possible. Stair walking was assessed on a series of steps 10, 20, 30, 40, and 50 cm in height. Sixty-two percent of the women and 68% of the men had no physical impairments to ambulation. The rest of the sample comprised individuals who had cardiovascular, neurological, or musculoskeletal disease that altered walking ability. Walking aids were used by 27% of the women and 25% of the men. The recommended speed to cross intersections in Sweden is 1.4 m/s. No women or men in this study achieved this speed when walking at their preferred speed. At their maximum walking speed only 32% of the women and 72% of the men reached 1.4 m/s. All subjects climbed up and down a 10 or 20 cm step with the handrail as needed. Twenty percent of the women and 6% of the men were unable to climb up the 40 cm step height even with use of the handrail. The authors concluded that public transportation vehicles and the timing of lights at intersections in Sweden are not in accordance with the functional capacity of older persons.

The studies just reviewed indicate that foot fall patterns are sensitive indicators of aging. If foot fall variables are used as a standard by which a person's performance is evaluated, then this brief review of some the literature also emphasizes the importance of ensuring that the standard is age-matched. If performance of an 80-year-old person with a recent total knee replacement is compared to the performance of a youthful standard, the walking of the 80-year-old person may be erroneously labeled abnormal.

Maturation   Level of maturation is another factor to consider when evaluating walking performance. The time frame for the acquisition of the adult foot contact pattern in children is an area in which normal standards are still being developed.[5,8,37,49,51] An adequate sample has not been described to date. Research, however, indicates that the gait pattern is age-dependent. If the quality of walking performance is used as a tool for monitoring treatment progress, as well as an indication of delayed motor development, the following must be considered: (1) the foot fall variables dependent on central nervous system (CNS) maturation should be distinguished from those that are stature dependent, and (2) gait pattern changes that occur because of therapeutic intervention must be distinguished from those that are dependent on maturation.

Beck et al. examined foot fall patterns in 51 healthy children.[5] Children less than 4 years of age demonstrated growth-related pattern changes when the test-retest interval was longer than 3 months. The interval between growth-related changes is relevant to the clinician who uses gait analysis to assess children before and after treatment. Changes in foot fall patterns may be inappropriately attributed to treatment when they result, in fact, from maturation. The investigators reported the effect of maturation on walking velocity, stride length, cadence, stance time, and double and single support times. Some of the variables were, however, also related to stature. For example, when normalized to the child's height, the length of the stride was 76% of the child's height regardless of age. Therefore, normalized stride length may serve as an outcome measure that does not reflect maturation of the CNS. On the other hand, the development of a heel strike rather than a foot-flat or toe-first initial contact to begin stance appears to be a sensitive indicator of CNS maturation.[20] Depending on the purpose of the evaluation, one gait variable may be more sensitive than another for measuring changes in foot fall patterns.

Velocity   The velocity-dependence of gait variables has been documented.* The relationship between other gait variables and velocity depends on the velocity range examined. For example, cadence or step length with velocity demonstrates direct linear relationships when the range of velocities is within 0.8 through 2.0 m/s. On the other

---

* Refer to these sources: 2, 12, 16, 25, 31, 38, 43, 46.

hand, the relationships between cadence or step length and velocity are curvilinear when the lower end of the velocity range is extended to 0.3 m/s. Single and double support are inversely proportional to velocity and demonstrate a curvilinear relationship when actual or "raw" time is used. These relationships become linear when single and double support are normalized to the gait cycle.

The percentage of the gait cycle spent in stance and swing appears to hold true for the moderate-fast and fast walking velocities.[45] Double support time, however, decreases with increasing velocities nearing zero with race walking. In running there is no double support time and the percentage of the cycle spent in swing exceeds the time spent in stance. During very slow walking, on the other hand, the stance phase may occupy as much as 80% of the gait cycle, leaving only 20% of the time for single support. As walking velocity increases, the percentage of time spent in stance and double support decreases.

When healthy young individuals are asked to walk slowly, features including a shortened step length, decreased cadence, and diminished single support time are evident. The characteristics reported to accompany aging are seen in the healthy young person who is walking slowly. Since gait variables demonstrate velocity-dependence, investigators should account for the effect of velocity in research or in clinical practice when comparing performance of a particular group to some "gold" standard.

Gillis et al. asked their young and old subjects to walk at three speeds: slow, medium, and fast.[24] The only variables measured were the phases of foot contact. Older subjects walked more slowly than the young subjects at the medium and fast speeds so differences in the gait variables were not examined. Velocities were the same between the two samples at the slow speed. Step length was not measured. At the slow speed there was no difference in stance or single or double support times expressed as a percentage of stride time. The only difference was stride time or its inverse, cadence. This study illustrates the advantage of controlling velocity. Instead of concluding that the older subjects walked more slowly, this study indicates that cadence was significantly slower in the older subjects despite velocity control. Cadence, therefore, may be a variable sensitive to walking ability between age groups.

Crowinshield, Brand, and Johnston approached the velocity-dependence of gait variables by developing regression lines for velocity and age and such other gait variables as stride length and sagittal hip excursion.[12] Twenty-six subjects demonstrated walking speeds ranging from 0.3 to 1.5 m/s. The authors squared the velocity terms, which produced a linear relationship between the squared velocity and stride length. The mean regression equations were again significantly different between the two age groups. The authors concluded that the older subjects walked with shorter strides and less sagittal hip excursion and that the differences in the kinematic parameters are apparently of increased significance at the higher velocities. Studies of this type conducted with large samples, which also control for such factors as stature, weight, and sex, may help unravel the age, velocity, and walking pattern issues.

The velocity-dependence of gait variables is too often neglected in studies that select a data base of nondisabled subjects to examine the effect of disease on walking performance. Many reports in the literature indicate that disabled persons walk more slowly than healthy subjects. For example, Gabel et al. reported that, prior to total hip replacement, patients walked more slowly, with a slower cadence and a shorter stride length and swing time, than age-matched nondisabled individuals.* A velocity-matched standard may have provided a more sensitive indication of the effect of hip disorders on walking ability.

The results of a study by Smidt suggest that matching the standard and the patient walking speeds aids in separating the velocity-dependence of gait variables from other indications of disease.[46] The walking patterns of patients with hip disease were compared to the walking patterns of healthy subjects of similar sex, height, and weight. The author concludes that the patients had a higher cadence and shorter step length at velocities that matched the standards. However, the healthy subjects were an average 32 years of age while the patients were an average of 63 years. The effect of age and hip disease or disorder are confounding variables in this data analysis. Moreover, the variables selected to describe walking performance do not distinguish hip disorder from other lower extremity disability. The same performance may occur in any patient who has pain in the lower extremity and walks with an antalgic gait. If the gait assessment is to yield information that guides treatment, the standard must be appropriate, that is, age and velocity-matched.

Andriacchi et al. examined the effect of disease on the walking ability of 16 patients with total

---

* Refer to these sources: 4, 11, 15, 21, 42, 50.

knee replacements or high tibial osteotomies.[1] Using a velocity-matched standard, it was observed that the patients walked with a shorter step length and a higher cadence. Among the temporal parameters measured, swing time was the best indicator of gait abnormalities; 84% of the swing time observations for the patients were "abnormal." Repeated observations of the patients after surgery indicated a shift in the step length and swing time toward "normal." The improved gait was related to another measure of clinical improvement of the knee joint. The results indicate that controlling extraneous variables such as the walking speed and monitoring clinical changes increases the usefulness of the gait evaluation. By considering the effect of walking velocity, the examiner has measures that can indicate the effect of disease on performance, which may suggest specific forms of therapeutic intervention.

DISABLED STANDARDS

An investigator who is interested in describing the effect of CNS disease on the control of movement may select a nondisabled sample for comparison. The use of this type of standard for clinical gait evaluation may not describe functional deficits. For example, the goal of the treatment for a patient with rheumatoid arthritis who has just received pharmacologic relief of acute knee pain is often restoration of the function that was lost due to the acute pain. Gait evaluation is one means of evaluating the efficacy of the treatment. The standard used to examine the effect of the treatment on managing acute pain should not be derived from an age-matched nondisabled group. Because the patient had rheumatoid arthritis, gait deviations were probably present before the acute episode. If nondisabled performance is the standard, the scale may not be sensitive enough to detect changes in abnormal function. Changes in the patient's performance may not be noticed when inappropriate standards are used for comparisons. The patient's pretreatment ambulatory status, if known, may be a more useful standard for the evaluation of the treatment's effect. Appropriate comparisons can also be made with data collected from patients with similar disabilities.

An example to illustrate the potential use of a disabled standard can be found in a study by Holden et al., which investigated the use of foot fall parameters in a sample of subjects with multiple sclerosis or hemiparesis.[23] An inked footprint record and ambulation time were used to calculate velocity, cadence, step and stride lengths, stride

length to lower extremity length ratio, and derived step and stride times. In addition, the clinician rated the functional ambulation ability of the subject with a scale developed at Massachusetts General Hospital. The scale assesses the amount of human assistance, rather than devices, needed for ambulation. Interrater reliability (range, $r = 0.9$ to 1.0) and test-retest reliability (range, $r = 0.9$ to 1.0) were high for all measures (except stride-time) for the total sample and within diagnostic categories. Test-retest reliability was examined by comparing walking performance on two trials separated by a 15-minute rest period. The functional ambulation ability scale divided subjects into five categories: Physical Assistance Level II, Physical Assistance Level I, Supervision, Independent on Level, Independent. All measures except stride and step times displayed a strong linear relationship to a functional ambulation scale, which suggests that the foot fall measures were sensitive enough to distinguish among categories. The linear relationship between the foot fall variables and the ambulation scale is noteworthy considering the other variables that affect the foot fall variables such as age, height, types of assistive devices, and types of clinical symptoms. The results of this study suggest that comparison of performance among patients with disability, rather than between disabled and nondisabled performance, may serve as the basis for developing a functional and sensitive classification of walking ability. Such classification may in turn suggest different avenues of intervention or no intervention.

Diamond and Ottenbacher reported the usefulness of foot fall parameters in evaluating a prefabricated plastic molded ankle-foot orthosis and a tone-inhibiting dynamic ankle-foot orthosis in a single subject with right hemiparesis.[14] Using a single-subject alternating-treatment design, they reported a significant improvement in walking velocity, step length, and stance time on the hemiparetic limb and significant decrease in cadence with either orthosis compared to barefoot walking. Again, this study exemplifies the potential use of the disabled standard—in this case, the patient himself—as a sensitive indicator for treatment efficacy.

Additional research is necessary before we can conclude that foot fall patterns using disabled standards are sensitive indicators of functional change. The research to date suggests that the selection of the appropriate standard is dependent on the purpose of the gait evaluation and the goal of treatment. The use of a "normal" standard may be inappropriate if the goal of the evaluation is to describe functional deficits or if the goal of treatment is functional gait rather than cosmetic gait. Gait deviations are often adaptive. Use of the normal standard may label the patient's adaptive strategy for improving mobility as a gait deviation in need of correction. Use of a standard derived from patients may lead to a ranking or classification of the degree of adaptive behavior achieved and suggest additional adaptive strategies to the clinician and to the patient.

SUMMARY

The studies just cited indicate that foot fall patterns may be useful in distinguishing among various populations. A difference in foot fall patterns has been reported related to age, stature, weight, and between disabled and nondisabled populations. Although the effects of aging, height, and weight on walking are still unknown, these variables do not rule out the use of apparently nondisabled subjects as standards to examine the effects of disability on walking behavior in this population. One purpose of a gait evaluation is to describe how a patient's performance differs from "normal." An accurate assessment requires that all differences between the patient's performance and the standard result from the patient's disability. Therefore, the standard used to judge performance should match the patient in terms of anthropometric characteristics, sex, age, and walking velocity.

Normative foot fall data for both the nondisabled and disabled populations are still needed. Careful attention must be given to certain criteria when developing a normative data base. An effort must be made to use an appropriate sample size to ensure adequate representation. An adequate sample size is necessary in order to generalize the results thus allowing comparisons between the client and the appropriate normative data. With this comparison of the client's gait to the appropriately matched normative data, goals of treatment and treatment interventions can be determined.

The gait variables selection should be based on a model of locomotion that will yield meaningful information. An attempt to relate specific walking variables and clinical symptoms may assist in addressing the following issues: (1) the specific effect that pathology has on ambulation, (2) the severity of involvement, and (3) the ability to differentiate among different types of pathology.

Investigators interested in examining the effect of aging or pathology on walking may find the use of foot fall variables intriguing. The variables can be collected without encumbering the individual.

They also indicate that foot fall patterns are sensitive to the process of aging and disease. It is important, however, to consider the limitations of foot fall measures alone. Foot fall patterns represent the final outcome between the neuromuscular system and the environment, but we do not believe that the variables are sensitive enough to identify specific mechanisms responsible for producing the gait pattern.

While descriptive studies have provided a range of normally expected behaviors across ages, they have not identified underlying mechanisms. The causal relationship among the foot fall variables presented in various studies is unknown.[43] For example, researchers cannot conclude that a person with Parkinson's disease demonstrates a shortened step length because of less hip flexion. The diminished step length may relate to diminished pelvic rotation, decreased knee extension at heel strike, diminished plantarflexion at toe off, or a combination of these factors. Therefore, the use of foot fall parameters alone does not definitively indicate that weak musculature or slowed reaction time leads to diminished joint motion resulting in slower walking velocity. The scientist does not gain insight into the effect of cellular changes on behavior by studying foot fall parameters. The clinician does not learn from foot fall patterns where to intervene to improve behavior or if intervention will change behavior.

Collection of foot fall variables accompanied by data on neuromuscular integrity and physical activity level may yield results that suggest avenues for measuring and analyzing additional kinematic and kinetic variables, which may, in turn, assist in the development of causal relationships. Examination of the coordination among the joints and EMG activity and correlation of the timing of the EMG with foot fall variables may help address the motor control issue. A multiple regression or discriminant analysis may indicate the degree of relationship among gait variables and the amount of variance that is accounted for by these relationships. In this way, such research may aid ultimately in developing a theoretical model that suggests mechanisms responsible for a pattern of locomotion altered by aging or disease. The data available on foot fall patterns suggest that the variables may serve as sensitive indicators to describe the final outcome of the collective motions of the whole body as it attempts to move through space. Many exciting avenues for future clinical and basic research are offered through additional study of these variables. Examination of foot fall parameters alone distinguishes between disabled and nondisabled walking performance. Examination of foot fall parameters in combination with other variables may provide insight into the mechanisms responsible for the production of walking.

REFERENCES

1. Andriacchi T, Galante J, Fermier R: The influence of total knee-replacement design on walking and stair-climbing, *J Bone Joint Surg* 64-A:1328, 1982.
2. Andriacchi T, Ogle J, Galante J: Walking speed as a basis for normal and abnormal gait measurements, *J Biomech* 10:261, 1977.
3. Azar G, Lawton A: Gait and stepping as factors in the frequent falls of elderly women, *Gerontologist* 4:83, 1964.
4. Barron RC: Disorder of gait related to the aging nervous system, *Geriatrics* 22:113, 1967.
5. Beck R, Andriacchi T, Kuokn, et al: Changes in the gait patterns of growing children, *J Bone Joint Surg* 63-A:1452, 1981.
6. Blanke DJ, Hageman PA: Comparison of gait of young men and elderly men, *Phys Ther* 69:144, 1989.
7. Boenig D: Evaluation of a clinical method of gait analysis, *Phys Ther* 57:795, 1977.
8. Burnett CN, Jr: Development of gait in childhood: part II, *Dev Med Child Neurol* 13:207, 1971.
9. Chao E, Laughman R, Schneider E, et al: Normative data of knee joint motion and ground reaction forces in adult level walking, *J Biomech* 16:219, 1983.
10. Colaso MJ, Singh N: Variation of gait patterns in adult hemiplegia, *Neurology India* 19(4):212, 1971.
11. Critchley M: On senile disorders of gait, including the so-called "senile paraplegic," *Geriatrics* 13:364, 1948.
12. Crowinshield R, Brand R, Johnston R: The effects of walking velocity and age on hip kinematics and kinetics, *Clin Ortho* 132:140, 1978.
13. Cunningham D, Rechnitzer P, Pearce M, et al: Determinants of self-selected walking pace across ages, *J Gerontol* 37:560, 1982.
14. Diamond M, Ottenbacher K: Effect of a tone-inhibiting dynamic ankle-foot orthosis on stride characteristics of an adult with hemiparesis, *Phys Ther* 70:423, 1990.
15. Drillis R: The influence of aging on the kinematics of gait. In *Geriatric amputee* (NAS-NRC Pub. No. 919), Washington, D.C., 1961, NAS-NRC.
16. Eberhart HD, Inman VT, Saunders JB, et al: Fundamental studies of human locomotion and other information relating to design of artificial limbs. A Report to the National Research Council, Committee on Artificial Limbs, University of California, Berkeley, 1947.
17. Ferrandez AM, Pailhous J, Durup M: Slowness in elderly gait, *Exp Aging Res* 16(2):79, 1990.
18. Finley F, Cody K: Locomotive characteristics of urban pedestrians, *Arch Phys Med Rehabil* 51:423, 1970.
19. Finley F, Cody K, Finizie R: Locomotion patterns in elderly women, *Arch Phys Med Rehabil* 70:140, 1969.
20. Forssberg H: Ontogeny of human locomotor control I: infant stepping, supported locomotion and transition to independent locomotion, *Exp Brain Res* 57:480, 1985.
21. Gabel R, Johnston R, Crowinshield R: A gait analyzer/trainer instrumentation system, *J Biomech* 12:543, 1979.
22. Gabell A, Nayak USL: The effect of age on variability in gait, *J Gerontol* 39(6):662, 1984.
23. Gifford G, Hughes J: Gait analysis system in clinical practice, *J Biomed Eng* 5:297, 1983.
24. Gillis B, Gilroy K, Lawley H, et al: Slow walking speeds in healthy young and elderly women, *Physiother Can* 70:350, 1986.
25. Grieve D, Gear R: The relationships between length of stride, step frequency, time of swing, and speed of walking for children and adults, *Ergonomics* 5(9):379, 1966.
26. Hageman P, Blanke D: Comparison of gait of young and elderly women, *Phys Ther* 66(9):1382, 1986.
27. Himann J, Cunningham D, Rechnitzer P, et al: Age-related changes in speed of walking, *Med Sci Sports Exerc* 20(2):161, 1987.
28. Holden MK, Gill KM, Magliotti MR: Clinical assessment in the neurologically impaired: reliability and meaningfulness, *Phys Ther* 64:35, 1984.
29. Inman VT, Ralston HJ, Todd F: *Human walking,* Baltimore, 1981, Williams & Wilkins.
30. Jansen E, Vittas D, Hellberg S, et al: Normal gait of young and old men and women: ground reaction force measurement on a treadmill, *Acta Orthop Scand* 53:193, 1982.
31. Lamoreux L: Kinematic measurements in the study of human walking, *Bull Prosthet Res* 10:3, 1971.
32. Larish DD, Martin PE, Mungiole M: Characteristic patterns of gait in the healthy old, *Ann NY Acad Sci:* 18, 1988.
33. Larsson L, Odenrick P, Sandlund B, et al: The phases of the stride and their interaction in human gait, *Scand J Rehab Med* 12:107, 1980.
34. Lehmkuhl L, Smith L: Standing and walking. In Lehmkuhl L, Smith L, editors: *Brunnstrom's clinical kinesiology,* ed 4, Philadelphia, 1983, F.A. Davis.
35. Leiper C, Craik R: Relationships between physical activity and temporal-distance characteristics of walking in elderly women, *Phys Ther* 71:791, 1991.
36. Lundgren-Lindquist B, Aniansson A, Rundgren A: Functional studies in 79 year olds. III: Walking performance and climbing ability, *Scand J Rehab Med* 12:107, 1983.
37. McGraw M: Neuromuscular development of the human infant as exemplified in the achievement of erect locomotion, *J Pediatr* 17:741, 1940.
38. Molen HH: *Problems on the evaluation of gait,* Amsterdam, 1973, Free University.
39. Murray MP, Kory RC, Clarkson BH: Walking patterns in healthy old men, *J Gerontol* 24:169, 1969.
40. Murray MP: Gait as a total pattern of movement, *Am J Phys Med* 46(1):290, 1967.
41. Murray MP, Drought AB, Kory RC: Walking patterns of normal men, *J Bone Joint Surg* 46(2):335, 1964.
42. Murray M, Kory R, Sepic S: Walking patterns of normal women, *Arch Phys Med* 51:637, 1979.

43. Rosenrot P, Wall J, Charteris J: The relationship between velocity, stride time, support time, and swing time during normal walking, *Human Movement Studies* 6:323, 1980.

44. Schwartz R, Heath A, Misick W: The influence of the shoe on the gait, *J Bone Joint Surg* 17-A:406, 1935.

45. Smidt GL: *Gait in rehabilitation, clinics in physical therapy,* New York, 1990, Churchill Livingston.

46. Smidt G: Hip motion and related factors in walking, *Phys Ther* 51(1):9, 1971.

47. Soderberg G: Posture and gait. In Soderberg G, editor: *Kinesiology: application to pathological motion,* Baltimore, 1986, Williams & Wilkins.

48. Speilberg PI: Walking patterns of old people: cyclographic analysis. In Bernstein NA, editor: *Investigations on the biodynamics of walking, running and jumping, part II,* Moscow, 1940, Central Scientific Institute of Physical Culture.

49. Statham M, Murray M: Early walking patterns of normal children, *Clin Orthop* 79:8, 1971.

50. Steinberg F: Gait disorders in old age, *Geriatrics:* 134, 1966.

51. Sutherland D, Olshen R, Cooper L, et al: The development of mature gait, *J Bone Joint Surg* 62-A:336, 1980.

52. Waters RL, Hislop HJ, Perry J, et al: Comparative cost of walking in young and old adults, *J Orthop Res* 1(1):73, 1983.

CHAPTER 14

KINEMATICS THEORY

Ge Wu

KEY TERMS

Acceleration

Differentiation

Displacement

Euler angles

Integration

Reference frame

    Absolute

    Joint

    Local

    Segmental

Rigid body

Signal to noise ratio

Transformation

Velocity

Rigid Body Model of the Lower Limb

The structure of a human body is extremely complicated, yet well organized. Basically, it is articulated with hundreds of bones that are covered by soft tissue consisting of muscles, tendons, ligaments, and skin. Such structural complexity makes the exploration of human movement a great challenge.

Fortunately, the primary properties of gross body movement, such as gait, are represented by the bones, although soft tissues undergo various kinds of motions such as stretch, compression, or contraction. Therefore, in this regard, the soft tissues can be ignored and the human body can be considered as a structure that consists only of bones. It should be stressed that soft tissue movement is an important issue in some aspects of gait analysis. However, it is beyond the focus of this book.

Let's take a look at this skeletal body as illustrated in Figure 14-1A. Anatomically, it is still complicated by the facts that (1) every bone has its unique shape, and (2) two adjacent bones are mainly connected through a complicated arrangement of ligaments. Functionally, however—kinematics in particular—it is quite simple. That is, the primary function of the bones is for the transformation of movement from one point of the body to the other, and the function of the connections between the bones is to form a center of rotation so that the two coupled bones can undergo relative rotational movement. Clearly, such functions can be easily replaced by a mechanical structure. For example, a bone could be represented conceptually, without loosing generality, by a rigid mechanical structure, such as a nondeformable cylinder that has identical inertial properties to the bone (see Figure 14-1B), and the articulations could be represented by mechanical joints, such as hinges, ball and socket joints, or universal joints (see Figure 14-1C). Thus, a sophisticated human skeletal structure can be superseded by a simple mechanical system that consists of multiple rigid segments, or links, and joints. Such a mechanical system is called the *rigid body model of the human body.*

For various reasons, a rigid body model of the human body could include different numbers of rigid segments. As an example, a fifteen-segment model is illustrated in Figure 14-2. It includes fifteen links: two feet, two shanks, two thighs, one pelvis, one trunk, two upper arms, two forearms, two hands, and one head; and fourteen joints: two ankles, two knees, two hips, one spinal disc, two shoulders, two elbows, two wrists, and one neck. The model can have more segments by adding flexibility to the foot and the trunk, or have fewer segments by restricting joints such as the ankle or the knee in the lower limb, the elbow or the wrist in the arm, or the spinal disc and the neck in the upper body.

Reference Systems

In order to describe the movement of body segments, it is essential to establish a reference space so that all the description is referred to that space. In general, the reference space is represented by a set of three orthogonal unit vectors, called the Cartesian coordinate system, that is rigidly attached to the space. For gait analysis there are commonly four reference systems: Absolute Reference System, Local Reference System, Segmental Reference System, and Joint Reference System. In the following sections, the definition as well as the determination of these systems will be discussed. It should be noted that no unique, consistent definitions presently exist for these systems. The ones introduced in this chapter are based on the "Recommendations for Standardization in the Reporting of Kinematics Data" proposed by the International Society of Biomechanics.[5]

Absolute Reference System

The Absolute Reference System is also called the Inertial Reference System or Global Reference System.

> *Definition:* A right-handed orthogonal triad $<X, Y, Z>$ fixed in the ground. While a person is standing in an anatomically defined neutral posture, each of the axes is defined as:
> $+X$ axis pointing anteriorly (forward)
> $+Y$ axis pointing superiorly (upward) and in parallel with the field of gravity
> $+Z$ axis pointing rightward

The Absolute Reference System is depicted in Figure 14-3. The directions of the X, Y, and Z axes are chosen so that for those conducting two dimensional studies, X, Y will lie in a sagittal plane. This will be consistent with the three dimensional convention.

Local Reference System

The Local Reference System is also called the Body-Fixed Reference System. It is a Cartesian coordinate system that is fixed to and moves with the body. The three axes in this system may or may not have anatomical meanings. Such a

FIGURE 14-1 **A,** skeletal body structure (From: Gosling JA et al: *Human Anatomy.* 2d ed., 1990, Gower Medical Publishing, 1.11).

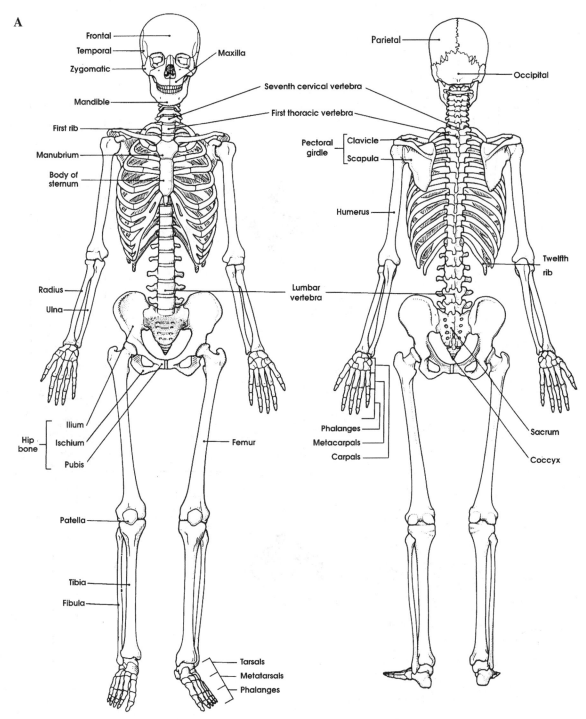

Continued

FIGURE 14-1—CONT'D **B,** a femur and a rigid cylinder. **C,** a knee joint and its mechanical model, a hinge joint.

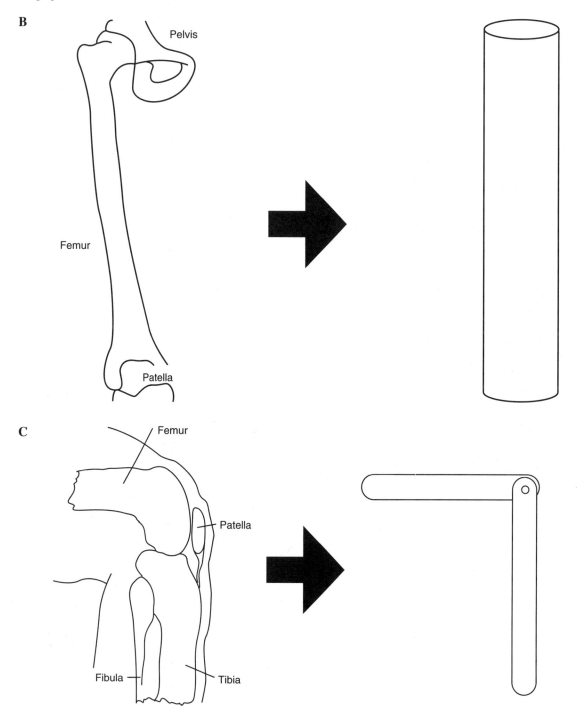

system is needed to describe segmental position and orientation with respect to the Absolute Reference System.

Definition: A right-handed orthogonal triad $\langle X_{Li},$ $Y_{Li}, Z_{Li} \rangle$ fixed to a point on the ith body segment. Although it may seem trivial to define the exact directions of

the axes, we have defined the exact directions of all the axes to keep them consistent throughout the chapter. Thus, the directions of the axes are recommended as:

$+X_{Li}$ axis pointing forward
$+Y_{Li}$ axis pointing upward
$+Z_{Li}$ axis pointing rightward

FIGURE 14-2 A 15-segment rigid body model that includes feet, shanks, thighs, pelvis, trunk, forearms, upper arms, hands, and head.

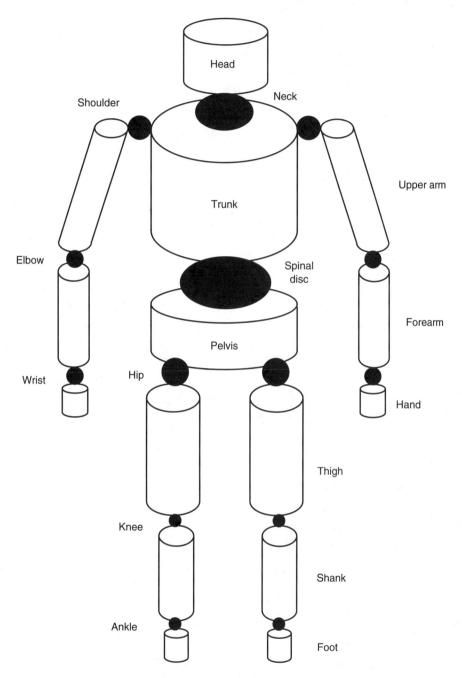

Obviously, the anatomical directions used in the preceding definition refer to the individual body segment, rather than the whole body. Usually, the Local Reference System is established by a group of markers that are attached to the body. They can be attached directly to the body at various locations, or connected to each other to form a rigid segment and then attached to the body segment as a whole. This latter method is called rigid-segment approach. Since the former method is the same as the anatomi-

cal landmark approach, which will be discussed in detail in the section entitled "Segmental Reference System" on page 165, only the rigid-segment approach is described here. Figure 14-4 illustrates a rigid segment i that includes three markers (1, 2, and 3). An Absolute Reference System $<X, Y, Z>$ is first established so that the coordinates of these three markers are known. That is:

$$R^1 = [x^1 \ y^1 \ z^1]^T \qquad (1)$$

Figure 14-3   Definition of Absolute Reference System.

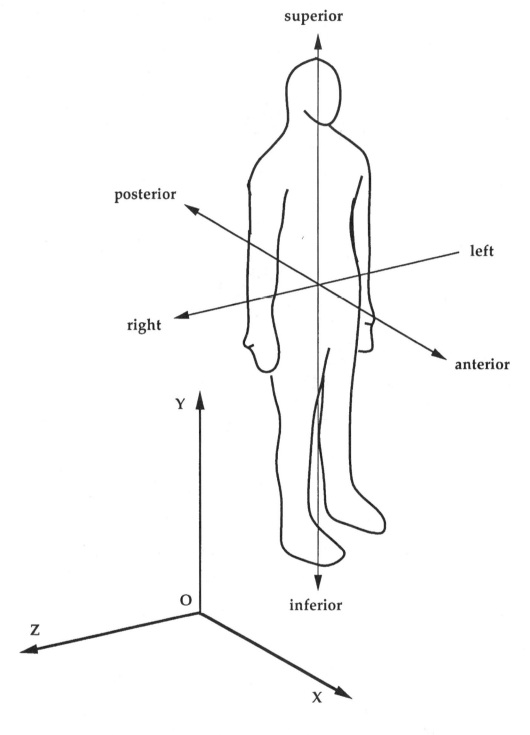

$$R^2 = [x^2 \, y^2 \, z^2]^T \qquad (2)$$

$$R^3 = [x^3 \, y^3 \, z^3]^T \qquad (3)$$

where T denotes the transpose operator to the matrix. Based on these three position vectors the Local Reference System $\langle X_{Li}, Y_{Li}, Z_{Li} \rangle$ can be determined as:

$$R^{1,2} = R^1 - R^2 \qquad (4)$$

$$R^{1,3} = R^1 - R^3 \qquad (5)$$

and

$$Z_{Li} = R^{1,2} / |R^{1,2}| \qquad (6)$$

FIGURE 14-4 Rigid segment with three markers.

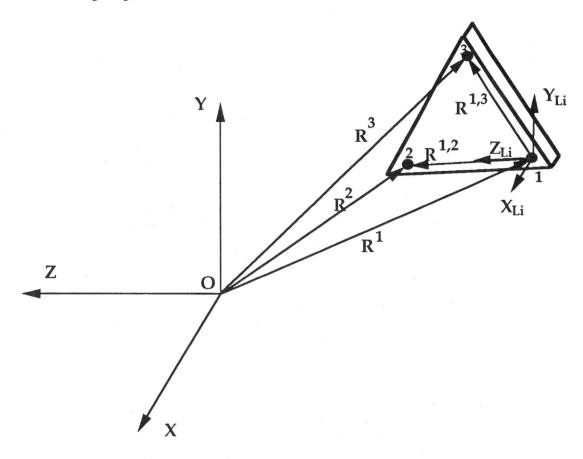

$$X_{Li} = (R^{1,3} \times R^{1,2}) \, / \, |R^{1,3} \times R^{1,2}| \qquad (7)$$

$$Y_{Li} = Z_{Li} \times X_{Li} \qquad (8)$$

There are a few advantages to the rigid-segment approach. First, the rigid segment may include as many markers (more than three) as necessary. Obviously, the more markers involved in the calculation of the Local Reference System, the less noise. Second, the arrangement of the markers can be arbitrary, as long as they are not all connected in a line. This advantage gives great freedom and flexibility to suit an individual's research need. Third, since the markers are rigidly connected, concern about the relative intermarker movement is eliminated. As a result, a relatively reliable and accurate Local Reference System is available. However, the reference system that is established by this approach may lack anatomical representations.

Segmental Reference System

The Segmental Reference System is also called Anatomical Reference System. This system uses Cartesian coordinates that are not only fixed to the body segment, but also have clear anatomical meanings such as proximal-distal, medial-lateral and anterior-posterior.

Definition: A right-handed orthogonal triad <X_{Si}, Y_{Si}, Z_{Si}> fixed to a point on the ith body segment. The directions of the axes are defined as:

  +X_{Si} *axis pointing anteriorly*
  +Y_{Si} *axis pointing proximally*
  +Z_{Si} *axis pointing laterally for the right side of the body segments, and medially for the left side of the body segments*

Needless to say, in order to have the axes represent the anatomical directions, markers that represent anatomical landmarks should be used to define the Segmental Reference System. For example, the landmarks on the shank may include medial and lateral malleoli, tibial turbercle, and femoral epicondyle, and the ones on the foot may include metatarsal heads (first through fifth), heel, and malleoli. Table 14-1 lists some widely used landmarks for pelvis, thigh, shank, and foot.

TABLE 14-1 Commonly used landmarks for the foot, shank, thigh and pelvis, for defining segmental reference systems.

Body segment	Landmarks
Foot	1. Metatarsal heads 2. Heel 3. Medial malleolus 4. Lateral malleolus
Shank	1. Medial malleolus 2. Lateral malleolus 3. Tibial turbercle 4. Lateral femoral epicondyle
Thigh	1. Medial femoral epicondyle 2. Lateral femoral epicondyle 3. Greater trochanter
Pelvis	1. Left anterior superior iliac spine (ASIS) 2. Right ASIS 1. Left posterior superior iliac spine (PSIS) 2. Right PSIS 3. Sacrum

Obviously, the definition of the Segmental Reference System depends heavily on how to choose the landmarks and on how to construct the three orthogonal unit vectors based on the chosen landmarks. Because there is no standard yet on these issues, a consistent reference system for every body segment is not available. Nevertheless, a rule of thumb is that no matter how the landmarks are chosen, *three* points are the minimum number for each body segment in a three-dimensional case, and the three unit vectors should be determined in such a way that they are perpendicular to each other.

Now, let us consider a free body segment *i* (e.g., a shank) moving in space with an Absolute Reference System $<X, Y, Z>$. Three landmark points *a, b,* and *c* are chosen from the segment: *a* is at medial malleolus, *b* is at lateral malleolus, and *c* is at tibial turbercle. Their locations in the Absolute Reference System are known as $R^a, R^b,$ and R^c (see Figure 14-5). Based on these three position vectors we are ready to establish a segmental Reference System $<X_{Si}, Y_{Si}, Z_{Si}>$ in the following way:

$$R^{a,b} = R^a - R^b \qquad (9)$$

$$R^{a,c} = R^a - R^c \qquad (10)$$

and

$$Z_{Si} = R^{a,b} / |R^{a,b}| \qquad (11)$$

$$X_{Si} = (R^{a,c} \times R^{a,b})/|R^{a,c} \times R^{a,b}| \qquad (12)$$

$$Y_{Si} = Z_{Si} \times X_{Si} \qquad (13)$$

Based on Equations 9 through 13 and the landmarks as listed in Table 14-1, a set of Segmental Reference Systems for the pelvis, thigh, shank, and foot can be established.

Overall, the main advantages of the anatomical landmark approach are that some of the axes may have anatomical meanings (i.e., along the anatomical directions of the bones) and that the localization of landmarks is less dependent on personal judgment.

Joint Reference System

A Joint Reference System is a system that is fixed to a joint. It is needed in order to describe the relative movement of the body segments with respect to each other. It allows rotations about axes with anatomical meanings such as flexion-extension, inversion-eversion and adduction-abduction, which are in common usage in clinical medicine. However, such a system may consist of nonorthogonal axes, but as long as force and moment are not resolved along these nonorthogonal axes, this does not present a problem.

Definition: A right-handed triad $<X_{Ji}, Y_{Ji}, Z_{Ji}>$ fixed to a point in the ith joint that connects the ith and the $(i + 1)^{th}$ segments. The axes are defined as:

X_{Ji} axis representing an axis of the $(i + 1)th$ Segmental Reference System

Z_{Ji} axis representing an axis of the ith Segmental Reference System

Y_{Ji} axis representing a floating axis that is the cross product of Z_{Ji} and X_{Ji}.

The Joint Reference System is defined for each joint individually. The most well-known examples of such systems are those developed for the knee by Grood and Suntay[4] and Chao[2] (see Figure 14-6). Two axes in the Segmental Reference Systems are established relative to anatomical landmarks, one in each body segment on opposing sides of the joint. The third axis, or the floating axis, that is perpendicular to each of the two segmental axes is then determined.

TRANSFORMATION BETWEEN REFERENCE SYSTEMS

Reference systems are established for the purpose of describing the movement of a body segment. In general, the same movement may look completely

Figure 14-5 Conceptual diagram of determining the Segmental Reference System via landmark approach.

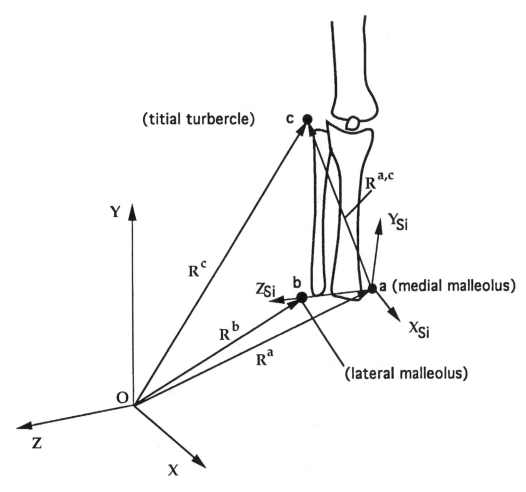

different when it is observed in different reference systems. However, these different descriptions of a single movement are related by the transformation between the reference systems.

Linear Transformation

Without loosing generality, let us assume that a body segment i, with a Local Reference System $<X_{Li}, Y_{Li}, Z_{Li}>$, is moving in a space with Absolute Reference System $<X, Y, Z>$ (see Figure 14-7A). Originally, both reference systems coincide with each other. That is, the origins of the Absolute system (O) and the Local system (O_{Li}), as well as the corresponding axes in both systems overlap. Given an arbitrary point p on the segment, its position in the Absolute Reference System R^p and the Local Reference System R^p_{Li} can be described as:

$$R^p = [x^p \ y^p \ z^p]^T \qquad (14)$$

and

$$R^p_{Li} = [x^p_{Li} \ y^p_{Li} \ z^p_{Li}]^T \qquad (15)$$

Clearly, at time $t = t_0$, we have:

$$R^p = R^p_{Li} \qquad (16)$$

or

$$\begin{bmatrix} x^p \\ y^p \\ z^p \end{bmatrix} = \begin{bmatrix} x^p_{Li} \\ y^p_{Li} \\ z^p_{Li} \end{bmatrix} \qquad (17)$$

Now, let us further assume that the segment i is only moving translationally, that is there is no rotational movement. At time $t = t_n$, the segment, along with the Local Reference System, moves to another location which is represented by the position vector of O_{Li} ($R^{O_{Li}}$) (see Figure 14-7B):

$$R^{O_{Li}} = [x^{O_{Li}} \ y^{O_{Li}} \ z^{O_{Li}}]^T \qquad (18)$$

Figure **14-6** Joint Reference System of the knee.

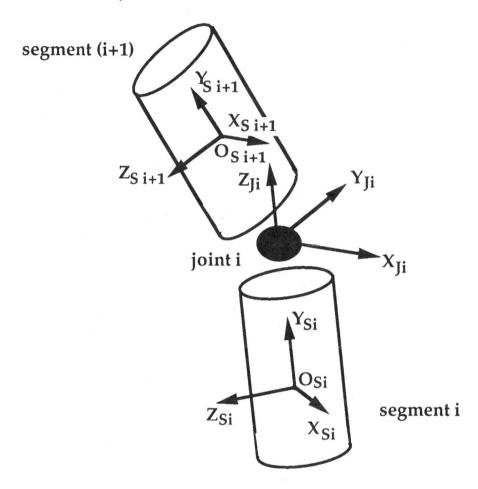

Based on vector algebra, the position of point p that is described in the Local Reference System is related to the one in the Absolute Reference System in the following way:

$$R^p = R_{Li}^p + R^{O_{Li}} \qquad (19)$$

or

$$\begin{bmatrix} x^p \\ y^p \\ z^p \end{bmatrix} = \begin{bmatrix} x_{Li}^p \\ y_{Li}^p \\ z_{Li}^p \end{bmatrix} + \begin{bmatrix} x^{O_{Li}} \\ y^{O_{Li}} \\ z^{O_{Li}} \end{bmatrix} \qquad (20)$$

In order to generalize the description of the linear transformation, it is now necessary to introduce the quatrain or quaternion quantities method. A quatrain is a four-element vector including a spatial vector (three elements) and a scalar (one element). In general, the scalar is taken to be 1. For example, the quatrain form of vector R^p is:

$$R^p = [x^p \; y^p \; z^p \; 1]^T \qquad (21)$$

Now, rearranging Equation 21 in a quaternion format, we obtain:

$$\begin{bmatrix} x^p \\ y^p \\ z^p \\ 1 \end{bmatrix} = \begin{bmatrix} 1 & 0 & 0 & x^{O_{Li}} \\ 0 & 1 & 0 & y^{O_{Li}} \\ 0 & 0 & 1 & z^{O_{Li}} \\ 0 & 0 & 0 & 1 \end{bmatrix} \begin{bmatrix} x_{Li}^p \\ y_{Li}^p \\ z_{Li}^p \\ 1 \end{bmatrix} \qquad (22)$$

We define a 4×4 matrix $\Im_{Li}$ as:

$$\Im_{Li} = \begin{bmatrix} 1 & 0 & 0 & x^{O_{Li}} \\ 0 & 1 & 0 & y^{O_{Li}} \\ 0 & 0 & 1 & z^{O_{Li}} \\ 0 & 0 & 0 & 1 \end{bmatrix} \qquad (23)$$

which is called the linear transformation matrix from the Local Reference System i to the Absolute Reference System.

Expanding the preceding example into a general case, the linear transformation from Reference System II to Reference System I is:

FIGURE 14-7   Linear transformation: **A** at $t = t_0$, both Absolute and Local Reference Systems coincide with each other; **B** at $t = t_n$, Local Reference System translates to another location.

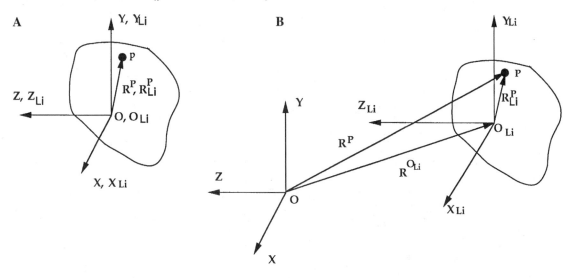

$$\begin{bmatrix} x_I^p \\ y_I^p \\ z_I^p \\ 1 \end{bmatrix} = \begin{bmatrix} 1 & 0 & 0 & x_I^{O_{II}} \\ 0 & 1 & 0 & y_I^{O_{II}} \\ 0 & 0 & 1 & z_I^{O_{II}} \\ 0 & 0 & 0 & 1 \end{bmatrix} \begin{bmatrix} x_{II}^p \\ y_{II}^p \\ z_{II}^p \\ 1 \end{bmatrix}$$

$$= \mathfrak{I}_{I,II} \begin{bmatrix} x_{II}^p \\ y_{II}^p \\ z_{II}^p \\ 1 \end{bmatrix} \qquad (24)$$

where $[x_j^k \quad y_j^k \quad z_j^k \quad 1]^T$ represents the coordinates of point k (k is either an arbitrary point p or the origin of the J Reference System O_J) in the J Reference System (J = I or II).

Rotational Transformation and Euler Angles

Considering the same body segment as shown in Figure 14-8, *A*. Again, at $t = t_0$, two reference systems coincide so that Equations 16 and 17 hold. At $t = t_n$, however, the body segment (or Local Reference System i) has rotated around an axis of the Absolute Reference System, say **Z**, an angle of α (see Figure 14-8B). The coordinates of point p in both reference systems have the following relations:

$$x^p = x_{Li}^p \cos\alpha - y_{Li}^p \sin\alpha \qquad (25)$$
$$y^p = x_{Li}^p \sin\alpha + y_{Li}^p \cos\alpha \qquad (26)$$
$$z^p = z_{Li}^p \qquad (27)$$

or

$$\begin{bmatrix} x^p \\ y^p \\ z^p \\ 1 \end{bmatrix} = \begin{bmatrix} \cos\alpha & -\sin\alpha & 0 & 0 \\ \sin\alpha & \cos\alpha & 0 & 0 \\ 0 & 0 & 1 & 0 \\ 0 & 0 & 0 & 1 \end{bmatrix} \begin{bmatrix} x_{Li}^p \\ y_{Li}^p \\ z_{Li}^p \\ 1 \end{bmatrix}$$

$$= \mathfrak{R}_{Li}^Z \begin{bmatrix} x_{Li}^p \\ y_{Li}^p \\ z_{Li}^p \\ 1 \end{bmatrix} \qquad (28)$$

where

$$\mathfrak{R}_{Li}^Z = \begin{bmatrix} \cos\alpha & -\sin\alpha & 0 & 0 \\ \sin\alpha & \cos\alpha & 0 & 0 \\ 0 & 0 & 1 & 0 \\ 0 & 0 & 0 & 1 \end{bmatrix} \qquad (29)$$

is the rotational transformation matrix from the Local Reference System i to the Absolute Reference System about the **Z** axis. Similarly, the rotation matrices about the **Y** and **X** axes for an

FIGURE 14-8   Rotational transformation.

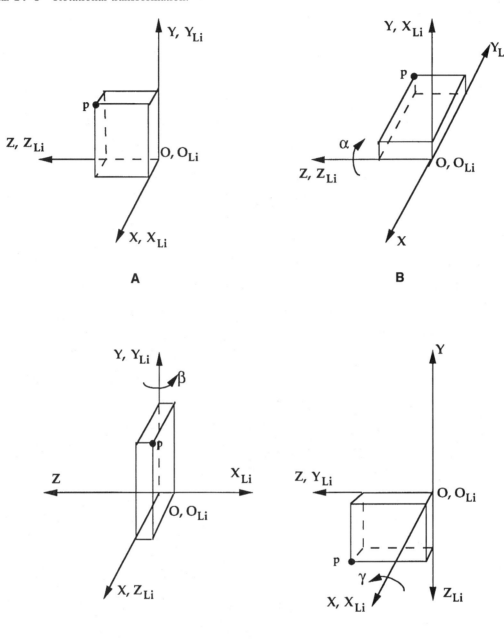

angle of β and γ, respectively, are (see Figures 14-8C and D):

$$\mathfrak{R}_{Li}^{Y} = \begin{bmatrix} \cos\beta & 0 & \sin\beta & 0 \\ 0 & 1 & 0 & 0 \\ -\sin\beta & 0 & \cos\beta & 0 \\ 0 & 0 & 0 & 1 \end{bmatrix} \quad (30)$$

$$\mathfrak{R}_{Li}^{X} = \begin{bmatrix} 1 & 0 & 0 & 0 \\ 0 & \cos\gamma & -\sin\gamma & 0 \\ 0 & \sin\gamma & \cos\gamma & 0 \\ 0 & 0 & 0 & 1 \end{bmatrix} \quad (31)$$

We are now ready to introduce the concept of Euler angles. The Euler angles are three successive rotations φ, θ and ϕ with respect to the Z, the resulting axes X_{Li}, and Z_{Li}, respectively. The final rotational transformation matrix between the Local Reference System $<X_{Li}, Y_{Li}, Z_{Li}>$ and the Absolute Reference System $<X, Y, Z>$ is the product of these three single axis rotational matrices. That is

$$\Re_{Li}^{ZX_{Li}Z_{Li}} = \Re_{Li}^{Z_{Li}}\Re_{Li}^{X_{Li}}\Re_{}^{Z_{}}$$

$$= \begin{bmatrix} c\phi c\varphi - s\phi c\theta s\varphi & -c\phi s\varphi - s\phi c\theta c\varphi \\ s\phi c\varphi + c\phi c\theta s\varphi & -s\phi s\varphi + c\phi c\theta c\varphi \\ s\theta s\varphi & s\theta c\varphi \\ 0 & 0 \end{bmatrix}$$

$$\begin{bmatrix} s\phi s\theta & 0 \\ -c\phi s\theta & 0 \\ c\theta & 0 \\ 0 & 1 \end{bmatrix} \quad (32)$$

where $c\alpha = cos\alpha$ and $s\alpha = sin\alpha$. It should always be kept in mind that such a rotational transformation matrix is sequence dependent. That is, a rotation about Z, X_{Li}, Z_{Li} is different from a series of rotations about X, Z_{Li}, X_{Li} or Y, X_{Li}, Z_{Li}, etc.

Expressing Equation 32 in a generalized form, a sequential rotation of Reference System II to Reference System I about Z_I, Y_{XI}, and Z_{II} axes for an angle of φ, θ and ϕ, respectively, can be described by the following rotational transformation:

$$\begin{bmatrix} x_I^p \\ y_I^p \\ z_I^p \\ 1 \end{bmatrix} = \Re_{I,II}^{Z_IX_{II}Z_{II}} \begin{bmatrix} x_{II}^p \\ y_{II}^p \\ z_{II}^p \\ 1 \end{bmatrix} = \Re_{I,II}^{Z_{II}}\Re_{I,II}^{X_I}\Re_{I,II}^{Z_I} \begin{bmatrix} x_{II}^p \\ y_{II}^p \\ z_{II}^p \\ 1 \end{bmatrix}$$

$$= \begin{bmatrix} c\phi c\varphi - s\phi c\theta s\varphi & -c\phi s\varphi - s\phi c\theta c\varphi \\ s\phi c\varphi + c\phi c\theta s\varphi & -s\phi s\varphi + c\phi c\theta c\varphi \\ s\theta s\varphi & s\theta c\varphi \\ 0 & 0 \end{bmatrix}$$

$$\begin{bmatrix} s\phi s\theta & 0 \\ -c\phi s\theta & 0 \\ c\theta & 0 \\ 0 & 1 \end{bmatrix}\begin{bmatrix} x_{II}^p \\ y_{II}^p \\ z_{II}^p \\ 1 \end{bmatrix} \quad (33)$$

Now, let us consider briefly the inverse transformation, or a transformation from Reference System I to Reference System II in the same sequence of rotation. According to Equation 33, this transformation can be written as:

$$\begin{bmatrix} x_{II}^p \\ y_{II}^p \\ z_{II}^p \\ 1 \end{bmatrix} = \Re_{II,I}^{Z_{II}X_IZ_I} \begin{bmatrix} x_I^p \\ y_I^p \\ z_I^p \\ 1 \end{bmatrix}$$

$$= (\Re_{I,II}^{Z_IX_{II}Z_{II}})^{-1} \begin{bmatrix} x_I^p \\ y_I^p \\ z_I^p \\ 1 \end{bmatrix} \quad (34)$$

or

$$\Re_{II,I}^{Z_{II}X_IZ_I} = (\Re_{I,II}^{Z_IX_{II}Z_{II}})^{-1} \quad (35)$$

Since the rotational transformation matrix is orthogonal, that is, its inverse equals its transpose, therefore, we have:

$$\begin{aligned}\Re_{II,I}^{Z_{II}X_IZ_I} &= (\Re_{I,II}^{Z_IX_{II}Z_{II}})^T \quad (36) \\ &= (\Re_{I,II}^{Z_{II}} \Re_{I,II}^{X_{II}} \Re_{I,II}^{Z_I})^T \\ &= (\Re_{I,II}^{Z_I})^T (\Re_{I,II}^{X_{II}})^T (\Re_{I,II}^{Z_{II}})^T\end{aligned}$$

The relation between the transformation matrices $\Re_{I,II}^{Z_IX_{II}Z_{II}}$ and $\Re_{II,I}^{Z_{II}X_IZ_I}$ as described in Equation 36 is important. It will provide economic computation time.

Transformation Matrix for Both Translation and Rotation

If both translation and rotation occur between two reference systems, as illustrated in Figures 14-7 and 14-8, the transformation matrix is as follows:

$$T_{I,II}^{Z_IX_{II}Z_{II}} = \begin{bmatrix} c\phi c\varphi - s\phi c\theta s\varphi & -c\phi s\varphi - s\phi c\theta c\varphi \\ s\phi c\varphi + c\phi c\theta s\varphi & -s\phi s\varphi + c\phi c\theta c\varphi \\ s\theta s\varphi & s\theta c\varphi \\ 0 & 0 \end{bmatrix}$$

$$\begin{bmatrix} s\phi s\theta & x_I^{O_{II}} \\ -c\phi s\theta & y_I^{O_{II}} \\ c\theta & z_I^{O_{II}} \\ 0 & 1 \end{bmatrix} \quad (37)$$

Determination of Rotational Transformation Based on Markers

In most of the cases of gait analysis study, the angular movement between two reference systems (i.e., the angles α, β and γ) is unknown, whereas the coordinates of a few points on the body segment are known with respect to the Local and Absolute Reference Systems. Now the question is how to calculate the transformation matrix based on these known coordinates. Since translational transformation is straightforward, this section will focus only on the derivation of rotational transformation.

According to Equation 33, the coordinates of an arbitrary point p on a body segment in Reference Systems I and II that undergo a pure rotation with respect to each other are related by a transformation matrix $\mathfrak{R}_{I,II}^{Z_I X_{II} Z_{II}}$. That is,

$$
\begin{bmatrix} x_I^p \\ y_I^p \\ z_I^p \\ 1 \end{bmatrix} = \mathfrak{R}_{I,II}^{Z_I X_{II} Z_{II}} \begin{bmatrix} x_{II}^p \\ y_{II}^p \\ z_{II}^p \\ 1 \end{bmatrix} \tag{38}
$$

In fact, Equation 38 holds for any point on the body. Given a total of n points, the relations between their coordinates in both reference systems can be written as

$$
\begin{bmatrix} x_I^1 & x_I^2 & \dots & x_I^i & \dots x_I^n \\ y_I^1 & y_I^2 & \dots & y_I^i & \dots y_I^i \\ z_I^1 & z_I^2 & \cdots & z_I^i & \dots z_I^n \\ 1 & I & \cdots & 1 & \dots 1 \end{bmatrix}
$$

$$
= \mathfrak{R}_{I,II}^{Z_I X_{II} Z_{II}} \begin{bmatrix} x_{II}^1 & x_{II}^2 & \dots & x_I^i & \dots x_{II}^n \\ y_{II}^1 & y_{II}^2 & \dots & y_{II}^i & \dots y_{II}^i \\ z_{II}^1 & z_{II}^2 & \cdots & z_{II}^i & \dots z_{II}^n \\ 1 & I & \cdots & 1 & \dots 1 \end{bmatrix} \tag{39}
$$

or

$$
\Gamma_I = \mathfrak{R}_{I,II}^{Z_I X_{II} Z_{II}} \Gamma_{II} \tag{40}
$$

where Γ_I and Γ_{II} represent the position matrices on the left and the right sides of the equation, respectively. Since these two position matrices are known (usually through direct measurements), the rotational transformation matrix $\mathfrak{R}_{I,II}^{Z_I X_{II} Z_{II}}$ can then be determined. Two restrictions, however, are imposed in order to attain unique solution: (1) there should be a minimum of three points (i.e., $n \geq 3$); and (2) these points are not linearly connected (i.e., in a line).

Usually, $\mathfrak{R}_{I,II}^{Z_I X_{II} Z_{II}}$ in Equation 40 is solved by the least square approach, or it can be solved by the following equation:

$$
\mathfrak{R}_{I,II}^{Z_I X_{II} Z_{II}} = \Gamma_I \Gamma_{II}^T (\Gamma_{II} \Gamma_{II}^T)^{-1} \tag{41}
$$

Concept of Screw Theory

The transformations between coodinate systems that are described in the preceding sections are based on the Cartesian coordinates. It should be mentioned that such transformations can also be described using Plücker coordinates. Similar to the Cartesian coordinate, which describes the motion of an arbitrary point in space by vectors, the Plücker coordinate describes the motion of a point in space by screws, called screw motion or helical motion. Accordingly, the theory that concerns the operations of screws is called screw theory.

Occasionally, the screw theory is applied to gait analysis. Since its use is rare, a detailed discussion on this topic is not provided in this book. Interested readers can refer to the references by Shiavi et al.[13] and by McCarthy.[7]

DEFINITION OF KINEMATIC VARIABLES

A free rigid body moving in a three-dimensional space has a total of six degrees of freedom: three linear movements and three rotational movements. The status of such movement can be completely described by the following variables: displacement, velocity, and acceleration.

Displacement

Displacement describes the change in position of the body relative to a reference system. The change that is in a translational fashion is called linear displacement, whereas the change that is in a rotational fashion is called angular displacement.

When the displacement of a body segment is presented relative to the Absolute Reference System, it describes the absolute movement of the body. However, such a description rarely has anatomical meanings. Usually, in gait analysis, the displacement of a body segment is presented either with respect to another body segment to describe their relative movement, or in a Joint Reference System to describe the joint movement. Nevertheless, no matter which reference system is used to present the displacement, it should be kept in mind that these representations are interrelated and transformable.

Velocity

The velocity of a movement describes the speed of the change in position. For example, when a person moves from point A to point B in space, it could take 1 minute to complete the move if the person moves quickly or 10 minutes if the person moves slowly. The velocity is defined as the amount of change in position per unit time. If the position change is linear, the velocity is called the linear velocity. Likewise, if the position change is in rotation, the velocity is called angular velocity.

It should be stressed that the linear velocity depends on the location on the body segment, whereas the angular velocity does not. For example, during gait, the velocities at the proximal and distal ends of the shank are, for most of the time, different. However, the linear velocities at two different locations are closely related. The relation is expressed by the following equation:

$$V_L^p = V_L^q + \Omega_L \times R_L^{p,q} \qquad (42)$$

where V_L^p and V_L^q are the absolute linear velocity vectors at points p and q on one body segment, respectively; Ω_L is the angular velocity vector of the body segment; and $R_L^{p,q}$ is the position vector between these two points. The subscript L indicates that the variable is expressed in the Local Reference System. Of course, Equation 42 also holds if all the variables are expressed in the Segmental Reference System. Therefore, as long as the velocity at one point of the rigid body is known, the velocities at other locations of the body can be determined.

Acceleration

Acceleration describes the speed of change in velocity. It is defined as the change in velocity per unit time. As with displacement and velocity, there are linear and angular accelerations as well. Also, the linear acceleration is location dependent. The relation between the linear accelerations at two arbitrary points on a body segment is as follows:

$$a_L^p = a_L^q + \alpha_L \times R_L^{p,q} + 2\Omega_L \times \frac{dR_L^{p,q}}{dt} + \Omega_L$$
$$\times (\Omega_L \times R_L^{p,q}) \qquad (43)$$

where a_L^p and a_L^q are the linear accelerations at points p and q, respectively, and α_L is the angular acceleration of the body segment.

DIRECT MEASUREMENT OF KINEMATIC VARIABLES

Direct Measurement of Displacement

Perhaps the direct measurement of displacement of body segment (including linear and angular displacement) is the most popular approach in the field of gait analysis.[1,11,15] There are many commercially available kinds of equipment, such as goniometry and video imaging techniques, for such purposes. The chapter by Koff will discuss imaging systems in detail.

Direct Measurement of Acceleration

Direct measurement of acceleration requires the use of accelerometers. Although some accelerometers measure angular acceleration, most of them are for linear acceleration measurement.[3,8,11,17]

Although the measurements of both linear displacement and linear acceleration are location dependent, the linear acceleration measurement is also orientation dependent under the influence of the field of gravity. For example, while an accelerometer is held stationary with its sensitive axis pointing vertically downward (i.e., along the direction of the gravity), its reading corresponds to 9.8 m/s^2 (or 1g). If it is rotated 90° so that its sensitive axis is perpendicular to the line of gravity, its reading is 0. Clearly, the output from the accelerometer depends heavily on its orientation.

Of course, such a problem may be avoided by using an accelerometer with a dynamic range above $0 \, Hz$ so that it is not sensitive to constant acceleration. However, this implies that not only the constant gravity acceleration will be eliminated, but some other constant accelerations that might be important in describing the movement of a body segment will be eliminated as well.

In addition to the orientation problem, the accelerometry approach is also concerned with the weight and size of accelerometers and with the vibration of soft tissue. Therefore, its application in the field of gait analysis is limited.

Direct Measurement of Multiple Variables

Each of the two previously mentioned direct measurements involves either displacement or acceleration. In order to derive other kinematic variables (such as velocity, etc.) based on these measurements, either differentiation or integration computation is needed (see the following section on Calculation of Kinematic Variables). Another approach, called the Integrated Kinematic measurement,[6,12,17] has been used to directly measure a set of kinematic variables such as displacement, angular velocity, and linear acceleration.

The goal of the Integrated Kinematic measurement is to make necessary direct measurements of certain kinematic variables in order to achieve maximal accuracy in defining completely the status of movement of a rigid body segment. It was proposed that the following variables be measured: the displacements of at least three points on a rigid body segment, the angular velocity of the segment, and the linear acceleration of one point on the body. For detailed derivation of the complete set of kinematics, refer to the publication by Wu and Ladin.[17]

CALCULATION OF KINEMATIC VARIABLES

Direct Approach

Linear Displacement   Usually, the direct measurement of linear displacement is via imaging, which records and then determines the coordinates of certain points on a rigid body in the Absolute Reference System. That is, given a total of n points on a body segment, their coordinates are directly measured as $[x^i, y^i, z^i]^T$ $(i = 1, 2, \ldots, n)$.

At a location j other than those n points (i.e., $j \neq i$), its linear displacement can be determined as:

$$R^j = R^i + R^{i,j} \qquad (44)$$

where $R^{i,j}$ is the displacement vector of point j with respect to point i in the Absolute Reference System (see Figure 14-9). On the other hand, since we model body segments as rigid, that is, there is no deformation or relative movement between any points on the body, the position vector from points i to j is constant in the Local Reference System, say, k. That is, $R_{Lk}^{i,j}$ is constant. According to Equations 39 and 41, as long as $n \geq 3$ and noncolinearly arranged, the transformation matrix T_{Lk} from Local Reference System, k, to the Absolute Reference System can be calculated. Thus, the position vector $R^{i,j}$ can be determined based on Equation 38. Finally, Equation 44 is rewritten as

$$R^j = R^i + T_{Lk}R_{Lk}^{i,j} \qquad (45)$$

where R^i is directly measured, T_{Lk} is calculated based on R^i $(i = 1, 2, \ldots, n; n > 3)$, and $R_{Lk}^{i,j}$ is given or known.

Angular Displacement   The most direct method of obtaining angular displacement of a body segment with respect to another body segment is the measurement by goniometer, a transducer whose output is proportional to the relative angular movement of two linkages. In gait analysis, such measurement is commonly done around joints. Therefore, the measured angular movement is in the Joint Reference System.

Another method of obtaining angular displacements of a rigid body is based on the direct measurement of displacements at multiple points on the body (as discussed in linear displacement in the previous section). The procedure is as follows: (1) to determine the rotational transformation matrix from the Local Reference System (e.g., k) to the Absolute Reference System (Equation 41), as long as there are three or more noncolinear points on this body segment whose coordinates are known; (2) to define a sequence of rotation from the Local Reference System, k, to the Absolute Reference System and calculate the final transformation matrix based on single axis transformations that are given by Equations 28, 30, and 31. For example, Equation 32 gives the final transformation for the rotation sequence of Z, X_{Li} and Z_{Li} axes, respectively; and (31), to determine the angular displacements of the body segment $\{\varphi, \theta, \phi\}$ with respect to the axes in the Absolute Reference

---

FIGURE 14-9   Linear displacement at point j based on point i.

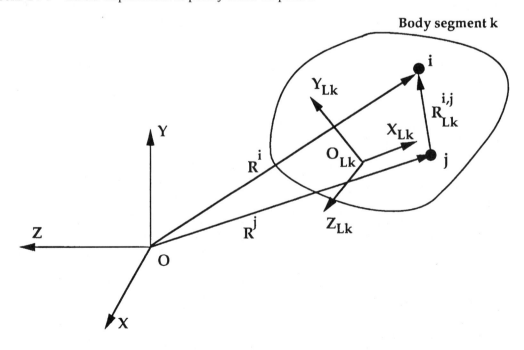

System. Taking Equation 32 as an example, the Euler angles {φ, θ, φ} are determined as:

$$\varphi = \arctan\left[\frac{\Re^{ZX_{Lk}Z_{Lk}}_{Lk}(1,3)}{\Re^{ZX_{Lk}Z_{Lk}}_{Lk}(2,3)}\right] \tag{46}$$

$$\theta = \arccos[\Re^{ZX_{Lk}Z_{Lk}}_{Lk}(3,3)] \tag{47}$$

$$\phi = -\arctan\left[\frac{\Re^{ZX_{Lk}Z_{Lk}}_{Lk}(3,1)}{\Re^{ZX_{Lk}Z_{Lk}}_{Lk}(3,2)}\right] \tag{48}$$

where $\Re^{ZX_{Lk}Z_{Lk}}_{Lk}(l,m)$ is an element that is located at the lth row and mth column of matrix $\Re^{ZX_{Lk}Z_{Lk}}_{Lk}$. Euler angles φ, θ and φ are the angular displacements of the body segment around the Z, X_{Li}, and Z_{Li} axes, respectively. Note that the above derivation can be easily modified so that the calculated angular displacements can be expressed not only in the Absolute Reference System, but also in the Segmental Reference System or in the Joint Reference System.

So far, we have discussed the calculation of the three-dimensional angular displacements of a body segment in space. For a plane motion, however, the calculation can be simplified. Let us now consider a case in which the knee flexion-extension angle is to be calculated. One can, of course, use the procedures that are described in the previous paragraph and Equations 46 through 48. But there are other alternatives.

Let us assume that, without losing generality, the shank and the thigh are moving in a plane defined as $<X, Y>$, and each of the segments is modeled by a line that connects the distal and proximal joints of the segment (i.e., the ankle and knee joints for the shank and the knee and hip joints for the thigh). Also, each of the three joints can be represented by a single marker that is directly attached to the lateral malleolus, tibial turbercle, and greater trochanter, respectively (see Figure 14-10). Given that the positions of these three markers are known through direct measurement, they are

at ankle: $\boldsymbol{R}^a = [x^a\ y^a\ z^a]^T \tag{49}$

at knee: $\boldsymbol{R}^k = [x^k\ y^k\ z^k]^T \tag{50}$

and at hip: $\boldsymbol{R}^h = [x^h\ y^h\ z^a]^T \tag{51}$

Then, the angular displacement of the knee joint, θ^k, that is defined as the relative angle between the shank and the thigh segments can be calculated as

$$\theta^k = 180° - \theta \tag{52}$$

FIGURE 14-10 Illustration of calculation of knee joint angular displacement in the X,Y plane.

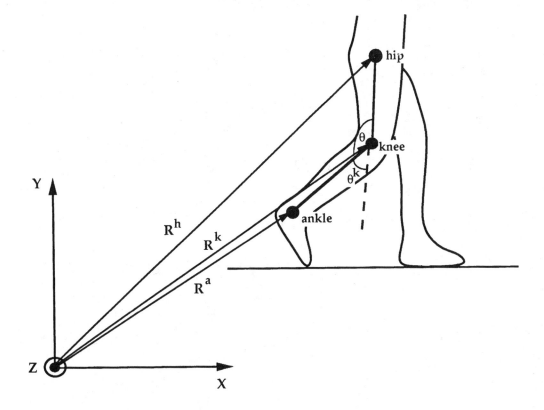

where

$$\theta = \arccos\left(\frac{|R^{a,k}|^2 + |R^{k,h}|^2 - |R^{a,h}|^2}{2|R^{a,k}||R^{k,h}|}\right) \qquad (53)$$

and

$$|R^{i,j}| = \sqrt{(x^j - x^i)^2 + (y^j - y^i)^2} \qquad (54)$$

It is important to note that most kinematic data collected until recently utilized this joint marker approach.[8,13]

Angular Velocity   The angular velocity of a body segment with respect to the Absolute Reference System can be directly measured by a transducer, called angular rate sensor.[17] Arranging three single axis sensors in such a way so that their sensitive axes are orthogonal to each other, three orthogonal components of the angular velocity are attained.

There are two important aspects that one should keep in mind. First, one should remember that unlike linear movement, which is location dependent, the angular movement is independent of location. That is, one rigid body has only one angular velocity vector regardless of where the observation point is. This characteristic implies that it does not matter where the sensors are located on the body segment. Second, since the sensors are attached to and moving with the body segment, the outputs from the three orthogonal

axes correspond to three components that are along the axes of either the Local or the Segmental Reference System. The components along the absolute axes can be calculated when the rotational transformation from either the Local or the Segmental Reference System to the Absolute Reference System is known.

Linear Acceleration   The direct measurement of linear acceleration is accomplished through accelerometers. However, unless one uses the kind of accelerometer that has a dynamic range of above 0 Hz (i.e., not sensitive to constant or slow-changing acceleration), the direct output from a single accelerometer is always contaminated by the gravity acceleration.

One of the methods of eliminating the gravity acceleration component in the measurement is to use multiple (at least two) accelerometers. Let's take a look at the situation along one direction. Assume that two single axis accelerometers are located at points 1 and 2, respectively, with their sensitive axes arranged in such a way that they are parallel with respect to each other, but have an angle of η with respect to the field of gravity (see Figure 14-11). Then, the outputs from these two accelerometers ($\hat{a}^1$ and $\hat{a}^2$) are

$$\hat{a}^1 = a^1 + g\cos\eta \qquad (55)$$

$$\hat{a}^2 = a^2 + g\cos\eta \qquad (56)$$

Figure 14-11   Two accelerometers that are arranged in parallel.

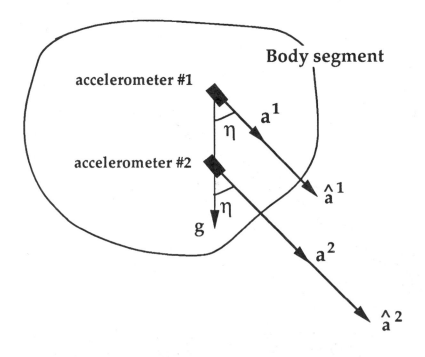

where a^i is the true acceleration at point i ($i = 1$, 2), and g is the gravity acceleration. Subtracting Equation 55 from Equation 56, the acceleration difference between points 1 and 2 is obtained as:

$$\Delta \hat{a}^{1,2} = \hat{a}^2 - \hat{a}^1 = a^2 - a^1 \tag{57}$$

As a result, the gravity acceleration term is crossed out. Clearly, this acceleration difference depends heavily on where those two points are located. If one of the points (say, point 1) is chosen at the center of rotation of the body segment (pure rotation), then $\Delta \hat{a}^{1,2} = a^2$. On the other hand, if those two points are located too close to each other in distance, then $\Delta \hat{a}^{1,2} \to 0$ might occur.

Differential Approach

This approach refers to the calculation of kinematic variables that utilizes the differentiation or time derivative technique. That is, given a time series $x(t)$, its first time derivative results in another time series $y(t)$ as:

$$y(t) = \frac{dx(t)}{dt} \tag{58}$$

Or in a discrete form:

$$y(n) = \frac{\Delta x(n)}{\Delta t} = \frac{x(n) - x(n-1)}{\Delta t} \tag{59}$$

where n stands for the nth sample at Δt interval each.

According to the definition of velocity and acceleration, they are either the first order or the second order derivatives of the displacements. That is

linear velocity: $\quad V^i = \dfrac{dR^i}{dt} \tag{60}$

linear acceleration: $\quad a^i = \dfrac{dV^i}{dt} = \dfrac{d^2 R^i}{dt^2} \tag{61}$

angular velocity: $\quad \Omega = \dfrac{d\Theta}{dt} \tag{62}$

angular acceleration: $\quad \alpha = \dfrac{d\Omega}{dt} = \dfrac{d^2\Theta}{dt} \tag{63}$

where R^i, V^i and a^i are the position, linear velocity, and linear acceleration vectors at point i; and Θ, Ω, and α are the angular rotation, angular velocity, and angular acceleration vectors of the body segment. If, for example, the displacement vector, R^i, is known via direct measurements, the rest of the kinematic variables, such as velocities and accelerations, can be easily obtained. However, one should keep in mind that the differentiation process tends to amplify high frequency noises. As a

result, an additional process such as low-pass filtering is always necessary. This point will be discussed in detail in the section on noise analysis and treatment in the kinematic data.

Integral Approach

The integral approach refers to the calculation of kinematic variables via integration. The inverse process of integration is differentiation. Thus, given a time series $x(t)$, its time integral results in another time series $y(t)$ as:

$$y(t) = \int_{u=t_0}^{t} x(u)du = \int x(t)dt + y(t_0) \tag{64}$$

Or in a discrete form:

$$y(n) = \sum_{i=0}^{n} x(i)\Delta t = y(n-1) + x(n)\Delta t \tag{65}$$

where n stands for the nth sample at Δt interval each, and $y(t_0)$ is called the initial condition.

Given the angular acceleration vector of a body segment α and the linear acceleration vector at point i on the body a^i, one can calculate the velocity and displacement vectors through integration:

linear velocity: $\quad V^i = \int a^i \, dt + V^i(t_0) \tag{66}$

linear displacement: $\quad R^i = \int V^i dt + R^i(t_0)$
$$= \iint a^i \, dt^2 + V^i(t_0)t + R^i(t_0) \tag{67}$$

angular velocity: $\quad \Omega = \int \alpha \, dt + \Omega(t_0) \tag{68}$

angular displacement: $\quad \Theta = \int \Omega dt + \Omega(t_0)$
$$= \iint \alpha \, dt^2 + \Omega(t_0)t + \Theta(t_0) \tag{69}$$

Likewise, the integration process also amplifies noise. However, the low frequency noise, rather than the high frequency noise, is amplified. Again, this point will be discussed in more detail in the following section on noise analysis.

It is worth mentioning here that the integration process requires the knowledge of initial status of the movement, or initial condition. This could be a problem in gait analysis because it is difficult to estimate the status of velocity and displacement of a body segment in the middle of a gait unless assumptions are made.

NOISE ANALYSIS AND TREATMENT IN KINEMATIC DATA

Differentiation

Given that a signal $\hat{x}(t)$ represents the measurement of a time varying variable $x(t)$ that changes sinusoidally with frequency of ω_0, usually there are noises from the measurement chain that tend to contaminate the measurement. Assuming that, without loosing generality, the noise $n(t)$ has one frequency component ω_n, therefore, $\hat{x}(t)$ has two components:

$$\hat{x}(t) = x(t) + n(t) = A_0\sin(\omega_0 t) + N_n\sin(\omega_n t) \quad (70)$$

where A_0 is the magnitude of the variable to be measured, and N_n is the magnitude of the noise. The signal-to-noise ratio of the measurement $\hat{x}(t)$, denoted as $S/N|_{\hat{x}}$, is defined as the ratio of the magnitude of the signal $x(t)$ to the magnitude of the noise $n(t)$. That is

$$S/N|_{\hat{x}} = \frac{A_0}{N_n} \quad (71)$$

Taking the first time derivative of the signal $\hat{x}(t)$, we have:

$$\hat{x}'(t) = x'(t) + n'(t)$$
$$= A_0\omega_0\cos(\omega_0 t) + N_n\omega_n\cos(\omega_n t) \quad (72)$$

It can be seen that the magnitudes of both the signal and the noise are changed by a factor of the corresponding frequency. Hence the S/N ratio becomes:

$$S/N|_{\hat{x}'} = \frac{A_0\omega_0}{N_n\omega_n} = \left(\frac{\omega_0}{\omega_n}\right)S/N|_{\hat{x}} \quad (73)$$

which is $\left(\dfrac{\omega_0}{\omega_n}\right)$ times of the S/N ratio for the original measurement $\hat{x}(t)$. In general, the S/N ratio

after taking the kth time derivative of signal $\hat{x}(t)$ has the following relation with that of the original measurement:

$$S/N|_{\hat{x}(k)} = \left(\frac{\omega_0}{\omega_n}\right)^k S/N|_{\hat{x}} \quad (74)$$

In the situation where the frequency of the noise is higher than that of the signal (i.e., $\omega_n > \omega_0$), the S/N ratio after differentiation would be smaller than that of the original measurement. For example, if we assume that for the original measurement the S/N ratio is 0.1 and that the frequency of the noise is 10 times higher than that of the signal, then the magnitude of the noise will equal the magnitude of the signal after first time derivative and will be 10 times larger than the signal after second time derivative. Figure 14-12 shows the time trajectories of these signals. Clearly, this high frequency noise amplification after the differentiation process is a serious problem in gait analysis and should be treated cautiously.

The most popular approach to treating this problem is low-pass filtering. That is, prior to any differentiation process, apply a filter to the measured signal that allows only the low frequency components to pass through. One of the filters that are commonly used in gait analysis is the higher order (e.g., 4th order) Butterworth filter. In order to compensate for the phase shift, the filter is usually applied twice to the signal, i.e., once

FIGURE 14-12   Time trajectories of three signals: original signal $\hat{x}(t) = x(t) + n(t) = \sin(t) + 0.1\sin(10t)$ and its first and second time derivatives.

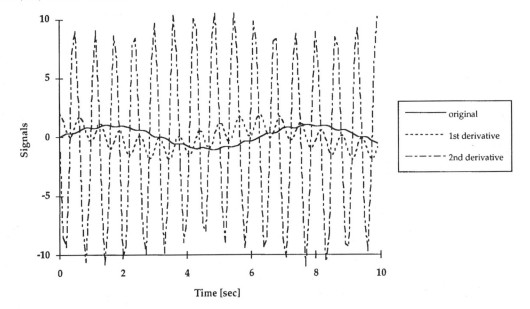

forward and once backward. The bandwidth of the low-pass filter should be chosen carefully so that the output from the filter includes as many of the frequency components as possible in the variable that is measured and as few as possible of the frequency components in the noise. Since the topic on filtering technique is beyond the scope of this book, interested readers should refer to other books that deal with signal processing. A few recommmended books are Oppenheim and Schafer[10] and Winter.[16]

Integration

Now, let us take a look at the integration process. Taking the same measurement $\hat{x}(t)$ as in Equation 70, the time integration is:

$$\int \hat{x} = \int x + \int n = -\frac{A_0}{\omega_0} \cos(\omega_0 t)$$
$$-\frac{N_n}{\omega_n} \cos(\omega_n t) \tag{75}$$

and the S/N ratio becomes:

$$S/N_{\int \hat{x}} = \left(\frac{\omega_n}{\omega_0}\right) S/N_{\hat{x}} \tag{76}$$

Clearly, the S/N also depends on the frequency ratio as the differentiation process does. In general, the S/N ratio after k^{th} integration can be expressed as

$$S/N_{\underbrace{\int ... \int \hat{x}}_{k}} = \left(\frac{\omega_n}{\omega_0}\right)^k S/N_{\hat{x}} \tag{77}$$

In contrast to the differentiation process, the integration process tends to amplify the low frequency noise. For example, if the noise frequency is 10 times smaller than the signal frequency, then the noise will be amplified 100 times compared to the signal after a double integration (see Figure 14-13). In fact, low frequency noise, such as DC drift, does exist in the direct measurement of acceleration by accelerometers. Therefore, particular attention should be devoted to this problem.

As with the differentiation approach, a filtering process is usually applied to the original signal before integration. However, instead of a low-pass filter that allows only the low frequency components to pass through, a high-pass or a band-pass filter is needed for integration. While a high-pass filter allows high frequency components to pass through, a band-pass filter passes through only those components whose frequencies are within the band of the filter. Again, the bandwidth of either the high-pass or the band-pass filter should be decided according to the gait activity that is under investigation as well as the quality of the measurement.

Optimal Design of Kinematic Measurement

Based on our previous analyses, it is clear that the differentiation process tends to amplify high frequency noise, whereas the integration process tends to amplify low frequency noise. It seems that the direct measurement is perhaps a best solution,

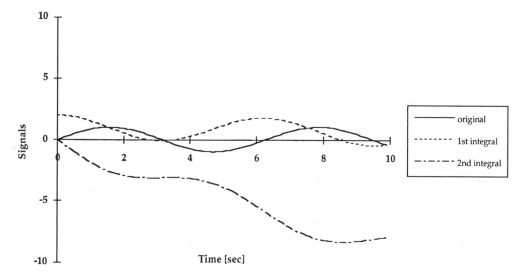

FIGURE 14-13 Time trajectories of three signals: original signal $\hat{x}(t) = x(t) + n(t) = \sin(t) + 0.1\sin(0.1t)$ and its first and second time integrals.

if the noise level can be controlled and if the direct measurement can be done. The latter condition is of particular concern in gait analysis since measuring all of the kinematic variables directly will be extremely expensive. Moreover, some of the variables cannot be directly measured because of physical constraints. For example, one of the important kinematic variables in studying gait dynamics is the acceleration at the center of mass (COM) of the body segment. Usually, this COM is located inside the body segment. Obviously, it is impossible to directly measure the acceleration at this point unless one is willing to drill a hole into the body so that an accelerometer can be mounted there. Now, a gait analyst might be challenged by at least one question: how to design an optimal measurement scheme so that the error in the desired kinematic variable is minimized?

To answer this question, let us continue to work on the COM acceleration problem. First, according to Equation 43, the acceleration at an arbitrary point p on a rigid body is related to the acceleration at the COM of the body by the following equation:

$$a_L^p = a_L^{COM} + \alpha_L \times R_L^p + 2\Omega_L \times \frac{dR_L^p}{dt} + \Omega_L \times (\Omega_L \times R_L^p) \qquad (78)$$

where R_L^p is the position vector from point p to COM that is expressed in the Local Reference System, Ω_L and α_L are the absolute angular velocity and the acceleration vectors, respectively, of the body segment that are expressed in the Local Reference System. Note that since all the variables in Equation 78 are expressed in the Local Reference System, the subscript L will be omitted in the following description.

Rearranging Equation 78 and taking into account that the body segment is modeled as rigid, thus, $\frac{dR_L^p}{dt} = 0$, the acceleration at the COM of the body segment is obtained as:

$$a^{COM} = a^p - \alpha \times R^p - \Omega \times (\Omega \times R^p) \qquad (79)$$

Now, we are at a position to evaluate the error in computing a^{COM} based on various approaches.

First, let us assume that each kinematic variable is either directly measured or calculated (except for R^p because it is a constant). Thus, each estimated variable has a noise component n. That is

$$\hat{a}^p = a^p + n_a \qquad (80)$$

$$\hat{\alpha} = \alpha + n_\alpha \qquad (81)$$

$$\hat{\Omega} = \Omega + n_\alpha \qquad (82)$$

Replacing these estimated variables into Equation 80, we have:

$$\begin{aligned}
\hat{a}^{COM} &= \hat{a}^p - \hat{\alpha} \times R^p - \hat{\Omega} \times (\hat{\Omega} \times R^p) \qquad (83) \\
&= (a^p + n_a) - (\alpha + n_\alpha) \times R^p - (\Omega \\
&\quad + n_\Omega) \times [(\Omega + n_\Omega) \times R^p] \\
&= a^p - \alpha \times R^p - \Omega \times (\Omega \times R^p) \\
&\quad + [n_a - n_\alpha \times R^p - \Omega \times (n_\Omega \times R^p) \\
&\quad - n_\Omega \times (\Omega \times R^p) - n_\Omega \times (n_\Omega \times R^p)] \\
&= a^{COM} + \Delta a^{COM}
\end{aligned}$$

where

$$\begin{aligned}
\Delta a^{COM} &= n_a - n_a \times R^p - \Omega \times (n_\Omega \times R^p) \\
&\quad - n_\Omega \times (\Omega \times R^p) - n_\Omega \\
&\quad \times (n_\Omega \times R^p) \qquad (84)
\end{aligned}$$

is the error in the calculation of COM acceleration. In the worst situation, the maximum error can be determined as

$$|\Delta a^{COM}| \leq |n_a| + |n_\alpha||R^p| + 2|\Omega||n_\Omega||R^p| \\ + |n_\Omega|^2|R^p| \qquad (85)$$

Second, let us consider the following cases:

Case 1: Direct measurement—all three kinematic variables that are listed in Equations 80 through 82 are directly measured. Assuming that the noises are white and identical, their magnitudes are constant and independent of frequency:

$$|n_\alpha| = |n_a| = |n_\Omega| = N \qquad (86)$$

Case 2: Differentiation—all three variables are obtained through first- or second-order differentiation based on the direct measurement of position, which has the same kind of white noise. Then, noises for the velocity and accelerations are, according to Equation 74, proportional to the frequency of the noise. That is:

$$|n_\Omega| = N\omega_n \qquad (87)$$

$$|n_a| = |n_\alpha| = N\omega_n^2 \qquad (88)$$

Case 3: Integration—the angular velocity is obtained by integration of the angular acceleration which, along with the linear acceleration, is directly measured. The noises for the accelerations are white, and the noise for the velocity is, according to Equation 76, inversely proportional to the frequency of the noise. That is

$$|n_a| = |n_\alpha| = N \qquad (89)$$

$$|n_\Omega| = \frac{N}{\varphi_n} \qquad (90)$$

FIGURE 14-14 Errors in computing the linear acceleration at the COM of a body segment.

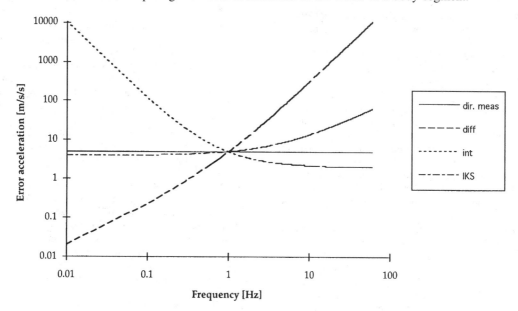

Case 4: Integrated approach—the angular velocity and linear acceleration are directly measured, along with white noise, and the angular velocity is obtained by differentiating the angular velocity. Therefore, the noises are

$$|\boldsymbol{n}_a| = |\boldsymbol{n}_\Omega| = N \tag{91}$$

$$|\boldsymbol{n}_\alpha| = N\omega_n \tag{92}$$

Now let us substitute Equation 85 with Equations 86 through 92 accordingly, the maximum error for each of the four cases is derived as following:

Case 1: $|\Delta a^{\text{COM}}| \leq (1 + |R^p| + 2|\boldsymbol{\Omega}||R^p|)N$
$$+ |R^p|N^2 \tag{93}$$

Case 2: $|\Delta a^{\text{COM}}| \leq 2|\boldsymbol{\Omega}||R^p|N\omega_n + (1 + |R^p|$
$$+ N|R^p|)N\omega_n^2 \tag{94}$$

Case 3: $|\Delta a^{\text{COM}}| \leq (1 + R^p|)N + \dfrac{2|\boldsymbol{\Omega}||R^p|N}{\omega_n}$
$$+ \dfrac{|R^p|N^2}{\omega_n^2} \tag{95}$$

Case 4: $|\Delta a^{\text{COM}}| \leq (1 + 2|\boldsymbol{\Omega}||R^p| + N|R^p|)N$
$$+ |R^p|N\omega_n \tag{96}$$

Clearly, these errors depend on the magnitudes of angular velocity, distance from point p to COM, the noise level, and the frequency of the noise. A graphical representation of these errors as a function of ω_n is shown in Figure 14-14 with all the magnitudes set at 1.

Overall, the error analysis as illustrated in this section provides a useful tool that allows one to design an optimal measurement scheme so that the estimated kinematic variables have as few errors as possible.

SUMMARY

This chapter is focused on the theories of describing the movement of a body segment. Firstly, our whole body is divided into multiple single body segments. Each body segment is considered as rigid based on the assumption that the gross movement of the body can be represented by the bones supporting the body. Secondly, various reference systems are established, including the Absolute Reference System, Local Reference System, Segmental Reference System, and Joint Reference System. The theory of transformation between these systems is discussed. In addition, a practical approach for determining the transformation matrix is introduced. Thirdly, the definitions of kinematic variables are presented and are followed by discussions of various approaches on how to obtain these kinematic variables. They include direct measurement, differentiation, integration, and integrated kinematic approaches. Lastly, a noise analysis and treatment for those previously mentioned approaches is presented, and an optimal design method is introduced through an example.

REFERENCES

1. Bresler B, Frankel JP: The forces and moments in the leg during level walking, *ASME Transactions* 27-36, 1950.
2. Chao EYS: *Biomechanics of human gait.* In Schmid-Schobein GW, Woo SLY, & Zweifach BW, editors: *Frontiers in biomechanics,* New York, 1986, Springer Verlag.
3. Gilbert JA et al: A system to measure the forces and moments at the knee and hip during level walking, *Journal of Orthopedic Research* 2:281-288, 1984.
4. Grood ES, Suntay WJ: A joint coordinate system for the clinical description of three-dimensional motions: Application to the knee, *Journal of Biomechanical Engineering* 105:136-144, 1983.
5. International Society of Biomechanics Newsletter: (1992), No. 45.
6. Ladin Z, Wu G: Combining position and acceleration measurements for joint force estimation, *Journal of Biomechanics* 24(12):1173-1187, 1991.
7. McCarthy JM: *An introduction to theoretical kinematics,* Cambridge, Mass, 1990, The MIT Press.
8. Morris JRW: Accelerometry—A technique for the measurement of human body movements, *Journal of Biomechanics* 6:729-736, 1973.
9. Murray MP: Gait as a total pattern of movement, *American Journal of Physical Medicine* 48: 290-333, 1967.
10. Oppenheim AV, Schafer RW: *Digital signal processing,* Englewood Cliffs, N.J., 1975 Prentice Hall.
11. Radin EL et al: Relationship between lower limb dynamics and knee joint pain, *Journal of Orthopedic Research* 9:398-405, 1991.
12. Seemann MR, Lustick LS: Combination of accelerometer and photographically derived kinematic variables defining three-dimensional rigid body motion, *SPIE Biomechanics Cinema* 291: 133-140, 1981.
13. Shiavi R et al: Helical motion analysis of the knee. I. Methodology for studying kinematics during locomotion, *Journal of Biomechanics* 20(5):459-469, 1987.
14. Simon SR, Deutsch SD, Nuzzo RM, et al: Genu recurvatum in spastic cerebral palsy, *Journal Bone and Joint Surgery* 60-A(7):882-894, 1978.
15. Winter DA et al: Kinematics of normal locomotion—A statistical study based on T.V. data, *Journal of Biomechanics* 7:479-486, 1974.
16. Winter DA: *Biomechanics and motor control of Human Movement,* 2d ed, New York, 1990, John Wiley & Sons.
17. Wu G, Ladin Z: The kinematometer—An integrated kinematic sensor for kinesiological measurements, *Journal of Biomechanical Engineering* 115(1):53-62, 1993.

JOINT KINEMATICS: CAMERA-BASED SYSTEMS

Dan Koff

KEY TERMS

Azimuth

Calibration

Centroid

Detector

Direct linear transformation (DLT)

Field height

Field of view

Focal length

Lens

Optical axis

Photogrammety

Pixel

The study of biomechanical function often relies on observation as the primary data-gathering method. Several different technologies and approaches are available in the collecting of observational data. A historical overview introduces the technological development of two- and three-dimensional measurement instrumentation with an emphasis on photogrammetic technology. Modern video-based data acquisition instrumentation is discussed in detail in terms of its principal components, operation, and the advantages and limitations to its use. Finally, performance standardization, comparative analysis techniques, and a view into the future are discussed.

HISTORY

Human motion has been investigated since the time of Aristotle. The first graphic recordings of human gait were published by Carlet in 1872. Also in that same year, the first photographic analysis was performed by Eadweard Muybridge, an American photographer.[12] Summoned to California by Leland Stanford, Muybridge began an extensive study on horse locomotion. Utilizing electrical switches to activate sequentially the shutters on a linear array of cameras, Muybridge provided the evidence that as a horse gallops at top speed, there is a period during which all four feet are off the ground simultaneously. In addition to completing this historical analysis, Stanford won a substantial bet. Muybridge then proceeded to apply his technique coined *chronophotography* to the study of human motion.

Chronophotography is directly responsible for the development of **cinematography,** and although similar in principle they are quite distinct in nature. The object of chronophotography is to present a series of still pictures for detailed study, each picture capturing a particular phase of the motion. In cinematography the object is to produce a moving picture of the whole event. In truth, cinematographic techniques are used to obtain data for chronophotographic analysis as Muybridge suggested. Concurrently, E.J. Marey, professor and member of the Academy of Medicine at the College of France, studied locomotion of animals and humans.[10] Developing techniques for studying the interaction between the human body and its environment using pneumatic sensors and pressure chambers connected to the soles of shoes, Marey measured the pressure, timing, and amplitudes of the signals. Marey concluded that running should be viewed as a controlled falling process as opposed to an intentional jumping process.

With innovations such as a dynamic tracking camera, a rotating photographic plate, and the first passive kinematic markers (white strips against a black suit), Marey was able to follow moving targets at a frequency of 12 Hz. Thus was born the first two-dimensional passive photographic motion tracking system.

Starting in 1895, a series of publications by Wilhelm Braune and Otto Fisher described the advent of the active marker motion tracking system.[5] Attaching tethered electrically activated light tubes to the body segments, Braune and Fisher captured discrete body positions from multiple synchronized cameras at rates up to 26 Hz. Two-dimensional coordinate digitization accuracy was claimed to be 10 μm. By reconstructing the three-dimensional coordinates of the markers to an accuracy on the order of a few millimeters, and utilizing simplified assumptions regarding the locations of the markers with respect to the joint centers, both the spatial orientation and the time derivatives were studied. As a benchmark for modern systems, data acquisition, processing, and analysis of a single set of tests required up to 3 months to complete compared to only minutes that it takes today.

Published in 1926, Bernstein and his collaborators in Moscow improved upon both the sampling frequency and upon the accuracy in identifying corresponding points from stroboscopically exposed multiple photogrammetry by the use of mirror cinematography with a rotating shuttered single camera observing the direct field of view and a mirrored field of view simultaneously. Multiple camera synchronization problems could thus be avoided and an increase in depth resolution provided. Sampling frequencies ranging between 50 and 150 Hz provided increased temporal resolution compared to that of Braune and Fisher's system; however, with a two-dimensional coordinate digitization accuracy of 500 μm Bernstein's system accuracy fell substantially short of the 10 μm claimed by Braune and Fisher.

In Berkeley, California, Dr. Levens used a simpler method to obtain the frontal, lateral, and transverse views. In contrast to reconstructing the 3-D movements from projected cameras, three orthogonally positioned cameras were used. While this method provided adequate segment angle accuracy, calculated joint angles were susceptible to gross inaccuracies due to the assumption of being perpendicular, or normal, to each camera.

This historical survey describes the basis of most currently available video and optoelectric systems. Technological innovation has played a vital role in promoting studies in kinesiology. Modern instrumentation for two- and three-dimensional measurement includes: goniometers,[7,11] electromagnetic[2] and acoustic sensors,[3] and accelerometers.[10] The most common imaging devices, however, are optoelectric and video-based systems. A detailed discussion of these two technologies will follow along with a view into the future.

PHOTOGRAMMETRY: A BASIS FOR IMAGING ANALYSIS

General Principles

Photogrammetry consists of obtaining measurements of three-dimensional (3-D) objects based on two-dimensional (2-D) images of the object while stereophotogrammetry consists of two or more 2-D spatially unique images, or targets, producing a 3-D object. Typical close-range stereophotogrammetric systems consist of two or more imaging devices positioned at fixed locations in a globally referenced coordinate system (GRCS) with the imaging devices' axes forming mutually

oblique angles (see Figure 15-1). Determination of the 3-D location, or 3-D coordinates, of an object from multiple 2-D images can be broken into three specific tasks: (1) identification of the object or target, (2) determination of the center or centroid, of the target, and (3) triangulation using the multiple 2-D images to identify the 3-D coordinates of the target. The 3-D reconstruction of the target's location utilizes the azimuth and elevation angles from each of the two or more cameras to extract the three spatial coordinates. The most popular 3-D reconstruction method is the Direct Linear Transformation (DLT), which uses the azimuth and elevation angles and the 2-D coordinates from each 2-D image (that is, from each camera) to derive the 3-D coordinates of the target. The DLT determines the relative camera locations and orientations, but does not correct for image distortions.[1] A simplified introduction to Abdel-Aziz and Karara's DLT is presented in the appendix to this chapter. In addition to the "standard" DLT which typically uses 11 parameters, several modified DLTs exist each trying to avoid the nonlinear or nonorthogonality problems.

FIGURE 15-1   Globally referenced coordinate system (GRCS).

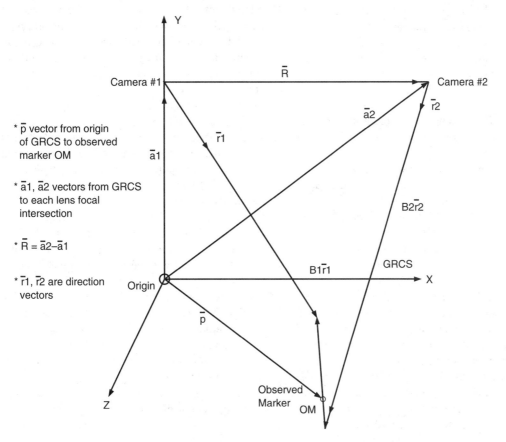

Components

Imaging-based data acquisition systems are comprised of many intertwined hardware and software components. Each must be carefully integrated if the total system performance is to be optimized. These components and their integration will be discussed in detail. A typical imaging system consists of the following:

1. Front-end optics consisting of a lens and detector

2. 2-D image acquisition, storage medium, and processing components consisting of either an online real-time analog-to-digital converter or an analog storage medium, such as a tape recorder, to an off-line digital converter, such as a frame grabber.

3. Image processing and geometric scaling component consisting of both hardware and software to convert the 2-D data into 3-D data. An abundance of off-the-shelf two- and three-dimensional systems exists, varying from inexpensive tape-recorded 2-D manual digitization to expensive, automated real-time 3-D systems. Imaging systems are either video-based or optoelectric. These systems are distinguished from each other by the kind of targets used. Video systems use passive targets, while optoelectric systems use active markers. The issues surrounding these markers are discussed later in this chapter. A table of current manufacturers provides a list of many commercially available systems on a variety of computer platforms. (see Table 15-1.)

The Front End: Lens, Detector, and Intrinsic Calibration   A typical video-imaging device, or camera, consists of two major components, the lens and the detector. It is assumed that these two components are held together in a fixed relative position by the detector housing.

The lens gathers and focuses light. In close-range stereophotogrammetry, these lenses vary in thickness, curvature, and quality-dependent factors, such as the positional relationship between the detector and the subject, detector size, and manufacturer. The more common thick lenses are described here while a thorough discussion of all lens types may be found in Moffit and Mikhail.[13] Perfect optics will produce a linear relationship between spot location in the image plane and the marker location in an object plane. Deviations from this linear relationship are referred to as image distortions. The principal type and source of optical image distortions is lens distortions. Cox classified lens aberrations into six primary categories according to their distortional effects: coma, spherical distortion, astigmatism and curvature of field, oblique spherical distortions, chromatic, and optical distortion.[9] The first five categories cause a reduction in the quality of an image. Optical distortion, however, causes a geometric change in the image, which is of greater importance than image quality. Optical distortion deforms an image away from, or toward, the point of symmetry. The geometric changes produced in a square image when influenced by optical distortion result in the commonly observed edge distortions of the "barrel" or "pincushion" type. While barrel distortion has the effect of enlarging the object's image, pincushion distortion has the effect of shrinking the image. Because a perfect lens that is distortion-free and suitable for the consumer market is unlikely, the design of the lens can be adjusted to produce a lens optimized for a particular application.[9] Given an optimized lens with minimal distortion and given the distortion in the form of a calibration curve, optical corrections are possible. Optical distortion of off-the-shelf lenses has been investigated by Olsen who concluded that typical image deformation levels attributable to optical distortion are less than 20 μm in a 9×9 inch square image. In addition, Olsen stated that the maximum relative distortion of a lens can be below 0.01 percent, but the maximum relative distortion of some lenses may be less than 0.005 percent. In general, localized image deformations are primarily manufacturing based. Grinding precision, accuracy, and in some cases thermal stress contribute to localized nonuniformities.

Lens distortions can be either lens aberrations, such as barrel or pincushion distortion, or lens decentering distortion. Lens decentering distortion results from misalignment of the lens elements of a compound lens, resulting in tangential or asymmetric radial distortions. Lens decentering distortion, unlike optical distortion, is construction based, not design based. Decentering distortion can be eliminated when the glass elements of a lens are perfectly aligned with their centers of curvature on a single straight line, commonly called the "optical axis" of the lens. In practice, manufacturers strive to align their lenses; however, perfect alignment is almost impossible to achieve. In general, a direct correlation between decentering alignment and the cost of the lens exists with expensive Swiss lenses minimizing the decentering distortion.

Decentering distortion consists of two components: tangential distortion and asymmetric radial distortion. Brown compared two independent

TABLE 15-1 Current Manufacturers.

1. Arial Performance Analysis Systems, Inc.
    6 Alicante
    Trabuco Canyon, CA 92679
    (714) 858-4216

2. Ascension Technology Corp.
    P.O. Box 527
    Burlington, VT 05402
    (800) 655-7879

3. BioEngineering Technology & Systems—Elite
    Via Capecelatro, 66
    1-20148 Milano
    ITALY
    39-2-40092116
    02/4046819-4047896

4. Charnwood Dynamics, Ltd.—CODA
    63 Forest Rd.
    Loughbourgh, Leics. LE11 3NW
    ENGLAND
    44-0509-233224

5. Columbus Instruments Inc.
    950 North Hague Ave.
    Columbus, OH 43204
    (614) 488-6176

6. CSP Inc., Scanalytics Division
    40 Linnell Circle
    Billerica, MA 01821
    (617) 272-6020

7. Eastman Kodak Company
    11633 Sorrento Valley Road
    San Diego, CA 92121
    (619) 535-2909

8. HCS Vision Technology B.V.
    Hurksestraat 18 D
    5652 Eindhoven
    THE NETHERLANDS
    31-40-521637

9. Hentschel Systems—GMBH
    Franische Strasse 62
    3000 Hannover 91
    GERMANY
    49-511-494099

10. Innovativ Vision—AB
    Teknikringgen 1
    S-583 30 Linkoping
    SWEDEN
    46-1321-4060

11. Loridan Biomedical, Inc.
    3650 Industrial Blvd.
    West Sacramento, CA 95691
    (800) SAY-LIDO

12. Motion Analysis Corp.
    3650 N. Laughlin Rd.
    Santa Rosa, CA 95403
    (707) 579-6500

13. Northern Digital Corp.
    403 Albert Street
    Waterloo, Ontario N2L 3V2
    CANADA
    (519) 884-5142

14. Optron Corp.
    30 Hazel Terrace
    Woodbridge, CT 06525
    (203) 389-5384

15. Osteokinetics Inc.
    82 Stuart Rd.
    Newton, MA 02159
    (617) 332-5954

16. Oxford Metrics, LTD
    Unit 8, 7 West Way
    Botley, Oxford OX2 0JB
    ENGLAND
    44-0865-244656

17. Peak Performance Inc.
    7388 S. Revere Parkway, Suite 601
    Englewood, CO 80112
    (303) 799-8686

18. Pixsys
    1727 Conestoga Street
    Boulder, CO 80301
    (303) 447-0248

19. Primas—Delf System
    N.A.

20. Selspot Selective Electronics, Inc.
    P.O. Box 250
    Valdese, NC 28690
    (704) 874-4102

21. Sartis One
    N.A.

22. TAU Corp.
    485 Alberto Way
    Los Gatos, CA 95032
    (408) 395-9191

23. Qualisis
    Ogardesvagen 2
    S-433
    30 Partille, SWEDEN
    46-031-36-3010

24. YAMAN Ltd
    2005 Hamilton Ave
    San Jose, CA 95125
    (408) 559-9100

models, which fully represented the type of distortion caused by decentering.[6] In the first so-called "thin prism" model, there was an assumption that the image deformations produced by a decentered lens could be duplicated by placing a thin prism in front of a perfectly centered lens. This assumption and method was the accepted standard prior to Brown's work. Brown concluded that the thin prism model only partially corrects for tangential distortion and that the radial distortion component remains a major deformation factor. The second model, the "Conrady" model was investigated by Brown to mathematically resolve the radial component of decentering distortion.[8] The Conrady model is based on analytical ray tracing through a decentered lens and is exact to the number of terms carried out. The assumption by Conrady that the reference point is also the principal point, as opposed to Brown's assumption that the reference point for optical distortion is the point of symmetry, was investigated by Abdel-Aziz and Karara.[1] They reported that this error could be corrected using expressions identical to those used by Conrady describing decentering distortion. In conclusion, if both expressions are included in the final

model, the model will compensate for the error in the reference point, thus justifying the use of the principal point as the reference point for both tangential and asymmetric radial distortion. Manufacturers who provide lens correction packages with their systems utilize some form of the Abdel-Aziz and Karara DLT.

A perfect detector will produce a linear relationship between spot location and the resulting data. Neither perfect optics nor perfect detectors exist, hence an introduction of nonlinear factors as in the preceding lens-detector calibration scheme must be undertaken to extract the full capacity of the front-end system. For purposes of this discussion, modern charge coupled device (CCD) detectors or optoelectric line scan detectors are assumed to be linear with respect to modern lenses since the major distortion component resides in the optics or lens. However, to optimize the effectiveness of the calibration, both the lens and detector should be considered as a single unit (see Figure 15-2). Both extrinsic parameters (those related to the global and relative camera locations and orientations) and intrinsic parameters (those related to a single camera's angle measurement accuracy) must be

Figure 15-2   Single camera view with GRCS.

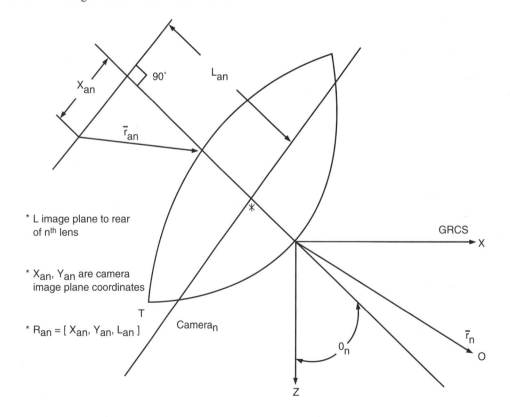

considered independently with respect to the calibration process. The issues of extrinsic calibration will be addressed later in this chapter.

A variety of methods for intrinsic calibration exist but it is essential to recognize that intrinsic calibration is most accurate and effective when used in conjunction with a lens correction software package. A review of contemporary techniques are detailed by Tasi with a new technique introduced.[16] Tasi's method uses 60 calibration points for a 388×480 CCD camera. Other techniques using over 400 points are available from a variety of modern commercially available data acquisition systems as well as a far more detailed study with 12,000 points by Antonsson and Mann.[4] Antonsson and Mann's data show that one of Tasi's assumptions of purely radial intrinsic errors for TV lenses is not warranted. However, given the complexity of Antonsson and Mann's lens calibration test, a correction for edge, parallax, and some "localized" distortion corrections can be obtained with 400 to 500 points.

A relatively inexpensive method of correcting for localized distortions that utilizes a 21×21 point photo-plotted polyurethane film, used by Motion Analysis Corporation, provides suitable digitizing accuracy and ease of calibration. Other calibration devices include machined plates used by Vicon Corp., Elite Corp., and Motion Analysis Corp., and the rotary table driven calibration bars used by E.K. Antonsson and R.W. Mann.[4] These and other calibration devices and associated software are available from several manufacturer's either as a standard product or on a custom basis. Each of these intrinsic calibration devices has its unique advantages and inherent disadvantages that should be considered. These include user misalignment of calibration device to detector, marker to marker cross-talk, intensity dependencies, and calibration algorithm accuracy. Misalignment of calibration device to detector can introduce greater errors than the process may correct, hence extreme care must be taken to ensure accurate detector-device positioning. In addition, marker to marker cross-talk, a function of the detector resolution, must be avoided. Marker to marker cross-talk occurs in plate calibration devices due to an inadequate detector resolution to marker separation distance. A general rule of twice the marker diameter separation between any adjacent marker minimizes this problem. Passive marker calibration plates utilizing retroreflective markers require uniform lighting to eliminate intensity inaccuracies. The Computer Aided Motion Analysis in a Rehabilitation Context (CAMARC) society suggests that proper adherence to correcting these intrinsic properties will produce subpixel accuracies. Actual accuracy and precision specifications will be discussed in a later section; however, directly related to the accuracy and precision is the resolution of the detector.

Specifics About the Detector Element   The detector element of the camera is the charge coupled device or CCD chip. The resolution of the camera is determined by the resolution of this CCD chip. Resolution is defined by the number of pixel, or video, units, in the horizontal view and the number of scan lines in the vertical view. The greater the number of pixels and scan lines, the greater is the resolution. The following information was assembled based on literature provided by various manufacturers or acquired during 1993. Due to the changes in manufacturing specifications, continuous improvements and upgrading of equipment, and outdated or lack of timely response from some manufacturers, this information may not contain the latest manufacturers' specifications. CCD-based cameras are universally used for video-based data acquisition systems due to the factory deposited highly linear, stable imaging geometry inherent in their design and manufacture. Since accuracy and precision are a function of the detector's resolution, modern CCD camera manufacturers strive for an even balance between the highest resolution and the lowest cost. Typical off-the-shelf black and white CCD cameras vary in resolution and cost, from 240 Vertical (v) by 256 Horizontal (h) using 1/2″ sensors to over 486v × 1134h in NTSC, RS-170 format, which is a television transmission standard that supports 30 frames per second (FPS) interlaced, established by the National Television Standards Committee and used in the United States, Canada, and Japan. Other non-NTSC based CCD cameras, such the Phase Alternation Line, or PAL, standard offer slightly better resolution at the basic level. PAL is a color video broadcast standard that supports 25 FPS, used in China and European nations including England and Germany. In addition to manufacturers offering higher and higher resolution cameras, both NTSC- and PAL-based CCD manufacturers are offering increased frequency or higher frames per second (FPS). These high speed video-based cameras offer speeds of over 200 FPS allowing for the accurate capture of quick motions typical in sports applications. Several off-the-shelf nonstandard video-based camera/recorder systems by Kodak, NAC, and others offer speeds of over 1,000 FPS. Presently, most high speed video cameras offer greater frames per second at the expense of lower resolution. This tradeoff, however, is becoming less evident in today's exponentially advancing video market.

In deciphering modern manufacturers' specifications, each function must be understood and compared relative to its identical counterpart. Camera performance specifications involve various descriptions of the imager, the pickup area, number of picture cells or pixels, active picture elements, resolution, sensitivity, contrast variation, shuttering speeds, signal-to-noise ratio, and synchronization. The major comparative factors for use with data acquisition systems are the horizontal and vertical resolution, image pickup area, and synchronization. In general, resolution should be as high as possible in both horizontal and vertical directions and should be compared in units of usable TV lines, not total pixel or total elements since these are often inaccurate representations of the camera's true performance. Image pickup area is typically either 6.4v × 4.8h mm (1/2 inch format) or 8.8v × 6.6h mm (2/3 inch format). Both provide equal linear performance but affect the camera field of view (*W*) and camera-to-subject or object distance (*U*). The object-distance is measured along the camera axis, orthogonal (at 90 degrees) to the imaging array sensor in the camera. The field of view (*W*) is measured orthogonal to the camera axis and parallel to the field height (*H*), that is the long side of the image. The field height is measured orthogonal to the camera axis and parallel to the short side of the image. In video-based motion capture, the total event must "fit" within the camera's active field of view or window. Due to laboratory factors such as size limitations, light reflectivity, and control, the camera-to-subject distance or object distance (*U*) is a critical factor and is a function of the image pickup area and lens focal length used as shown in Equations (1) and (2). Optimally both equations should be satisfied. Restrictions on laboratory size result in the need for a small focal length (*F*) lens that incorporates large distortions. Under such conditions there is more reason to utilize lens linearization techniques.

$$U = F[(\phi \times W) + v]/v \tag{1}$$
$$U = F[(\infty \times H) + h]/h \tag{2}$$

where *F* is the focal length of the lens; *H* is the image height; *W* is the field of view; ø is derived from the proportion of the horizontal scan cycle actually used to draw the active horizontal region

of a single scan line; and ∞ is derived from the active or true ratio of the number of lines used to generate the active window to the number of available lines. Additionally, *v* and *h* are the width and height of the camera's CCD imaging array in mm.

Synchronization of multiple cameras should have the standard NTSC/PAL-EIA, RS-170, Genlock, external sync, phase adjustable line lock and/or external horizontal and vertical drive capability. Cameras with all or most of these synchronization methods offer added flexibility in synchronizing multiple cameras for 3-D analysis.

As camera technology improves providing greater resolution and increased linearity at a decrease in consumer costs, it will be up to the specialized analog-to-digital (A/D) processor to stay abreast of this fast-moving market. Ultimately, these A/D processors will be the key factor in determining the speed, accuracy, and flexibility of optically based data acquisition systems.

Processor: The Image Converter   Modern processors convert electrically based continuously variable signals called analog data into a set of discrete numerical binary values called digital data. Various unique innovative features for obtaining the digital data form the core of most motion analysis data acquisition systems. The conversion of raw analog information into binary digitally processed data occurs through a variety of hardware devices. Video-based systems may convert the analog "picture" into digital form at real-time speeds directly into a computer for immediate viewing, analysis, and feedback control or may utilize an analog storage medium, such as a video tape recorder. If the latter storage medium is used, the analog-to-digital (A/D) process must occur through sometimes tedious means. At the low end of the market, tape recorded manual digitization via a digitizing pad may provide a useful, flexible analysis tool. However, the process is highly labor intensive, inaccurate, and unreliable due to the lack of repetitiveness. These factors limit the utility of manual digitization to specific applications where environmental factors prevent the application of external markers or an automated digitization process. Despite limitations, there are a number of companies that offer equipment requiring manual digitization. Manufacturers such as Arial, Motion Analysis Corp., Peak Performance, Loridan Biomedical, and other off-the-shelf systems offer manual digitization systems, which usually include the necessary cameras, tape recorders, frame grabber, tape recorder control interface, digitizing hardware, and computer for data storage and analysis. Prices start at about $20,000 for a basic two-camera complete 3-D system.

The next level in motion analysis performance is the addition of an automated video A/D processor. These processors require a differential either in color or gray-scale between the required markers and the background. The majority of today's video-based systems use black and white cameras due to the increased resolution these cameras offer. Black and white A/D conversion is accomplished by comparing the brightness of the incoming video signal with a threshold value or values. When the video signal exceeds the threshold value, the X and Y coordinates of the processor array are recorded. The most common and widely used edge detection method uses the Sobel operator for gray-scale threshold differential. A typical video signal representation and video processing unit are shown in Figures 15-3, 15-4, and 15-5. Several recently

developed color-based systems by Columbus Instruments Corp. and others use the color differential to distinguish between desired information and background noise. The digitized color information is scanned on a per frame basis and the corresponding information is recorded into computer memory. Once the desired digitization has occurred either by gray-scale edge detection or full gray-scale or color scanning, this pixel X, Y position information is ready to be converted into accurate marker centroidal positions.

Calculation of marker centroid positions from pixel X, Y positions is accomplished by a variety of methods, none of which has been proven experimentally to be the most accurate, most precise, and fastest. Centroidal processing, 2-D or 3-D, has recently become a major factor in modern data acquisition technology due to its increased acceptance and duration of today's applications. While real-time 3-D processing is desired, many factors prevent this from becoming readily available at an

FIGURE 15-3   Video signal representation of marker.

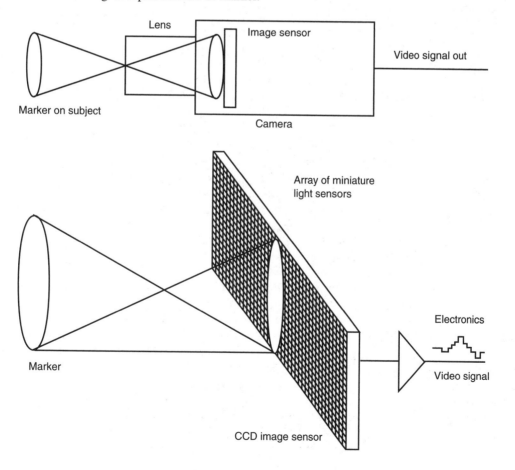

FIGURE 15-4   Video signal representation of marker.

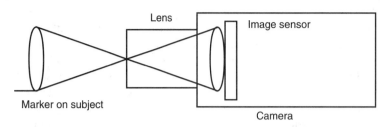

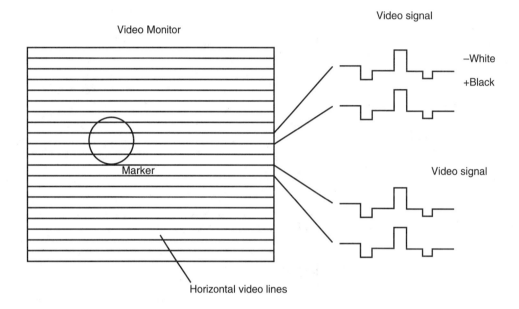

affordable price in the immediate future. These factors include marker type (passive or active), frequency of acquisition, number of markers, and working volume.

Active markers, used in optoelectric systems, are generally light-emitting diodes that flash at given frequencies. Therefore, each marker can be uniquely identified in both the spatial and time domains and can be processed in real-time. These real-time processors are presently limited in bandwidth to around 3500 Hz. Practically speaking, this provides the user with 35 markers at 100 Hz or FPS, which is sufficient in most applications when displacements of a walking or moderately active person are to be analyzed. However, when fast movements, velocities, and particular accelerations and forces are to be analyzed, 100 Hz may not be adequate. Several real-time active marker systems are currently available with both tethering and telemetry connections to the processing unit.

(Optotrack, Selspot, Polhemas, Ascension). Due to the inherent uniqueness in both the spatial and time domains, these active marker systems simplify the marker identification, 2-D centroid, and 3-D triangulation processes significantly but at the expense of cumbersome active tethering or complex telemetry hardware.

Active marker identification is simplified since only one unique marker is at the measured threshold at any point in time and space. If the external environment is sufficiently darkened such that the usually LED-based light marker is brighter, the processor identifies a single marker above the required cutoff threshold from all time synchronized sensors and the 2-D centroid, and the 3-D triangulation process can be resolved instantly.

Under laboratory conditions where reducing environmental noise while optimizing the desired marker contrast differential is strictly adhered to, these active systems can provide extremely accu-

FIGURE 15-5 Video signal processor function.

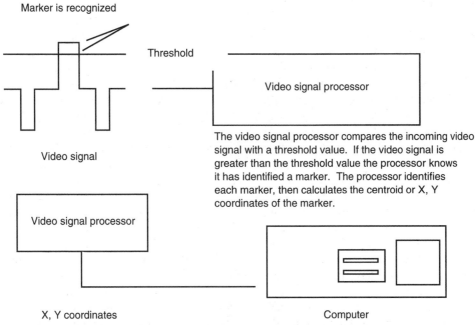

Marker is recognized

Threshold

Video signal processor

Video signal

The video signal processor compares the incoming video signal with a threshold value. If the video signal is greater than the threshold value the processor knows it has identified a marker. The processor identifies each marker, then calculates the centroid or X, Y coordinates of the marker.

Video signal processor

X, Y coordinates

Computer

After finding the threshold markers and calculating the X, Y coordinates of each, the video signal processor passes the coordinates to the computer for further processing and display.

rate data in real time. On the negative side, the tethering, frequency, and noise levels may be unacceptable for the application desired.

Recent advances in telemetry have been incorporated into some of these active marker systems in the form of a portable power, synchronizer, and sending unit. This enables the user to eliminate the tethering to the receiving unit with only the individual marker wires to deal with. As telemetry systems improve, the noise problems typically found in frequency transmission systems should make this marriage of technologies an exciting prospect for real-time, accurate 3-D data acquisition.

At the current time, the passive marker alternative is the other viable option. The problems with passive markers are twofold: (1) each marker must be uniquely identified and in each of the 2-D camera's views; and (2) an accurate centroid must be calculated. Since each camera views only a 2-D projection of the actual 3-D space, markers are not held by the 3-D spatial uniqueness rule whereby no two objects may lie in the same 3-D space. Hence in the camera's viewing perspective, markers merge, occlude, disappear, and distort. Each of these problems presents complications in the

marker identification, 2-D centroid, and ultimately in the desired 3-D centroid calculations. In the past, passive 3-D marker systems have utilized two substantially different methods to obtain 3-D data. The level of complexity, accuracy, and applicability depends on which methodology is used. The two methods differ in the 2-D marker centroid acceptance and in the 3-D triangulation calculation. Although both methods may utilize the same edge detection, 2-D centroid, and 3-D DLT mathematics, the methodologies differ significantly.

The basics of these two passive systems are multiple time-synced video cameras, incorporating a thresholding gray-scale processing unit and a 3-D triangulation DLT algorithm. Both systems digitize each of the incoming video signals, either serially using tape recorded data and a single video frame grabber or in parallel, simultaneously digitizing all incoming video signals using specialized real-time digitizing hardware. Since the markers are passive and neither spatially nor temporally unique, the digitized information must be reduced to 2-D centroids utilizing several methods. In contrast to active marker systems, each passive marker does not have its own unique characteristic. Therefore, passive marker systems must deal with single "perfect" markers, occluded markers, merged markers, noise, and marker variations all during a single instant in time. The 2-D centroid processing procedure has resulted in producing two significantly different 3-D processing methodologies utilizing a variety of centroid calculation algorithms. The first 3-D processing method calculates the 3-D path from 2-D centroids (2C-3P). The second 3-D method calculates the 3-D path from 3-D centroids (3C-3P). Two-dimensional centroid algorithms include subpixel geometric averaging from dual and quad edge marker outlines, leading-trailing edge algorithms, circle fitting, pattern recognition, and ring fitting techniques. Depending on the A/D processing type, each of these centroid calculation methods has advantages or disadvantages with respect to speed, accuracy, and precision. To date, no direct experimental comparison has proven which method is more accurate.

Geometric averaging involves the equal weighting average of each X and Y pixel coordinate associated with each marker. This association may, however, include pixels corresponding to other merged markers or extraneous noise. This method, while mathematically simple, requires a neighborhood searching algorithm to include the associated pixels and is slow in processing the data. Geometric averaging techniques are based on either the leading-trailing edges of the digitized marker or on all four edges generated by specialized quad edge detection hardware (Motion Analysis Corporation). While quad edge detection using geometric averaging is inherently more accurate than dual edge, both methods are processed after data acquisition, which prevents real-time centroidal processing. Many systems utilize this geometric averaging technique. A faster, potentially more accurate 2-D centroidal method uses the leading-trailing edges in conjunction with fitting algorithms via specialized hardware to process real-time 2-D centroids. These fitting algorithms include the previously mentioned circle, and ring fitting iterative methods are used by manufacturers such as Vicon and Primas.

Pattern recognition techniques such as those used in the Elite system, Qualisis system, and others provide additional digital information, which may minimize the contribution of noise from cross-correlation. Computing the center of mass (COM) by comparing the digitized 6-bit information with a reference shape is yet another method of obtaining 2-D information. This and other recently introduced 2-D centroid algorithms

may increase both the accuracy and precision; however to date, no direct comparison has been made.

The 2-D centroid to 3-D positions (2C-3P) system typically utilizes video tape recorders to capture the analog image. Several real-time capture systems use this methodology of a computer-based frame grabber board and tape recorder controller to accurately advance the recorder one frame or field at a time and associated software to grab and process each frame of data. The digital data are then processed either automatically through the use of threshold gray-scale marker detection or manually via mouse and crosshair location software producing a 2-D "named" centroid for each observable marker in time for each camera.

The manual method of marker identification and 2-D centroid calculation, although extremely laborious and inaccurate, solves several difficult 2-D marker identification and 2-D centroid calculation problems that plague these systems. The ability or level of software intelligence presently available in these 2C-3P systems in a purely automated mode is insufficient to accurately solve for unique marker identification and 2-D centroid calculation in all but the simplest of 3-D applications.

Many algorithms and methods have been implemented by the 2C-3P data acquisition manufacturers with good but not perfect results. Due to the independence or separation of the 2-D centroid calculation from the 3-D centroid calculations, the method assumes that the 2-D data are "perfect." These "perfect" 2-D time series data are then passed through an unforgiving 3-D DLT, and the resulting 3-D centroids are assembled into 3-D trajectories. Reiterating, the 2-D time series data for each observed marker are used to calculate the desired 3-D trajectories without any 3-D data check or user interface since these 2-D data are assumed "perfect." This assumption is the cause of many inaccuracies and in some cases the inability to acquire accurate 3-D data. In simple limited marker set applications with numerous and properly oriented cameras, the use of these 2C-3P systems may provide accurate data if the operator of such a system is knowledgeable of the pitfalls, the limitations, and the solutions. Problems caused by the disappearance, distortion, occlusion, or merging of markers in the camera's 2-D view have prompted the development of more intelligent 2-D and 3-D algorithms and more user-friendly interfacing software.

Data acquisition systems that employ the 3-D centroids to 3-D positions (3C-3P) use 3-D algorithms dependent on, not independent of, the 2-D marker centroid calculations. These 3C-3P systems threshold and calculate the 2-D centroidal positions in a manner similar to many of the 2C-3P systems. However, this is as far as the similarities go. Whereas the 2C-3P methodology assumes the 2-D data are independent of the 3-D data and are "perfect," the 3C-3P methodology assumes that the 3-D centroids are dependent on the 2-D centroids and that the projected 2-D data may contain imperfect data.

The 3C-3P algorithms calculate the 2-D centroids for each unnamed marker using various centroidal algorithms that may deal with marker merging, occluding, distorting, or disappearing for every camera at each instance in time. From the 3-D calibration information, a ray from each of these 2-D centroids is projected normal to each camera's image plane and through each camera's observed objects. Given perfectly linear optics, infinite resolution, and absolute spatial and temporal calibration accuracies, the projected rays should intersect. This is seldom the case, however. Typically, a best fit averaging method assembles this intersection point into each marker's 3-D centroidal position. During this complicated, elaborate 3-D ray tracing process, several accuracy checks occur. Since a best fit 3-D intersection is calculated within either a user-specified or manufacturer's preset error tolerance, any inaccuracies at any stage in the marker identification or 2-D centroid calculation process can be eliminated given an overspecified system containing more than two cameras. The final step in obtaining 3-D data using the 3C-3P methodology is to initialize or identify the 3-D centroid or 3-D trajectory. As opposed to the 2C-3P system, which identifies the 2-D centroids or 2-D trajectories prior to the 3-D triangulation (DLT) process and accepts and retains this identity as the 3-D trajectory, the 3C-3P procedure requires the user to initialize or identify the accepted 3-D *after* the 3-D triangulation process on either the 3-D centroids or on the 3-D trajectories.

In the previous case, the 3-D centroids are often identified by the user at a particular point in time and all subsequent marker identifications are automatically identified either forward or backward in time. By using algorithms that incorporate length between markers, previous position, velocity, and acceleration, this automatic identification can, in the best case, be a fast, accurate, faultless process. In the worst case, however, the process simply does not work and the user must reidentify every marker at each point in time. On average, this automatic identification process can be optimized

by overspecifying the number of cameras, by minimizing the environmental background noise, and by optimally positioning the cameras to minimize marker merging, occluding, disappearing, and distorting.

The other method of identifying 3C-3P data is to identify the 3-D trajectories after all 3-D centroids are assembled into their correct paths. This identification procedure, again, can be easy and produce fast, accurate, 3-D named trajectories, or be so difficult and inaccurate as to produce no data within a reasonable amount of time.

The main problem with this method of 3-D data identification is in automating the 3-D centroids to 3-D trajectories processing. Again the effectiveness depends on careful setup, calibration, noise minimization, camera number, and camera placement. Given optimal conditions, the number of 3-D trajectories processed and available for user identification is the same as the number of markers used. Under poor conditions, the number of 3-D trajectories may be many times the actual number of markers used. These 3-D trajectory segments must then be identified spatially and the temporal gaps or missing data be interpolated to obtain continuous 3-D trajectories.

Clearly, 3C-3P systems have inherent advantages in producing accurate, precise, fast 3-D data over 2C-3P systems if accurate calibration, camera positioning, camera quantity, noise reduction, and marker identification are performed. However, while 2C-3P systems can usually produce 3-D data of some sort, 3C-3P systems may not be able to resolve the 2-D projected rays within the error requirements, and they do not produce 3-D data. Increasing the error tolerance beyond acceptable may produce 3-D data, but the accuracy and precision may be unacceptable as may be the accuracy and precision of the data produced from merged, occluded, distorted 2-D markers in the 2C-3P system.

Solutions to the many problems plaguing passive gray-scale data acquisition systems can be as simple as understanding the process at hand. Unfortunately, this requires both a trained experienced expert in optics, dynamics, and photogrammetry. In the clinical environment where the data acquisition system is to be a tool used by many, the latter solution is not acceptable. On the other hand, software "artificial intelligence"—software with user-friendly interfaces—are improving the performance, speed, and ease of these passive black and white systems.

An interesting solution to the nondiscriminatory black and white passive data acquisition system is in the use of colored markers and color image detection. Although still passive, this method provides uniqueness in both the spatial and temporal domains. Marker merging, occluding, distorting, disappearing, and identification problems, difficult to solve in the black and white domain, become simple in the color domain. Several systems are either in the prototype phase or are available for limited numbers of markers. The prototypes are providing real-time data acquisition, with automated 3-D data processing of over 60 markers at 30 FPS. The limiting factor at present is the frequency and resolution of the color video cameras. Typically color cameras and digitizing hardware provide differentiation up to 256 colors but only at 30 FPS. Specialized color systems provide frequencies up to 1000 FPS but at lower resolutions and at a cost of more than $30,000 per camera (NAC, KODAK).

It should now be evident that standardization of equipment performance must be established in order to compare and contrast each data acquisition system. The Computer Aided Motion Analysis in a Rehabilitation Context (CAMARC) society, a primarily European-based society has proposed standards for comparing data acquisition system performance. However, no international standards have been established to include both NTSC and PAL-based passive and active motion capture systems. In addition, CAMARC is focused more towards PAL video-based systems and not the computer-aided motion analysis field as a unique entity. Standards must include all aspects of data acquisition including 2-D and 3-D spatial and temporal calibration, data acquisition frequency specifications, as well as 2-D and 3-D data analysis.

SPATIAL CALIBRATION TECHNIQUES

Two-dimensional spatial calibration converts digital pixel-based X,Y positions into real world units. Assuming the camera imaging array is normal to the plane of movement, two calibration points may be used. This 2-D distance scale factor calculates a pixel to a real-world ratio as shown in Figure 15-6. In addition to assuming a normal camera plane

FIGURE 15-6 Distance scale factor.

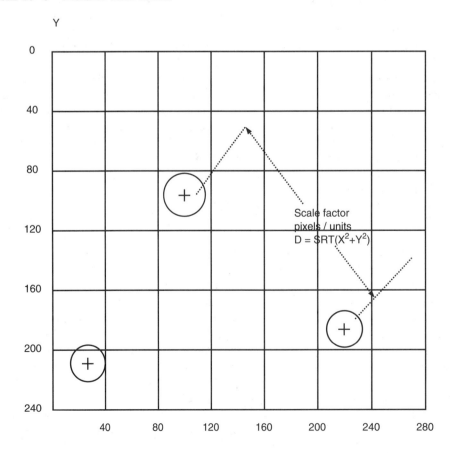

with respect to the movement plane, an aspect ratio scaling may be required. The aspect ratio scaling corrects for differences in the horizontal and vertical scaling since most cameras have rectangular rather than square imaging arrays. Additionally, the normal camera plane assumption may not be valid; hence, the two-point scaling factor may be modified to a three- or four-point scaling process to compensate for skewed movement orientation and skewed X and Y aspect ratio scaling. Figure 15-7 shows the aspect ratio scaling for a three-point spatial calibration process.

The four-point spatial calibration technique is the basis for all 3-D calibration techniques used in most optically based data acquisition systems. Most 3-D systems, however, use a spatial calibration process using a minimum of six noncollinear points. These six points provide the $X, Y,$ and Z scaling and aspect ratio variables required to calculate each camera image position and orientation necessary for the DLT process. See Equations

DLT-10 through DLT-13 for details. While a minimum of six calibration points is required for solving the standard DLT equations, most optically based systems use more. The advantage of utilizing more than six points is redundancy. The possibility of actual calibration measurement errors and optical errors makes a redundant system more robust.

The evolution of calibration devices from hanging plumb bobs (see Figure 15-8) to rigid robotically measured cubes or structures has increased the accuracy while reducing the time required for calibration. The plumb bob calibration method, although flexible in nature, resulted in point-to-point accuracies seldom greater than 0.25 inches. The plumb bobs were positioned at the boundaries of the required volume and each hanging marker was measured using a tape measuring device and a transit site. This boundary calibration method attempted to linearize the working field of view but failed in most cases to accurately correct the true

---

FIGURE 15-7 Vertical/horizontal scale factor.

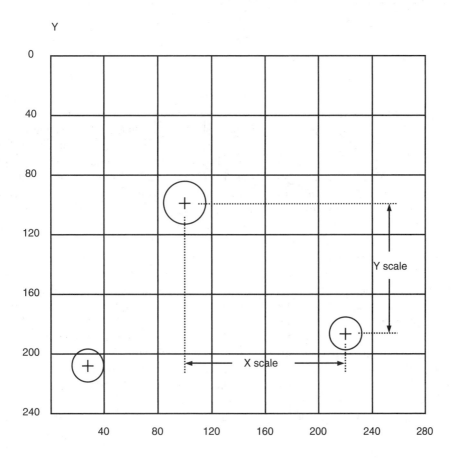

FIGURE 15-8 Hanging bob calibration.

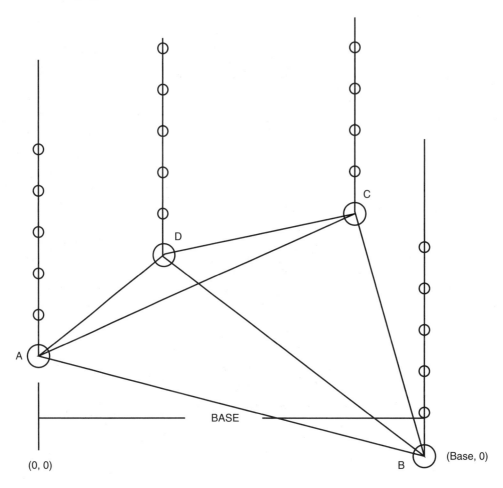

optical distortions, since the number of calibration points used was not more than 32. The solution to optical linearization and accurate and fast calibration was solved using both a 2-D per camera optical distortion plate and a highly accurate rigid 3-D calibration structure with as many points as possible. Given these recent calibration devices and optical correction software, present optically based data acquisition systems are among the most accurate methods of obtaining position data.

As previously discussed, CAMARC has attempted to prescribe measurement standards using experimental methods. While most major data acquisition system manufacturers are including both their systems' theoretical and experimental performance specifications, the lack of standardization renders most of this information useless in direct comparison testing between different manufacturers. CAMARC and others are attempting to offer the industry comparative accuracy and preci-

sion testing protocols and recommendations. Three topics should be included in any testing protocol: (1) the protocol or definitions of all tests and mandatory conditions applying to them for repeatability; (2) the equations or algebraic definitions of how the results from each test are calculated and presented; and (3) procedures or tasks for performing the tests. The following discussion details these three topics.

A performance protocol for testing 3-D data acquisition systems for kinematic analysis of human movement must begin with calibration of the measured volume. Typical volumes for human motion analysis vary based on current technology and analysis requirements. A volume of not less than 2.5 meters length by 1.5 meters width by 2.0 meters height should be used. Larger measurement volumes may be used, but it must be possible to determine the 3-D position of a target marker continuously throughout this volume. The measurement area is defined as the horizontal floor level area within the measurement volume. The field of view of the measurement volume is defined as the longest corner-to-corner diagonal of the enclosed cuboid. Finally, the calibration must be performed using the recommended manufacturers' procedures and equipment. Cameras and/or sensors may not be moved or recalibrated at any time during the performance protocol tests. Calibration performance accuracy testing must include a comparison between the known calibration marker positions obtained using a third party measurement system and the experimentally obtained calibration marker positions using the motion measurement system. For all tests, prior measurements of all devices must be obtained using third party, certified measurement test equipment. All experimental data must be presented in the raw form where smoothing and interpolation are not permitted.

CAMARC has described a static accuracy test to determine the mean radial accuracy. In this test a stiff rod of 2 m in length is fixed to a spherical hinge. Markers are attached at nominal distances of 0.45 m, 1.20 m, 1.40 m, and 1.95 m from the hinge. The distances are measured from the center of the marker to the center of the hinge. The hinge is fixed with its center of rotation at a precisely known position on the floor on the center of the measurement area. The rod is moved sequentially through eight horizontal positions within the measurement area. These positions include parallel to the long or greatest axis providing two measurements, 30 degrees to either side of the long axis providing four measurements, and perpendicular to the long axis providing a final two measurements. From each of the reference directions, the free end of the rod is raised to 0.75 m, 1.65 m, and finally vertical. In each of the 25 rod orientations, the positions of all markers are measured with a minimum of 50 consecutive samples or frames recorded. For analysis, all data outside the measurement volume are excluded, thus providing 96 marker positions at 50 samples per position for a total of 4,800 samples.

Similarly, dynamic noise testing can be accomplished by using a rigid pendulum constructed of two horizontal rods of 0.50 m each. Attached to their centers is a third vertical rod also of 0.50 meters. Four markers are attached to the ends of the horizontal rods, and two markers attached to the vertical rod with at least 0.40 m separation. The exact locations of these markers are not required, only approximations. The pendulum is

suspended with the ability to swing freely. The horizontal crosspieces should be approximately aligned with the major axis of the measurement volume. The movement of the pendulum should be in a symmetrical circular motion of approximately 30 degrees about the vertical axis. The three-dimensional coordinates of all six markers should be recorded for at least 100 consecutive samples of frames. Analyzing the distances between pairs of markers on each of the three rods results in 300 intermarker distance samples, which are used to calculate the standard deviation of the intermarker distances.

A sample full volume noise test consists of a stiff rod approximately 1 m in length with markers fixed at each end. The length between the centers of these two markers is accurate completely through the measurement volume. The velocity of the rod movement should be kept steady between 0.5 and 2 m per second. A minimum of 50 consecutive samples or frames of three-dimensional coordinates of each marker moving throughout the measurement volume are calculated and recorded for each test. The data consisting of a minimum of 4,500 samples are used to calculate the RMS (root means square) error between the experimentally calculated and the known intermarker distances, σv.

Finally, a gravity test consists of a marker projected upward from near the floor into a trajectory that is entirely contained within the measurement volume. An odd number of at least 21 samples is selected from the free flight period of the trajectory. Impact with the ground and maximum height should be excluded. The vertical coordinates of the marker are measured and recorded. The acceleration due to gravity, g, is then calculated.

Equations for these tests are as follows:
The *Mean Radial Accuracy, αr,* is defined by the formula

$$\alpha r = [1/n \sum_{k=1}^{n}(Rc_k - Rt)^2]^{1/2}$$

where
n = number of qualifying samples (4,500)
Rc = computed radius (distance between measured marker position and known hinge center)
Rt = true radius (known distance between marker and hinge center).

Mean Dynamic Noise, σd, is defined by

$$\sigma d = [1/2m(n - 1) \sum_{i=1}^{m}\sum_{j=1}^{n}(D_{ij} - D_i)^2]^{1/2}$$

where

D_{ij} = sample distance between the marker pair on the ith rod

$D_i = 1/n \sum_{j=1}^{n}, D_{ij}$ mean intermarker distance on the ith rod

m = number of marker pairs (three)

n = number of samples (100).

Full Volume Noise, σv, is defined by

$$\sigma r = [1/2n \sum_{k=1}^{n}(Lc_k - Lt)^2]^{1/2}$$

where

n = number of rod length samples (≥ 450)

Lc = computed length of rod

Lt = true measured length of rod.

The gravity test uses the vertical coordinates recalculated to lie about a mean value of zero such that

$$Z_k = Z_k - 1/2n + 1 \sum^{+n} Z_j; k = -n, \ldots, +n$$

where

Z_k = kth free fall vertical coordinate.

Thus acceleration due to gravity, g, is calculated using

$$g = 2a/(\tau \times \tau)\sum_{k=1}^{n} K \times K (Z_{+k} + Z_{-k})$$

where

$a = 45/[n(n + 1)(2n - 1)(2n + 1)(2n + 3)]$

τ = sample interval

Z_k = kth zero mean free fall coordinate

and where the odd number of samples n is from $n = 2n + 1$.

It should be noted that the preceding tests are only several from the unlimited possibilities available. Each of the above tests, however, results in a comparative estimation of a system's accuracy and precision for both a static and dynamic case suitable for human movement such as gait analysis. Many high-speed sports applications or extremely small movements may require modifications to the measurement volume and to the intermarker distances.

Future

With exponential processing power, real-time video compression, increasingly high-definition video resolution, and the video market booming, the future of optically based passive data acquisi-

tion instrumentation and analysis will provide fast, accurate, inexpensive processing. Already, prototype 3-D real-time totally passive motion analysis systems are being tested. Some of these state-of-the-art systems utilize 3-D tracking DLTs, digital cameras, and 3-D solid model graphical analysis and visualization. Other prototypes are utilizing real-time digital color cameras, multiple 3-D lasers, and 3-D acoustic systems providing full body analysis at unprecedented speeds and accuracy. Although most of these prototypes are several years away from full production, present systems are providing processing speeds and accuracies Eadweard Muybridge and fellow innovators never dreamed of.

Summary

The history of motion analysis spans more than one hundred years. The rapid expansion of computer and camera technology has wrought dramatic changes in image-based motion analysis in the last 20 years. The purpose of this chapter has been to review the methods used in imaging and current motion analysis systems. The basic hardware elements of current technologies have been presented. The problems of image distortion and calibration schema have also been presented. The goal has been to provide an explanation of the underlying technologies best suited for the user's purpose. In addition, the chapter has addressed the basic questions of accuracy and resolution, which users should consider as they implement motion analysis in specific applications.

References

1. Abdel-Aziz YI, Karara HM: Direct linear transformations into object space coordinates in close range photogrammetry. In *Symposium on close range photogrammetry,* Urbana, Ill, 1971, University of Illinois at Urbana-Champaign.
2. An KN, Jacobsen LJ, Chao EYS: Application of a magnetic tracking device to kinesiologic studies, *J Biomech* 21:613-620, 1988.
3. Andrews JG, Youm Y: A biomechanical investigation of wrist kinematics, *J Biomech* 12:83-89, 1979.
4. Antonsson EK, Mann RW: Automatic 6-D.O.F. kinematic trajectory acquisition and analysis, *Journal of Dynamic Systems, Measurement, and Control* 111: 34-35, 1989.
5. Braune W, Fischer: *The human gait,* Berlin, 1987, Springer.
6. Brown DC: Decentering distortion of lenses *Photogrammetric Engineering* 32:444-462, 1966.
7. Chao EYS, Hoffman RR: Instrumented measurements of human joint motions, *ISA Transactions* 17:13, 1977.

8. Conrady AE: Decentered lens systems, *Monthly Notices of the Royal Astronomical Society* 79:384-390, 1919.

9. Cox A: *Photographic optics,* 15th ed Garden City, N.Y., 1974, Amphoto.

10. Hayes WC, Gran JD, Nagurka ML et al: Leg motion analysis during gait by multiaxial accelerometry: Theoretical foundations and preliminary validations, *J Biomech Eng* 105:283-289, 1983.

11. Lamoreaux L: Kinematic measurements in walking, *Bulletin of Prosthetics Research* 10:3-84, 1971.

12. Marey EJ: Animal mechanism: A treatise on terrestrial and aerial locomotion. In *Vol. XI of the International Scientific Series,* New York, 1887, D. Appleton and Company.

13. Moffit FH, Mikhail EM: *Photogrammetry,* 3rd ed, New York, 1980, Harper & Row.

14. Muybridge E: Animal locomotion. In Brown LS, editor: *Animal in Motion,* London, 1975, Chapman & Hall.

15. Quinn TP, Mote CD: A six degree of freedom acoustic transducer for rotation and translation measurements across the knee, *J Biomech Eng* 112:371-378, 1990.

16. Tasi RY: An efficient and accurate camera calibration technique for 3D machine vision, *Proceedings of the 1986 IEEE Computer Society Conference on Computer Vision and Pattern Recognition,* 364 374.

APPENDIX: INTRODUCTION TO DLT

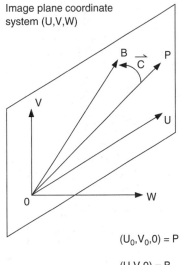

Image plane coordinate system (U,V,W)

$(U_0, V_0, 0) = P$

$(U, V, 0) = B$

Refer to the figure at right and to the figures on page 202.

$$\vec{C} = \vec{PB} = (U - U_0, V - V_0, 0)$$

$$\vec{NP} = (0, 0, -\vec{f})$$

$$\vec{b} = \vec{NB} = \vec{NP} + \vec{C}$$

$$= (0, 0, -\vec{f}) + (U - U_0, V - V_0, 0)$$

$$= (U - U_0, v - v_0, -\vec{f})$$

Since *A, B, N* form a single line due to collinearity, then

$$b = \begin{bmatrix} U - U_0 \\ V - V_0 \\ -f \end{bmatrix}, r = \begin{bmatrix} r_{11} & r_{12} & r_{13} \\ r_{21} & r_{22} & r_{23} \\ r_{31} & r_{32} & r_{33} \end{bmatrix}, a = \begin{bmatrix} X - X_0 \\ Y - Y_0 \\ Z - Z_0 \end{bmatrix} \quad OR \quad a = \begin{bmatrix} \Delta X_0 \\ \Delta Y_0 \\ \Delta Z_0 \end{bmatrix}$$

and

$$b = K \times r \times a$$

where

K = constant

r = rotational matrix.

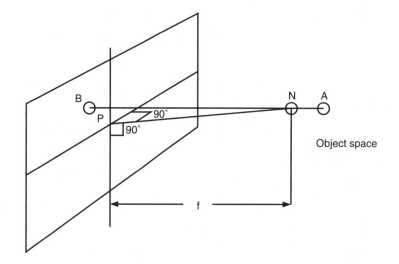

Object - image mapping

Object space

Image Plane

A = Object
B = Image
N = Camera Node
P = Principal point
f = Principal distance

Where A, N, B are colinear

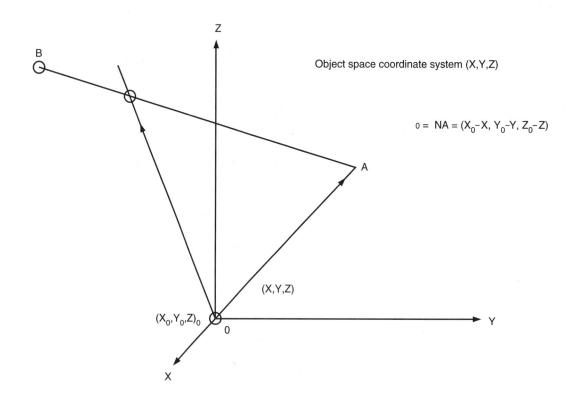

Object space coordinate system (X,Y,Z)

$$0 = NA = (X_0 - X, Y_0 - Y, Z_0 - Z)$$

Thus

$$
\begin{bmatrix} U - U_0 \\ V - V_0 \\ -f \end{bmatrix} = K \cdot \begin{bmatrix} r_{11} & r_{12} & r_{13} \\ r_{21} & r_{22} & r_{23} \\ r_{31} & r_{32} & r_{33} \end{bmatrix} \cdot \begin{bmatrix} \Delta X_0 \\ \Delta Y_0 \\ \Delta Z_0 \end{bmatrix}
\qquad (DLT\text{-}1)
$$

From Equation DLT-1

$$U - U_0 = K\left[r_{11}(X - X_0) + r_{12}(Y - Y_0) + r_{13}(Z - Z_0)\right] \qquad (DLT\text{-}2)$$

$$V - V_0 = K\left[r_{21}(X - X_0) + r_{22}(Y - Y_0) + r_{23}(Z - Z_0)\right] \qquad (DLT\text{-}3)$$

$$-f = K\left[r_{31}(X - X_0) + r_{32}(Y - Y_0) + r_{33}(Z - Z_0)\right] \qquad (DLT\text{-}4)$$

From Equation DLT-4

$$K = \frac{-f}{r_{31}(X - X_0) + r_{32}(Y - Y_0) + r_{33}(Z - Z_0)} \qquad (DLT\text{-}5)$$

Similarly for Equations DLT-2 and DLT-3, substituting in Equation DLT-5

$$
\begin{aligned}
\Delta U_0 &= U - U_0 \\
&= -f\left[\frac{r_{11}(\Delta X_0) + r_{12}(\Delta Y_0) + r_{13}(\Delta Z_0)}{r_{31}(\Delta X_0) + r_{32}(\Delta Y_0) + r_{33}(\Delta Z_0)}\right]
\end{aligned}
\qquad (DLT\text{-}6)
$$

$$
\begin{aligned}
\Delta V_0 &= V - V_0 \\
&= -f\left[\frac{r_{21}(\Delta X_0) + r_{22}(\Delta Y_0) + r_{23}(\Delta Z_0)}{r_{31}(\Delta X_0) + r_{32}(\Delta Y_0) + r_{33}(\Delta Z_0)}\right]
\end{aligned}
\qquad (DLT\text{-}7)
$$

Solving for U and V

$$U = \frac{A_x + B_y + C_z + D}{I_x + J_y + K_z + 1} \qquad (DLT\text{-}8)$$

where

$$V = \frac{E_x + F_y + G_z + H}{I_x + J_y + K_z + 1} \qquad (DLT\text{-}9)$$

$$A = \frac{U_0 \times r_{13} - f \times r_{11}}{R}$$

$$B = \frac{U_0 \times r_{23} - f \times r_{21}}{R}$$

$$C = \frac{U_0 \times r_{23} - f \times r_{31}}{R}$$

$$D = \frac{(U_0 \times r_{13} - f \times r_{11})X_0 + (U_0 \times r_{23} - f \times r_{21})Y_0 + (U_0 \times r_{33} - f \times r_{31})Z_0}{R}$$

$$E = \frac{V_0 \times r_{13} - f \times r_{12}}{R}$$

$$F = \frac{V_0 \times r_{23} - f \times r_{22}}{R}$$

$$G = \frac{V_0 \times r_{33} - f \times r_{32}}{R}$$

$$H = \frac{(V_0 \times r_{13} - f \times r_{12})X_0 + (V_0 \times r_{23} - f \times r_{22})Y_0 + (V_0 \times r_{33} - f \times r_{32})Z_0}{R}$$

$$I = \frac{r_{13}}{R}$$

$$J = \frac{r_{23}}{R}$$

$$K = \frac{r_{33}}{R}$$

$$R = (r_{13} \times X_0 + r_{23} \times Y_0 + r_{33} \times Z_0)$$

Applying Equations DLT-8 and DLT-9

$$A_x + B_y + C_z + D - U_x \times I_x - U \times J_y - U_y \times K_z = U_z \qquad (DLT\text{-}10)$$

$$E_x + F_y + G_z + H - V_x \times I_x - V_y \times J_y - V_z \times K_z = V \qquad (DLT\text{-}11)$$

The calibration step X, Y, Z, U, and V are known while A through K are unknown. Consequently from Equations DLT-10 and DLT-11

$$\begin{bmatrix} X & Y & Z & 1 & 0 & 0 & 0 & 0 & -U_x & -U_y & -U_z \\ 0 & 0 & 0 & 0 & X & Y & Z & 1 & -U_x & -U_y & -U_z \end{bmatrix} \begin{bmatrix} A \\ \cdot \\ \cdot \\ \cdot \\ K \end{bmatrix} = \begin{bmatrix} U \\ V \end{bmatrix} \qquad (DLT\text{-}12)$$

For n control points where $N \geq 6$,

$$\begin{bmatrix} X_1 & Y_1 & Z_1 & 1 & 0 & 0 & 0 & 0 & -U_1 \times Y_1 & -U_1 \times Y_1 & -U_1 \times Z_1 \\ 0 & 0 & 0 & 0 & X_1 & Y_1 & Z_1 & 1 & -V_1 \times X_1 & -V_1 \times Y_1 & -V_1 \times Z_1 \\ & & & & & \cdot & & & & & \\ & & & & & \cdot & & & & & \\ & & & & & \cdot & & & & & \\ X_n & Y_n & Z_n & 1 & 0 & 0 & 0 & 0 & -U_n \times X_n & -U_n \times Y_n & -U_n \times Z_n \\ 0 & 0 & 0 & 0 & X_n & Y_n & Z_n & 1 & -V_n \times X_n & -V_n \times Y_n & -V_n \times Z_n \end{bmatrix} \cdot \begin{bmatrix} A \\ \cdot \\ \cdot \\ \cdot \\ K \end{bmatrix} = \begin{bmatrix} U_1 \\ V_1 \\ \cdot \\ \cdot \\ \cdot \\ U_n \\ V_n \end{bmatrix} \qquad (DLT\text{-}13)$$

Using known values A through K, then X, Y, and Z can be obtained. Similarly, from Equations DLT-10 and DLT-11

$$\begin{bmatrix} A - U \times I & B - U \times J & C - U \times K \\ E - V \times I & F - V \times J & G - V \times K \end{bmatrix} \begin{bmatrix} X \\ Y \\ Z \end{bmatrix} = \begin{bmatrix} U - D \\ V - H \end{bmatrix} \qquad (DLT\text{-}14)$$

Expanding for m cameras

$$\begin{bmatrix} A_1 - U_1 \times I_1 & B_1 - U_1 \times J_1 & C_1 - U_1 \times K_1 \\ E_1 - V_1 \times I_1 & F_1 - V_1 \times J_1 & G_1 - V_1 \times K_1 \\ & \cdot & \\ & \cdot & \\ & \cdot & \\ A_m - U_m \times I_m & B_m - U_m \times J_m & C_m - U_m \times K_m \\ E_m - V_m \times I_m & F_m - V_m \times J_m & G_m - V_m \times K_m \end{bmatrix} \begin{bmatrix} X \\ Y \\ Z \end{bmatrix} = \begin{bmatrix} U_1 - D_1 \\ V_1 - H_1 \\ \cdot \\ \cdot \\ \cdot \\ U_m - D_m \\ V_m - H_m \end{bmatrix} \qquad (DLT\text{-}15)$$

where $m \geq 2$.

A Review of Body Segmental Displacement, Velocity, and Acceleration in Human Gait

Ge Wu

Key Terms

Angular acceleration

Angular displacement

Angular velocity

Body-fixed reference frame

Global reference frame

Linear acceleration

Linear displacement

Linear velocity

The movement of the human body can be considered a system of articulated rigid links connected through joints. The study of the kinematics of these links is important not only for objectively and accurately quantifying the motion, but also for investigating the control mechanism of human movement—that is, to estimate the joint force and moment associated with the motion. After all, it is the joint force and moment applied through the muscles and passive tissues around the joint that control the desired movement of the adjacent links. Over the years, investigators have attempted to measure the joint loading in vivo by directly instrumenting certain joints.[2,18,39] Such an approach provides valuable insight into the joint functions; however, it requires highly invasive procedures and, therefore, is limited in its applicability. More often, the joint loading is estimated by the inverse dynamics approach based on the externally measured kinematics of body segments.[3,13,46] Therefore, the kinematic information of the moving links is essential for dynamic estimation.

Factors Influencing the Kinematics of Gait

Human gait is a complicated movement, making a quantitative description of human gait even more intricate. Over the years, a great number of researchers have studied the kinematics of human gait. Their findings, however, have been inconsistent, if not contradictory, and have made comparisons between various groups and the establishment of the normative data impractical. The differences among various reports might stem from the following factors: different measurement approaches used to obtain the gait kinematics; the varied number, age, and gender of the subject population; different gait speeds; different footwear on the subjects; different reference frames used to present the kinematics variables; etc. In the following sections, each of these factors will be discussed.

Reference Frames

Kinematic variables describing the body motion in the following sections can be represented in two reference frames: the global reference frame and the body-fixed reference frame.

Angular Displacement   Angular displacement (ϑ) describes the rotational component of the motion of a body segment moving in space. Usually, ϑ is a vector. When ϑ is represented in the global reference frame, it is called the segmental angular displacement, because it describes the absolute angular motion of the segment with re-

spect to the globe. However, when ϑ is represented in the body-fixed reference frame of the adjacent body segment (e.g., the distal segment), it is often referred to as the joint angular displacement (e.g., the distal joint of the segment being described), because it describes the relative angular motion of the segment with respect to another.

It should be noted that the components of the segmental and joint angular displacement vectors are, in general, not identical. However, the segmental angular displacement can be determined based on the joint angular displacement, or vice versa, once the relation between the global and body-fixed reference frames is known. The joint angular displacement is often used in the literature to describe body motion, whereas the segmental angular displacement is used to determine the rotation matrix between the body-fixed and the global reference frames.

Linear Displacement   Linear displacement (Γ_p) describes the translational component of the motion of a body segment moving in space. It can be represented in either the global or the body-fixed reference frame to define the absolute or the relative translation, respectively. In particular, the linear displacement of a segment relative to the body-fixed reference frame of an adjacent segment often describes the translational motion in the joint.

Different from the angular motion, the linear displacement is location dependent (as the subscript p indicates)—that is, the linear displacements at different locations of a rigid body vary. Therefore, the term *linear displacement* should be location specific and be defined as linear displacement at ankle, knee, or center of mass of the shank for clarity.

Angular Velocity and Acceleration   Angular velocity (Ω) describes the rate of change of the rotational motion (i.e., the first derivative of ϑ), while angular acceleration (α) describes the rate of change of the angular velocity (i.e., the second derivative of ϑ). As with angular displacement, both the angular velocity and acceleration can be represented in global or body-fixed reference frames to describe the segmental or joint angular velocity and acceleration, respectively. Note, however, that the segmental angular velocity and acceleration are not the same as the joint angular velocity and acceleration.

Limited data on angular velocity and acceleration during gait are available. Furthermore, those data have been presented inconsistently with respect to the reference frame, thus making the comparison difficult.

Linear Velocity and Acceleration   Linear velocity (V_p) describes the rate of change of the translational motion, while linear acceleration (A_p) describes the rate of the linear velocity. As with linear displacement, both the linear velocity and acceleration can be represented in global or body-fixed reference frames to describe the segmental or joint linear velocity and acceleration, respectively. Furthermore, the linear velocity and acceleration are also location specific.

Measurement Approaches

Body segmental kinematics during locomotion include the linear and angular displacements, velocities, and accelerations. These variables have been studied in the past using one of the following approaches: (1) differentiation approach, which directly measures the displacement and calculates its time derivatives by numerical differentiation; (2) accelerometry approach, which directly measures the acceleration and calculates the velocity and displacement by numerical integration; and (3) integrated approach, which directly measures the displacement, velocity, and acceleration.

Those groups using either the differentiation or accelerometry approaches tended to report the directly measured kinematic data (i.e., the displacement or the acceleration), while those groups using the integrated approach covered a broader range of kinematics. Table 16-1 lists examples of biases in the reports on kinematic data from different investigators. These differences in measuring techniques might create incompatible results that make the comparisons between the kinematic variables difficult. For this reason, the advantages and disadvantages of each of these techniques will be discussed.

Differentiation Approach   This approach requires a direct measurement of either the spatial position of the body segment by utilizing, for example, markers on the body segment, or the joint rotation by using multi-degree of freedom goniometers. The time trajectories of both the segmental position and the joint rotation define the complete rigid body motion and form the basis for the calculation of other kinematic variables such as velocity and acceleration. These values are obtained by taking the first and second time derivatives of the displacement measurements. The direct measurement of displacement was first developed by Marey in 1873 as the quantitative tool to study locomotion and is still the basic approach in modern motion analysis laboratories that use the photogrammetric, goniometric, and optoelectronic approaches.[7,15,24,41,43]

The reliability of the velocity and acceleration estimates depends on both the displacement measurement and the differentiation technique. Although the accuracy, reliability, and efficiency of displacement measuring systems have been increased substantially in the last decade by utilizing computer technology, the inherent problem in the differentiation procedure—the amplification of the high frequency components of noise in the position signal—still prevents accurate estimates of the velocity and acceleration of moving links and, therefore, of joint loading. The differentiation process is usually associated with the use of low-pass filters, which can distort some of the original signal contents. Therefore, the interpretation of force estimates generated by this process requires some information on the inherent accuracy of such a computational approach.

Some studies have been conducted in an attempt to assess the accuracy of estimating second time derivatives from noisy data. Those studies include experimental systems that measure both the position and acceleration of mechanical devices,[22,37] theoretical algorithms that quantify the expected noise in second time derivatives,[25,26] differentiation techniques to minimize that noise,[6,47] and low-pass filtering techniques to eliminate the noise.[11,50,51,54] Studies by Pezzack et al.,[37] Ladin et al.,[22] and Lanshammar[25,26] describe the dependence of the acceleration estimates on the nature of the smoothing and differentiating algorithms, the frequency content of the displacement data, and the cut-off frequencies selected for the low-pass filters. However, studies have shown that the frequency content of different activities varies widely from 8 Hz for normal walking[49] to 200 Hz or higher for hurdling.[20] This wide range of frequency content of signals sometimes makes it impossible to separate signal and noise completely and achieve meaningful signal-to-noise ratio in the corresponding derivatives. In addition, because of the nonideal characteristics of the smoothing or filtering techniques, the signal itself may be distorted by the filter if the filter's cutoff frequency and the signal's highest frequency are close.

Accelerometry Approach   The accelerometry approach requires the direct measurement of the kinematic derivatives such as acceleration using accelerometers.[14,30,40,42] The velocity and displacement are then calculated through integration of the acceleration. There are two major concerns regarding the integration process. First, although the integration procedure attenuates the high frequency noise, the derived velocity and

TABLE 16-1   Examples of the kinematics reported by various investigators.

Approach	Investigator	Technique	Displacement	Velocity	Acceleration
Differentiation	Bresler & Frankel (1950)	photography	lin. at ankle, knee, hip	none	none
	Murray (1967)	photography	lin. and ang. at various locations	none	none
	Winter et al (1974)	photography	sagittal lin. and ang. at various loc.	sagittal lin. and ang. at various loc.	sagittal lin. and ang. at various loc.
	Crowninshield et al (1978)	photography	sagittal ang. at ankle, knee, hip	none	none
	Patriarco et al (1981)	optoelectronic technique	ang. at ankle, knee, hip	none	lin. and ang. at shank, thigh, pelvis
	Cavanagh (1987)	optoelectronic technique	sagittal ang. at ankle, knee, hip	none	none
	Shiavi et al (1987)	6 dof goniometer	lin. and ang. at knee	none	none
	Apkarian et al (1989)	optoelectronic technique	ang. at ankle, knee, hip, pelvis	none	none
Accelerometry	Morris (1973)	accelerometer	lin. at mid-shank during swing	sagittal and coronal ang. lin. at mid-shank during swing	lin. at mid-shank during swing
	Light et al (1980)	accelerometer	none	none	sagittal lin. at shank
	Gilbert et al (1984)	accelerometer	none	none	sagittal lin. at shank, thigh
Integrated	Seemann & Lustick (1981)	accelerometer, photography	lin. and ang. at head	lin. at head	ang. at head
	Wu (1991)	integrated kinematic sensor	lin. at foot, shank, thigh	ang. at foot, shank, thigh	lin. and ang. at foot, shank, thigh
	Radin et al (1991)	accelerometer, optoelectronic technique	lin. and ang. at ankle, knee	sagittal ang. at shank	sagittal lin. and ang. at shank

displacement result in increasing sensitivity to low frequency accelerometer error. Secondly, initial conditions for velocity and displacement have to be available for the completion of the integration process. This information can be either *assumed*, as was done by Morris,[30] Gilbert et al.,[14] and Hayes et al.,[17] or *measured*, as was done by Seemann and Lustick.[42] In both cases the integration process introduces errors that increase with time, leading to significant errors in the calculated orientation of the rigid body.[42]

Some researchers have tried to overcome these difficulties by using multiple accelerometers to resolve the full segmental kinematics. For example, Morris used six accelerometers;[30] Padgaonkar et al. described a system based on nine accelerometers;[34] and Kane et al. described a 12 accelerometer system.[19] More recently Hayes et al. described a four-accelerometer system for studying the kinematics of gait;[17] and Gilbert et al. described a system of eight uniaxial accelerometers for the study of the sagittal plane kinematics of gait.[14] Nevertheless, these authors still acknowledged the need to identify an initial orientation that could serve as the initial condition for the integration process. Overall, because of the above difficulties with the accelerometry approach, the direct measurement of human body acceleration during locomotion has been limited to a planar analysis of the swing/stance phase.[14,27,30]

Integrated Approach   The integrated approach combines the direct measurements of segmental displacement, linear acceleration, and/or angular velocity using a special sensor unit that contains multiple (at least three) markers, a triaxial linear accelerometer, and/or a triaxial angular rate sensor. Coupled with the six degrees of freedom analysis of the rigid body, the integrated approach is able to provide the complete three-dimensional kinesiological information of the moving body. This integrated approach was first introduced by Seemann and Lustick[42] and Ladin and Wu,[21] and was enhanced later by Wu and Ladin.[53]

Seemann and Lustick conducted experiments on human subjects and compared the externally applied known kinematic variables with those estimated using either the integrated approach, the photographic approach, or the accelerometry approach. They have demonstrated high consistency in the displacement data using the integrated and photographic approaches. Furthermore, using a well-controlled two degrees of freedom mechanical pendulum, Wu and Ladin demonstrated a high degree of correlation between the joint loads estimated by the integrated kinematic sensor approach and those directly measured by the strain gauges, whereas the estimates based on the differentiation approach were less accurate and noisier.[53]

The integrated approach eliminates the low-pass filtering process required by the differentiation approach, substantially increasing the frequency range of the kinematic observations during transients and during high-speed activities. It also eliminates the existing problems in the current accelerometry approach, so that neither the multi-accelerometry scheme nor the time integration process (which amplifies the low frequency error) is necessary. As a result, the derived joint loading is independent of any assumptions of the initial conditions and any artifacts in the data processing scheme.

Number of Subjects

The difference in the total number of subjects being tested will certainly affect the statistical outcome of the results. While searching through the literature we were surprised to find that the subject population in most of the studies was very limited. Table 16-2 summarizes the subject information found in the studies that are listed in Table 16-1. The most comprehensive investigation was done by Murray in which 60 men were tested.[31] However, keep in mind that this large population also covered a broad range of life span (from 20 to 65 years of age), which might bias the normative data of the young adult.

Age

Age is an important factor affecting body kinematic patterns during locomotion. A number of functional changes accompany the normal aging process in the sensory, neurological, and musculoskeletal systems. These changes ultimately express themselves as changes in the biomechanics of physical task performance, including gait. We can easily observe, for example, that gait postures of children and the elderly are distinctively different from those of young adults. However, this factor has often been neglected in the past (see Table 16-2).

Gait Maturation in Childhood   While there have been a few studies on gait maturation in children, very few quantitative measurements on the kinematics of the body have been included.[5,44] In 1980, Sutherland et al. first reported, among other variables, the angular kinematics of the lower limb of 186 normal children between the ages of 1 and 7 years.[45] They reported similar sagittal plane angular rotations in the subjects from 2 years of age and older. Subjects less than 2 years old showed greater knee flexion and dorsiflexion during stance, diminished knee flexion wave, and pronounced external rotation of the hip. Nevertheless, Sutherland et al. recognized five important determinants of mature gait: duration of single limb stance, walking velocity, cadence, step length, and the ratio of pelvic span to ankle spread. These parameters were found well established at the age of 3 years.

Later, Marino and McDonald reported the running gait patterns in 63 children between the ages of 6 and 12.[29] The results indicated that many parameters in the running gait pattern have been developed by the age of six and do not change significantly between the ages of 6 and 12. However, slow horizontal running velocity and short stride length are primarily the two distinguishable characteristics among children at the ages of 6 and 7.

Gait Patterns in the Elderly   Similarly, there has been limited research on gait patterns in the elderly. Among a few leading researchers, Murray

TABLE 16-2   Subject information in various investigations.

Investigator	# Subjects	Age (yrs)	Gender	Health
Bresler & Frankel (1950)	4	unknown	unknown	normal
Murray (1967)	60	20-65	male	normal
Winter et al (1974)[48]	12	adult	unknown	normal
Crowninshield et al (1978)	4	unknown	unknown	normal
Patriarco et al (1981)	2	19 and 27	female	normal
Cavanagh (1987)	1	unknown	unknown	normal
Shiavi et al (1987)	1	unknown	unknown	normal
	1	unknown	unknown	knee injury
Apkarian et al (1989)	2	21 and 26	male	normal
	1	21	female	normal
Morris (1973)	unknown	unknown	unknown	unknown
Light et al (1980)	unknown	unknown	unknown	unknown
Gilbert et al (1984)	12	unknown	unknown	normal
	9	but matched	unknown	amputee
Seemann & Lustick (1981)	unknown	unknown	unknown	unknown
Wu (1991)	4	25-32	male	normal
Radin et al (1991)	14	unknown	unknown	normal
	18			preosteoarthrotic

et al. reported gait patterns in elderly men[32]; and Finley et al. reported gait patterns in women, respectively.[12] Recently, Nigg and Skleryk conducted a biomechanical study investigating the aging effect on gait.[33] Changes in gait patterns do occur when people age. In general, as people become older, they tend to walk with shorter and broader stride dimensions, slower cadence, and lower swing-to-stance time ratios.[12,32,33] These changes have been reported to occur as early as 60 years old.[32]

Gender

Studies have shown that there is a difference in the gait pattern changes between elderly men and women. For example, using the photography technique, Murray et al. studied the gait patterns of 64 healthy men aged 20 to 87 years.[32] They found that the amplitudes of the sagittal plane angular rotations at the joints in the lower limb were less for the older men than for the younger men, resulting in less vertical oscillation of the head in the elderly. Finley et al.[12] and Hageman and Blanke,[16] on the other hand, studied the gait patterns of both young and elderly women. They concluded that no significant difference exists in the joint rotations in the lower limb between young and elderly women. Nevertheless, gender difference has again been often neglected in the past as evidenced by the list in Table 16-2.

Speed

The kinematic measurements on the lower limb during locomotion provide valuable information for a quantitative characterization of gait differences at different speeds. It has been widely reported that the lower limb kinematics are dependent on walking speed.[4,8,31,48] For example, the stride length increases and the ratio of the time duration between swing and stance phases decreases as the speed of the locomotion increases.

Angular Displacement   Winter et al. conducted a statistical study on a group of normal subjects walking at slow, normal, and fast cadences.[48] They reported the average maximum values of the sagittal plane segmental rotations of the foot, shank, and thigh segments (see Table 16-3). While the angular motions of the thigh increased with an increase in walking speed, they showed only a slight increase for the foot and shank segments at normal speed. Such a slight difference as 2 to 3 degrees is not significant judging by the associated standard deviations.

Cavanagh[8] studied the biomechanics of the human lower limb during distance running. Among many kinematic variables, the sagittal plane angular displacement at the ankle, knee, and hip joints was calculated and presented. Figure 16-1 illustrates these angular trajectories during treadmill running at a speed of 4.2 m/s. Compared

TABLE 16-3   Maximum mean (S.D.) angular displacement (in degrees) of the foot, shank, and thigh.

Speed	Foot	Shank	Thigh
Slow (82 cad/min)	203 (5)	107 (3)	115 (3)
Normal (93 cad/min)	205 (6)	110 (3)	116 (5)
Fast (114 cad/min)	203 (8)	108 (3)	118 (4)

Modified with permission from Winter DA et al: *J. Biomech,* 7:479, 1974.

to the sagittal plane angles at the ankle, knee, and hip joints during level walking (as shown later in Figure 16-4), the temporal patterns are quite similar between walking and running except for the difference in the swing/stance time ratio. Moreover, the maximum magnitude of the hip flexion-extension during running is on the same order of magnitude as during walking. The significant difference observed is the increase in the knee and ankle flexion-extension angles in running. It should be kept in mind, however, that the results presented in Figure 16-4 were from free walking, whereas the ones in Figure 16-1 were from treadmill running.

Angular Velocity and Acceleration   In the same study by Winter et al. cited above, the angular velocity and acceleration of the lower limb during walking at three different speeds were also reported.[48] Table 16-4 lists the average maximum values. There are two observations based on these data. First, both the angular velocity and accelera-

tion tended to increase with the increase in speed. Second, at each speed, the values of the distal segment(s) were larger than those of the proximal segment(s).

Recently, Wu conducted a series of experiments using the integrated kinematic sensor approach in an attempt to quantify the lower limb kinematics during gait at various speeds.[52] Three walking speeds and one running speed were tested on four healthy young male subjects. They included slow walking (1.13 ± 0.06 m/s), normal walking (1.36 ± 0.05 m/s), fast walking (2.15 ± 0.13 m/s), and running (3.87 ± 0.16 m/s). Three-dimensional angular velocities of the foot, shank, and thigh segments were directly measured. Both the temporal pattern and maximum magnitude of these variables were compared.

One of the most interesting and important phenomena observed in the angular velocity measurements was the heel strike impact. Such impact increased significantly from slow walking to running. In general, the increase of the peak impacts was on the order of tenfold, while the increase of the speed was only three. Such a dramatic increase could perhaps explain why the injury rate in the lower limb is much higher during high-speed activities.

The maximum range of the angular velocity of the foot, shank, and thigh during walking and running were extracted and are shown in Figure 16-2. The following observations are made: (1) the peak values of all three body segments increased as the speed of the gait increased; (2) the rate of such increase was similar for both the shank and thigh, and yet it was much faster for the foot; and

FIGURE 16-1   Flexion-extension (in degree) at the hip, knee, and ankle joints during treadmill running at 4.2 m/s. Two complete cycles are shown. From Cavanagh, PR: *Foot and Ankle,* 7(4):197, 1987.

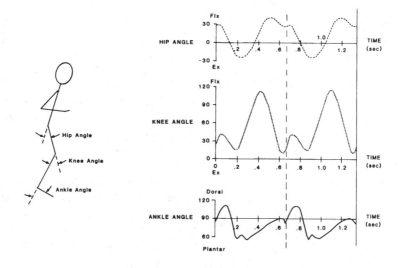

Table 16-4   Maximum mean (S.D.) angular velocity (in deg/sec) and acceleration (in deg/sec^2) of the foot, shank, and thigh.

Speed	Angular Velocity			Angular Acceleration		
	Foot	Shank	Thigh	Foot	Shank	Thigh
Slow (82 cad/min)	356 (62)	273 (45)	136 (26)	5150 (1060)	2930 (750)	1210 (240)
Normal (93 cad/min)	446 (42)	337 (21)	164 (17)	7100 (1090)	3916 (590)	1760 (320)
Fast (114 cad/min)	520 (97)	405 (91)	195 (36)	8600 (2730)	4710 (2010)	1970 (530)

Modified with permission from Winter DA et al, *J Biomech,* 7:479, 1974.

(3) the more distal segment experienced higher peak values at all the speeds than the more proximal segment did.

Although the general observations on the data by Winter et al.[48] are similar to those on the data by Wu,[52] the maximum values are smaller. This discrepancy could be accounted for in part by the differences in the speeds being tested and in part by the smoothing process adopted by Winter et al.[48] They applied a low-pass filter with 5 Hz cutoff to the angular velocity data. This process often results in a reduced peak magnitude in the filtered signal.

Linear Acceleration   In the study by Wu, three-dimensional linear accelerations of the foot, shank, and thigh segments were also directly measured.[52] The maximum magnitudes are shown in Figure 16-3. The general observations on the temporal patterns as well as on the maximum values are similar to those on the angular velocity values.

Footwear

The kinematics of gait are altered by different footwear. Although limited data are available to quantify such kinematic change, many studies have been conducted to measure the foot pressure distribution change in relation to different footwear. Recently, Perry et al. measured in 39 individuals the in-shoe plantar pressures during walking in an oxford shoe and a running shoe, respectively, and compared the results to the in-shoe pressures during walking in socks on a hard surface.[36] In the oxford shoe, plantar pressures in all but one anatomical region were not significantly different from those measured during walking without shoes. Inexpensive running shoes provided an average plantar pressure relief of 30% in the forefoot compared to the oxford, with the greatest relief of pressure occurring in those feet with the greatest unshod pressures.

Unfortunately, the effect of footwear on gait kinematics has not been given enough attention. For example, in some of the literature the type of footwear worn by the subjects is never mentioned. In addition, the variation of the footwear used in each study is so large (including bare footed, soft cushioned, hard cushioned, high heeled, rocker bottomed, etc.) that it makes the comparison between different studies difficult.

Normative Data

The kinematics of the body segments during gait has been studied by many investigators. However, the total number of parameters that can be presented to quantify the motion of the whole body is tremendous. Taking one body segment, such as shank, for example, the complete three-dimensional kinematics of the shank includes linear and angular displacements (six variables), velocities (six), and accelerations (six), totaling 18 variables. If three body segments in one lower limb are considered, there would be a total of 54 variables. Consequently, all these variables during one single task (such as gait) have not been reported by one research group. Table 16-1 is an example of how scattered the reports on the kinematic data are from different investigators. As a result, a complete view of the kinematics of the human body during gait can only be obtained by putting together the pieces from numerous reports. Unfortunately, each study was conducted under specific, nonstandard conditions. Therefore, one should be careful when "normative" kinematic data are to be established.

Angular Displacement

The angular displacement at the lower limb joints during normal gait has been documented by various investigators. For example, Crowninshield et al.[9] and Cavanagh[8] reported the time trajectories

Figure 16-2   The peak value (mean + standard deviation) of the angular velocity of the foot, shank, and thigh segments during gait at four speeds. Total of eight trials for walking and 12 trials for running from three subjects. From Wu G: *Dynamic estimation of human joint loading during locomotion,* 1991.

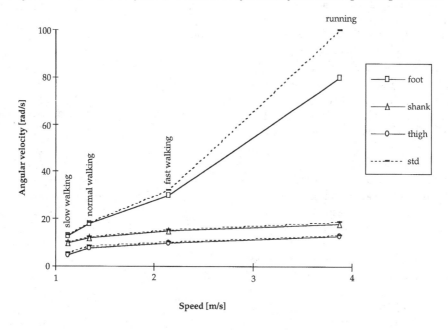

Figure 16-3   The peak value (mean + standard deviation) of the linear acceleration at the center of mass of the foot, shank, and thigh segments during gait at four speeds. Total of three trials for walking and four trials for running from a single subject. From Wu G: *Dynamic estimation of human joint loading during locomotion,* 1991.

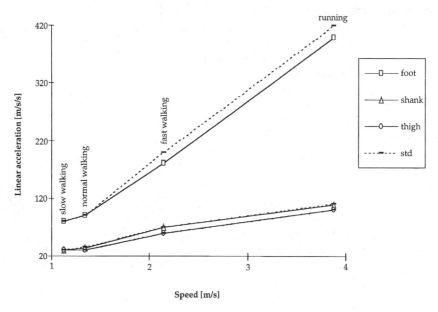

of the flexion-extension angles at the ankle, knee, and hip joints during walking and running, respectively. Shiavi et al. reported the time trajectories of the three-dimensional angular displacements only at the knee joint.[43] The complete measurement of the three-dimensional angular displacements at the ankle, knee, and hip joints during gait can be found from the reports by Patriarco et al. and Apkarian et al., respectively.[1,35] For most of the investigators, the angular displacement variable has been presented with respect to the body-fixed reference system, that is, the joint angular motion has been mostly reported.

Because the primary movement of normal gait occurs in the sagittal plane, the flexion-extension motion of the lower limb joints is the dominant component in the overall angular displacement measurement. The reports from various investigators on the time trajectories of the flexion-extension angles at the ankle, knee, and hip joints are fairly consistent. One of the representative time trajectory plots of these angles is shown in Figure 16-4. This set of data was based on 30 normal men in free speed walking.

The representative data on the maximum magnitude of sagittal joint rotation can be found in the literature by Murray[31] and by Winter et al.[48] Table 16-5 summarizes their results, which correspond well.

The other components of the angular displacements (i.e., the adduction-abduction and axial rotation) at the lower limb joints are found to be less consistent among different investigators. In fact, Apkarian et al. have demonstrated intersubject variation in both the patterns and maximum magnitudes.[1] They pointed out that such variation might be due to interindividual repeatable artifacts such as skin movement or limited system resolution. A three-dimensional time trajectory of the angular displacements at the ankle, knee, and hip joints is shown in Figure 16-5. The data were based on one subject during level walking with unspecified speed. Note that the data presented in Figure 16-5 were in the global reference system, whereas the data presented in Figure 16-4 were in the body-fixed reference system.

Linear Displacement

Different from the angular displacement, which is location independent, the linear displacements at different locations of the lower limb vary during gait. Using markers, Bresler and Frankel made the direct measurement of the global linear displacement at the toe, ankle, knee, and hip joints.[4] Later, Murray[31] and Winter et al.[48] reported the linear displacement measurement at various locations of the body (e.g., at the toe, heel, head, and neck). Using accelerometers or the integrated approach, Morris[30] and Radin et al.[38] reported the linear displacement at mid-shank, or at ankle and knee. Recently, Wu, using the integrated approach, calculated and reported the linear displacement at the center of mass of the foot, shank, and thigh during normal gait.[52] In general, the linear displacement variable has been mostly described in the global reference frame.

FIGURE 16-4   Sagittal plane angular displacements (in degree) at (**A**) the ankle, (**B**) the knee, and (**C**) the hip joints during free speed walking, based on 30 subjects. From Murray MP: *American J Physical Medicine,* 46(1)290, 1967.

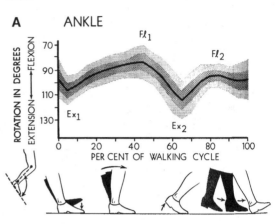

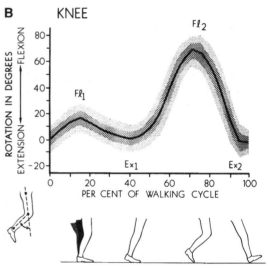

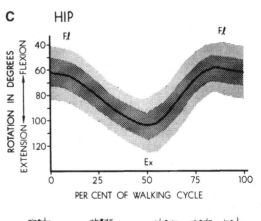

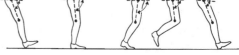

TABLE **16-5**   Maximum mean (S.D.) joint rotation (in degrees).

Investigator	Number of subjects	Speed	Ankle	Knee	Hip
Murray (1967)	30	free	30	73	44
	8	82 cad/min	31	71	*
Winter et al. (1974)	12	93 cad/min	35	67	*
	8	114 cad/min	34	76	*

*Indicates no data were reported.

FIGURE **16-5**   Angular displacements (in degrees) at (**A**) the ankle, (**B**) the knee, and (**C**) the hip joints during level walking, based on one subject. From Apkarian J et al.: *J Biomech* 22(2):143, 1989.

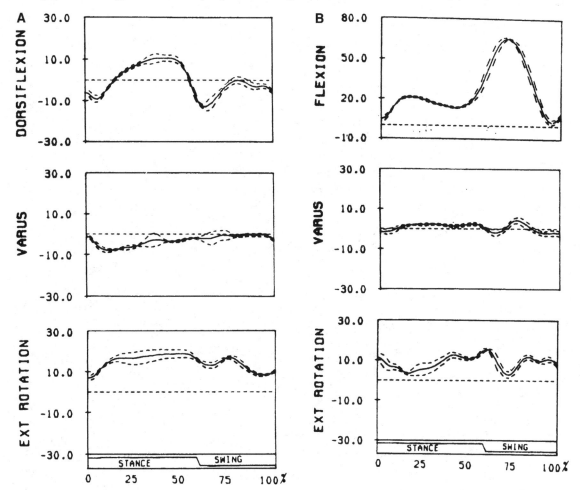

The representative time trajectory of the linear displacement at the toe, ankle, knee, and hip joints is shown in Figure 16-6. Keep in mind, however, that the actual displacement as indicated in the figure does not represent the motion at the center of rotation of each joint. In fact, the location of the center of rotation of lower limb joints, especially the knee joint, is not fixed with respect to the bony landmark during joint movement.

The representative time trajectories of the linear displacement at the center of mass of the foot, shank, and thigh during level walking is shown in Figure 16-7. A systematic medial shift from the first toe off to the successive one, as observed in the foot, shank, and thigh segments, was due to data presented in the global reference system whose axes were not aligned exactly with the travel direction of the subject.

Figure 16-5—Cont'd

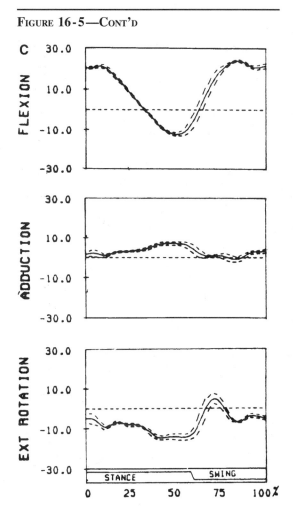

Figure 16-6 Linear displacements at the toe, ankle, knee, and hip during walking: (A) Y component, (B) Z component, and (C) X component. Single trial from one subject. From Bresler B, Frankel JP: *ASME Trans,* 27, 1950.

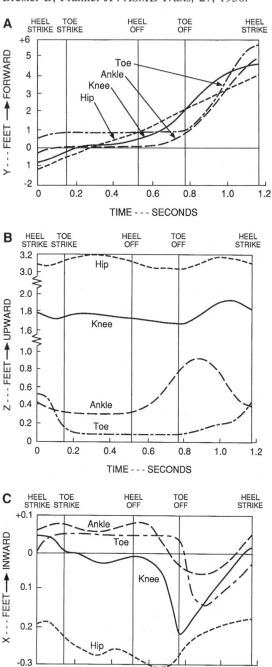

The results as shown in Figures 16-6 and 16-7 are, in general, in agreement except for the vertical foot/ankle displacement. The vertical displacement at the center of mass of the foot (Figure 16-7) clearly showed a double peak pattern during swing phase of the gait while the one at the toe and ankle (Figure 16-6b) showed only a single peak. A closer examination reveals that if the two trajectories of the ankle and the toe were combined—that is, if a line was formed by connecting these two points—the resulting displacement at the mid-point of this line (close to the center of mass of the foot) would yield double peaks within the swing phase. The first one reflected the toe off period, when the heel (or ankle) was raised higher than the toe, and the second one reflected the heel strike period, when the toe was raised higher than the heel (or ankle).

While the above studies were based on a few subjects, the study done by Winter et al. presents the mean maximum range of vertical displacement at seven locations of the lower limb based on eight or 12 subjects.[48] They demonstrated larger vertical movement at the heel (about 25 cm) than at the toe (about 11 cm) and at the proximal joints

(about 6 to 7 cm). No significant differences were found between three different walking speeds.

Angular Velocity

Reports on the angular velocity of the lower limb during normal gait have been limited. Using the

Figure 16-7 Linear displacements at the center of mass of the foot, shank, and thigh segments during walking at speed of 1.35 m/s vs. one complete gait cycle. Single trial from one subject. From Wu G: *Dynamic estimation of human joint loading during locomotion,* 1991.

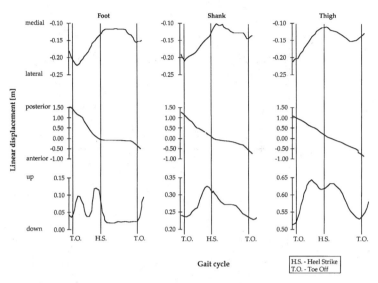

differentiation approach, Lamoreux was perhaps the first who reported the sagittal plane angular velocities of the lower limb joints based on data from one subject walking on a treadmill.[24] Later, Winter et al. reported the mean sagittal plane angular velocities of the lower limb segments and joints based on data from eight to 12 subjects during walking at three different speeds.[48] The results from the above two studies were within the same range.

Using the accelerometry approach, Morris first calculated and reported the angular velocity of the shank in the sagittal and coronal planes.[30] The data were based on only one subject, and the speed of the gait was not specified. Later, Radin et al., using the integrated approach, also calculated and reported the sagittal plane angular velocity of the shank during gait on a total of 14 normal subjects.[38] The first direct measurement of three-dimensional angular velocity in the human lower limb during gait was done by Wu using the integrated kinematic sensor approach.[52] The results from these three studies were in good agreement. The maximum mean ranges of the angular velocities of the foot, shank, and thigh during movement from slow walking to fast walking and running are summarized in Figure 16-2. As an example, the time trajectories of three components of the angular velocity of the foot, shank and thigh of three trials from a single subject during level walking at a speed of 1.3 m/s are shown in Figure 16-8. The angular velocity was considered as a vector whose direction was determined using the right-handed rule. That is, the sagittal component was defined as a vector along the medial-lateral direction;

the frontal component was defined as a vector along the anterior-posterior direction; and the transverse component was defined as a vector along the vertical direction. The results indicated that the temporal patterns of all the components were repeatable within individual subjects. The variability between subjects was mainly in the foot and during phase transitions (such as from swing to stance or vice versa). In general, the dominant angular velocity for all three segments was in the sagittal plane, and the angular velocity of the more distal segment was larger than that of the more proximal segment.

The results obtained by either the acceleration or integrated approach were larger than the results obtained by the differentiation approach. This difference can be attributed to the low-pass filtering process that was associated with the differentiation approach. For example, Winter et al. used a low-pass filter with 5 Hz cutoff frequency.[49] This process might smooth or partially cut the signals.

Linear Velocity

Although, as indicated by Morris, the angular and translational velocities can "reveal most about the gait of the subject," there have been inadequate reports on linear velocity data during gait.[30] Three publications have included linear velocity data: Morris, Winter et al., and Seemann and Lustick. Morris, who used multiple accelerometers and appropriate initial conditions, calculated the three-dimensional linear velocities at a point near the mid-shank region during the entire stance phase of gait.[30] Winter et al., who used the differentiation approach as described in the previous sections,

FIGURE 16-8   Angular velocity of the foot, shank, and thigh segments during walking at speed of 1.35 m/s vs. one complete gait cycle. Total of three trials from single subject. From Wu G: *Dynamic estimation of human joint loading during locomotion,* 1991.

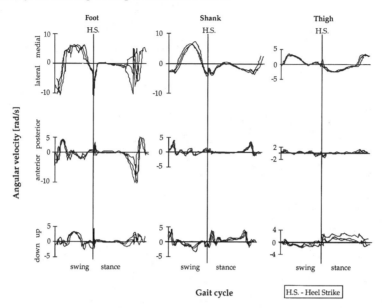

reported the sagittal plane linear velocities at seven locations of the body.[48] Seemann and Lustick integrated the accelerometers and photographic technology to calculate the horizontal linear velocity of the head during a simulated test.[42]

Based on the available information, the linear velocity of the mid-shank during swing phase of the gait is shown in Figure 16-9. As observed by Morris, "a small positive angular velocity in the sagittal plane, in conjunction with a low vertical velocity, prepares the leg for a low energy heel strike. These are clear characteristics of normal gait."[30] It should be pointed out that the data shown in Figure 16-9 were based on only one subject, and the exact speed of the gait was not clear.

The maximum mean sagittal linear velocities of the lower limb during walking at three speeds

were reported by Winter et al. (Table 16-6).[48] Clearly, the results demonstrate the increase in the velocities with the increase of speed. However, they fail to indicate exactly where these maximum velocities occur within the gait cycle. Also, the velocities were calculated using the differentiation approach with a 5 Hz cutoff low-pass filter. Thus, the actual maximum velocities in the lower limb might be larger.

Angular Acceleration

To date, no direct measurement has been done on the angular acceleration of human lower limb during gait. The reported data have been calculated either by double differentiation of the angular displacement, or by single differentiation of the angular velocity.[24,35,48,52] Consequently, this variable

TABLE 16-6   Maximum mean (S.D.) linear velocity (in cm/sec) of the lower limb.

Marker Location	82 cad/min		93 cad/min		114 cad/min	
	Vertical	Horiz.	Vertical	Horiz.	Vertical	Horiz.
tubero. greater trochanter	25(5)	104(15)	31(4)	126(12)	34(7)	154(35)150
tibial tubercle	29(8)	167(26)	38(8)	204(17)	49(9)	244(57)
lat. malleolus of fibula	87(14)	239(34)	99(9)	294(27)	120(33)	346(82)
heel	125(19)	266(38)	147(13)	323(28)	176(46)	378(93)
ball	85(19)	277(42)	91(11)	338(29)	96(14)	408(103)
toe	87(16)	286(42)	98(18)	351(30)	106(23)	425(108)

Modified with permission from Winter DA et al, *J Biomech,* 7:479, 1974.

FIGURE 16-9 Linear velocity at the mid-shank during swing phase of walking. The rows, from the top, show fore-backward, sideways, and vertical directions. From Morris JRW: *J Biomech* 6:729, 1973.

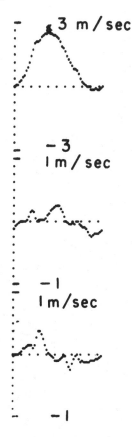

comparable data were very limited. In the four studies, the angular acceleration of the ankle reported by Lamoreux[24] was more than double of that by Winter et al.[4]; and the angular acceleration of the shank reported by Winter et al.[48] was higher than that by Patriarco et al.[35] Moreover, the angular accelerations by both Winter et al.[48] and Patriarco et al. were much smaller than those reported by Wu.[52]

There are many factors that might result in such large discrepancies between different studies. These factors include, but are not limited to, footwear, such as low soft-heeled shoes by Winter et al.,[48] higher-heeled leather shoes by Lamoreux,[24] and bare foot by Wu[52]; instrumentation, such as photograph technique by Winter et al.[48] and Patriarco et al.,[35] and integrated kinematics approach by Wu[52]; and walking surface, such as level floor by Winter et al.,[48] Patriarco et al.,[35] and Wu,[52] and treadmill by Lamoreux.[24] Taking the footwear for example, the study by Wu[52] was done on barefoot subjects (the hardest interface), whereas the study by Lamoreux[24] was with leather shoes and the one by Winter et al.[48] was with soft-heeled shoes (the softest interface). Therefore, it is not surprising to find the largest angular accelerations by Wu[52] and the smallest angular accelerations by Winter et al.[48] Furthermore, all the studies listed in Table 16-7 except for the one by Wu[52] applied second order time derivative to the displacement data and low-pass smoothing process in calculating the angular accelerations. Such a process might have reduced the magnitude of the signal, resulting in smaller maximum angular acceleration readings.

Regardless of the differences in the maximum values, the time trajectories of the angular accelerations of the shank, thigh, and pelvis as reported by Patriarco et al. are shown in Figure 16-10.[35] The trajectories covered one entire gait cycle from heel strike to the successive heel strike. The data

was the noisiest among other kinematic variables, and no consistent results have been reported. Table 16-7 summarizes the maximum range of angular accelerations of the lower limb from four different studies. Clearly, considering the speed factor, the

TABLE 16-7 Maximum mean sagittal angular acceleration (in rad/sec^2) of the lower limb during walking from four different studies.

Investigator	Speed	Foot	Shank	Thigh	Pelvis	Ankle	Knee	Hip
Lamoreux (1981)	normal	—*	–	–	–	333	150	33
	slow	170	97	36	–	100	112	–
Winter et al. (1974)	normal	228	134	30	–	150	150	–
	fast	282	163	60	–	169	190	–
Patriarco et al. (1981)	slow	–	60	40	20	–	–	–
	slow	250	180	120	–	–	–	–
Wu (1991)	normal	400	230	150	–	–	–	–
	fast	600	400	250	–	–	–	–

*Indicates no data were reported.

FIGURE 16-10   Angular acceleration (in rad/s^2) of the shank, thigh, and pelvis during gait at 1.2 m/s. The x (solid), y (dash), and z (dot) components are flexion-extension, medial-lateral rotation, and adduction-abduction. From Patriarco AG et al.: *J Biomech* 14:513, 1981.

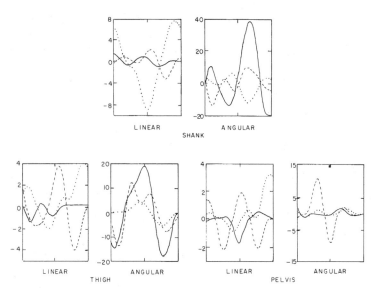

were for one subject and were representative of the set of six individuals. The speed of the gait was about 1.2 m/s (slow walking).

Linear Acceleration

In the past, there have been a number of direct measurements of the linear acceleration of the human lower limb during gait using either the accelerometry or the integrated approach. However, because of the complexity of the accelerometer arrangement, the acceleration measurement has been done mainly in the limited fashion. For example, Light et al.[27] and Radin et al.[38] reported the *sagittal* plane linear acceleration (i.e., the forward-backward and vertical accelerations) at the *shank;* Gilbert et al. reported similar components at both the *shank* and *thigh;*[14] and Morris[30] made the three-dimensional measurement on the *shank* only. All the accelerations reported by these investigators were at the actual measurement site. Recently, the complete three-dimensional linear acceleration at the center of mass of the foot, shank, and thigh segments during normal gait was presented by Wu using the integrated approach.[52]

The time trajectories of the lower limb linear acceleration during normal speed walking are shown in Figure 16-11. Although they are based on one subject, they are representative of a set of four young male subjects. It is important to note that all the components of the linear accelerations showed distinct impulses around heel strike. This characteristic has been observed in all other reports in which the accelerometers were used for direct measurement.[14,27,30,38] Furthermore, the

peak values of the medial-lateral acceleration at all three body segments were comparable to the ones in the sagittal plane, although the major movement of the gait was in the sagittal plane.

Using the differentiation approach, very little has been reported for the calculated linear accelerations of the lower limb during gait. Eberhart and Inman calculated the horizontal accelerations at the ankle, knee, and hip based on one subject.[10] Winter et al. calculated, based on a maximum of twelve subjects, the sagittal plane linear accelerations at seven locations on the lower limb.[48] The data from both studies were in good agreement. Later, Patriarco et al. presented the linear acceleration at the shank, thigh, and pelvis, although no detailed information was given with respect to the specific locations at which the accelerations were presented.[35]

This is perhaps a good time to bring attention to the difference in the linear acceleration data that are obtained through differentiation and direct measurement. This difference can be easily demonstrated by examining the time trajectories of the acceleration based on these two approaches. For example, the horizontal acceleration of the toe marker calculated directly from the second derivative of the horizontal trajectory of the toe marker with low-pass filtering at 5 Hz is presented in Figure 16-12. Comparing these data with the anterior-posterior (A-P) acceleration at the center of mass of the foot (as shown in Figure 16-11), the overall patterns and the maximum values throughout the gait cycle were in considerable agreement except around heel strike (or heel contact), where a rather smooth transient was observed by using the

FIGURE 16-11   Linear acceleration (in m/s²) at the center of mass of the foot, shank, and thigh segments during walking at speed of 1.35 m/s vs. one complete gait cycle. Single trial from one subject. From Wu G: *Dynamic estimation of human joint loading during locomotion,* 1991.

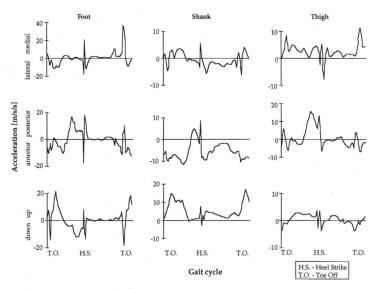

FIGURE 16-12   Linear acceleration (in cm/s²) of the toe marker during normal walking. From Winter DA et al.: *J Biomech* 7:479, 1974.

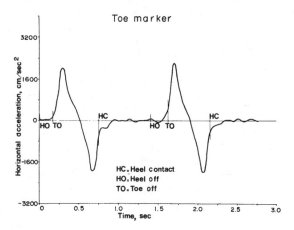

differentiation approach. This lack of impact acceleration at the transient from swing to stance phase was clearly due to the low-pass smoothing process that was applied to the differentiated data. Although it is not quite clear yet how important the impact acceleration at the transition is to the biomechanics of human gait, it is at least a piece of information that deserves a factual representation.

SUMMARY

The existing normative data on the kinematics of the body during gait are not conclusive, not standardized, and not consistent. The majority of the

data is within the sagittal plane, and the velocity and acceleration information is very limited. There is also debate on the existence of impact acceleration during transition of the gait.

Whenever the kinematic data of gait from literature are to be used as references, it is wise to be cautious about a few important factors that are likely to affect the results: the measurement approaches used to obtain the gait kinematics (in particular, whether an additional process such as low-pass filtering is applied); the total number of subject; subject's age and gender; speed of gait; footwear; and reference frames to present the kinematic variables.

REFERENCES

1. Apkarian J et al: A three-dimensional kinematic and dynamic model of the lower limb, *J Biomech* 22(2):143, 1989.
2. Bergmann G et al: Five month in vivo measurement of hip joint forces, *Proceedings of the Twelfth International Congress of Biomechanics,* Abstract No. 43, 1989.
3. Bernstein NA et al: Biodynamics of locomotion, *VIEM,* vol. 1, Moscow, 1935.
4. Bresler B, Frankel JP: The forces and moments in the leg during level walking, *ASME Trans:* 27, 1950.
5. Burnett CN, Johnson EW: Development of gait in childhood: I and II, *Methods Devel Med Child Neurol* 13:196, 1971.
6. Busby HR, Trujillo DM: Numerical experiments with a new differentiation filter, *J Biomech Eng* 107:293, 1985.
7. Cappozo A: Considerations on clinical gait evaluation, *J Biomech* 16(4):302, 1983.
8. Cavanagh PR: The biomechanics of lower extremity action in distance running, *Foot Ankle* 7(4):197, 1987.

9. Crowninshield RD et al: A biomechanical investigation of the human hip, *J Biomech* 11:75, 1978.

10. Eberhart HD, Inman VT: Evaluation of experimental procedures in fundamental study of human locomotion, *Ann NY Acad Sci* 51(7):1213, 1951.

11. Ferrigno G, D'Amico M: The assessment of first and second derivatives from noisy kinematic data, *Proceedings of the Twelfth International Congress of Biomechanics,* Abstract No. 75, 1989.

12. Finley FR et al: Locomotion patterns in elderly women, *Arch Phys Med Rehabil* 50:140, 1969.

13. Fischer O: Human gait, *Abhandlunsen der Seachs,* vol. 21, 1898, Gesellschaft der Wissenschaft.

14. Gilbert JA et al: A system to measure the forces and moments at the knee and hip during level walking, *J Orthop Res* 2:281, 1984.

15. Goldbranson FL, Wirta RW: The use of gait analysis to study gait patterns of the lower limb amputee, *Bull Prosth Res* 18(1):153, 1981.

16. Hagemen PA, Blanke DJ: Comparison of gait of young women and elderly women, *Phys Ther* 66(9):1382, 1986.

17. Hayes WC et al: Leg motion analysis during gait by multiaxial accelerometry: theoretic foundations and preliminary validations, *ASME Trans J Biomech Eng* 105:283, 1983.

18. Hodge WA et al: Contact pressures in the human hip joint measured in vivo, *Proceedings of the National Academy of Sciences,* 1986.

19. Kane TR et al: Experimental determination of forces exerted in tennis play, *Biomech* IV:284, 1974.

20. Kerwin DG, Chapman GM: The frequency content of hurdling and running, *Biomech in Sports:* 107, 1988.

21. Ladin Z, Wu G: Combining position and acceleration measurements for joint force estimation, *J Biomech* 24(12):1173, 1991.

22. Ladin Z et al: A quantitative comparison of a position measurement system and accelerometry, *J Biomech* 22(4):295, 1989.

23. Lamoreux LW: Kinematic measurements in the study of human walking, *Bull Prosth Res:* 3, 1971.

24. Lamoreux L: Exoskeletal goniometry, *Bull Prosth Res* 18(4):288, 1981.

25. Lanshammar H: On practical evaluation of differentiation techniques for human gait analysis, *J Biomech* 15(2):99, 1982.

26. Lanshammar H: On precision limits for derivatives numerically calculated from noisy data, *J Biomech* 15(6):459, 1982.

27. Light LH et al: Skeletal transients on heel strike in normal walking with different footwear, *J Biomech* 13:477, 1980.

28. Marey EJ: Terrestrial locomotion of bipeds and quadrupeds, *J de l'anat et de la Physiol* 9:42, 1873.

29. Marino GW, McDonald M: A biomechanical analysis of children's running patterns. In Watkins J et al, editors: *Sports Science,* London, 1986, E & FN Spon Ltd.

30. Morris JRW: Accelerometry: a technique for the measurement of human body movements, *J Biomech* 6:729, 1973.

31. Murray MP: Gait as a total pattern of movement, *Am J Phys Med* 46(1):290, 1967.

32. Murray MP et al: Walking patterns in healthy old men, *J Gerontol* 24(2):169, 1969.

33. Nigg BM, Skleryk BN: Gait characteristics of the elderly, *Clin Biomech* 3:79, 1988.

34. Padgaonkar AJ et al: Measurement of angular acceleration of a rigid body using linear accelerometers, *J Appl Mech* 42:552, 1975.

35. Patriarco AG et al: An evaluation of the approach of optimization models in the prediction of muscle forces during human gait, *J Biomech* 14:513, 1981.

36. Perry JE et al: Non-therapeutic footwear can play a role in reducing plantar pressure in the diabetic foot. Submitted.

37. Pezzack JC et al: An assessment of derivative determining techniques used for motion analysis, *J Biomech* 10:377, 1977.

38. Radin EL et al: Relationship between lower limb dynamics and knee joint pain, *J Orthop Res* 9:398, 1991.

39. Rydell N: Forces acting on the femoral head prosthesis, *Acta Orthop Scand* 88 Suppl:9, 1966.

40. Sabelman EE et al: Accelerometric body-motion detection in spinal injury patients, *Human-Machine Integration,* Report 68, 1988.

41. Scholz JP: Reliability and validity of the WATSMART three-dimensional optoelectric motion analysis system, *Phys Ther* 69(8):1989.

42. Seemann MR, Lustick LS: Combination of accelerometer and photographically derived kinematic variables defining three-dimensional rigid body motion, *SPIE Biomech Cinema* 291:133, 1981.

43. Shiavi R et al: Helical motion analysis of the knee. I. Methodology for studying kinematics during locomotion, *J Biomech* 20(5):459, 1987.

44. Statham L, Murray MP: Early walking patterns of normal children, *Clin Orthop* 79:8, 1971.

45. Sutherland DH et al: The development of mature gait, *J Bone Joint Surg* 62A(3):336, 1980.

46. Thunnissen JG et al: Determining muscle force and energy in the leg during walking using the inverse dynamics method. *Proceedings of the Twelfth International Congress of Biomechanics,* Abstract No. 322, 1989.

47. Usui S, Amidror I: Digital low pass differentiation for biological signal processing, *IEEE Trans Biomed Eng* 29(10):686, 1982.

48. Winter DA et al: Kinematics of normal locomotion: A statistical study based on T.V. data, *J Biomech* 7:479, 1974.

49. Winter DA et al: Measurement and reduction of noise in kinematics of locomotion, *J Biomech* 9:253, 1974.

50. Winter DA: *The biomechanics and motor control of human gait,* Waterloo, Ontario, 1990, University of Waterloo Press.

51. Woltring HJ: An optional smoothing and derivative estimation from noisy displacement data in biomechanics, *Human Movement Science* 3:229, 1984.

52. Wu G: *Dynamic estimation of human joint loading during locomotion,* 1991.

53. Wu G, Ladin Z: The kinematometer: an integrated kinematic sensor for kinesiological measurements, *ASME Trans J Biomech Eng* 115(1):53, 1993.

54. Yeadon MR: Numerical differentiation of noisy data, *Proceedings of the Twelfth International Congress of Biomechanics,* Abstract No. 125, 1989.

CHAPTER 17

THE THEORY OF KINETIC ANALYSIS IN HUMAN GAIT

Rami Seliktar
Lin Bo

KEY TERMS

Acceleration	Moment
Angular momentum	Moment of inertia
Deformable body	Position
Dynamics	Rigid body
Energy	Scalar
Equations of motion	Statics
Free body diagram	Vector
Impulse	Velocity
Inertia tensor	Work
Modeling	

The objective of this methodological discussion is to provide those readers who are not fully acquainted with the basic dynamic methods employed in gait analysis with a somewhat clearer understanding of the relevant terminology. It is not to serve as a substitute for a textbook. If one wants to follow and perform an actual kinetic analysis of the locomotor system, this discussion should serve as a guide to the subjects that need to be covered more thoroughly with the aid of textbooks and relevant publications.

Kinetics is the part of mechanics that deals with the study of forces and the way they affect motion of objects and systems. Kinetics can be studied either by solving the direct dynamic problem—e.g., measuring the forces and substituting them in the "equations of motion" to obtain the resulting motion—or by solving the inverse dynamic problem, which involves substitution of measured motion data, to obtain the forces responsible for the motion. The direct dynamic problem is often complicated to solve as will be seen in the discussion that follows, while the inverse solution can be relatively simple if kinematic information is readily and accurately available.

Human motion (kinematic) studies have been performed for some time in a variety of improvised ways, although the objective was not always a kinetic one. In 1887, Eadweard Muybridge published a set of sequential photographs of the human figure in action performing different activities. This was probably the first artistic attempt to resolve human motion into its kinematic composition. Evidence of attempts to study human gait as a diagnostic tool can be found in the late part of the 19th century. Braune and Fisher recognized the need to know about the mass properties of the human body and were among the first known to have performed a mass distribution study on cadavers.[2] Greater interest in the subject began in the middle of the twentieth century at the outset of the Second World War and continues to the present. Although the drive for studying locomotion originated from clinical demand, the bulk of the studies focused on the improvement of existing methodology rather than development of clinically viable methods. Some of the most notable early contributions to the study of locomotion are the works by Elftman,* Inman, and Brestler.[5]

The latter recognized the need to develop scientific methods of monitoring locomotion. As a result, some kinetic attitudes towards gait analysis evolved, and these remain almost unchanged to the present day. The recognition that motion, forces, and muscle activity are the fundamental variables in monitoring locomotion is traced back to these early studies. With the advent of modern technology, these techniques have been refined and somewhat adapted for clinical use. Studies were further expanded to cover human performance in a more general sense such as in athletics, rehabilitation, orthopedics, and vocational task performance.

The Objectives of Locomotion Studies

Besides satisfying our curiosity as to how we function and execute motion, we study locomotion for some very practical purposes. The following are examples of the applications of locomotion studies:

- In certain instances we study gait for the evaluation of performance in people who undergo physical rehabilitation to follow their progress and optimize treatment. In such an event we need not be too detailed with regard to the variables that we monitor; it may be sufficient to measure just one or two variables that will provide an integrated picture of overall performance. Usually we refer to such analysis as "Lumped Parameter Modeling." Our variables in such an event could be for example: metabolic energy consumption, overall mechanical work done, impulses of the ground reaction forces and many other parameters.

- In other instances we may be studying gait to establish design criteria and quality control methods for prosthetic devices. In such an event we may want to draw correlations between certain variables of the prosthetic device and "gait patterns" of the individual. Then, a greater degree of detail may be required in the simulation at the same time less "lumping" of parameters is permissible.

- On other occasions, we may want to develop some data to be used in the design of implanted orthopedic appliances such as joint prostheses or even for the study of load-related degenerative joint disease such as osteoarthritis. In such studies internal muscle and joint forces have to be assessed. Since invasive measurements of forces are not acceptable, we need to model the musculoskeletal system to determine the muscle forces and in turn, the joint reaction forces. Such an analysis requires a physical model of the joint and its constituents; such a model then becomes representative of the physical structure and function.

---

* References 11, 12, 13, 14, 15, 16.

Some other examples of application of gait studies are:

- Establishment of a data base used to identify pathological conditions and in the investigation of their causes (could be a statistical model).
- Optimization of the socket fit and alignment of lower limb prosthetic devices.
- Development of methods for detection and evaluation of functional disorders associated with the use of limb prostheses, orthopedic corrective surgery, and neuromuscular lesions.
- Development of methods for evaluation and refinement of athletic activities.
- Evaluation of the role of the musculoskeletal system, muscular activity and effort, joint and connective tissue mechanics, and energy cost of task performance.

In order to understand the kinetics of human motion let us first review some basic mechanical principles.

CLASSICAL MECHANICS

Classical mechanics deals with the relationship between force, position, and time. We usually distinguish between a static state of a system and a dynamic state, or statics and dynamics. **Static** systems are those for which time has no effect, and hence they maintain a constant position at all time, while **dynamic** systems are dependent on time. Although such a distinction need not be made, it is chosen as a matter of convenience.

The Basic Variables

Force is a fundamental variable that is responsible for causing motion. Force is a **vector** and therefore both its magnitude and orientation determine its effects. **Mass** is a basic substance property and is representative of the inertia properties of the system in linear motion. Mass is a **scalar,** which means that it takes only one value to represent it. **Position** in mechanical terms represents the instantaneous state of the system in a three-dimensional space. Position is also a vector; its variation with time is what we call **velocity,** and the variation of the velocity with time is the **acceleration.** In mathematical terminology, such variations are called **derivatives.** The velocity is the first derivative of the position with respect to time, and acceleration is the second derivative of the position with respect to time, or the first derivative of the velocity:

$$\vec{v} = \frac{d\vec{r}}{dt}; \vec{a} = \frac{d\vec{v}}{dt}; \text{ or } \vec{a} = \frac{d^2\vec{r}}{dt^2} \qquad (1)$$

where $\vec{r}$ designates the position vector, $\vec{v}$ is the velocity vector, and $\vec{a}$ designates acceleration.

Newton's Equations of Motion

Isaac Newton, when formulating the basic laws of mechanics, chose to distinguish between the "first law," the law of inertia, and the "second law," although for all practical purposes, the first law is only a particular case of the second law.

Newton's second law constitutes a simple relationship between the forces acting on a system and the resulting acceleration:

$$\sum \vec{F} = m\vec{a} \qquad (2)$$

This formulation is referred to as the **Equation of Motion** because if solved, the resulting equations will describe the pattern of motion of an object and its dependence on time. However, this simple relationship does not guarantee simplicity of the resulting equations of motion, once the forces and the accelerations have been explicitly substituted into Newton's formula.

Under static conditions, the system is said to be in equilibrium, and the sum of all the forces acting on it is zero. The static situation is therefore only a particular case of the $\sum \vec{F} = m\vec{a}$, when $\vec{a} = O$. In general, when the forces add up to zero, the implication from Newton's second law is that the acceleration is zero, and hence the velocity is constant. In other words, in order for an object to be at rest, the forces acting on it must add up to zero. However, the opposite is not necessarily correct, e.g., if the forces are zero, the object is not necessarily at rest.

The Fundamental Tools of Kinetic Modeling

In order to physically represent and understand a dynamic system, we apply a method called **modeling.** The object or the system is graphically described with the aid of schematic mechanical symbols, which have distinct physical properties that can be expressed mathematically. When we model a dynamic system, we distinguish between several representations of objects or systems. The simplest one is the **particle.** The particle is any object (no matter what its size is) that for the purpose of the analysis can be treated as a point concentrated mass. A **system of particles** is literally a medium containing an unlimited number of independent particles. These particles however, may or may not be subjected to internal constraints. A **rigid body** is basically a system of particles that have been constrained in such a way that the distance between the particles remains constant at all times. We can progress further and define a **system of rigid bodies,** which is the basic tool most commonly used to represent the human body.

The analysis of a system of particles is beyond the scope of the present discussion. However, it is important to note that very often when dynamics of the system are analyzed, we apply rigid body modeling principles even though the body may otherwise be a **deformable body.**

Application to Modeling of the Human Body

None of the models described can be fully representative of the mechanics of the human body. Typically, in a kinetic analysis of the human body, one would attempt to divide the body into a finite number of segments. The segments are usually assumed to be rigid, despite the fact that they are deformable and their mass varies also with time due to fluid flow and mass transport. The higher the number of segments, the greater the reliability of the model. For example, if elements of the trunk were taken to correspond to individual vertebrae, the precision of kinetic representation would be higher than with segments representing portions of the trunk containing several vertebrae. However, when such fine resolution is chosen, it is impossible to ignore the deformability of the soft tissues and relative motion of the internal organs. A system of particles would therefore be an "ideal" model of the human body; however, such a model is impractical due to the complexity involved in formulating the constraints. In other words, in order for such a model to be determinable, one has to describe the constraining relationship of the microcomponents of the various tissues and fluids, and then formulate the interactive relationships between the different anatomical components.

As an example, a schematic description of one such model of the human body represented by 14 interconnected segments, is illustrated in Figure 17-1.

Under certain circumstances, when interaction between objects exists—in a form of contact forces transmitted through the surfaces—or the object's flexibility is notable, the deformation characteristics of the body have to be considered in the analysis. For example such conditions exist at the exoprosthetic stump/socket interface that form a "constrained joint," which in turn influences the kinetics of the prosthetic gait.

The difference between the treatment of the modeling of a particle and a rigid body arises from the geometrical fact that a particle, whose physical

FIGURE 17-1 A schematical 14-segment mechanical model of the human body.

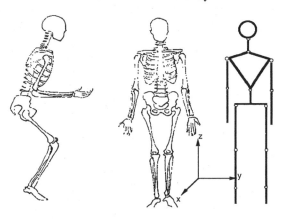

dimensions are minimal, does not perform any rotation, while a body can both translate and rotate. The distinction between the different mechanical models is made in order to facilitate a relatively simple approach to solving problems that don't require a comprehensive set of forces and conditions. In other words, if all we want to do is analyze the motion of the center of mass of the body of a walking person, all we need to do is model the person as a mass particle concentrated at the center of mass. Applying rigid body or system of particles analysis of the dynamics of the person's body would, given our objectives, lead to a large amount of redundant analysis.

Kinetics of Rigid Bodies

When a rigid body model is considered, the rotational motion of the body has to be accounted for in addition to the translational motion. For this purpose we have to define two new variables, the moment $\vec{M}$ and the angular velocity $\vec{\omega}$ (or alternative vector notation $\{\omega\}$). Both the angular velocity and the moment are vectors. Analytically, the moment is defined as the vector (cross) product between the position vector $\vec{r}$ and the corresponding force $\vec{F}$:

$$\vec{M} = \vec{r} \times \vec{F} \qquad (3)$$

In other words, the moment is a product of the magnitude of force and its distance (perpendicular) from a reference point.

The angular velocity is the variation of the angular position with time and can be written as:

$$\vec{\omega} = \{\omega\} = \begin{Bmatrix} \omega_x \\ \omega_y \\ \omega_z \end{Bmatrix}$$

Similar to translational displacement and velocity, the angular velocity can be further differentiated to obtain the angular acceleration, often designated by $\vec{\alpha}$. However, unlike translation, angular displacements are not vectors and cannot be added in a **commutative** way. In other words, if we rotate an object about an axis and subsequently rotate it about another axis, the final position will depend on the sequential order that these rotations were performed. Changing the order will produce a different result.

The equations of motion representing the translational motion of the body's center of mass via acceleration ($\vec{a}_G$) remain the same as for the particle, e.g.,

$$\sum \vec{F} = m\vec{a}_G \qquad (4)$$

The rotational equations of motion are derived from another variable called the angular momentum. Unlike in a translational motion where the dynamic behavior of the body depends on its mass alone, in a rotational motion, the distribution of the mass is important. In order to understand the angular momentum term, we need to acquaint ourselves with a mass distribution property called the **inertia tensor**, usually designated by **I**. The inertia tensor contains two types of components: moments of inertia and products of inertia. By using a certain fixed quantity of substance and distributing it in different geometrical forms, we would produce different moments of inertia. Moreover, moments of inertia about different reference locations on the body are different. Due to the dependence of the inertia of the body on geometrical distribution, the rotational inertia is represented by nine components, which, due to a law of symmetry, can be reduced to six. This overall inertial variable is referred to as the inertia tensor.

The basic definition of the components of the inertia tensor can be seen by using an x, y, z coordinates and defining moments of inertia

$$I_{xx} = \int_M (y^2 + z^2)dm, \qquad (5a)$$

$$I_{yy} = \int_M (x^2 + z^2)dm, \qquad (5b)$$

$$I_{zz} = \int_M (x^2 + y^2)dm, \qquad (5c)$$

and products of inertia

$$I_{xy} = \int_M (xy)dm \qquad (6a)$$

$$I_{xz} = \int_M (xz)dm \qquad (6b)$$

$$I_{yz} = \int_M (yz)dm \qquad (6c)$$

Certain properties are apparent from these definitions: (1) moments of inertia can never be negative or zero unless the object reduces to a point concentrated mass; (2) distributing the mass of the system far from the origin of the coordinates will increase the moment of inertia quadratically without any change in the mass; which is the basic feature utilized when designing a flywheel.

On the other hand, the products of inertia can be negative or zero, depending on the mass distribution. The existence of nonzero products of inertia is often regarded undesirable in engineering but sometimes unavoidable. The process of elimination of products of inertia, either through alignment of the axes (x, y, z), or through redistribution of the mass is referred to as **dynamic balancing.** The perception of a dynamic imbalance in a lower limb prosthetic system resulting from nonzero products of inertia about the knee axes will be a lateral "throw" of the shank of the prosthesis as it swings forward.

The rotational inertia of the system (the inertia tensor) is usually described in a form of a 3×3 symmetric matrix of the form:

$$[I] = \begin{bmatrix} I_{xx} & -I_{xy} & -I_{xz} \\ -I_{xy} & I_{yy} & -I_{yz} \\ -I_{xz} & -I_{yz} & I_{zz} \end{bmatrix}$$

For computational purposes it is desirable to diagonalize this matrix, which means setting all the products of inertia to zero. This is done by identification of a specific set of axes (x', y', z') about which the products of inertia vanish. Such axes are referred to as *principal axes* and the matrix obtains the form:

$$[I] = \begin{bmatrix} I_1 & O & O \\ O & I_2 & O \\ O & O & I_3 \end{bmatrix}$$

The angular momentum can then be described as:

$$\{H\} = \begin{bmatrix} I_{xx} & -I_{xy} & -I_{xz} \\ -I_{xy} & I_{yy} & -I_{yz} \\ -I_{xz} & -I_{yz} & I_{zz} \end{bmatrix} \begin{Bmatrix} \omega_x \\ \omega_y \\ \omega_z \end{Bmatrix}$$

Differentiation of the angular momentum (relative to the center of mass) with respect to time, yields Euler's equations of motion:

$$\sum \vec{M} = \frac{d\vec{H}}{dt} \tag{7}$$

where $\vec{M}$ is the corresponding moment exerted by the external forces relative to the center of mass.

Euler's equations can be written in different variations, and corresponding adjustments have to be made when the equations of motion are written with respect to a point that does not coincide with the center of mass. The explicit form of Euler's equations relative to the center of mass (or any other nonaccelerating point of the body) and with respect to coordinates that coincide with **principal axes of inertia** obtains the form:

$$
\begin{aligned}
M_x &= I_{xx}\dot{\omega}_x + (I_{zz} - I_{yy})\omega_y\omega_z \\
M_y &= I_{yy}\dot{\omega}_y + (I_{xx} - I_{zz})\omega_x\omega_z \\
M_z &= I_{zz}\dot{\omega}_z + (I_{yy} - I_{xx})\omega_y\omega_x
\end{aligned}
$$

The combined set of equations resulting from both the force equation and the moment equation constitute a set of six scalar equations that define the nature of the spatial motion of the object. These equations are referred to as the Newton-Euler equations and are often quite complicated to formulate and particularly difficult to solve. They are differential equations and may be highly nonlinear.

$$\sum F_x = ma_{Gx} \tag{8a}$$

$$\sum F_y = ma_{Gy} \tag{8b}$$

$$\sum F_z = ma_{Gz} \tag{8c}$$

$$\sum M_x = I_{xx}\dot{\omega}_x + (I_{zz} - I_{yy})\omega_y\omega_z \tag{8d}$$

$$\sum M_y = I_{yy}\dot{\omega}_y + (I_{xx} - I_{zz})\omega_x\omega_z \tag{8e}$$

$$\sum M_z = I_{zz}\dot{\omega}_z + (I_{yy} - I_{xx})\omega_y\omega_x \tag{8f}$$

It is important to understand though, that these equations are in no way to be considered as the general equations of motion, and they are subjected to the restrictions specified.

Dynamic Modeling

A first step in any mechanical modeling is to draw a **free body diagram** (F.B.D.) of the "particle" or the "rigid body" or a segment of the system of rigid bodies. The free body diagram is intended to specify all the forces that act on the system in order to facilitate the formulation of the equations of motion. The forces represented in the F.B.D. are the applied forces, such as gravitation and the

interactive (reactive) forces, that are exerted through interaction with the environment. For example, ground reaction forces applied to the feet of a walking person are reactive forces. Figure 17-2 depicts a free body diagram of the shank of the lower limb. For simplicity, it was chosen to describe a two-dimensional configuration in the coronal plane. The shank was separated from the rest of the body by an imaginary section, and the forces at the knee joint are representative of the interaction between the shank and the rest of the body. In a three-dimensional representation, we would have to add two more moments at the knee about each of the other axes, add one more force at the knee in the anterior-posterior (A-P) direction, and modify the ground reaction force to include the A-P shear component.

Once the free body diagram has been drawn, the forces and the moments are resolved into components of the corresponding coordinates and substituted into the Newton-Euler equations to form the equations of motion.

The corresponding dynamic equations would be

$$\sum F_x = S - R_x = ma_{Gx} \tag{9}$$

$$\sum F_y = -N - W + R_y = ma_{Gy} \tag{10}$$

$$
\begin{aligned}
\sum M_{Gz} &= -R_x \times Y_G + R_y \times f - \\
& \quad S \times Y_K + N \times e - M \\
&= \textit{the corresponding component} \\
& \quad \textit{of the expanded Euler's equations}
\end{aligned} \tag{11}
$$

FIGURE 17-2 A free body diagram of the shank: *left,* general; *right,* with a corresponding coordinate system.

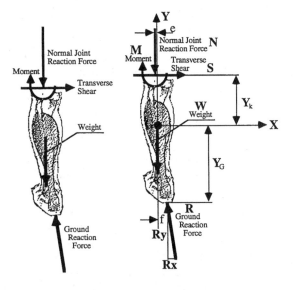

Work, Energy, Impulse, and Momentum

We often use the terms *work, energy,* and *impulse* in dealing with locomotor biomechanics. These terms have to be used with caution since their mechanical definitions are complicated and their use requires familiarity with the restrictions that apply to each one of them.

Work/energy and impulse/momentum relationship are tools derived from the basic variables and principles of mechanics. Work is defined as the force-displacement integral, $W = \int \vec{F} \cdot d\vec{r}$. More explicitly, if a force is acting on an object and during the course of action this force progresses along a certain path of motion, then the force is doing work. The amount of work done equals the product between the force component, which acts in the direction of the path, and its displacement. Hence, a force that does not move does not do any work. When looking at this definition of work from a different perspective, expressing the force as mass times acceleration according to Newton's law, it can easily be shown that the work done by the forces equals the change of kinetic energy of the system, e.g.:

$$W = \frac{mv_2^2}{2} - \frac{mv_1^2}{2} \qquad (12)$$

where W represents the work done, and v_2 and v_1 are the velocities of the object, which correspond to the beginning and end of the path interval under consideration.

The term *potential energy* relates only to a category of forces said to be conservative. Description of the basic principles of potential energy is complicated and may be too distracting in the present discussion. In general terms, however, we can say that if the nature of the system is such that the work done is not dissipated, then the forces are conservative and there is a conservation of energy in the system. A system of forces acting on a body may be composed of conservative and nonconservative forces. The work of the conservative forces alone can then be represented by potential energy as follows:

$$W_{\substack{conservative \\ forces}} = -(E_{p2} - E_{p1}) \qquad (13)$$

where E_p is the potential energy pertaining to the conservative forces only at the corresponding position (1 or 2). In other words:

The work done by the conservative forces only equals the negative of the difference between the potential energies at the corresponding positions of the system as the body is moved from position 1 to position 2.

If we now combine the conclusions of the work–kinetic energy relationship with the potential energy, we can demonstrate that, for a conservative system of forces, the sum of potential and kinetic energy remains constant at all times.

$$W_{\substack{conservative \\ forces}} = -(E_{p2} - E_{p1}) = \frac{mv_2^2}{2} - \frac{mv_1^2}{2} \qquad (14)$$

or alternatively, the principle of conservation of energy:

$$E_{p1} + \frac{mv_1^2}{2} = E_{p2} + \frac{mv_2^2}{2} = Constant. \qquad (15)$$

This expression of conservation of energy can be expanded further to represent kinetic energy of rigid body and systems of rigid bodies.

Work and energy are scalar values and are often easier to deal with than the equations of motion. However, there is an inherent risk in using potential energies for analytical purposes because the forces have to be examined very thoroughly in order to determine whether they are conservative or nonconservative. Typical conservative forces are gravitational forces (weight) and spring forces, while friction forces are nonconservative.

Examples of potentials (potential energies):

Gravitation: $\quad E_{p-gravity} \quad = mgh \qquad (16)$

Spring: $\qquad\qquad E_{p-spring} = \dfrac{kx^2}{2} \qquad (17)$

where g is the value of the gravitational acceleration, h is the altitude of the object, k is the spring constant (coefficient of elasticity), and x is the extension of the spring relative to its relaxed position.

The **impulse momentum** relationship is obtained from the summation of the products of the force and infinitely small time intervals and equating those with the product of mass-velocity, e.g., integration of Newton's law with respect to time:

$$\vec{I} = \int \vec{F} dt = \int m\vec{a} dt = m(\vec{v}_2 - \vec{v}_1) \qquad (18)$$

This impulse momentum equality can be quite useful in the analysis of certain aspects of locomotion and performance. The impulse, $\vec{I}$ and the momentum $m\vec{v}$ are vectors, and therefore they can be represented either by an ambiguous vector notation or by an explicit resolution of the quantity into three independent components.

If we consider, for instance, the ground reaction forces during locomotion as a variable for assessment of performance, then the impulse would be represented by the area enclosed between the baseline and the curve. Figure 17-3 depicts the

FIGURE 17-3   A typical anterior-posterior ground reaction force during normal locomotion.

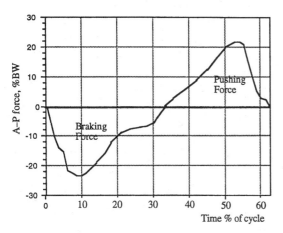

anterior-posterior component of the ground reaction force during locomotion. This A-P force component is responsible for the forward progression of the body as a whole; therefore any irregularities in it would be indicative of ambulation problems. The negative area (under the base line) represents the braking impulse while the positive area represents the pushing action of the leg. Since the impulse in this case represents a certain specific action of the leg by a single quantitative value, it is apparent that such a representation, if consistent, can be convenient to assess the quality of functioning of the leg. The method was described by Seliktar in 1979.[40] For example, in the gait of a subject with an above-knee amputation, one would expect to detect a considerable reduction in the braking impulse due to problems of knee instability and a slight reduction in the pushing impulse. However, if we accept the notion that gait is cyclical, then all the events are repeated within every cycle. Since during one complete cycle of gait the velocity of the body center of mass is equal to that of the previous cycle, then based on the impulse-momentum equality, the total impulse per cycle must add up to zero. This concept serves as the basis for the development of the Gait Consistency Test by Seliktar et al.

Lagrange's Formulation of the Equations of Motion

An alternative formulation of the equations of motion can be achieved through a less illustrative method called the Lagrangian method. Lagrange's formulation is more suitable for assembling the equations of systems made up of multiple bodies

than the Newtonian approach. The equations appear to be simpler to use, but there is a greater risk of erroneous application as a result of misunderstanding of the basic theory underlying these equations. Lagrange's equations are based on a principle of virtual work, and their derivation is obtained by using a concept of generalized coordinates rather than a vector approach. The theoretical derivation of these equations is complicated, and the equations are subject to restrictions imposed during the course of the derivation. However, if one understands the basic limitations of the Lagrangian analysis, the use of these equations becomes considerably simpler than the Newton-Euler formulation.

A feature giving Lagrange's equations superiority over the Newton-Euler formulation is the omission of the constraint forces from the analysis. This results from the premise that the constraint forces (reactive forces) do not do any work and need not be included in the computation of the virtual work. The absence of the reactive forces from the equations of motion provides substantial relief from computation of a number of complicated force variables. This, however, can turn into a major limitation of Lagrange's equations with regard to certain biomechanical models when joint reaction forces need to be computed. It is therefore often necessary to apply both Lagrange's equations and the Newton-Euler equations in order to simplify the solution. Lagrange's equations are then used to obtain the kinematics of the system, and Newton Euler's equations are applied in an inverse dynamic solution to obtain the reactive forces.

Unlike the Newtonian approach where the forces and the position (and its derivatives) are described by vectors, the Lagrangian analysis transforms the position coordinates into generalized coordinates and the forces into generalized forces. The transformed coordinates and forces are collinear (have the same direction), and work (or virtual work) results from a simple scalar product between the generalized coordinates and the generalized forces. As a result, the equations of motion obtained are scalar equations, and the coordinates used do not necessarily correspond to a Cartesian set, nor do they have to be of a lineal geometrical nature.

The understanding of Lagrange's equations requires some definitions with regard to the characteristics of the system. The system is characterized by the *generalized coordinate, degrees of freedom,* and *constraints.*

Generalized coordinates were briefly discussed above. One can select any number of generalized coordinates to describe the state of a system. **Degrees of freedom** are the minimum number of coordinates required to define the configuration of the system. In such an event all the coordinates are independent coordinates. For example, to define the position of a point in space, three coordinates are required. These coordinates can be ordinary Cartesian coordinates (x,y,z) or they can be any other set. For instance, a spherical coordinate system will utilize two angular coordinates and one lineal (radial) coordinate. However, no matter what kind of coordinates are used, the number of degrees of freedom does not change. Often we choose more coordinates than the degrees of freedom of the system. For instance, if we want to describe the state of a line in a plane (see Figure 17-4), we may choose to use x,y for one end of the line and another x,y for the other end. Such description utilizes four coordinates, but the line only has three degrees of freedom because its state in the plane can be defined by the position of one of its points (x,y) and the angle with respect to one axis. In other words, we can say that the coordinates we selected are not all independent but are related by one **constraint,** which is

$$\sqrt{((X_2 - X_1)^2 + (Y_2 - Y_1)^2)} = l^2 \qquad (19)$$

In general we can say that *the number of degrees of freedom equals the number of coordinates less the number of constraints of the system.*

Constraints are not always as simple as the previous example of the line. A constraint that can be described as a direct relationship between the coordinates is referred to as **holonomic.** However, some constraints can only be described by the relationship between the derivatives of the generalized coordinates (generalized velocities). In such an event the constraint is called **nonholonomic.** The principal difference between the two types of constraints is that in a system containing only holonomic constraints, redundant variables can be eliminated through substitution. Also, the number of variables can be reduced to the number of degrees of freedom. The same cannot be done in a system containing nonholonomic constraints.

The nature of the constraints has a direct bearing on the formulation of Lagrange's equations. The standard form of the equations cannot be used in order to formulate equations of motion of a nonholonomic system.

The simplest form of Lagrange's equation is

$$\frac{d}{dt}\left(\frac{\partial L}{\partial \dot{q}_k}\right) - \frac{\partial L}{\partial q_k} = Q_k \qquad (20)$$

where q_k represents the kth generalized coordinate, $\dot{q}_k$ is the time derivative of this same coordinate, also referred to as the generalized velocity, and Q_k is the *nonconservative* generalized force. These forces are often zero and the equation reduces to a zero on the right-hand side. The corresponding conservative forces are already contained in the Lagrangian L. For instance if our generalized coordinate is an angle θ, then the corresponding generalized velocity is the angular velocity $\dot{\theta}$ and the generalized force would be torque τ. L is called the Lagrangian and is made up of the difference in kinetic and potential energies of the system:

$$L = T - V \qquad (21)$$

where T represents the kinetic energy and V is the potential energy term.

The above Lagrange's equation can be written only for a system in which the number of coordinates does not exceed the number of its degrees of freedom (a holonomic system). Different variations can be applied to Lagrange's equation in order to adapt it to the different applications and readers can supplement their knowledge in this area by using a text in advanced dynamics such as Greenwood.[19]

One of the major advantages of the Lagrangian approach is that often a free body diagram is not required, and as stated above, the reactive forces (constraint forces) do not need to be considered in this procedure because they usually do not do work. Friction, however, poses a problem in such analysis.

LUMPED PARAMETERS MODELING OF HUMAN LOCOMOTION

Biped locomotion can be regarded as a mechanical task during which the bulk of the body performs a spatial oscillation while the legs alternately as-

FIGURE 17-4 Coordinates and constraints of a straight line in a plane.

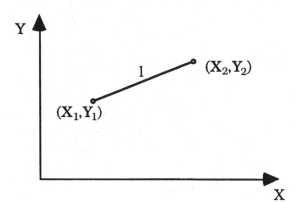

sume a supporting role. The complexity of the control of motion is evident from the complicated pattern of firing of the muscles involved in the activation of the pertinent joints. However from the mechanical point of view, a steady state gait is rather ballistic in nature and the motion can be grossly represented by an inverted pendulum model.[42]

We presented the preceding list of clinical objectives of gait analysis, some of which can be achieved without explicitly dealing with a detailed modeling of the system. For instance, the ground reaction force characteristics represent the gross outcome of the general kinetic activity of the musculoskeletal system. The kinetic activity of the musculoskeletal system can be modeled as a multivariable system. However, if the objective is to monitor performance in order to detect differences between individuals or the progress of an individual undergoing physical rehabilitation, then an integrated approach may be appropriate. One such integrated approach was previously described with respect to the gait-impulse variable. Engineers refer to such an integrated approach as a lumped parameters modeling, where all the variables are lumped together into a significantly smaller number of ambiguous inputs and outputs.

Lumped parameters modeling is useful in the development of clinically viable methods of gait monitoring. Consider a situation in which a person wears a prosthesis, and the resulting performance is not satisfactory. Assuming that a modification to the alignment of the prosthetic foot will correct the problem, this modification is performed and the resulting performance is evaluated by the changes that occur in the motion patterns of the different body segments, center of mass, etc. (dependent variables). Such documentation of changes of dependent variables due to the administration of a change to a single independent variable is extremely complex and totally unsuitable for clinical use. On the other hand, the net result of the change in the independent variable is a change in the ambulation pattern, which could be represented by the ground force impulses. In such an event, measuring the overall impulse (say in the A-P direction) could give a sufficient measure of achievement of the objective. In other words, if the subject with the amputation is not using the prosthesis sufficiently and as a result of the change of alignment, the ground reaction force impulses have increased, then the objective of increasing the utility of the prosthetic limb has been achieved. This objective is then reflected in a single (lumped) quantitative value, which is easy enough to comprehend and use in the clinic.

Another common lumped parameter model is one that utilizes work or energy as its main dependent variable. Although work is done by the individual muscles that are active about the joints, it is impractical to deal with a resolved work-energy model. Typically the work done at the joint is computed as a whole rather than by individual muscles. Such computation is done by utilization of the external moments about the joint M, multiplied incrementally by the joint displacement $d\theta$ such that

$$W_{(work)} = \int M d\theta, \tag{22}$$

or in terms of power

$$H_{(Power)} = \int M d\omega \tag{23}$$

where ω is the angular velocity of the joint.

Often in clinical application, the overall energy expenditure of the whole body is used as a measure of the efficiency of the system. This work is obtained either by lumping the mechanical work done by all the joints or by measuring the metabolic energy consumption. However, it is apparent from the preceding computation that if no displacement occurs at the joint, no work is done. This conclusion is in disagreement with the metabolic energy cost, which is based on the activity of the muscles whether they are in an isometric state or in motion. Yet for comparative purposes both mechanical work and metabolic energy assessments can be used while their limitations are kept in mind.

MUSCULOSKELETAL MODELING

The musculoskeletal system can be regarded as an unstable chain of elements due to the nature of the articulations between these elements and the way gravity applies to the corresponding body segments. One can visualize this instability by considering a puppet made of articulated wooden links, connected to one another by pins that are totally unconstrained. Such a puppet collapses to the ground if placed on its feet. The only body parts that are mechanically stable are the arms, which are suspended from the shoulders and do not require a constant muscle tone in order to maintain their posture. The relatively unconstrained articulation between the joints of the lower limbs within their normal range of motion permits complex movements; on the other hand it is responsible for persistent muscle and joint loading, which results in fatigue and may produce overuse trauma under certain conditions.

Basic Characteristics of the Locomotor System

Human motion involves a complex control mechanism. For most of the musculoskeletal system, muscles exert force, which produce moments about the joints and, in turn, rotational motion of the joint. In many functions however, muscles contract only to counteract external forces and maintain the joint in static equilibrium. In a static upright posture for instance, the quadriceps muscle group may be active for the sole purpose of maintaining extension in the knee that in turn will require antagonistic activity in the hip muscles in order to maintain stability at that level. Due to the large number of muscles involved in the control of the joints, from the purely mechanical point of view, the system is highly redundant. In mechanical terms, redundancy means duplication of tasks by different muscles, which in turn means that function or equilibrium of the system could be achieved with fewer muscles.

In engineering terms, there are practically no reasons for the musculoskeletal system to be as complicated as it is. In engineering we refrain from applying *multijoint actuators:* actuators applying extension in one joint and simultaneously flexion about another joint (such as the two joint muscles), or actuators that will apply simultaneously torsion and flexion about a joint. Moreover, mechanically, exerting antagonistic forces would be considered a waste and is quite uncommon unless required by control demands of the system. Such control demands may arise from the need to maintain "alertness" or stability. In the design of an alternative mechanical system, we would attempt to design the actuators totally uncoupled from each other, e.g., one actuator per one independent axis of rotation (degree of freedom).

The mechanical redundancy, however, attests to the "smartness" of the evolutionary process. In mechanical design we rely on replacement of failed components. In the biological system, this duplication of tasks by the multiple muscle system safeguards continuous function of the system even under partial neuromuscular failure as a result of injury or disease. Moreover, the system utilizes different muscles for different levels of effort and/or different extents of motion. Computationally this mechanical redundancy implies that the forces in the muscles cannot be computed unless some assumptions are made in order to eliminate the redundancy. This problem will be discussed at a later stage.

During locomotion, some of the joints actively rotate but many joints remain in an isometric configuration. In mechanics we use a quasi-static situation to mean that the motion is small and slow (negligible velocity and acceleration). For instance, during the stance phase of locomotion, when the leg is load bearing and major effort is invested in propelling the body forward, the knee joint remains immobile for a considerable part of this phase. The quasi-static configuration of a joint does not necessarily imply that the muscles about that joint are inactive. On the contrary, these muscles often bear much of the burden of ambulation and are responsible for a great part of the metabolic energy consumed. For instance, during a considerable part of the stance phase of normal gait, the foot lies flat on the ground, the ankle joint rotates almost passively (as a pivot point), the knee is maintained in extension, and the hip actively rotates into extension. Past mid-stance the ankle joint stiffens and begins to perform an active pushoff. However most of the energy consumed at this stage by the ankle is due to its isometric stresses rather than mechanical work (torque-displacement) done at this site.

Although ambulation is obtained via such active stabilization and rotations of the different joints, from the mechanical point of view, the forces that produce the end result of progression of the whole body are the ground reaction forces. With exception of the weight, the ground reaction forces are the only external forces that act on the body. Hence, according to Newton's law, the ground forces combined with the gravitational force (the external forces) cause the center of mass of the whole body to translate. Concurrently, the moments of these forces relative to the center of mass produce the gross swaying (rotational) motion. The ambiguity of the position of the center of mass due to the changing instantaneous configuration of the whole body, however, makes it impossible to draw analogy between the whole body sway and a rotational motion of a rigid body.

Biomechanical Methodology of Gait Analysis

The fundamental information used in the analysis of human gait is composed of motion (e.g., displacement and its derivatives), the ground reactions forces, and electromyography. Motion variables and ground forces provide the basic information needed in order to compute the moments exerted about the joints and in turn facilitate the computation of the internal joint forces and muscles' contractions. Electromyography, at this point, is used primarily to determine which muscles are active and hence reduce the number of unknown muscle forces that need to be determined.

The computation of the moments also provides an insight into the mechanical work the muscles do in order to perform the motion under consideration. However, it is important to note that the mechanical work would at best be equal to the minimal amount of energy required in order to produce the motion. In other words, if one compares metabolic energy consumption with computed mechanical work, the metabolic energy will always be greater than the mechanical work. Moreover, no linear relationship (simple proportionality) exists between the two. This is due to the muscles' consumption of metabolic energy even when the joint is immobile during contraction. Furthermore, metabolic energy measurements reflect, in addition to mechanical work, metabolism and consumption of the nonmusculoskeletal and nonmuscular systems.

Determination of the internal moments about the joints and forces in the muscles is of major importance to the understanding of the biomechanics of the bones, joints, and connective tissues. These forces are often responsible for degenerative conditions in bones and joints and also contribute to expected loading in implanted orthopedic appliances and prosthetic devices.

Basic Modeling Approach and the Redundancy Problem

General dynamic modeling of the musculoskeletal function can be formulated as a two-stage solution.[3,8] The first stage of the solution is often referred to as the inverse dynamic problem and the second stage is a force distribution problem.

In the first stage of the computation, inertial properties of body segment (mass, moments of inertia) of the subject are estimated, and body segment displacement histories are recorded by using an appropriate motion analysis technique. Segment velocities and accelerations are calculated by analytical differentiation. Foot-floor reactions are measured with dynamic force plates. The body segment inertial properties, segment accelerations and foot-floor reactions are substituted into the equations of motion to obtain the intersegmental resultant forces and moments. These resultants represent the forces and moments that need to be transmitted between adjacent segments in order to sustain the motion or the configuration. They do not, however, represent the forces in the anatomical structure (muscles, ligaments, joint surfaces), and further analysis is required in order to obtain the actual muscle and joint forces. These are obtained in the second stage.

In the second stage of the solution, the intersegmental resultants are distributed or apportioned to the anatomical structures. However, in a three-dimensional configuration, the equations of motion can only solve for six unknown variables. Since there are more unknown muscle forces and joint contact forces than the number of equations of motion that can be written, the problem of calculating individual force is indeterminate.[3]

Figure 17-5 illustrates the modeling and force distribution concept in a rather schematic way. Unlike Figure 17-2 where the moments and forces about the knee represent the ambiguous values depicted in Cartesian coordinates, these moments and forces have already been distributed to represent actual forces of the muscles, tendons, and joint elements. On the left in Figure 17-5A, the line of action of the calf muscles is illustrated by the two **Fm** vectors and the joint forces in this case are made up of two parts: the tibio-femoral joint reaction and the patello-femoral force. Usually, for the computation of the joint reaction forces, the proximal end of the gastrocnemius is released from the femur and a free body diagram of the shank is drawn, where the direction of the **Fn** force is reversed and applied to the tibia. The corresponding free body diagram of the shank is depicted on the right. Note that the shank force of the patellar tendon is represented by the subpatellar force of the tendon.

This representation of the knee structure is oversimplified and in most situations many more muscles act concurrently.

FIGURE 17-5 **A,** A schematic representation of internal forces acting about the knee joint; **B,** a free body diagram of the shank, with the knee forces and moments distributed into actual muscle, tendon, and joint forces.

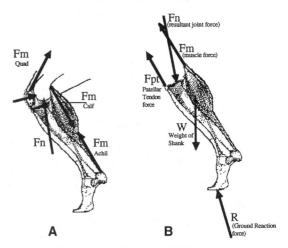

The problem of having more unknown muscle forces than equations (the redundancy) may be solved by making some assumptions based on physiological or logical criteria, which have been tested and reasonably validated by a mathematical technique of optimization. One of the most commonly used criteria for force distribution is the principle of equal muscle stress. The assumption in the equal stress concept is that the muscles share the burden of the force transmission in a way that is proportional to their cross-sectional area. In other words, if the forces exerted by several concurrently acting muscles produce a moment about a particular joint, then the total force is resolved into individual muscle forces that should yield a constant value when divided by the muscle cross section. Analytically this concept can be expressed in the following form:

$$\sigma_i = \frac{F_i}{A_i} = constant \qquad (24)$$

where σ_i is the stress in the muscle, F_i is the force in the individual ith muscle, and A_i is the effective cross-sectional area of the corresponding muscle. By combining the constant stress criterion with the knowledge of which muscles are inactive (derived from EMG) and the information derived from the equations of motion, the muscle forces can be determined uniquely. Although evidence does exist that the principle of constant stress is a sound one within reasonable limits of accuracy, it has not been physiologically substantiated; other techniques are selectively applied and explored by different researchers.

Optimization is a process that assumes that the function under consideration is subjected to some ground rules, which aim at achieving the objective in a "maximal" way, considering the circumstances (variables). In other words, if there are several ways of reaching a conclusion, none of these ways utilizes its best course, but the combined outcome is best for the specified set of constraints.

The key step in optimization is to establish a criterion—i.e. an objective function. According to the type of objective function, we can divide optimization methods into linear optimization and nonlinear optimization. A more thorough consideration of the principles of optimization is beyond the scope of the present discussion. However, some examples of simple objective functions could help the reader to understand the general approach.

One optimization concept that could be applied is to aim at minimization of the algebraic sum of the forces in all the muscles that activate a certain joint while performing a function. Analytically we can write

$$\sum F_i = G \qquad (25)$$

where F_i are the scalar values of the individual muscle forces, and G represents the algebraic sum of these forces. The objective is to minimize G—e.g., $G \rightarrow Minimum$—while observing the rest of the constraints of the system.

Whether or not such a concept is valid needs to be weighed very carefully. We have already seen that forces are vectors, and their directional properties are as important as their magnitudes. From the mechanical point of view, therefore, such summation of the scalar values of the forces is meaningless. However, if one thinks in terms of overall metabolic "effort," such a minimization of overall muscle tensions may be reasonable.

Another common objective is to minimize the mechanical work (or energy consumption). In such an event, a proper product of the muscle forces with their corresponding displacements has to be performed:

$$\sum_{i=1}^{n} \int \vec{F}_i \cdot d\vec{r}_i = W \qquad (26)$$

where $\vec{F}_i$ is the force in the ith muscle, n is the number of active muscles involved, W is the total work done by the muscles about the joint under consideration, and $d\vec{r}_i$ is the displacement vector pertaining to the ith muscle. Here the "objective" is to minimize the work, eg.,

$$W \rightarrow Minimum$$

This is a sound mechanical criterion. But despite the logical appeal, there has been no proof that the musculoskeletal physiology utilizes such an energy-efficient mechanism.

The above criteria are only two examples of objective considerations. One could make an unlimited number of such assumptions, provided that reasonable proof of the validity of the assumptions can be shown.

Anatomical Information

In order to perform such a force distribution as described previously, the location of the individual muscles relative to any joint center (i.e., the moment arm) at any given time must be known. This information can be specified by a straight-line muscle model or by using alternative methods. Information on the configuration of the anatomical structure is available in the relevant literature.

History of Biomechanical Modeling

Mechanical modeling of the musculoskeletal system is performed in order to determine how motion is produced and in order to assess the forces acting on the different hard and soft tissue elements. Once the forces have been determined, stress analysis can be performed, and the pattern of distribution of the forces through the bone, cartilage, tendons, ligaments, and muscles can be computed.

Scientific interest in biomechanics and the initial mechanical modeling can be traced back to Galileo.[18] The relationship between the load bearing capability of bone, specifically the femoral neck and its architecture, was initiated over a century ago by Bourgery.[3] Koch performed an extensive stress analysis of the femur using beam theory.[28] Some more recent studies using conventional stress analysis methods such as the work of Burstein et al., Minns et al., Piotrowski and Wilcox, and Toridis are noteworthy.[6,30,36,44]

With the advancement of the computational methods, finite element analysis was introduced into the biomechanical modeling for the purpose of evaluation of stresses in the tissues. Rybicki et al. proposed the first finite element model of a long bone (femur).

Most of the early studies were concerned with the lower extremities because of the importance of the walking function for independent living. In the 1930s Elftman did a considerable amount of work on human locomotion, taking into account the external force in walking,[15,16] the distribution of pressure in the human foot,[11] forces and energy changes in the leg during walking,[14] the function of muscles in locomotion,[13] and the dynamics of human walking.[12] Bresler and Frankel[5] were also among the pioneers in studying the forces and moments in the human leg during walking.[5]

In 1960s and 1970s numerous models of the knee joint and the hip joint were developed. Morrison computed muscle and ligament forces at the knee during normal gait.[31,32] Concurrently, Paul studied the forces of the hip muscles and the joint reaction forces during normal locomotion.[33] Harrington followed up on these studies and investigated the same variables as applied to pathological gait.[20] Other models of the knee were proposed by Kettlekamp and Chao, Engin and Korde, Crowninshield et al., Andriacchi et al., Hight et al., Chand et al., Wisman et al., and Minns, to name a few.*

Seireg and Arvikar proposed a one-legged static model, which represented one of the early thorough attempts at a mathematical model of the musculoskeletal system.[38] In this model, linear optimization was used for solving the static indeterminate problem. Seireg and Arvikar reported another model, which used a dynamic optimization, as an extension of their previous work in 1973.[39] In 1978 Pedotti et al. reported a nonlinear optimization technique, which produced patterns of muscle activity that agreed more closely with EMG recordings than the linearly optimal solutions.[34]

In 1981 Crowninshield and Brand summarized the modeling method and proposed a two-step process.[9] They introduced a new nonlinear optimization technique, which is based on the inversely nonlinear relationship of muscle force and contraction endurance.[9] They also suggested that muscle activity based on maximized activity endurance is physiologically reasonable during many normal activities, particularly prolonged and repetitive activities, such as gait. The results obtained through the use of their criteria agreed more closely with known patterns of muscle activity (revealed by EMG), as compared with most linear optimization techniques.

By using a simple planar model of the elbow with three potentially active flexor muscles, Crowninshield and Brand demonstrated the behavior of optimization solutions obtained for indeterminate problems of muscle force prediction.[9] The solution space for this problem can be conveniently illustrated as a plane in three-dimensional space with each axis representing the stress in one of the three muscles. They found that the optimum solution is where only one elbow flexor muscle is predicted active. As the number of muscles increases, the optimal solution produces an equal stress in each muscle, that is muscle acting proportional to their average cross-sectional area.

Davy and Audu applied the optimal control analysis (i.e. dynamic optimization)—in contrast to the static optimization—to solving the muscle force distribution problem.[10]

Models of lower extremities are quite numerous. The objective of most models is to determine joint reactions and moments during gait. Brand et al. reported a model of the lower extremity and provided the basic information on the locations of all muscles of the lower extremity.[4] Hoy et al. developed a musculoskeletal model of the lower extremity, which incorporates the salient features of muscle and tendon and defines the active isometric moment of these actuators about the hip, knee, and ankle joints in the sagittal plane.[24] They

---

found that tendon slack length, optimal muscle-fiber length, and moment arm are different for each actuator, thus each actuator develops peak isometric moment at a different joint angle. The joint angle where an actuator produces peak moment does not necessarily coincide with the joint angle where (1) muscle force peaks, (2) moment arm peaks, or (3) the in-vivo moment developed by maximum voluntary contraction peaks.

Hogfors et al. proposed a biomechanical model of the human shoulder.[22] In this modeling, they defined four coordinate systems for the main bones of shoulder and the basic data of the location of 21 main muscles that involve the motion of the shoulder. Tumer and Engin reported a three-dimensional kinematic model of the human shoulder.[45] In these two papers, they demonstrated the basic method of computing the motion of each part of the shoulder and the optimization solution.

A number of models of the shoulder have been also developed, such as the models proposed by Hogfors et al.[22] and Karlsson and Peterson.[26] Snijders et al. did impressive work in developing a kinematic and dynamic model of the cervical spine.[43] However, their method can only be used in a special case in which there are only three or fewer unknown forces.

SUMMARY

This chapter reviews the basic principles of kinetic analysis including the formulation of equations of motion using classical Newtonian and Lagrangian mechanics. The limitations of these approaches are discussed, and the reader is warned of areas that lead to frequent confusion and misinterpretation. Finally, examples from the literature are presented to provide a historical perspective on this form of analysis.

REFERENCES

1. Andriacchi TP, Mikosc RP, Hampton SJ et al: A statically indeterminate model of the human knee joint," *Proceedings of the Biomechanics Symposium,* AMY-Vol. 23, ASME, 1977.
2. Braune CW, Fisher O: Der Gang Des Menschen, i teil Versuche Unbelasten und Belasten Menschen. Abhandl, *J Math Phys* 21:153, 1895.
3. Bourgery: *Traite complet de l'anatomie de l'homme,* Paris, 1832.
4. Brand RA, Crowninshield RD, Wittstock CE et al: A model of lower extremity muscular anatomy, *J Biomech Eng* 104:304, 1982.
5. Bresler B, Frankel JP: The force and moment in the leg during walking, *Trans ASME:* 27, 1950.
6. Burstein AH, Shaffer BW, Frankel VH: Elastic analysis of condylar structures, ASME Paper No. 70-WA/BHF-1, 1970.
7. Chand RJ, Haug E, Rim K: Stresses in the human knee, *J Biomech* 9:417, 1976.
8. Crowninshield R, Pope MH, Johnson RJ: An analytic model of the knee, *J Biomech* 9:397, 1976.
9. Crowninshield RD, Brand RA: A physiologically based criterion of muscle force prediction in locomotion, *J Biomech* 14:793, 1981.
10. Davy DT, Audu ML: A dynamic optimization technique for predicting muscle forces in the swing phase of gait, *J Biomech* 20:187, 1987.
11. Elftman H: A clinematic study of the distribution of pressure in the human foot, *Anta Rec* 59:481, 1934.
12. Elftman H: Experimental studies on the dynamics of human walking, *Ann NY Acad Sci* 6:1, 1943.
13. Elftman H: Forces and energy changes in the leg during walking, *Am J Physiol* 125:339, 1939.
14. Elftman H: *Forces and energy changes in the leg during walking,* New York, 1938, Columbia University.
15. Elftman H: Scientific apparatus and laboratory methods: the measurement of external force in walking, *Science* 88: 1938.
16. Elftman H: The measurement of the external force in walking, *Science* 88:152, 1938.
17. Engin AE, Korde MS: Biomechanics of normal and abnormal knee joint, *J Biomech* 9:397, 1976.
18. Galileo G: *Discorsi e dimostrazioni mathematiche,* translated by H. Crew and A. de Salvio, Evanston, Ill, 1638, Northwestern University Press.
19. Greenwood DT: *Principles of dynamics,* New York, 1965, Prentice Hall.
20. Harrington JB: A bioengineering analysis of force actions at the knee in normal and pathological gait, *Biomed Eng* 11:167, 1976.
21. Hight TK, Piziali RL, Nagle DA: A dynamic, non-linear finite-element model of a human leg, *J Biomech Eng* 112:176, 1979.
22. Hogfors C, Peterson B, Sigholm G et al: Biomechanical model of the human shoulder joint. II. The shoulder rhythm, *J Biomech* 24:699, 1991.
23. Hogfors C, Sigholm G, Herbers P: Biomechanical model of human shoulder. I. Elements, *J Biomech* 20:157, 1987.
24. Hoy MG, Zajac FE, Gordon ME: A musculoskeletal model of the human lower extremity: the effect of muscle, tendon, and moment arm on the moment-angle relationship of musculotendon actuators at the hip, knee, and ankle, *J Biomech* 23:157, 1990.
25. Inman VT, Eberhart HD, Saunders JB et al: Fundamental studies of human locomotion and other information relating to the design of artificial limbs. A Report to the National Research Council, Committee on Artificial Limbs, University of California, Berkeley, 1947.
26. Karlsson D, Peterson B: Towards a model for force prediction in the human shoulder, *J Biomech* 25:189, 1992.
27. Kettelkamp DB, Chao EY: A method for quantitative analysis of medial and lateral compression forces at the knee during standing, *Clin Orthop Res* 83:202, 1972.
28. Koch JC: The laws of bone architecture, *Am J Anat* 21:117, 1917.
29. Minns RJ, Bremble GR, Campbel J: A biomechanical study of internal fixation of the tibial shaft, *J Biomech* 10:569, 1977.

30. Minns RJ: Forces at the knee joint: anatomical considerations, *J Biomech* 14:633, 1981.

31. Morrison JB: Bioengineering analysis of force actions transmitted by the knee joint, *Biomed Eng* 3:164, 1968.

32. Morrison JB: Function of the knee joint in various activities, *Biomed Eng* 4:573, 1969.

33. Paul JP: Forces transmitted by joints in the human body, *Proceedings of the Institute of Mechanic Engineering* 181(3J)(8): 1967.

34. Pedotti A, Krishnan VV, Stark L: Optimization of muscle-force sequencing in human locomotion, *Math Biosci* 38:57, 1978.

35. Penrod DD, Davy DT, Singh DP: An optimization approach to tendon force analysis, *J Biomech* 7:123, 1974.

36. Piotrowski G, Wilcox GA: The stress program: a computer program for the analysis of stress in long bone, *J Biomech* 4:497, 1971.

37. Rybicki EF, Simonen FA, Weis EB: On the mathematical analysis of stress in the human femur, *J Biomech* 5:203, 1972.

38. Seireg A, Arvikar RJ: A mathematical model for evaluation of forces in lower extremities of the musculoskeletal system, *J Biomech* 6:313, 1973.

39. Seireg A, Arvikar RJ: The prediction of muscular load sharing and joint forces in the lower extremities during walking, *J Biomech* 8:89, 1975.

40. Seliktar R: Integrated information approach to clinical analysis of gait, *Proceedings of the Third ASCE Engineering, Mechanical Division,* Specialty Conference, Austin, Texas, 1979.

41. Seliktar R, Yekutiel M, Bar A: Gait consistency test based on the impulse momentum theorem, *Prosthetics & Orthotics International* 3(2):91, 1979.

42. Siegler S, Seliktar R, Hyman WA: Simulation of human gait with the aid of a simple mechanical model, *J Biomech* 15(6): 1982.

43. Snijders CJ, Hoek Van Duke GK, Roosch ER, A biomechanical model for the analysis of the cervical spine in static postures, *J Biomech* 24:783, 1991.

44. Toridis TG: Stress analysis of the femur, *J Biomech* 2:163, 1969.

45. Tumer ST, Engin AE: Three-dimensional kinematic modeling of the human shoulder complex. Part II: Mathematical modeling and solution via optimization, *J Biomech Eng* 111:113, 1989.

46. Wisman J, Veldpaus F, Janssen J et al: A three-dimensional mathematical model of the knee joint, *J Biomech* 13:677, 1980.

CHAPTER 18

MEASUREMENT OF KINETIC PARAMETERS TECHNOLOGY

Scott Z. Barnes
Necip Berme

KEY TERMS

Center of pressure

Cross talk

Force

Force plate

Gage factor

Ground reaction force

Piexoelectric crystal

Pressure

Strain gage

This chapter addresses technologies used in force and pressure measurement related to kinetic assessment of gait. It is appropriate to discuss force and pressure concurrently due to the similarity of the physical principles used in measuring them. This parallelism becomes obvious when one recalls that pressure is a derived scalar quantity defined as force per unit area:

$$p = \frac{F}{A} \tag{1}$$

where p is the pressure, F the component of the applied force normal to the area, and A the area over which the force is applied. Force itself is a derived quantity and is defined as a mass times acceleration. Force is a vector quantity and takes on the directional characteristic of the acting acceleration:

$$\vec{F} = m \cdot \vec{a} \tag{2}$$

where $\vec{F}$ is the force vector, m is the mass, and $\vec{a}$ is the acceleration vector acting on the mass.

These quantities and how they are measured are discussed in detail in this chapter. The chapter is broken down into two main sections: force measurement and pressure measurement. A brief, general discussion of each is presented followed by an analysis of measurement of these quantities as related to kinetic assessment of gait. The limitations and accuracy of these measurement techniques are explored, as well as the future direction of the technology. Brief reviews of the physics and mechanics involved are presented when necessary. However, it is not the scope of this chapter to serve as a primer in these areas.

FORCE MEASUREMENT

As stated above, force is defined as a mass times the acceleration of this mass. While mass is a fundamental quantity, acceleration is derived from length and time. The rate of change of length is, of course, velocity, while the rate of change of velocity is acceleration. Therefore, acceleration has the units of length divided by time squared. A force applied to a body causes acceleration, and similarly, a body subjected to acceleration experiences a force. The weight of an object is the force due to its mass being attracted by the Earth's gravitational field. The gravitational acceleration, g, is inversely proportional to the square of the distance between the location where it is measured and the center of the Earth. An average representative value of g is 9.81 m per second squared. With current technology, its actual value can be measured to an accuracy of 1 part in 1 million. The National Bureau of Standards' (NBS) mass and/or deadweight standards are based on the gravitational acceleration and, for the range of 10 lbs. to 1 million lbs. force, are accurate to approximately 1 part in 5000.

Basic methods of force measurement rely on the ability to calibrate according to NBS standards. These methods include balancing against standard weights, measuring or calculating the acceleration of a body of known mass, relating the deformation of an elastic member to the applied unknown force, measuring the change in precession of a gyroscope, transforming force to a fluid pressure then measuring the pressure, using a current coil to balance against an electromagnetic force and relating the magnet coil current to a force, or measuring the change in natural frequency of a wire tensioned by a force. This list, though incomplete, presents methods of varying complexity and feasibility. Depending on the specific circumstances of the force measurement application, some methods would have advantages over others.

Force Measurement Technology in Kinetic Assessment of Gait

The basic concept of load transducers is that of measuring some physical change that results from the deformation of the transducer due to the applied force. The common bathroom scale is a good example. Here, a deformable spring is calibrated to measure the weight applied to the scale. This is an acceptable transducer for measuring static loads applied within a relatively specific range. A system with better dynamic characteristics, finer resolution, and larger range is generally desirable for more sophisticated measurements. Strain gages and piezoelectric crystals are the sensing elements most commonly used in such transducers.

Although both strain gages and piezoelectric crystals produce electrical output signals, their principles of operation are totally different. Strain gages are bonded to the surface of a transducer element. As the transducer element deforms under the applied force, the gage deforms together with it. This deformation causes a change in the electrical resistance of the gage. Thus, monitoring the resistance change in the gage using an appropriate electrical circuitry results in an output proportional to the applied force. Details of transducer design will be discussed in the following sections. It is, however, worth noting here that strain-gaged transducer design is a compromise between the requirements of rigidity and flexibility. Flexibility of the transducer element is needed for increased sensitivity. On the other hand, rigidity of the element is required for desirable dynamic transducer characteristics.

Transducers utilizing piezoelectric crystals operate on the principle that an electrical charge develops on the surface of the crystal when the crystal is mechanically stressed. This charge is proportional to the applied force. Such transducers have the advantage of having a high sensitivity and high rigidity. However, under a constant load the charge developed decays by time, giving a false signal that the force is decreasing. Therefore, piezoelectric transducers are only capable of measuring transients, and are not suitable for measuring static forces.

Strain Gage-Based Biomechanical Load Transducers

In the late 1930s researchers at MIT and Cal Tech, working independently, found that a small-diameter wire made of an electrical resistance alloy could be adhesively bonded to a structure for measurement of surface strains. In the 1950s, as an offshoot to the printed circuit techniques that were introduced to the electronics industry, foil strain gages were developed. Foil gages are produced by etching or cutting the desired gage pattern into a thin sheet of metal foil. The foil and its plastic backing has a typical total thickness of 0.02 to 0.05 mm, depending on the type of foil alloy and the backing material used. The size of gages vary from a fraction of a millimeter up to several centimeters and longer. Their grid patterns also vary. Figure 18-1 depicts three different gages: a single gage and two two-gage rosettes, each for measuring strain in two orthogonal directions. Today, the vast majority of metallic strain gages used are of foil type; wire type gages are usually used for measurements at very high temperatures. Semiconductor gages differ from the metallic wire and foil strain gages. Their most significant differences are their small size and high sensitivity, i.e. the relative resistance change in the gage due to a given applied strain level. However, semiconductor gages also have serious limitations, including fragility, lack of ductility, and temperature sensitivity, among others. Therefore, use of semiconductor gages are usually limited to miniature transducers.

Strain gages measure the average strain over the entire grid length. The average strain is the change in length divided by the original grid length. Gages function on the principle that the resistance of the wire or foil changes as its cross-sectional area changes. This inverse relationship of

FIGURE 18-1   Three of the many different strain gage patterns depicting a single gage and two 90° rosettes. The longitudinal direction of the pattern is the sensitive direction of the gage.

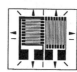

increasing resistance with decreasing area allows the deformation of the parent member to be quantified. As the member deforms, so does the gage, causing its cross-sectional area to change, and thus the resistance to change. Resistance changes can be related directly to the amount of deformation, which in turn can be related to the strain and eventually to the force applied to the loaded member. In practice, for strain gage-based force transducers the output voltage is proportional to the applied load.

The relationship of strain to resistance change is the sensitivity of the gage and defined by the *gage factor*, denoted by *GF*.

$$GF = \frac{\frac{\Delta R}{R}}{\frac{\Delta L}{L}} = \frac{\frac{\Delta R}{R}}{\varepsilon} \tag{3}$$

where ΔR is the change in gage resistance, R is the original gage resistance, ΔL is the change in gage length, L is the original gage length, and ε is the average strain. The *GF* is a function of the material used for the foil. A typical value is around 2. Gages are mainly sensitive to changes in length along their major axes, defined by the longitudinal direction of the foil pattern. Any sensitivity they may have in the orthogonal direction is known as the transverse sensitivity, which can be neglected for the purpose of the following discussion.

Since the resulting resistance changes in strain gages are so small, an ordinary ohmmeter is inadequate for measuring these changes. Most transducers are designed around 1,000 microstrain ($\mu\varepsilon$) deformation at full scale load, and for a 0.1 percent resolution the strain that needs to be measured would be around 1.0 $\mu\varepsilon$. From Equation 3, using a gage resistance of 350 ohms, and a gage factor of 2, the gage resistance change for 1.0 $\mu\varepsilon$ is at the order of 7×10^{-4} ohms. Thus, a Wheatstone-bridge circuit and/or signal amplification techniques are used to measure the small resistance variations. Figure 18-2 shows a Wheatstone bridge wired with four resistive legs and excited by a voltage V. The bridge legs, R_1 to R_4, represent the resistances that make up the bridge, and E is the output voltage.

From a simple circuit analysis it can be shown that a bridge is balanced when $E = 0$. This occurs when $\dfrac{R_1}{R_2} = \dfrac{R_4}{R_3}$.

Using the basic circuit analysis rules, it is a straightforward derivation to obtain the general relationship of excitation voltage, V, output voltage, E, and resistances. Note that the internal resistance of the voltage-measuring device is typically high and draws a negligible current, therefore the current in the bridge legs BAD and BCD can be written as

$$i_{BAD} = \frac{V}{R_1 + R_4} \tag{4}$$

$$i_{BCD} = \frac{V}{R_2 + R_3}. \tag{5}$$

Thus, the voltage loop equation is

$$
\begin{aligned}
E_{AC} &= E_{AB} + E_{BC} \\
&= E_{AB} - E_{CB} \\
&= i_{BAD} \cdot R_1 - i_{BCD} \cdot R_2. \tag{6}
\end{aligned}
$$

Now, substituting Equations 4 and 5 into Equation 6, the output voltage is obtained as

$$E_{AC} = \left(\frac{R_1}{R_1 + R_4} - \frac{R_2}{R_2 + R_3} \right) \cdot V. \tag{7}$$

If all the leg resistances are initially equal to R, and the bridge is wired such that R_1 and R_3 increase by ΔR, while R_2 and R_4 decrease by ΔR, then:

$$\Delta E = \left(\frac{\Delta R \cdot R}{(R + \Delta R)^2} \right) \cdot V \tag{8}$$

where ΔE is the change in output voltage. Note that the output voltage is linearly proportional to the excitation voltage, but nonlinear with the change in gage resistance. However, as ΔR is small compared to R, Equation 8 can be linearized as

$$\Delta E = \frac{\Delta R}{R} \cdot V. \tag{9}$$

For example, when a strain-gaged force transducer is loaded to full capacity, typically the gages are designed to experience a 0.1 percent resistance change. With $\Delta R/R$ equal to 0.001, Equations 8 and 9 show that, at full scale deflection, the transducer output will have a 0.2 percent deviation from linearity.

In most transducer designs each leg is chosen such that initial gage resistances are equal and all four gages contribute to the force measurement, which has several advantages. Each leg contributes to the transducer sensitivity, thus sensitivity is increased. Temperature compensation is achieved as each gage experiences the same thermally induced strain. Due to the properties of the Wheatstone bridge, strains from the opposite legs are added while the adjacent ones are subtracted, thus canceling the temperature effects. A further advantage of using full bridge circuits is that by suitable gage placement, any one of the combined loads can be isolated and measured separately. Mechanics principles are used to deduce these arrangements.

Similar application of mechanics principles and Wheatstone-bridge circuits can be applied to transducer design in order to decompose a general load into its Cartesian components. Consider the beam in Figures 18-3 through 18-6. It is subjected to a combined loading state that includes a bending moment about the x-axis, a y-shear force component, and a vertical or axial force component. The moment shown may represent either a vertical force acting at some distance along the y-axis or a pure couple applied as shown. By implementing the gage and bridge arrangement of Figure 18-4, the bridge output will only be sensitive to vertical forces. Any other loading effects will be canceled by this configuration. There are two options when

Figure 18-2 Wheatstone bridge.

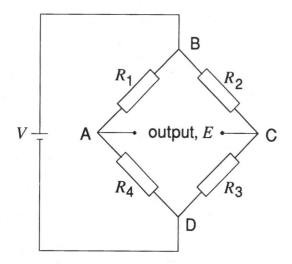

FIGURE 18-3 A cylindrical beam fixed at one end and subjected to combined loading at the other.

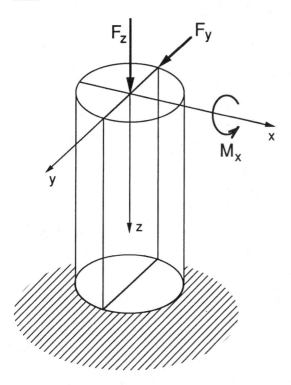

FIGURE 18-4 Axial force measurement. **A,** Gage locations on the beam. **B,** Gage connections in the Wheatstone bridge.

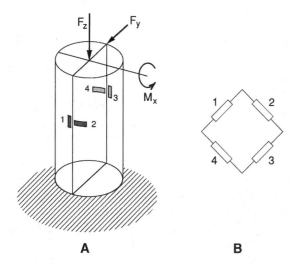

measuring shear forces. Figure 18-5 depicts the gage placement and bridge configuration that will measure shear by comparing the bending moment deformation of the column at two different levels

FIGURE 18-5 Shear force measurement by bending moment difference method. **A,** Gage locations on the beam. **B,** Gage connections in the Wheatstone bridge.

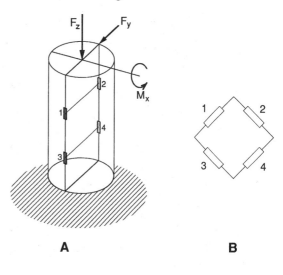

along the beam's long axis. The second shear force transducer layout utilizes gages placed at 45 degree angles with the long axis of the beam and measure the shear force directly from shear deformation of the beam. This is shown in Figure 18-6. By appropriate alignment of the gages the effects of any torsion that also causes shear deformation can be nullified. Now, the output will be a function of the shear force only. Since both shear methods have the desired effect of eliminating any other load measurement, the choice of which one to use defaults to space available for gaging and other practical matters of transducer design.

Keep in mind that all four bridge elements need not be on the same transducer element. In the same respect, more than one gage resistance can be placed in the same leg of the Wheatstone bridge. Also, the output of more than one bridge can be coupled to sum the effect of a force component acting on two or more transducer elements. This is demonstrated in Figure 18-7. When these techniques are implemented, care must be taken to preserve the advantageous properties of the bridge circuit. When bridges are split or combined, the gage sensitivities must be matched in order to maintain the independence of transducer output on load position. These rules apply to all three of the loading cases described above, and here lies the basis for force plate transducer design. This will be discussed further later in this chapter.

Figure 18-6 Shear force measurement using 45° gage orientation. **A,** Gage locations on the beam. **B,** Gage connections in the Wheatstone bridge. Gages 1 and 2 in the (**C**) unloaded and (**D**) loaded state.

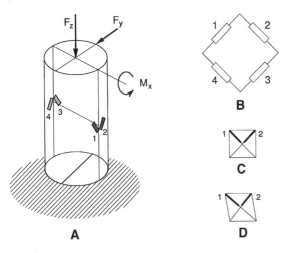

Figure 18-7 Combination of two shear bridges into one. **A,** Gage locations on individual beams. **B,** Gages connected inone bridge.

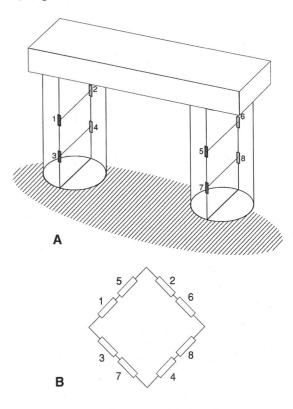

Piezoelectric Crystal-Based Biomechanical Load Transducers

Electrical charge develops within certain solid materials when they are mechanically stressed. This effect is reversible in that if a charge is applied, the material will mechanically deform in response. These actions are given the name piezoelectric effect. Quartz is a piezoelectric material with high stability and is normally used in load transducers.

The properties of the crystal are directional, and axial and shear force components can be isolated by orienting the material in the transducer. Figure 18-8 depicts disks cut out of a piezoelectric crystal with their sensitive axes oriented as shown. When a disk is sandwiched between metal electrodes and subjected to a force, the crystal deflects and a charge, *q,* is produced. This charge is proportional to the deflection. Simultaneously, a voltage is developed between the electrodes. The voltage output can be amplified and calibrated to measure the applied force. Normally, a pair of disks are used to measure one load component. Using the quartz disks in pairs doubles the sensitivity and permits simple electrical contact by a central electrode. By stacking three pairs of disks, one pair for the axial load and two pairs for the two orthogonal shears, a three-component force transducer is obtained. These types of transducers must be assembled with a compressive preload holding the disks together, which prevents the crystal from separating from the metal plate electrode sandwich

Figure 18-8 Orientation of piezoelectric disks in a quartz crystal.

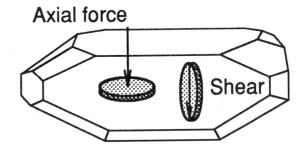

during tensile loading. Six-component transducers are built by placing four such three-component transducers at four corners of a platform.

Piezoelectric transducers have the advantage of having high sensitivity and high rigidity. Typical stiffness properties of these crystals result in natural frequencies as high as 30,000 Hz. When six-component load transducers are built however, the governing natural frequency is normally that of the platform supporting the individual three-component transducers, and the stiffness advantage of quartz crystals is lost.

On the other hand, the piezoelectric transducers have the disadvantage of not being suitable to measure static loads. The charge developed when the quartz crystal that is loaded gradually leaks, causing a decay in the signal, which eventually goes to zero. If the load is now released, the transducer will indicate application of a load in the opposite direction.

In order to fully understand the dynamics of a piezoelectric force transducer the following analysis is necessary. As stated above, an input force, f, is applied to a piezoelectric sensor causing a deflection, x. The resulting charge buildup produces a potential voltage, E, between the capacitive plates. This voltage can be expressed as

$$E = \frac{q}{C_{cr}} \tag{10}$$

where C_{cr}, is the crystal capacitance, defined as

$$C_{cr} = \frac{\varepsilon \cdot A}{t} \tag{11}$$

where ε is the dielectric constant of the crystal, A is the area of the plates, and t is the distance between the plates. Figure 18-9 depicts a piezoelectric sensor. The applied force, f, causing the deformation and charge, q, can be related by means of a piezoelectric constant, k:

$$q = k \cdot f. \tag{12}$$

A typical value of k for quartz is 2.3 picocoulombs per newton (pC/N). Substitution of Equations 11 and 12 into Equation 10 yields

$$E = \frac{k \cdot f \cdot t}{\varepsilon \cdot A}. \tag{13}$$

The induced voltage, E from above must be measured in order to quantify the force. Due to the magnitude of the voltage created, a charge amplifier is typically used in conjunction with the crystal sensor. Another complication is due to charge leaking back through the crystal. If the charge generator is considered as a current generator, the circuits of Figure 18-10 can be used to calculate the behavior of the transducer. Here, the current source, i_s, is the time derivative of the charge generated, C_{cr} is the crystal capacitance, R_{leak} is the sensor leakage resistance, C_{cable} is the capacitance of the connecting cables, C_{amp} is the capacitance of the amplifier, and R_{amp} is the amplifier internal resistance. E_o is the resulting output voltage to be measured. Figure 18-10, A is the schematic of the crystal alone, while Figure 18-10, B represents the cabling and amplifier. Both Figures 18-10, A and 18-10, B are reduced to the equivalent circuit of Figure 18-11. In this circuit, i_s, C, and R can be expressed as follows:

$$i_s = \frac{dq}{dt} = k\frac{df}{dt} \tag{14}$$

$$R = \frac{R_{amp} \cdot R_{leak}}{R_{amp} + R_{leak}}. \tag{15}$$

The value of R_{leak} is typically on the order of 10^{11} ohms for the type of transducers used in force measurement. Systems with high amplifier input impedances and sensor leakage resistances also exist, providing approximately 10^{14} ohms of total system resistance, R. Such systems will have a very slow leakage rate, making almost static force measurement possible.[6]

The equivalent circuit of Figure 18-11 can now be analyzed. The current loop equation reduces to

$$i_s = i_C + i_R. \tag{16}$$

The output voltage can now be expressed as

$$E_o = E_C = \int \frac{i_c}{C}dt = \frac{\int (i_s - i_R)dt}{C}, \tag{17}$$

rearranging terms:

$$C \cdot E_o = \int (i_s - i_R)dt \tag{18}$$

and finally, differentiating and substituting gives the following:

$$C \cdot \frac{dE_o}{dt} = i_s - i_R = k\frac{df}{dt} - \frac{E_o}{R}. \tag{19}$$

This differential equation can be rearranged to a standard form and expressed in terms of the differential operator, D.

$$(R \cdot C \cdot D + 1)E_o = (R \cdot k \cdot D)f. \tag{20}$$

FIGURE 18-9   Piezoelectric crystal.

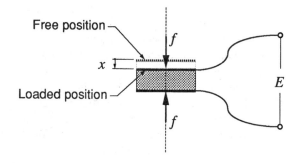

FIGURE 18-10   Equivalent circuit for the (A) piezoelectric transducer and (B) amplifier.

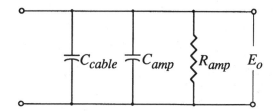

A   B

FIGURE 18-11   Equivalent circuit for the piezoelectric transducer and amplifier.

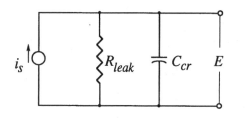

FIGURE 18-12   Response of piezoelectric transducer to a constant force: A, Applied force. B, Time response for a relatively high time constant. C, Time response for a relatively small time constant.

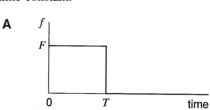

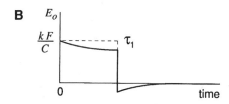

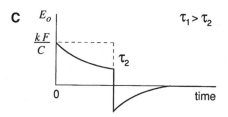

The terms of static sensitivity, $K = k/C$, and time constant, $\tau = RC$, can be defined. Now the equation can be written in the form of input over output. This is a first order system with "numerator dynamics."[6]

$$\frac{E_o}{f}(D) = \frac{K \cdot \tau \cdot D}{(\tau \cdot D + 1)} \qquad (21)$$

Consider a constant force input, F, for a time of T, as shown in Figure 18-12, A. The differential Equation 21 can be solved with these initial conditions for the time periods zero to T, and T to infinity. The resulting solutions are

$$E_o = \frac{k \cdot F}{C} e^{-t/\tau} \qquad (22)$$

and

$$E_o = \frac{k \cdot F}{C} (e^{-T/\tau} - 1) e^{-(t-T)/\tau}. \qquad (23)$$

Two qualitative responses, one for a relatively high time constant and one for a low one, are presented graphically in Figures 18-12, B and 18-12, C respectively. Note the effect of τ on the output signal decay. As τ decreases, the signal decays

more rapidly, and there is a considerable undershoot in the response of the sensor. Thus, for force-measuring piezoelectric transducers, it is desirable to have a high time constant that will allow for quasi-static calibration and measurements.

The physical properties and the dimensions of the crystal, as well as the amplifier properties determine the actual time constant for the system. There are, however, limited means to effectively increase τ. As previously defined, the time constant is the product of the effective capacitance and resistance for the transducer. Thus, increasing either R or C will increase τ. This can be achieved either with a shunt capacitor or a series resistor at the amplifier. As a result, however, the sensitivity of the transducer would decrease.

Force Measurement in Gait

The most common force-measuring instrument used in gait analysis is the force plate. Force plates are available in many configurations, sizes, and with various performance characteristics. They are six-component load transducers capable of measuring the three force and three moment components needed to completely describe the loading characteristics of a body in contact with a surface. One of the most common uses of force plates is the measurement of ground reaction loads produced during human ambulation, for clinical and research purposes.

Both strain gage and piezoelectric crystal technologies are used in force plate transducer design. Although the ultimate output is three forces and three moments, there is a difference in how the two methods arrive at these values.

Strain gage–based force plates typically have four load transducers separating two plates and arranged in a rectangular fashion. The principles of summation and superposition, described earlier, and illustrated in Figure 18-7, are utilized in order to sum the output of each transducer for each respective channel of total force plate output. It becomes obvious that the gage layout and wiring of a full six-component force platform is straightforward but elaborate. The precise placement of the gages is critical. The final result is that each output channel for a strain gage–based force plate represents a direct measurement of the respective force or moment. This is in contrast to the method of deducing the moments from the force components in piezoelectric-based force plates.

The typical transducers used in piezoelectric-based force plates are four identical three-component force transducers, one placed at each corner of the plate. This arrangement is depicted in Figure 18-13. The moments are deduced from the measured forces and relative transducer locations in the force plate, which is why there are eight output channels from a piezoelectric-based force plate instead of six as in strain gage-based platforms. The twelve outputs from the four three-component force transducers are connected such that eight outputs result from the force plate. The eight channels represent the four individual vertical forces measured, two shears in the x-direction,

FIGURE 18-13 Twelve individual force components measured by a piezoelectric force plate. The eight outputs from the force plate are $(F_{x1} + F_{x2})$, $(F_{x3} + F_{x4})$, $(F_{y1} + F_{y4})$, $(F_{y2} + F_{y3})$, F_{z1}, F_{z2}, F_{z3}, and F_{z4}.

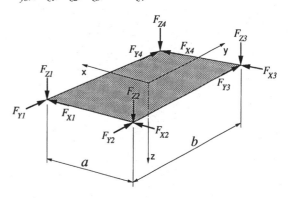

and two shears in the y-direction. In order to get the six ground reactions and moments, the data need to be further reduced as follows:

$$F_x = (F_{x1} + F_{x2}) + (F_{x3} + F_{x4}) \tag{24}$$

$$F_y = (F_{y1} + F_{y4}) + (F_{y2} + F_{y3}) \tag{25}$$

$$F_z = (F_{z1} + F_{z2}) + (F_{z3} + F_{z4}) \tag{26}$$

$$M_x = [(-F_{z1} - F_{z2}) + (F_{z3} + F_{z4})] \cdot \frac{b}{2} \tag{27}$$

$$M_y = [(-F_{z1} + F_{z2}) + F_{z3} - F_{z4})] \cdot \frac{a}{2} \tag{28}$$

$$M_z = [(F_{x1} + F_{x2}) - (F_{x3} + F_{x4})] \cdot \frac{b}{2} + [(F_{y1} + F_{y4}) - (F_{y2} + F_{y3})] \cdot \frac{a}{2}. \tag{29}$$

The loads transferred between the force plate and a body or bodies in contact with it can be expressed by a resultant force and a resultant moment. These are the quantities measured by a force plate. Figure 18-14 depicts a force plate with a force vector, $\vec{F}$, acting at a point (x, y). When only compressive forces are applied in the z-direction, the couple that can be transmitted to the force plate would be in the x-y plane. This couple is sometimes referred to as the *free moment*. The point of application of the resultant force and the free moment can be calculated from the measured force and moment components expressed in the Cartesian coordinate system using the following equations:

$$x = \frac{-h \cdot F_x - M_y}{F_z} \tag{30}$$

FIGURE 18-14   A force vector acting on a force plate. Components of the force vector, its point of application, and the distance from the force plate origin to the top surface are also shown.

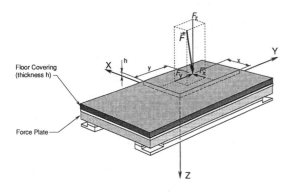

$$y = \frac{-h \cdot F_y + M_x}{F_z} \qquad (30)$$

$$T_z = M_z - x \cdot F_y + x \cdot F_x \qquad (31)$$

where, h is the distance from the x-y plane to the top surface of the force plate, and T_z is the couple.

Various parameters can be deduced from force plate data alone, as well as when a force plate is combined with motion measurement equipment. The point of application of the resultant force is often referred to as the center of pressure (COP). The variation in the COP as a function of time is typically used as a measure of stability of the subject standing on the force plate or in walking. By integrating and double integrating the measured force components, the respective change in velocity and change in position of the center of gravity of the body applying the force can be calculated. These are only relative changes in values, because integration constants and initial values are not known. However, when force plates are used with motion measurement systems, these constants can be determined from the position data collected.

There are a few concepts that require familiarity in order to implement force plates correctly and accurately. Although force plates are generally linear instruments (i.e., their output is linearly proportional to force input), several possible sources of error in the output signal exist. These include uncorrected cross talk between channels, transducer and amplifier nonlinearity, amplifier adjustable gain error, and imperfectly balanced initial bridge circuits, just to name a few. These are inherent in the force plate amplifier combination and are independent of the additional signal noise

and analog-to-digital conversion errors common to all data collection systems. A recent evaluation of the piezoelectric force plates has also shown that they have significantly larger errors than the strain-gaged devices in determining point of application of the force vector.[3]

Cross talk or cross sensitivity is the influence one load component has on another signal channel. This can result from imperfectly placed gages, machining tolerances, nonuniform transducer mounting, elastic deformations, and the like. Traditionally, cross talk has been regarded as undesirable. However, with the use of the digital computer in data acquisition and processing, a simple mathematical operation, as described below, is used to correct for cross talk. In fact, load transducer design can sometimes be simplified by allowing each output channel to be sensitive to more than one load component. For example, the triangular force plate designed by Gola measures two force components at each corner, and all six transducers contribute to each of the six output channels.[7]

In the case of a perfectly behaved six-component load transducer (i.e., no cross talk), each output would be directly proportional to the corresponding input. In vector notation the output load vector, $\vec{L}$, would be represented by the dot product of the calibration vector with the signal vector:

$$\vec{L} = \vec{c} \cdot \vec{S}. \qquad (32)$$

When cross talk is present, the equation takes on the following matrix form:

$$\vec{L_i} = [c_{ij}] \cdot \vec{S_j} \qquad (33)$$

where $\vec{L_i}$ is the load vector of forces and moments, $\vec{S_j}$ is the signal vector (amplifier signal output at any given instant), and $[c_{ij}]$ is the calibration matrix of the load transducer. The diagonal components of $[c_{ij}]$ are analogous to the elements of $\vec{c}$ in Equation 32, while the off-diagonal elements are the cross talk terms.

Each individual force plate will have its own unique calibration matrix. This calibration matrix is with respect to a point of origin, which can be at any specified point. It is obtained by applying various sets of known loads at known locations and solving backwards for the calibration matrix. This is detailed in the following equations:

$$[L] = [c_{ij}][S] \qquad (34)$$

where $[L]$ represents $[\vec{L_{i1}}, \vec{L_{i2}}, \ldots, \vec{L_{in}}]$, independent load sets of known and calibrated loads, and

$[S]$ represents $[\vec{S}_{j1}, \vec{S}_{j2}, \ldots, \vec{S}_{jn}]$, the corresponding signal outputs; then $[c_{ij}]$ can be found by post multiplying both sides of Equation 34 by the transpose of $[S]$:

$$[L][S]^T = [c_{ij}][S][S]^T. \tag{35}$$

Then, $[S][S]^T$ is inverted, and

$$[c_{ij}] = [L][S]^T\{[S][S]^T\}^{-1}. \tag{36}$$

Obviously the minimum number of load sets, n in Equation 34, must be at least six. It has been found through experimentation that if n equals 15, the result will be a calibration matrix $[c_{ij}]$ that will generate load values to an accuracy better than 1%.[2]

Force plate specifications vary widely depending on manufacturer, type of plate, and electronic amplifiers. Sensitivities of available plates also vary depending on their size, load capacity, signal conditioning and amplification capabilities, and stiffness of the plates. Vertical, or z-direction natural frequencies range from 350 Hz to 1800 Hz. Nonlinearity of these instruments varies from ± 0.2% to ±1.0% of full-scale range. Single force plate systems start in the $10,000 range and can climb to the $50,000 range for larger and/or an array of force plates.

With the emergence of high-power PC-sized computers, force plate applications are becoming more extensive. Faster computers allow for a more economical solution to the massive data collection and reduction problems encountered when using force plates. Therefore, it has now become possible to use a large array of force plates covering the walk path. Noting that outputs from several force plates can be resolved, either electronically or mathematically, to a single six-component output, it becomes possible to implement a larger array of smaller force plates covering gait laboratories. Problems of targeting a single force plate by the test subject can then be eliminated.[9]

PRESSURE MEASUREMENT

As defined in the introduction, pressure is the force per unit area, where p is the pressure, F is the normal component of force applied to an area, A (Equation 1). Pressure-measurement technologies vary widely. Suitable measuring methods are applicable dependent. For example, the technologies utilized in fluid pressure measurement are usually not applicable for measuring contact pressures, which is the type of pressure most often measured when studying gait and biomechanics.

Contact pressures arise when two bodies touch. Depending upon the material properties of the contacting bodies, these pressures can be high and have steep gradients. The resulting pressure distributions are then difficult to measure accurately. This is complicated further by the presence of a transducer. In many technologies used today, the pressure transducer itself might influence the pressure distribution and skew the measured data.

The physical size of a contact pressure sensor can have a profound effect upon the accuracy of pressures measured. Since pressure is area dependent, the smaller the area contacted by an individual sensor, the finer the resolution. In order to obtain a dense spatial resolution in pressure measurement, the individual sensors need to be miniaturized and closely packed together. This provides good resolution but significantly complicates the data collection tasks. Today's contact pressure transducers are generally a compromise between good spatial resolution and frequency, and complexity of data collection and reduction. This is a function of the size of the sensing element.

A simple illustration can be used to point out the significance of pressure measurement error due to inadequate sensor coverage. In Figure 18-15, the pressure distribution over 1 square unit area is shown with three different spatial resolutions. In each case, the applied pressure distribution and loading are identical. Thus, the average pressure over the total area for all three cases is identical (1 force unit per 1 squared area unit). This is shown by computing the individual force per sensor and summing to check vertical force equilibrium. In Figure 18-15A the sensor used is 1 square area unit in size. Four sensors, each one-quarter square unit area in size, are used to obtain the pressure distribution shown in Figure 18-15B. Similarly, Figure 18-15C depicts the pressure distribution obtained when the sensor length is halved once more. Note the significant difference in peak pressure in each case. Though this example is simplistic, it illustrates a real problem in pressure measurement. The intent of the pressure measurement must be kept in mind when selecting a measuring device and what impact its resolution may have on the data.

Pressure Measurement Technology in Kinetic Assessment of Gait

One common pressure parameter that is of interest to the biomedical researcher and clinician is the pressure distribution under the foot. The circumstances of this contact vary greatly in everyday activities. The ground surface can be regular and

FIGURE 18-15   Same pressure distribution measured using three different resolutions. Numbers indicate numerical values of the measured pressure. (See text.)

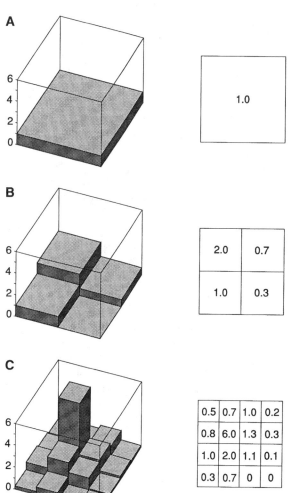

capacitive and resistive sensors used in pressure measuring mats.[8] This circuit provides a way to multiplex data from an $m \times n$ matrix of sensors with only $m + n$ acquisition channels.

Piezoelectric sensors are used in a pressure platform developed by Cavanagh and Hennig.[4] This platform consists of 1000 sensors, each being approximately 7 mm square and connected to a charge amplifier. The same techniques were also applied to a semiflexible in-shoe pressure sensor.[5]

Optical techniques utilizing refracted light leaving a glass plate have been developed. A plastic film layer on the glass provides a changing index of refraction in response to pressure. As a subject walks on the plate, the amount of light refracted and recorded by a video camera under the glass surface is proportional to the pressure. The video image is then digitized and the pressure distribution mapped. Problems with this method include the need for real-time calibration due to the variable properties of the plastic film and the inability to be used in-shoe or on curved surfaces.

The more recent trends in biomechanical pressure measurement require in-shoe, in prosthetic and orthotic, on mattress, and ambulation on flexible ground measurement capability.[1,10,11] Several of these issues have been addressed with thin foil capacitors with air gaps, fiber optic grids, resistive ink grids, as well as the more traditional methods.

Future developments in this area will benefit from the move toward miniaturization of electronics and computers. As the computing power increases, more and more sensors will be able to be used. The data collection capabilities will be the limiting factor here. As higher channel devices and telemetric systems improve, so will the ability to make these kinds of pressure measurements.

SUMMARY

The technology of force and pressure measurement as related to the kinetic assessment of gait has been discussed to provide the reader with the necessary background for instrument selection and usage. First, force and pressure are described and defined. Then, similarities in the principles used to measure force and pressure are discussed. After the association between the two is established, the general principles used in force measurement are presented. A detailed description of the strain-gaged transducers is followed by discussion of the piezoelectric type. Force plate technology, calibration, and measurement methodologies, including errors associated with these types of instruments, are detailed in each case. Finally,

hard or irregular and soft. The interest may be in foot-to-shoe contact, shoe-to-ground, or direct foot-to-ground contact. Current technology has not provided an ideal pressure transducer that is applicable for all biomechanical needs. A multitude of measurement techniques are currently being employed to quantify these pressures.

Some of the more prevalent principles used in commercially available devices include relating the change in capacitance between two surfaces, measuring resistances or monitoring a resistive grid, digitization of optical images, fiber optic transducers, piezoelectric principles, and thin film techniques.

Nicol and Hennig developed a multiplexing circuitry to interface with the high number of different methods used in pressure measurement and their advantages, disadvantages, and limitations are presented.

References

1. Babbs CF, Bourland JD, Graber GP et al: A pressure sensitive mat for measuring contact pressure distributions of patients lying on hospital beds, *Biomed Instr Tech* 24:363, 1990.
2. Berme N: Load transducers. In *Biomechanics of human movement: applications in rehabilitation, sports and ergonomics,* Worthington, Ohio, 1990, Bertec Corporation.
3. Bobbert MF, Schamhardt HC: Accuracy of determining the point of force application with piezoelectric force plates, *J Biomech* 23:705, 1990.
4. Cavanagh PR, Hennig EM: A new device for the measurement of pressure distribution on a rigid surface, *Med Sci Sport Exer* 14:153, 1982.
5. Cavanagh PR, Hennig EM, Bunch RP et al: A new device for the measurement of pressure distribution inside the shoe. In *Biomechanics VIII-B,* Baltimore, 1982, University Park Press.
6. Doebelin EO: *Measurement systems; application and design,* New York, 1990, McGraw-Hill.
7. Gola MM: Mechanical design, constructional details and calibration of a new force plate, *J Biomech* 13:113, 1980.
8. Nicol K, Hennig EM: Apparatus for time-dependent measurement of physical quantities, *U.S. Patent* No. 4,134,086, 1979.
9. Oaks WR: *Force measurement in closed loop biological systems* (Master's Thesis), The Ohio State University, Columbus, Ohio, 1984.
10. Saad I, Nicol K: Pressure distribution on soft surfaces: measuring systems and applications. In *Biomechanics XI,* Amsterdam, 1988, Free University Press.
11. Yücel M, Liebscher F, Nicol K: Pressure distribution in orthotic devices for treatment of the spine. In *Biomechanics IX-A,* 1985, Champaign, Ill, Human Kinetic Publishers.

A REVIEW OF KINETIC PARAMETERS IN HUMAN WALKING

David A. Winter
Janice J. Eng
Milad G. Ishac

KEY TERMS

Center of mass

Global reference system

Ground reaction force

Joint pressure

Joint reaction force

Mechanical energy

Moments of force

Power

Support moment

Work

Kinetics by definition deals with those variables that cause the specific walking pattern we observe or measure with our cameras. As such, we are concerned with the individual muscle forces, the net moments generated by those muscles (and other passive structures such as ligaments), and the mechanical power patterns (rates of energy generation, absorption, and transfer at each joint). At this point in time no reliable technique has been developed to decompose joint moments into individual muscle forces. This chapter focuses on the net muscle moments and powers and compares these profiles with the major muscle groups that must be involved. Theoretical approaches for resolving individual muscle forces are available and are discussed in some detail in Chapter 17.

INDETERMINACY AT THE MOTOR LEVEL

Walking involves the integration of signals at many different levels in a converging system as depicted in Figure 19-1. Every synaptic junction is an algebraic summation of all inhibitory and excitatory inputs. The convergence of all neural integration is seen in the final common pathways ①. However, beyond this neural integration we have three other levels of central nervous system (CNS) integration at the muscle and skeletal level. At the muscle level we see the net summation of all final common pathways innervating each muscle such that the tension signal ② is a CNS control variable, which reflects the neural summation of recruitment

and rate coding (modified by the length of the muscle and velocity of contraction of the muscle). A third level of musculoskeletal integration takes place at each joint where the moment of force ③ is the algebraic summation of all muscle force/moment-arm-length products. Finally, intersegment integration is evident where adjacent moments of force collaborate towards a common goal (synergy). One such synergy was reported over a decade ago, called the support moment ④, which quantifies the integrated defense of the total lower limb against a gravity-induced vertical collapse.[31]

The net result of these many levels of integration is that the motor level is considerably more variable than the kinematic level. This variability makes the diagnosis of pathological gait a major problem at the motor level, but it is also an early indicator of the tremendous adaptability (plasticity) of the CNS. Such adaptability is inherent in normal gait[32] as well as in pathological gait.[33]

INTERPRETATION OF 3-D MOMENTS OF FORCE DURING GAIT

With the advent of commercial 3-D movement analysis systems we now face a flood of 3-D kinematics and 3-D kinetics. It is important to look not only at how local axis systems (LAS) of each segment are defined from the external markers but also how to report joint angles, angular velocities, reaction forces, and moments of force.

FIGURE 19-1 Schematic of the four stages of neuromusculoskeletal integration that takes place in total body multisegment movements such as walking. The first integration ① is neural at the α neuron. The second integration ② is mechanical at the tendon where a summation of all motor unit forces is seen. The third integration ③ is mechanical at the joint where the sum of all agonist and antagonist moments of force appear. Finally, interlimb coupling and synergies ④ represents a fourth level of mechanical integration.

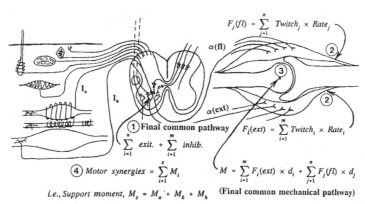

Lower Limb Considerations

In normal level gait a subject walks in a plane of progression defined by the average velocity of the total body center of mass over a stride period. In a gait laboratory this plane of progression is aligned with one of the planes in the global reference system (GRS). In many cases subjects walk with minimal internal or external rotation of the stance limb (see Figure 19-2), and in this situation the sagittal plane of each lower limb segment and the plane of progression will effectively be the same. Thus with less than 8 degrees out-of-plane rotation of the joint sagittal angles, the moments will have less than 1% difference from that calculated in the plane of progression defined by the GRS. However, the differences will not be insignificant when considering joint rotations and moments in the frontal and horizontal planes. The question remains, especially in the kinetics, how should the internal/external and abductor/adductor moments be reported? However, if the orientation of lower limbs is such that the sagittal plane of any segment does not agree with the plane of progression (i.e., because the lower limb is externally rotated during stance) then all three anatomical axes do not agree with the GRS. Figure 19-3 depicts this situation: should we report the joint moments in the anatomical axes or in the GRS?

The position we put forward is that the GRS moments are best to use rather than the anatomical axes, which change continuously over the gait cycle. This does not mean we do not carry out our inverse dynamics solution in the LRS of each segment. Our moments calculated at each joint are in the axes of the LAS of the distal segment, and they are then transposed into three orthogonal GRS components. The rationale behind this argument relates to our knowledge of the goal of gait, which is to transport the body's center of mass (COM) along a plane of progression with minor fluctuations out of the GRS. The plane-of-progression velocity ranges from 1 m/s for slow walking to 2 m/s for fast walking. The vertical velocity typically varies ± 0.3 m/s, and the medial/lateral velocity varies about ± 0.15 m/s. This plane-of-progression velocity is maintained in spite of varying orientations of limb segments. In Figure 19-3, for example, the foot, leg, and thigh are all externally rotated; however, their linear velocities are effectively in the plane of progression and not in their sagittal planes. Thus, to interpret the cause of acceleration/deceleration in the plane of progression we must have moments in an axis normal to that plane.

Pelvic, Trunk, and Total Body Center of Mass Considerations

Because the pelvis does not "belong" to either the right or left lower limb it must be treated separately. In Figure 19-2, for example, the pelvis is depicted during double support, and we cannot describe the pelvic translation with respect to either limbs; the right hip is internally rotated while the left hip is externally rotated. Because the major challenges to the head, arm, trunk segment (H.A.T.) are that of posture and balance, it makes sense to use gravity as the base reference vector and thereby use the GRS reference. Thus all

---

FIGURE 19-2 Orientation of the limb segments to illustrate situation when the lower limb segments will be oriented closely to the plane of progression and therefore dictate that the moments-of-force should be reported in axes normal to that plane of progression.

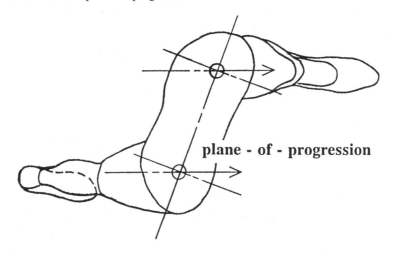

plane - of - progression

FIGURE 19-3   Illustrative situation to demonstrate that when lower limb segments are not oriented in the plane of progression their linear velocities are still closely oriented in the plane of progression. Thus the moments should be reported in the GRS, not in the LAS of each individual segment.

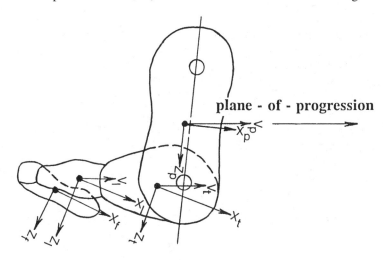

plane - of - progression

pelvic and trunk angles should be reported relative to the GRS. Pelvic tilt, obliquity, and rotation will represent the absolute angles of this segment as seen in the GRS. In a similar manner we see reports of the trajectory total body COM in 3-D space, with GRS as the reference system. Also, the location of the COM relative to the net center of pressure (COP) is critical in understanding body balance during steady-state gait as well as critical transition periods such as initiation and termination of gait.

Interpretation at the Muscle Level
In spite of the net interpretation we make at the level of moments of force, when we look for the muscles generating any given moment we must return to the anatomical axis. Figure 19-3 explains forward velocity changes of the leg segment occurring in spite of the fact that the foot is aligned well out of the plane of progression. The ankle moment responsible for decelerating or accelerating the leg would be a combination of that generated by the soleus and gastrocnemius with an above-normal assist from the peroneii. The peroneii are described as plantarflexors and evertors. However, with a large external foot rotation they will act more dominantly in the plane of progression. A similar interpretation would apply at the hip where the more posterior fibers of the gluteus medius would act in concert with the gluteus maximus and hamstrings to create the hip extensor moment in the plane of progression.

Ground Reaction Forces
The ground reaction forces as measured by a force platform reflect the net vertical and shear forces acting between the foot (shoe) and the force platform. As such as these three forces are an algebraic summation of the mass-acceleration products of all body segments while the foot is in contact with the platform. The vertical force reflects the accelerations due to gravity as well as the vertical acceleration (as seen by the cameras). The interpretation of these waveforms can lead to problems if the researcher is not reminded that these forces are an algebraic summation that give us no information as to what individual segments are doing. Clinically, these ground reaction forces may differ somewhat from those seen in normal walking; however, nothing in these waveforms yields specific information to the surgical or rehabilitation team regarding the management of their patient. Andriacchi et al. reported the magnitudes of three peaks in each of the vertical, anterior-posterior, and lateral forces as a function of walking velocity from 0.5 to 2.5 m/s.[1] Chao et al. looked at similar measures to see how they changed with age and sex and found that sex-related variation was more significant then age-related variation.[9] They reported the ensemble averaged waveforms as a % bw (body weight) for 26 normal subjects. The vertical and anterior-posterior patterns were quite consistent across subjects while the medial-lateral shear force averages were somewhat variable.

A plot of the vertical and anterior-posterior forces from our adult subjects walking their natural cadence is presented in Figure 19-4. Because we normalize these forces to body mass we show bw on the vertical force plot at 9.8 N/kg. The peaks of these forces change with cadence. The anterior-posterior shear force has a characteristic negative phase followed by positive phase. As this waveform represents the net acceleration of the total body mass in the plane of progression we would interpret that for the first half of stance the body was decelerating and for the latter half it was accelerating. If the subject walks at a "constant" velocity the negative area will equal the positive area. However, because no subject's gait is perfectly symmetrical we would look at separate records from both feet and integrate the area under both shear force curves. The vertical force has the characteristic double hump, and we interpret that curve relative to the body weight line. If this exceeds bw then the total body mass is accelerating upwards; when it is less than bw it is accelerating downwards. Again, over the stride period the area above bw should be equal to the area below (if the subject maintains the same height above ground). Such a situation will only be evident if we simultaneously record the forces under both feet, either with separate force plates or one big force platform.

The vertical and horizontal forces change with cadence. The maximum and minimum peaks increase with cadence. In Figure 19-4 the horizontal force had peaks of ± 2 N/kg for this natural cadence group (105 steps/min). The maximum and minimum vertical forces were 10.7 and 7.0 N/kg. For slow walkers (cadence ≈ 85 steps/min) the horizontal force peaks decreased to ± 1.5 N/kg, and for fast walkers the peaks increased to ± 2.5 N/kg. The vertical force maximum and minimum were 9.9 and 8.5 N/kg for the slow walkers and 12.5 and 5.5 N/kg for the fast walkers. These vertical force changes agree with the maximums and minimums reported by Andriacchi et al.[1] However, our horizontal force changes agree with Chao et al.[9] but do not agree completely with Andriacchi, et al.[1]; the positive peaks agreed but their negative peaks did not. Their data showed the negative peak to be at least twice the amplitude of their positive peak, which does not make sense for steady-state walking.

Joint Reaction and Bone-on-Bone Forces

In our inverse dynamic analyses we calculate the reaction forces at each joint starting at the ankle and continuing up to the hip. These reaction forces

Figure 19-4 Averaged intersubject horizontal and vertical ground reaction forces for 19 adult subjects walking their natural cadence. Forces here have been normalized by dividing by body mass prior to averaging, body weight (bw) is drawn at 9.81 N/kg. Published with permission: Winter, DA: *The biomechanics and motor control of human gait: normal, elderly and pathological.* 2d ed., Waterloo, Ont, University of Waterloo Press, 1991.

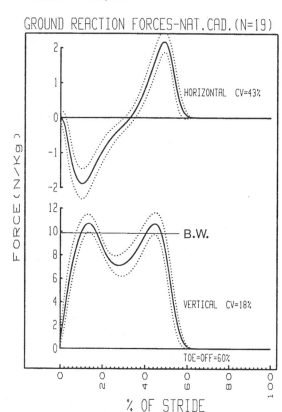

are not bone-in-bone forces because they do not reflect the compressive and shear forces due to our muscles and ligaments. Paul was first to make estimates of these contact forces.[16] The technique required the decomposition of the muscle moments into the individual muscle contributions followed by an estimation of the muscle force vector. The hip contact forces on one subject were estimated to reach peaks of four times body weight while the knee contact forces reached peaks of three times body weight.[17] Similar modelling yielded the ankle compressive and shear forces in normal and diseased ankles.[26] Direct measures of contact forces are not possible in normal circumstances; however, in the case of hip replacement surgery-suitable instrumentation can be installed in the prosthesis to record hip joint pressures.[27]

In normal walking the forces are small compared to running; it is at the more intensive level that we develop chronic injuries. The forces at the ankle and knee were estimated in five different running trials.[25] The ankle bone-on-bone compressive forces were estimated to range from 10 to 14 times body weight with minimal contribution ($\approx$ 2.3 bw) from the reaction force itself. The shear forces due to the muscles were in the opposite direction of the reaction forces; the net reduction was described as an antishear mechanism that prevents potential dislocation of the joint. Patellofemoral compressive forces were also estimated to be almost four times body weight while the knee joint reaction compressive forces were almost identical to that recorded at the ankle. One other variable calculated was the bending moment at the site along the tibia where stress fractures most often occur (about one third of the distance from the ankle to the knee). Ground reaction forces were responsible for about 180 Nm bending moment while the plantarflexor muscles (primarily soleus) countered with about 100 Nm in the opposite direction, reducing the net bending moment to about 80 Nm The estimation of these peak forces and moments relates closely to the sites of the more important chronic running injuries (Achilles tendonitis, chondramalacia, plantar fasciitis, stress fractures) and reveals that the cause of these injuries is dominated by the internal muscle forces, which peak during mid and late stance (and not at heel strike as inferred by many). However, the forces responsible for stress fractures are actually reduced by the internal muscle forces.

Normalization of Moment Patterns

Individual trials can be reported as the moment (Nm) versus time (sec) or versus stride period (%). When we compare intra- and intersubject patterns, the time bases are all slightly different. Thus, it makes sense to use the same time base and set the stride period to 100%. Even when we analyze walking at different cadences, necessary comparisons can be made only if the stride period is set to 100%.

The ordinate of our time-related pattern must also be normalized for intersubject comparisons especially when their masses vary drastically. Paul noted some years ago that the kinetic measures were linearly related to body weight.[18] Thus when intersubject ensemble averages are divided by body mass the intersubject variability is reduced. We therefore report moment patterns as Nm/kg and power patterns as W/kg. Current clinical assessments, which require comparisons of patients with normal subjects, routinely normalize their moment and power profiles by dividing by body mass or body weight.[20]

Convention for Plane-of-Progression Moments

Biomechanical convention sets a moment—which is clockwise as calculated—at the distal end of a segment to be positive. Then for the right limb of a subject walking to the right an ankle dorsiflex moment is positive. A knee extensor and hip flexor moment is also positive. Such convention appears to have been employed by a variety of researchers.[3,16,19] However, the left limb moments would have the opposite polarity. Thus we adopt a convention that reports all extensor moments as positive and all flexor moments as negative. This makes intuitive sense, especially during stance, because extensor moments at the ankle, knee, and hip will attempt to accelerate the body upwards in a positive direction. Similarly, negative (flexor) moments will attempt to collapse the body in a negative direction. A number of clinical gait laboratories involved in routine analysis of gait have adopted this convention.[24] However, until a universal convention is accepted it is critical that all moments are labelled flexor/extensor, dorsiflexor/plantarflexor, etc.

In the frontal plane all abductor (eversion) moments are positive and adductor (inversion) moments are negative. In the transverse plane external rotation moments are labelled positive and internal rotation moments negative. Again, these polarities are not universally adopted. However, several international societies and national organizations are currently discussing terminology and conventions used in gait.

Support Moment: Calculation and Interpretation

As a result of the analysis of scores of subjects and patients we have observed one basic pattern from the total lower limb during stance. In spite of large variations evident at individual joints, a net extensor (positive) pattern emerges during stance. We have called the algebraic summation $M_s = M_a + M_k + M_h$, the support moment, with all extensor moments reported as positive.[31] We have subsequently documented the reason why this pattern is so consistent.[32]

The reason for the consistency in the M_s profile goes as follows. The ankle plantarflexor pattern is quite large and has low variability. However, at the hip and knee, the variability is considerable and highly correlated. For example, in a given stride the knee extensors may be dominant in preventing collapse of the limb during weight bearing and will therefore contribute strongly to the support moment pattern. In a subsequent stride the same subject will downgrade his quadriceps activity and control the knee from the hip extensors (hamstrings + gluteus maximus). The decrease in knee extensor activity is replaced by a hip extensor increase such that the support moment remains about the same. The reason for the high variability at the hip and knee relates to the stride-to-stride control of balance of the H.A.T. In one stride the CNS senses that the H.A.T. is accelerating too fast anteriorly or is leaning forward too far; the regulating response is to increase activity of the posterior muscles at the hip and knee. In a subsequent stride the reverse may be true and the regulating response is to increase the activity of the anterior muscles at the hip and knee. This dynamic balance results in high variability in the hip and knee due to the anterior-posterior challenge.[33] Figure 19-5 contains the profiles taken from a study of nine repeat analyses of the same subject over a number of days. Knee and hip moment profiles are highly variable, as indicated by their coefficient of variation (CV) scores. The ankle patterns have a low CV of 24%. The support moment profile is almost as low (26%) in spite of the highly variable hip and knee moments included in the summation. In effect, what we have documented is a flexible stride-to-stride synergy between the hip and knee—a trade-off that is almost one-for-one during stance.[32]

SUMMARY OF MOMENTS AT THE ANKLE, HIP, AND KNEE

Figure 19-6 represents the moment of force profiles for 30 subjects walking their natural cadence (mean = 105.3 steps/min). These intersubject ensemble averages show almost double the variability at all three joints compared with the intrasubject profiles; this variability was reduced through normalization by dividing by body mass.

Functionally, each muscle group has a specific role. At the ankle from 0 to 5% a small dorsiflexor moment helps to achieve a controlled lowering of the foot to the ground. Then the plantarflexors dominate and increase almost as a ramp between 5% and about 50%. During most of this period (5 to 40%), they act eccentrically to control the forward rotation of the leg over the foot. Then from 40 to 60% they act eccentrically to cause rapid ankle plantarflexion and a forceful push off.

FIGURE 19-5   Ensemble average of joint moments of nine repeat walking trials across days for the same subject. Time base is normalized to 100% with toe off at 60%. See discussion regarding the support moment and the interpretation of variability. Published with permission: Winter, DA: *The biomechanics and motor control of human gait: normal, elderly and pathological.* 2d ed., Waterloo, Ont, University of Waterloo Press, 1991.

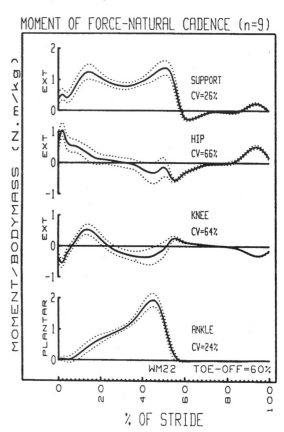

Immediately after toe off a miniscule dorsiflexor moment achieves rapid dorsiflexion to assist in toe clearance during mid-swing.

At the knee immediately after heel contact (HC) we see a momentary small flexor moment, which is a byproduct of the hamstrings that are involved in a strong hip extensor moment. From 5 to 25% the knee extensors dominate to control knee flexion during weight acceptance and, once reversed, to cause knee extension. During midstance and into the push off period (25 to 50%) a low knee flexor moment appears. This pattern is due to the increasing activity of the gastrocnemii. Such activity may be partially responsible for the knee beginning to collapse around 40% of the gait cycle. Then at about 50% the knee extensor be-

FIGURE 19-6 Ensemble average of moment-of-force patterns of 30 subjects walking their natural cadence. Moments are normalized by dividing body mass in order to reduce intersubject variability, which is still high, especially at the hip and knee.

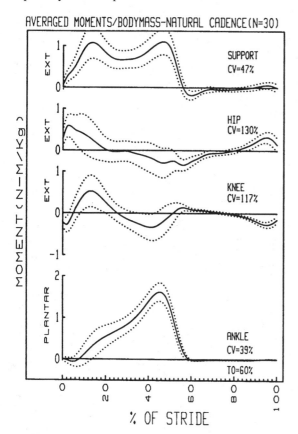

comes active to exert control of knee flexion during the period of rapid upward thrust from the ankle (push off). Then after toe off (TO) a small extensor activity continues to arrest the backward swinging leg and foot. Knee flexion reaches its maximum at about 70% where rapid extension begins and is controlled by the knee flexors (hamstrings), which decelerate the leg and foot prior to the next HC.

At the hip a strong extensor pattern develops at HC for two reasons. First, the hip extensors arrest the forward acceleration of H.A.T., which results from the sudden posterior hip reaction force that begins at HC and lasts for the first half of stance. Second, the hip extensors aid the knee extensors in controlling the collapse of the thigh and assist in controlling the total knee collapse ($\approx$ 20 degrees). Then at 20% of stride the pattern reverses to hip flexion; until about 50% these flexors act eccentrically to reverse the backward rotating thigh. From

50 to 70% of stride these same flexors act eccentrically to cause a pull off of the lower limb and add energy to the entire lower limb. Then at the end of swing a concentric contraction of the hip extensors occur as the thigh is accelerated backwards prior to HC.

The support moment pattern is seen to be positive from HC to about 55% of the stride indicating a net extensor pattern from all three joints of the lower limb. Then just prior to TO there is a small net flexor pattern characteristic of the limb unloading. The characteristic shape of the support moment profile is a double hump pattern similar to the vertical ground reaction force. This is not surprising when we realize that the support moment represents the net extensor push away from the ground, and the ground reaction force merely reflects that net push.

A comparison of these intersubject averages with other such averages is not possible because very few studies reported more than a few subjects and most of them report single subjects.[3,16,19] Also, many studies report only stance phase kinetics[2,19] while others report swing phase only.[2,8,13,19] However, if one were to compare the individual curves from these reports with the intersubject averages reported for 30 subjects in Figure 19-6 all the curves have the same general shape and most fall within the one standard deviation limit. Some individual profiles lie slightly outside the $\pm$ 1 s.d. bands but this should be expected for about one third of the normal subjects.

Changes of Moment Profiles with Cadence

Figures 19-7, 19-8, and 19-9 present a comparison of the mean moments at the ankle, knee, and hip respectively for three cadence groups: natural, fast, and slow. The slow-walking group had a mean cadence of 86.8 steps/min and the fast a cadence of 123.1 steps/min.

The ankle moment patterns (Figure 19-7) are particularly interesting in the way they change from early and mid-stance (5 to 40%) compared to pushoff (40 to 60%). During the eccentric phase as the leg rotates over the foot, the lowest moment was seen in the fast walkers, the largest moment in the slow walkers. The reverse was seen during push off. Such a reversal is strong evidence of a muscle synergy: in order to walk faster we use the "brakes" less and the "accelerators" more. Conversely, in order to maintain a slower cadence we increase the braking action and decrease the generator activity. The crossover of all three curves is seen to be at 40% of stride, which is precisely the transition from energy absorption to energy generation.

Figure 19-7 Averaged intersubject ankle moment-of-force patterns for three difference cadences. During eccentric phase (6 to 40%) the slow walkers have highest moment while fast walkers have the lowest moment. During concentric phase (push off) the reverse is seen.

Figure 19-8 Averaged intersubject knee moment-of-force patterns for three different cadences. Patterns are essentially the same with the largest amplitude being the fast walkers and lowest amplitude the slow walkers.

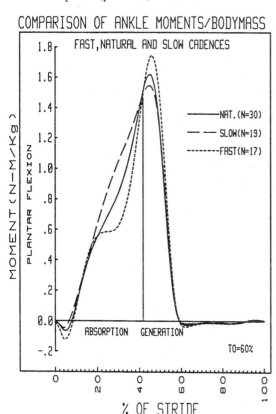

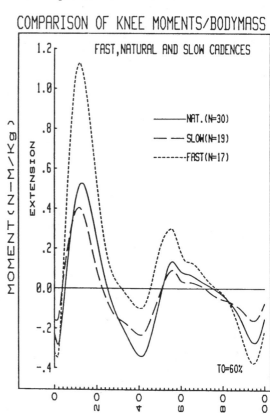

The knee moment patterns (Figure 19-8) show that the motor patterns remain essentially the same at all cadences, except "gain," which increases with cadence. In a similar manner the hip moment patterns (Figure 19-9) are also very similar in shape but show minor timing differences, especially for the fast cadence group. The initial hip extensor moment at slow and natural cadences lasts for 20% of the stride whereas the fast group had a short sharp extensor pattern lasting only 10% of the stride. Thus the hip flexor pattern in this fast cadence group began earlier and with double the amplitude of the natural cadence group, presumably to decelerate the faster rotating thigh and accelerate it more vigorously at pulloff.

Relationship of Muscle Motor Patterns with Joint Moment Patterns

The joint moment we estimate from an inverse dynamics analysis is a net moment, meaning it is

the algebraic sum of all muscle moments acting at that joint. If there is a cocontraction it is the sum of all agonist and antagonist muscle contributions. In fact, the polarity of the moment profile is what defines which muscles are agonists and which are antagonists: agonists are the same "polarity" as the moment, antagonists have the reverse polarity. Each time the moment profile crosses zero then the agonist muscles change.

The ankle patterns are not presented because the interpretation is quite simple. After heel contact and until flat foot, the tibialis anterior dominates over a small plantarflexor moment (as seen in a very small but increasing activation of the soleus and gastrocnemius muscles). Then at flat foot, plantarflexor activity rises as tibialis anterior decreases toward zero. For the balance of stance the plantarflexors are totally dominant culminating in the peak activity of the plantarflexor EMGs coinciding with the peak in the plantarflexor moment.

FIGURE 19-9 Averaged intersubject hip moment-of-force patterns for three cadence groups. Amplitude increases with cadence with a shortening of the initial extensor phase and lengthening of the flexor phase for the fast walkers.

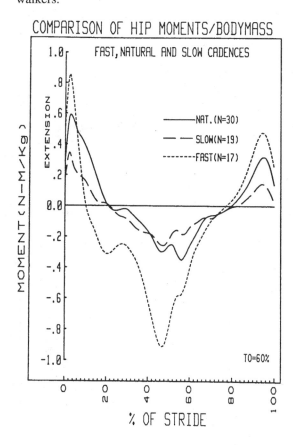

FIGURE 19-10 Ensemble-averaged knee moment plus ensemble-averaged EMG profiles of five major muscles responsible for the knee moment. See text for discussion of their contribution to the five different phases in the moment profile.

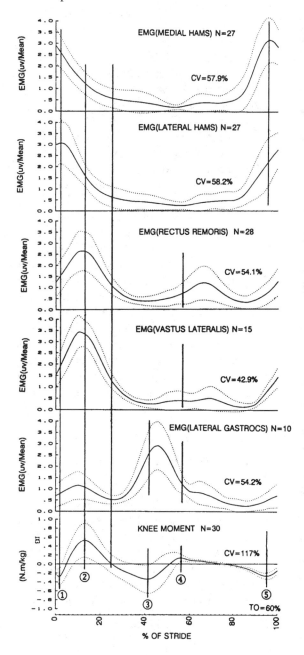

At the knee there are three major muscle groups that have the potential to create a significant moment. The four quadriceps muscles contribute to extension while hamstrings and gastrocnemius muscles oppose as flexors. With reference to Figure 19-10 we identify each phase in the moment curve by numbers ①, ②, etc. Just after heel contact a small short knee flexor moment occurs ①. At this time the hamstrings are active; the quadriceps are also active but increasing. Then after 5% of the gait cycle the quadriceps become dominant and are the agonists to produce a net extensor moment ② as the hamstrings decrease their activity. Note the peak of quadriceps activity (rectus femoris + vastus lateralis) virtually coincides with the peak of the knee extensor moment. This phasic agreement is largely due to the processing of the EMG as a linear envelope and the judicial choice of the low-pass filter (3 Hz, critically damped, second order) to closely match the twitch response of the

muscles.[35] During mid-stance the knee moment becomes flexor ③ primarily due to the simultaneous rise in gastrocnemii activity and fall in quadriceps activity. Again, there was close agreement (within 2% of gait cycle) between the peak flexor moment and peak activity of the lateral gastrocnemius. Then at the start of double support and continuing until mid-swing the knee moment becomes slightly extensor ④, which results from a sharp drop in gastrocnemii activity and a small increase in quadriceps activity (especially rectus femoris). Finally, during late swing the knee moment is flexor ⑤ primarily due to rising activity of the medial and lateral hamstrings. The peak moment coincides fairly well with that of the medial hamstrings.

At the hip in Figure 19-11 we see the hip moment plotted along with four major muscles responsible for that net motor pattern. One major muscle missing from these records is the iliopsoas; this major deep hip flexor cannot be recorded using surface electrodes. To date, only an isolated single-stride record of raw EMG taken with indwelling needle electrodes from one subject is the only data available on this flexor. The first hip moment phase is extensor ①, which is the weighted contribution of three hip extensors recorded here: gluteus maximus, medial and lateral hamstrings. Then during mid-stance, push off, and early swing, the hip pattern becomes flexor. Some of this flexor contribution comes from the rectus femoris; however, by the process of elimination we must attribute most of it to the iliopsoas. Then during the latter half of swing we identify a hip extensor pattern with the same phasic shape and timing as the knee flexor pattern already discussed in Figure 19-10. Obviously, the biarticulate hamstrings are a contributor along with a minor contribution of the gluteus maximus.

THREE-DIMENSIONAL ANALYSES: ANGLES AND MOMENTS

As indicated earlier in this chapter special considerations must be made when reporting and interpreting the three-dimensional variables that are now becoming available. We have made the argument that, in gait studies, we should report all kinetic variables in the global reference system (GRS) rather than the local axis system (LAS) of each segment.

Preliminary results from our laboratory are reported here from natural walking trials of five subject strides. The 3-D joint moment and angle profiles were initially averaged to produce five intrasubject averages. These averages were then ensemble averaged to yield intersubject averages. Both right and left limbs were analysed and were found to be symmetrical within each of the five subjects; thus only one limb (the right) is reported here.

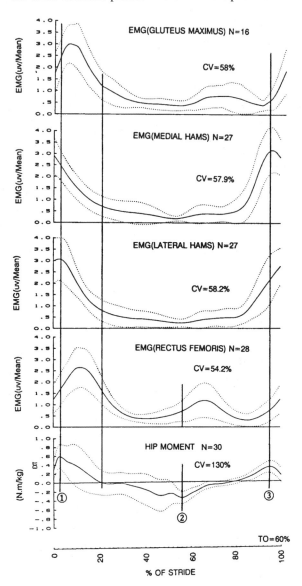

FIGURE 19-11 Ensemble-averaged hip moment plus ensemble-averaged EMG profiles of four major muscles responsible for the hip moment. See text for discussion of their contribution to the three different phases in the moment profile.

Hip Profiles

The 3-D hip profiles are presented in Figure 19-12; the discussion focuses on the patterns in the frontal and transverse planes because the previous sections have already interpreted the plane-of-progression moments (labelled here as sagittal plane).

A small angular change in the frontal plane occurs over the gait cycle. Immediately after heel contact there is a small (7 degrees) but rapid adduction mainly due to the drop of the pelvis as

FIGURE 19-12   Intersubject profiles of 3-D hip angles and moments for five adult subjects walking their natural cadence. Five repeat trials on each subject were averaged to reduce intrasubject variability, then the intersubject ensemble averages were calculated. Solid line indicates the average, and dotted line (plotted on one side of average only) is the standard deviation.

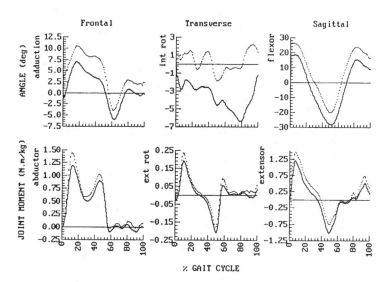

INTERSUBJECT HIP ANGLE AND MOMENTS (N=5, n=25)

one limb loads and the other limb unloads. Then during single support (10 to 50%) the adduction is reduced. During push off the hip rapidly abducts to about 6 degrees as swing begins. After toe off this small abduction reduces to a neutral position by mid-swing and maintains that angle until heel contact. The muscle moments responsible for this control are dominantly abductor and result from the need to control the large mass of HAT during stance against gravitational and balance demands.[14] The initial abductor burst peaks at 10% of the cycle when the limb is fully loaded and controls the drop of the pelvis to about 7 degrees. Then during the balance of single support the abductors return the pelvis to the horizontal position. During push off as the limb unloads, the pelvis drops in the opposite direction, and the abductors cause the thigh to abduct slightly in preparation for swing. A minor adductor burst at toe off results in a return of the hip to a neutral position by mid-swing.

In the transverse plane the hip angular changes are even smaller and are somewhat variable across these five subjects; most of the variability is due to small bias differences between the subjects—each subject walks with slightly different external rotation, which is evident in how they place their feet on the ground during stance. The subjects averaged about 5 degrees external rotation, which

increased slightly (2 to 6 degrees) during stance and an additional 2 degrees into mid-swing, then rapidly back toward the neutral position by heel contact. The moment patterns are much more consistent across these five subjects. These patterns are characterized by an initial external rotator pattern during the first half of stance followed by an almost equal internal rotator pattern. During all of stance the pelvis rotates forward around the stance limb; this initial external rotator burst serves to slow down the rotation, the second internal rotator burst serves to reaccelerate the pelvis (and HAT).

Knee Profiles

The 3-D knee profiles are presented in Figure 19-13. In the frontal plane the knee angle remains in the neutral position during most of stance. As the knee unloads prior to toe off, the knee abducts reaching a maximum of about 8 degrees during mid-swing. This abduction change is part of the general abductor pattern seen at the hip during swing. The knee moments during stance are essentially passive due to the internal anatomical structure and ligaments. The knee has a similar but smaller abductor moment compared to the hip reflecting the gravitational load of HAT located medial of the joint center. Mechanically such an internal moment reflects an increased loading of the medial

Figure 19-13 Intersubject profiles of 3-D knee angles and moments for the subjects described in Figure 19-12.

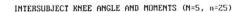
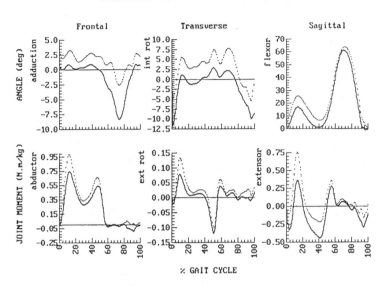

condyles and a similar unloading of the lateral condyles plus some possible tension in the lateral (fibular) collateral ligament. The abductor changes evident in swing appear to be passive as the pendular leg and foot swing outward and the leg "hangs" by the tendons and ligaments.

The transverse angular changes at the knee show the knee to be neutral for most of stance (10 to 60%) and into swing. At the end of swing the knee joint is externally rotated about 10 degrees. Immediately after HC the thigh rotates forward on the leg indicating a sliding action on the medial condyles as the limb bears weight (0 to 10%). Such an internal rotation is part of the forward rotation of the pelvis during the stance phase. The transverse knee moments are passive and are a reaction to the active hip moments—a reduced knee external moment for the first half of stance followed by a reduced internal moment during the latter half of stance. Internal structures such as the anterior and posterior cruciate and transverse ligaments act to create the small passive moments to constrain these transverse rotations.

Ankle Profiles

The ankle profiles are presented in Figure 19-14. At heel contact the ankle is inverted about 5 degrees. As it loads on the lateral border it rapidly everts almost 10 degrees and maintains about 5 degrees eversion until push off. Then during push off the foot rapidly inverts reaching about 10 degrees at toe off. The motor patterns associated with these rota-

tions are both small and variable. During weight acceptance they are evertor followed by invertor during mid-stance, then evertor during push off. The role of these muscles has been shown to be of minimal importance in the medial-lateral balance of the body during stance; at best the patterns on any given stance period represent a fine tuning of the medial-lateral acceleration of the body.

In the transverse plane the ankle will suddenly perform an external rotation during weight acceptance (0 to 15%) equal and opposite to the internal rotation of the leg segment, which presumably allows the leg to rotate forward in the plane of progression over the foot that is now flat on the ground. During swing the major dominant angular change in an external rotation at the knee simultaneous with an almost equal internal rotation of the thigh segment prior to heel contact. The moment patterns at the hip are characteristically external during the first half of stance followed by internal rotation during the latter half. Given that the pelvis is rotating forward over the stance thigh during this time, the moment pattern represents an eccentric contraction by the external rotators during 0 to 30% followed by a concentric contraction by the internal rotators during the latter half of stance. The knee moment is passive and is a reaction to the hip moment; it has the same shape but half the amplitude. The ankle motor pattern is a small but consistent external rotation increasing to a peak at push off, which results from active plantarflexors.

FIGURE 19-14.   Intersubject profiles of 3-D ankle angles and moments for the subjects described in Figure 19-12.

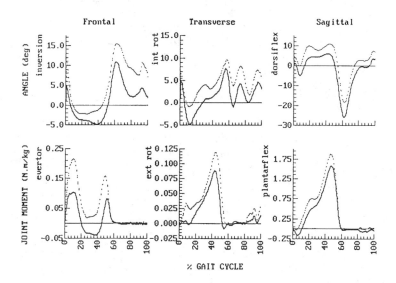

MECHANICAL ENERGY, POWER, AND WORK

Energetics of Walking

Considerable research has been reported on the energetics of walking and running. Unfortunately, much of the research has not properly recognized the laws of mechanics or has ignored certain energy saving phenomena that occur during various phases of the gait cycle. For example, Fenn in a study of runners ignored the potential and kinetic energy exchanges within each segment he analyzed, resulting in a much exaggerated assessment of internal work.[12] Likewise, Cavagna and co-workers introduced a series of papers focused on the potential and kinetic energies of the body's center of mass.[5-7] In doing so, they were looking at the *vector* summation of the mass-acceleration products of all segments and failed to realize that energies are *scalars*. Thus, movements of legs and arms in opposite directions would tend to cancel in spite of the fact that energy was required to accelerate and decelerate those limbs. Thus, all their analyses result in erroneously low values of internal work, giving results that cannot be traced to the source or sink of the energy. A major improvement was made by Ralston and Lukin, Winter et al., and Cappozzo et al. when they analysed the mechanical energy segment by segment.[4,22,28] They all concluded that the energy conservation of H.A.T. during walking was high and that the lower limbs dominated the work required. A comparison between this segment-by-

segment approach with the center-of-gravity approach confirmed predicted errors of the center-of-mass technique.[30]

The segment-by-segment approach still has some potential errors in it for the calculation of internal work and does not identify the source and sink of the energy. Only through a mechanical power analysis can we determine which muscle groups are generating energy and which are absorbing.

Mechanical Power

If pressed to give the most important role of muscles during any movement, one would have to consider the function of muscles as they shorten and lengthen under tension. During these concentric and eccentric phases muscles generate and absorb the mechanical energy necessary to accomplish the movement that we observe. Mechanical power is the single variable that summarizes the role of muscles, and it is the product of the joint moment of force and joint angular velocity.

$$P_j = M_j \cdot \omega_j \; watts \qquad (1)$$

where M_j is the joint moment of force (Nm) and ω_j is the joint velocity (r/s).

The convention of M_j and ω_j is such that P_j is positive if M_j and ω_j have the same polarity (i.e., a concentric contraction). Conversely, when M_j and ω_j have opposite polarities—an eccentric contraction—then P_j is negative. The assumption inherent in Equation 1 is that the torque generator at each joint is independent of what is happening at adjacent joints. However, it is possible with close scrutiny to see the influence of biarticulate muscles acting cross adjacent joints. For example, during a given phase of the gait cycle, we may note generation of energy at one joint and absorption at an adjacent joint. If the moment of force patterns at that time appear to be related to activity of biarticulate muscles, then those muscles have probably generated energy at one end and absorbed energy at the other end. In fact, they may be contracting in a near-isometric fashion and are merely transferring energy between the segments attached to the origin and insertion.

Intersubject Averages of Mechanical Power

Figure 19-15 reports the mechanical power profiles of the natural cadence subjects whose moment profiles were plotted in Figure 19-6. The labels, A1, A2, etc., identify the major consistent power patterns. The variability of the power curves is higher than the moment curves from which they were derived. This increased variability is due to the fact that power is a product of two variables, moments and angular velocities, and therefore reflects the variability of both.

The ankle has two major power phases. A1 is the power absorption by the plantarflexors as the leg rotates over the foot, while A2 is the most important push off power burst. A2 represents about two thirds of the new energy generated during the walking cycle. At the knee K1 is the power absorption by the eccentrically contracting quadriceps during weight acceptance. K2 is a small amplitude power phase resulting from the knee extensors shortening to reduce knee flexion during mid-stance. When the knee starts to flex rapidly as the leg unloads, the quadriceps absorb energy (K3) to control the speed of collapse. K3 continues into early swing to record the energy lost in decelerating the backward rotating leg. Finally, K4 quantifies the energy absorbed by the hamstrings late in swing as they decelerate the forward swinging leg and foot. At the hip considerable variability is associated with H1 generation phase by the hip extensors. Most of this variability results from high variability in the hip moment (Figure 19-6). H2 power phase comes from the hip flexors as they absorb energy in decelerating the backward rotating thigh. The H3 burst is the second most important energy generation phase beginning at the start of double support (50%) as the hip flexors achieve a pull off, which lasts into mid-swing.

FIGURE 19-15 Ensemble-averaged power patterns at the ankle, knee, and hip for 19 subjects walking their natural cadence. See text for function of each power phase, A1, A2, etc. Published with permission: Winter, DA: *The biomechanics and motor control of human gait: normal, elderly and pathological.* 2d ed., Waterloo, Ont, University of Waterloo Press, 1991.

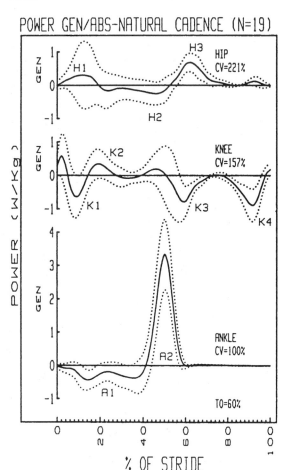

Transfers of Energy Within and Between Segments

Because gait involves a large number of segments whose trajectories must be simultaneously controlled by the CNS, how energy can be transferred between adjacent segments to contribute to the total body movement is an important concept. This transfer of energy relates to what is generally called *interlimb coupling*. During the gait cycle this mechanism is continuously used to advantage not only for improved efficiency but also as a means to compensate for lost function.[23, 34]

Elftman in his classic studies of human locomotion presented methods for calculating the rate of change of energy of the legs, the "rate of transfer due to joint forces," and the "rate at which the muscles do work on, or receive energy from each part of the leg."[10, 11] Unfortunately, the mathematical equations supporting his concepts were not clearly stated. It was not until 1975 that Quanbury et al. formalized the idea of a power balance within each segment and the mechanism of an active transfer of energy between segments via the muscles.[10]

The rate of work done (power) by the joint reaction forces can be calculated from

$$P_j(j,s) = F(j,s) \cdot V(j) \tag{2}$$

where $P_j(j,s)$ is the joint power done at joint j on segment s (watts); $F(j,s)$ is the joint reaction force acting at joint j on segment s (Newtons); and $V(j)$ is the absolute velocity of joint j (m/s).

This dot product is a scaler, which is positive or negative depending on the directions of the force and velocity vectors. For a given segment it will be positive, meaning energy flows into that segment at that joint. Because the reaction force for the adjacent segment is 180 degrees out of phase, the product for this adjacent segment will be negative but will have the same magnitude, which occurs because the rate of energy transfer between adjacent segments must be equal and opposite.

Segments can also receive mechanical energy from work done on them by attached muscles at both proximal and distal ends. If we assume that the joint reaction moments are caused by muscles

---

TABLE 19-1   Power generation, absorption and transfer functions

Description of movement	Type of contraction	Directions of segmental ang. velocities	Muscle function	Amount, type, and direction of power
Both segments rotating in opposite directions (a) joint angle decreasing	Concentric	ω_1, M, ω_2	Mechanical energy generation	$M\omega_1$ generated to segment 1; $M\omega_2$ generated to segment 2
(b) joint angle increasing	Eccentric	ω_1, M, ω_2	Mechanical energy absorption	$M\omega_1$ absorbed from segment 1; $M\omega_2$ absorbed from segment 2
Both segments rotating in same direction (a) joint angle decreasing (e.g., $\omega_1 > \omega_2$)	Concentric	ω_1, M, ω_2	Mechanical energy generation and transfer	$M(\omega_1 - \omega_2)$ generated to segment 1; $M\omega_2$ transferred to segment 1 from 2
(b) joint angle increasing (e.g., $\omega_2 > \omega_1$)	Eccentric	ω_1, M, ω_2	Mechanical energy absorption and transfer	$M(\omega_2 - \omega_1)$ absorbed from segment 2; $M\omega_1$ transferred to segment 1 from 2
(c) joint angle constant ($\omega_1 = \omega_2$)	Isometric (dynamic)	ω_1, M, ω_2	Mechanical energy transfer	$M\omega_2$ transferred from segment 2 to 1
One segment fixed (e.g., segment 1) (a) joint angle decreasing ($\omega_1 = O, \omega_2 > O$)	Concentric	M, ω_2	Mechanical energy generation	$M\omega_2$ generated to segment 2
(b) joint angle increasing ($\omega_1 = O, \omega_2 > O$)	Eccentric	M, ω_2	Mechanical energy absorption	$M\omega_2$ absorbed from segment 2
(c) joint angle constant ($\omega_1 = \omega_2 = O$)	Isometric (steitic)	M	No mechanical energy function	Zero

Source: Robertson DGE, Winter DA: Mechanical energy generation, absorption and transfer among segments during walking. *J Biomech*, 13:845–854, 1980. Reproduced with permission of *Journal of Biomechanics*.

alone, this work or power term must be considered active and with a metabolic cost. The muscle power at joint j acting on segment s is calculated from

$$P_m(j,s) = M(j,s) \cdot \omega(s) \qquad (3)$$

where $M(j,s)$ is the muscle moment at joint j acting on segment s (Nm), and $\omega(s)$ is the angular velocity of segment s (r/s).

Again, if $P_m(j,s)$ is positive, the muscle is doing mechanical work on the segment, while a negative rate shows the rate of mechanical work done by the segment on the muscle. Contrary to the situation for joint powers, the two segments connected at j do not necessarily have the same angular velocity. If the angular velocity is exactly the same there is a transfer of energy between adjacent segments. However, if the angular velocities differ, then the muscles can also generate or absorb as they contract concentrically or eccentrically.

Table 19-1 shows all the possible combinations of work functions that can occur between adjacent segments connected by active muscles that generate a net moment. The inherent assumption is that equivalent single joint muscles act at each joint

with a net effect at the joint quantified by $M(j,s)$, which we calculate from our inverse dynamics.

Figure 19-16 is a schematic diagram showing the net powers at all three joints of the lower limb over representative points of the gait cycle.[29] The straight arrows across the joint centers are the passive joint powers (Equation 2) while the curved arrows show the active muscle powers (Equation 3). The moment that generated these powers is indicated by the location of the arrows, either anterior or posterior of the joint. If two muscle powers are in the same direction, a power transfer occurs between segments; the smaller of the two values is the transfer component while the difference is either generation or absorption (indicated by the arrow direction). For example, at toe off at the hip there is a transfer of 5W from the pelvis to the thigh simultaneous to a 42W generation by the hip flexors.

Theoretically, according to the law of conservation of energy there should be a perfect power balance within each segment: the algebraic sum of all powers entering and leaving the segment should equal the rate of change of energy of that segment. For example, at toe off the sum of powers

---

FIGURE 19-16   Six phases of the walking cycle showing the passive and active flows of energy (W) across joints and muscles along with the active generation and absorption by the muscles. The rate of change of energy of each segment should equal the sum of all powers into and out of each segment. Published with permission: Winter, DA, Robertson, DGE: *Biol Cyber* 29:137, 1978.

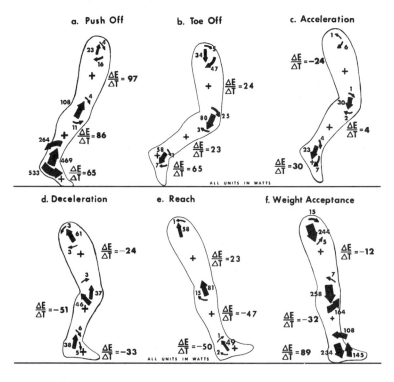

for the leg segment is $80 + 3 - 58 - 1 = 24W$. From our independent calculation of the rate of change of energy we calculate $\Delta E/\Delta t = 23W$. Any discrepancy in this balance is due to errors in any of the assumptions of our link segment model (i.e., that all segments are rigid with pin-joints at each end and with mass locations that are fixed).

The interpretation of Figure 19-6 allows us to determine the exact mechanism for the increase and decrease in energy of any segment. At push off the most important generation phase by the plantarflexors takes place. Here $533 - 264 = 269W$ are being generated at the ankle, which results in a major energy increase in the foot (65W), in the leg (86W), and in the thigh (97W). The major mechanism for that transfer to the leg and thigh is via passive transfers through the ankle and knee joints. Contrary to some claims, little energy is transferred to the upper body at this time. Virtually all the energy goes into accelerating the lower limb. At toe off and during early swing the dominant increase in foot and leg energy is passively via joint powers. The major source of this increase is a loss of energy in the thigh, some active generation by the hip flexors (47W at toe off), and some joint transfer from the pelvis. During late swing (deceleration and reach) the CNS again uses joint transfers to advantage. The reduction of energy of the swinging leg and foot is mainly removed passively, and much of it is conserved via a transfer across the hip to the upper body to increase the body's forward velocity. The only significant active absorption of energy at this time is via knee flexors (hamstrings), which absorbed at the rate of $46 - 3 = 43W$ during the deceleration phase.

The value of this type of analysis has not yet been exploited clinically. Power generation and absorption (Equation 1) is now being used by a number of clinical gait labs.[15,23,29] However, such analyses stop short of the full story, which involves major passive joint transfers and active muscle transfers.

SUMMARY

At the level of kinetic analyses and interpretation the apparently simple movement of level walking is extremely complex. Because of the large number of body segments, joints, and muscles acting in a three-dimensional space, interpretation of neuromuscular control requires a large number of integrated graphs. However, at the level of moments of force and mechanical powers sufficient neural integration has occurred to bring our task within reasonable bounds. The mode of presentation here

has been to focus initially on the plane of progression because the dominant neuromuscular patterns relate to that plane. The contribution of the individual muscles to these moment patterns can be seen from an overlay of suitably processed EMG profiles. The additional motor patterns in the other two planes are then added and show how these pattern elements contribute to forward progression or help maintain balance so that the body remains vertical in the plane of progression. Finally, the energetics (mechanical powers) of the muscles, joints, and segments demonstrate the tremendous interlimb coupling of which the CNS must be aware in order to maintain an efficient gait pattern.

REFERENCES

1. Andriacchi TP, Ogle JA, Galante JO: Walking speed as a basis for normal and abnormal gait measurements, *J Biomech* 10: 261, 1977.
2. Boccardi S, Pedotti A, Rodano R et al: Evaluation of muscular moments at the lower limb joints by an on-line processing of kinematic data and ground reaction, *J Biomech* 14: 35, 1981.
3. Cappozzo A: A general computing method for the analysis of human locomotion, *J Biomech* 8: 307, 1975.
4. Cappozzo A et al: The interplay of muscular and external forces in human ambulation, *J Biomech* 9: 35, 1976.
5. Cavagna, GA, Saibene FP, Margaria R: External work in walking, *J Appl Physiol* 18: 1, 1963.
6. Cavagna GA, Saibene FP, Margaria R: Mechanical work in running, *J Appl Physiol* 19: 249, 1964.
7. Cavagna GA, Kaneko M: Mechanical work and efficiency in level walking and running, *J Physiol* 268: 647, 1977.
8. Cavanagh PR, Gregor RJ: Knee joint torque during swing phase of normal treadmill walking, *J Biomech* 8: 337, 1975.
9. Chao EY, Laughman RK, Schneider E et al: Normative data of knee joint motion and ground reaction forces in adult level walking, *J Biomech* 16: 219, 1983.
10. Elftman H: Forces and energy changes in the leg during walking, *Am J Physiol* 125: 339, 1939.
11. Elftman H: The function of muscles in locomotion, *Am J Physiol* 125: 357, 1939.
12. Fenn WO: Frictional and kinetic factors in the work of sprint running, *Am J Physiol* 92: 583, 1929.
13. Judge G: Measurement of knee torque during swing phase of gait, *Eng Med* 4: 13, 1975.
14. MacKinnon C, Winter DA: Control of whole body balance in the frontal plane during human walking, *J Biomech* 26: 633, 1993.
15. Olney SJ et al: Work and power in gait of stroke patients, *Arch Phys Med Rehabil* 72: 309, 1991.
16. Paul JP: The biomechanics of the hip joint and its clinical relevance, *Proc Roy Soc Med* 59: 943, 1966.
17. Paul JP: Forces transmitted by joints in the human body, *Proc Instit Mech Eng* 181: 8, 1966.

18. Paul JP: The effect of walking speed on the force actions transmitted at the hip and knee joints, *Proc Roy Soc Med* 63: 200, 1970.

19. Pedotti A: A study of motor coordination and neuromuscular activities, *Biol Cybernet* 26: 53, 1977.

20. *Proceedings of the Eighth Annual East Coast Clinical Gait Laboratory Conference,* Mayo Clinic, Rochester, Minn, May 5–8, 1993.

21. Quanbury AO, Winter DA, Reimer GD: Instantaneous power and power flow in body segments during walking, *J Human Movement Studies* 1:59, 1975.

22. Ralston HJ, Lukin L: Energy levels of human body segments during level walking, *Ergonomics* 12: 39, 1969.

23. Robertson DGE, Winter DA: Mechanical energy generation, absorption and transfer among segments during walking, *J Biomech* 13: 845, 1980.

24. Rose SA, Ounpuu S, De Luca PA: Strategies for the assessment of pediatric gait in the clinical setting, *Phys Ther* 71: 961, 1991.

25. Scott SH, Winter DA: Internal forces at chronic running injury sites, *Med Sci Sports Exer* 22: 357, 1990.

26. Stauffer RN, Chao EYS, Brewster RC: Force and motion analysis of the normal, diseased and prosthetic ankle joint, *Clin Orthop Rel Res* 127: 189, 1977.

27. Strickland EM, Fares M, Krebs DE et al: In vivo acetabular contact pressures during rehabilitation. Part I: acute phase, *Phys Ther* 72: 691, 1992.

28. Winter DA, Quanbury AO, Reimer GD: Analysis of instantaneous energy of normal gait, *J Biomech* 9:253, 1976.

29. Winter DA, Robertson DGE: Joint torque and energy patterns in normal gait, *Biol Cybernet* 29: 137, 1978.

30. Winter DA: A new definition of mechanical work done in human movement, *J Appl Physiol* 46: 79, 1979.

31. Winter DA: Overall principle of lower limb support during stance phase of gait, *J Biomech* 13: 923, 1980.

32. Winter DA: Kinematic and kinetic patterns in human gait: variability and compensating effects, *Human Movement Sci* 3: 51, 1984.

33. Winter DA: Biomechanics of normal and pathological gait: implications for understanding human locomotor control, *J Motor Behav* 21: 337, 1989.

34. Winter DA: Foot trajectory in human gait: a precise and multifactorial motor control task, *Phys Ther* 72: 45, 1992.

35. Winter DA, Scott SH: Technique for interpretation of electromyography for concentric and eccentric contractions in gait, *J Electromyogr Kinesiol* 1: 263, 1991.

CHAPTER 20

EMG THEORY

Howard J. Hillstrom
Ronald J. Triolo

KEY TERMS

Action potential

Aliasing

Bode plot

Common mode rejection ratio

Cutoff frequency

Filtering

Frequency spectrum

Fundamental frequency

Motion artifact

Motor unit

Moving average

Nyquist frequency

Power Spectral density

Rectification

RMS

Signal to noise ratio

Stationary average

Transfer function

The Basics: What ,Who, Where, How, and Why

What is the EMG? The electromyogram (EMG) is the electrical manifestation of the contracting muscle.[1] It is not possible for a muscle to elicit a contraction without also producing the electrical signal known as the EMG. Because each contracting muscle generates its own EMG, studying these signals offers a unique opportunity to listen to the body's requests for functional movements.

Who would want to study the EMG? There are numerous professionals who are concerned with the functional status of the neuromuscular system. Many clinicians have the training and experience to deal quantitatively with the EMG. More often than not the signal is interpreted visually and qualitatively for its diagnostic and/or prognostic value. Individuals with research interests also study this signal to advance the clinical and/or scientific state-of-the-art through their research.

Where is the EMG measured? In the global sense the EMG is measured within a clinician's office, clinic, hospital, or human performance laboratory. Procedurally, the signal is measured either noninvasively with skin surface electrodes or invasively with wire or needle electrodes. The resulting EMG signals are very different for reasons to be discussed later in the chapter.

How is the EMG measured? Following the application of either surface or indwelling electrodes the signal is preamplified, amplified, and conditioned to yield a format that is most convenient for answering the clinical or scientific question of concern. Since a variety of different output formats are utilized, both clinically and scientifically, it is important to understand the rationale for the selection of a particular signal processing method for a given application.

Why is the EMG measured and studied? Numerous neuromuscular disorders present with aberrant EMG signals either on the examination table (i.e., the open kinetic chain) or while performing functional tasks such as posture and locomotion. A wide range of mild to severe myopathies, neuropathies, and central nervous system pathologies can be characterized through measurement and study of the EMG. Engineers may wish to derive volitional control of an artificial limb or electronic brace through interpretation of this signal. Scientists may wish to understand the mechanism by which humans maintain postural stability in the presence of various perturbations or descend stairs without *a priori* knowledge of the stair height. The precise control of the musculo-skeletal system for complex human movements such as gait is the subject of much current research.

There are a number of controversial issues that do not enjoy a unified position from the diverse group of electromyographers. Can the EMG signal be processed to yield quantitative information about muscle force or contraction level? How can one assess if a muscle is fatiguing? What are the optimum parameters of processing a myoelectric signal for a given signal processing method? What are the clinical correlates to an aberrant EMG signal? Will EMG-based, volitionally controlled prosthetic limbs become practical?

Many methods have been employed to extract a signal proportional to muscle force from the raw surface EMG. Most methods have been developed for isometric contractions at moderate force levels. However, all bets are off when examining contractions more like those employed in everyday activities (anisometric, anisotonic, and anisokinetic). Whether it is possible to obtain a signal proportional to muscle force under any circumstances is still a matter of debate. Most experts maintain that the EMG can be extremely useful to describe temporal events and to obtain timing information for various muscles.

It is impossible to measure anything perfectly in the real world. Wherever there's a signal, there's also noise or artifact that corrupts the measured quantity. The manner in which a myoelectric signal is processed depends upon the intended use of the information. The appropriate processing method is designed to yield a signal that contains a minimum amount of noise. What makes the field of electromyography so interesting is how the specific definitions of signal and noise can change pending the application.

To appreciate these controversial topics one must explore the origin of the electromyogram, how the signal is modeled, related engineering concepts, and how the signal is processed. Understanding several basic engineering concepts will help clarify the underlying physiology giving rise to the EMG signal. It will also provide a foundation for selecting appropriate processing techniques. The discussion will continue with an introduction to the fundamentals of electrical signals and signal processing.

Basic Engineering and Signal Processing Concepts

Fundamental Physical Principles

The fundamental terms are the essential words of the electromyographer's language and describe the relevant basic principles of physics, the foundation of electrical engineering.[14] The central concept is that of **current:** the flow or movement of charge. Charge is a fundamental property of matter that represents its electrical state and can be either positive or negative. In most solids, negative charge is represented by the electron. A material whose structure allows electrons to move freely is a good **conductor** of electricity. Materials in which the electrons are tightly bound and unable to flow or vibrate are poor conductors or **insulators.** A useful class of materials called semiconductors have special properties that put them somewhere in between.

In solutions, liquids, and some biological tissues, charges can be carried by ions. Negatively charged ions (anions) have a surplus of electrons and positive ions (cations) have too few electrons. In this instance, the movement of the charged particles themselves also represents an electrical current. More complicated molecules can be negative if they have excess negatively charged or too few positively charged elements. Charge is measured in units called **coulombs.** A single electron carries only a tiny amount of charge (approximately 1.6×10^{-19} coulombs). Current is defined as the rate of change (velocity or flow) of charge and is measured in units called **amperes.** The movement of 1 coulomb of charge in 1 second's time is defined as 1 ampere of current.

In electricity, as is often the case in life, opposites attract. That is, forces that act on oppositely charged particles tend to bring them together. Conversely, similar charges repel each other and forces act on them to drive them apart. It takes energy to separate opposite charges or to bring together similar charges. The situation is analogous to stretching an elastic band or compressing a spring; it takes the application of an external force to keep the rubber band in its elongated position or to keep the spring squeezed tight. The driving force to separate similar charges or bring together opposite charges is called **voltage.** One volt is the electromotive force required to separate one coulomb of positive charge from one coulomb of negative charge. Voltage is also referred to as **potential difference.** If dissimilar charges are kept apart and allowed to accumulate, the potential for current to flow between them will increase. The larger the difference in the potential between the two areas, the larger the driving force for current flow. As shown in Figure 20-1A, the accumulation of similar charges establishes the potential for current flow. If the leads of a voltmeter are held to each area, the potential difference

FIGURE 20-1 Current and Ohm's Law **A,** The distribution of charge accumulation known as potential difference drives the flow of current, **B,** Ohm's Law: $V = I \times R$, relates resistance, current, and voltage.

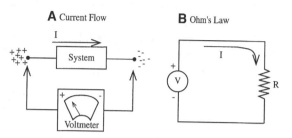

will be measured as a voltage. Only the *potential* for flow exists between the two regions because some conductive medium has to exist between them in order for the charges to relocate. It is one more example of how much nature abhors a vacuum.

As current flows through a system, biological or otherwise, it will generally encounter some resistance. The **resistance** of a material is a measure of how difficult it is for charges to flow in the form of an electric current. In a solid, resistance is a function of the type of material (its resistivity), its cross-sectional area, and its length. Materials with high resistivity are insulators and do not allow charge to move through them, while materials with low resistivity are generally good conductors. Electrical resistance increases with the length of an object and decreases as its cross-sectional area grows. This is analogous to the resistance offered by a pipe to the flow of water. It's more difficult to pass water through a long, narrow pipe than a short wide one. It would therefore take more force (or pressure) to drive the same amount of water through the high resistance pipe. This same relationship holds true for electricity. As shown in figure 20-1B, resistance *(R)*, voltage *(V)*, and current *(I)* are all related to each other by **Ohm's Law:**

$$V = I \times R \tag{1}$$

For a constant driving voltage, more current will flow through a path with lower resistance. Similar, if a constant current is desired, voltage must increase or decrease with resistance. Any two quantities will determine the third. Electrical resistance is expressed in units referred to as **ohms.**

Power is a measure of the ability to perform work and is expressed in units of **watts.** Power represents the rate of change of energy and 1 watt is equal to the use or generation of 1 joule of energy per second. When energy is being used or dissipated, the power is given a negative sign. Positive power implies that energy is being generated. The relationship between voltage, current, and power is given in Equation 2a. Power (energy/sec) is the product of voltage (energy/coulomb) and current (coulomb/sec). By applying Ohm's Law, power can also be expressed in terms of voltage or current and resistance, as given in Equations 2b and 2c.

$$P = VI \qquad (2a)$$
$$P = V^2R \qquad (2b)$$
$$P = I^2R \qquad (2c)$$

Capacitance is the ability of a material to store charge. If positive and negative charges are separated by an insulator, their tendency will be to gravitate towards each other. The separating insulator prevents the flow of current. Objects consisting of layers of conductive or insulating material act as capacitors. Capacitors pass current through them only when the voltage across them is changing. This happens not because of an actual physical movement of charges or charge carriers, but by variations in the electric field established between the two areas of different charge concentrations. The faster the voltage changes, the more current will flow. If the voltage across the capacitor is constant, a constant amount of charge will remain separated and no current will flow through it. Electrical capacitance is expressed in units referred to as **farads.**

A constant flow of charge is called **direct current** or (DC). One that changes over time is referred to as an **alternating current** (AC). A signal may be a current, voltage, or any parameter being measured across time. The myoelectric signal is a voltage, but varies across time just the same.

As Equations 2b and 2c show, the power in a signal is a function of the square of the voltage or the square of the current. The Root Mean Square (RMS) value of a time-varying signal is an indirect measure of power. It corresponds to the amplitude of a constant (DC) signal that produces the same average power and represents the effective amplitude of the AC waveform. The RMS measure is defined as the *square root* of the average (or *mean*) of the *squared* amplitude of a signal over a prescribed period of time (usually one cycle of a periodic signal). This relationship is given in Equation 3,

$$\text{RMS} = \sqrt{\frac{1}{T}\int_0^T x^2(t)\,dt} \qquad (3)$$

where $x(t)$ is a time varying signal and T is the period of time over which the signal will be averaged (e.g., the time duration of one complete cycle of a sine wave).

Time and Frequency Domain Analysis

The most common way to think about or represent a signal is to plot its time course—for example, a simple sine wave as it might be viewed on an oscilloscope. But representing a signal with respect to time is not the only way to describe it uniquely and unambiguously. Consider the sine wave. The following expression represents its time history:

$$y(t) = A\,\sin\!\left(\frac{2\pi}{T}(t)\right) \qquad (4)$$

where A is the amplitude of one peak of the sine wave. The time it takes to make one complete repetition of itself is the period of the signal and is represented by the symbol T. The units of the period are seconds per cycle. A reciprocal relationship exists between the period and the frequency of a signal. The frequency, f, of a periodic signal like the sine wave has units of cycles per second, or hertz (Hz). From the beginning, one must realize that time and frequency are inversely related and represent different aspects of the same phenomenon.

If all the signals of interest were sine waves, only two pieces of information would be needed to identify them completely and tell them apart. They are the signal's amplitude (A) and frequency (f). If the signal is assumed to follow the shape of a sinusoid, it can be reconstructed completely without loss of any information and without confusing it with any other signal from just its amplitude and frequency. This affords a powerful shorthand for thinking about sine waves. But the sine wave can also be represented in the frequency domain. If the X axis represents all the possible frequencies, while the Y axis represents the amplitude of the pure sine wave signal, a sinusoidal curve when plotted against time would then be represented as a point in this new amplitude versus frequency space. A sine wave of a higher frequency would be located farther to the right along the X axis, and signals that repeat themselves more slowly would be located closer to the origin. A signal represented by a point on the Y axis has magnitude only, and no frequency. A sine wave of "zero frequency" never repeats itself and is a constant value, or DC signal.

The graphs in Figure 20-2 are both equally valid and accurate ways to plot a sine wave. They

FIGURE 20-2   Time and Frequency Domains. A sinusoidal waveform is depicted in the time domain, and its frequency domain representation is shown immediately below it.

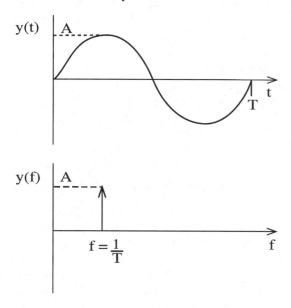

FIGURE 20-3   Fourier Approximation of a Square Wave. Sine waves of different amplitudes and frequencies may be summed to approximate any signal; **(A)** the first three sinusoids required to represent a square wave, **(B)** the composite approximation of the square wave.

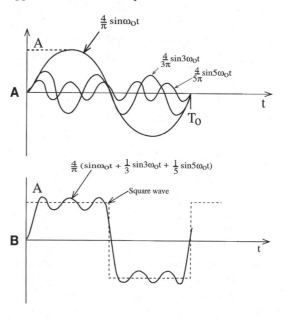

merely represent two different views of the same phenomenon. They contain exactly the same information and uniquely identify the sine wave.

All this would be fine if the EMG, or any other real-world signal behaved like a pure sine wave. But a French mathematician named Fourier discovered that a periodic signal of any shape can be expressed as the sum of sine waves of different frequencies and amplitudes. The first three sinusoids necessary to produce a square wave are illustrated in Figure 20-3. If they are added together, they result in a signal that approximates a square wave. It would take a lot of sine waves of higher frequencies to produce all the sharp edges and corners associated with a square. As a rule, the more abruptly a waveform changes in time, the higher the frequencies of sinusoids used to construct it. In the frequency domain, this square wave would look like an infinite series of points, each of which represents one of the sinusoidal components of the square wave. Each additional sinusoid occurs at a multiple of the underlying frequency of the square wave. The largest and slowest component occurs at the **fundamental** frequency. The higher frequency components are called **harmonics.** In the frequency domain, the square wave would look like Figure 20-4. The frequency domain representation of a signal (such as the example in Figure 20-10) is often called a **spectrum.**

FIGURE 20-4   Spectrum of a Square Wave. The frequency domain representation of the fundamental and harmonic sinusoidal components of the square wave estimate depicted in Figure 20-3b.

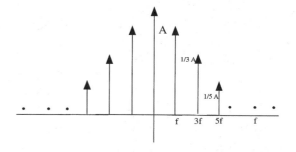

All this would be fine if the EMG was always periodic, like a square wave. But the concept extends to all signals, periodic or otherwise. If a signal is not periodic, its spectrum is continuous rather than made up of a series of discrete points as in Figure 20-4. So any signal, including the EMG, can be represented in the frequency domain.

The **power spectral density** (psd) is a plot of the squared magnitude of the frequency components of a signal and is useful in illustrating how the power in the signal is distributed. Operations can be performed on signals in the frequency domain, just as they can in the time domain. When frequencies are manipulated, the operations represent a **filtering.** Just as a filter for a camera lens blocks certain frequencies of light and lets other colors through, filters can exclude certain frequency components of a signal and pass on only those of interest. The human ear filters out very high-pitched (high frequency) and very low-pitched (low frequency) sounds. It passes a band of frequencies between 20 and 20,000 Hz, acting like a **band-pass filter.** Dogs can hear higher-pitched sounds because the **bandwidth** of their ears is wider and lets higher frequencies through. If all the high frequencies of a square wave were filtered out with a **low-pass filter** so that only the first three components got through, the resulting signal would look exactly like Figure 20-4. Mechanical systems can also act like filters and amplify or attenuate certain frequencies. Consider the parallel spring and shock absorber system in a car suspension. These components smooth out the high frequency vibrations and bumps, acting as a low-pass filter. Similarly, undesirable low frequencies can be removed by a **high-pass filter.** The **band-pass filter** is in essence a combination of a high-pass and low-pass filter. Filters of many different characteristics can be constructed electronically.

The filtering characteristics of a mechanical or electronic system can be represented by a **Bode plot,** which graphs the magnitude of the output of the system against frequency, as opposed to the psd, which shows the distribution of power. The Bode plot describes the **transfer function** or filtering action of mechanical or electrical systems. If a single impulse, or a stream of completely random "white" noise containing energy at all possible frequencies, were input into a system, the

Bode plot of the resulting output would be a picture of the system response or transfer function. (An example of a Bode plot of a low pass filter is given in Figure 20-16*B.*)

Sampling Theory

In order to process the EMG or any other signal with a computer it is first necessary to sample it at regular intervals and convert these values to a digital form. The sampling process is illustrated schematically in Figure 20-5 and can be modeled as a rapidly closing and opening switch leading to a measuring device. While the switch is open, the measuring device sees no signal. Only the value of the signal when the switch is closed is registered by the meter. Usually the switch is opened and closed at a fixed frequency (the sampling frequency, f_s) resulting in a sequence of samples evenly spaced in time. The act of sampling results in a repetition of the spectrum of a signal in the frequency domain at multiples of the sampling rate. Because of this fact, if signals with wide bandwidths are not sampled often enough (at too low a sampling frequency), the original spectrum will overlap with one of the duplicates, as illustrated in Figure 20-6. If this happens, it will be impossible to reconstruct the shape of the original signal in the time domain from the corrupted spectrum in the frequency domain. When the corrupted spectrum is converted into its time domain equivalent, it will resemble some other signal, rather than the one originally sampled. Because the sampled data is masquerading as a totally different signal, overlapping spectra caused by sampling at too low a rate is called **aliasing.** The new, corrupted signal can be mistaken for the original. Sampling at a rate in excess of twice the highest frequency component of a signal would insure that the spectra generated by the sampling process do not overlap, as illustrated in Figure 20-7.

Figure 20-5   Sampled Data. A continuous time sine wave is sampled at integer time intervals to yield a digitized or discrete representation of the signal.

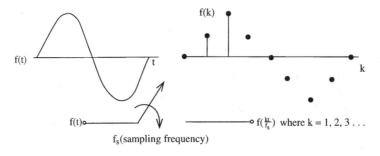

FIGURE 20-6 Aliasing in the Frequency Domain. The frequency spectrum of a given signal repeats at multiples of the sampling rate. Because this signal is under sampled (s $< 2f_{max}$), the spectra overlap, hence distorting or aliasing the data.

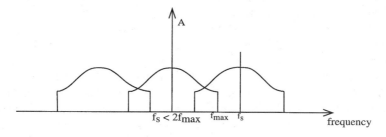

FIGURE 20-7 Unaliased Proper Sampling. The signal is properly sampled ($f_s \geq 2f_{max}$) as indicated by the spectra not being overlapped, and hence the data is not distorted or aliased.

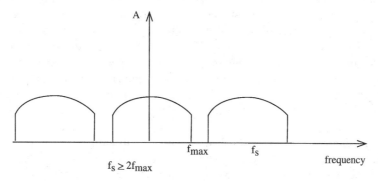

At least two samples are needed from each cycle of a sine wave to represent all the information in the signal. If the 5 Hz sine wave were sampled twice every period (an effective rate of 10 Hz), there is no way that it would be mistaken for another signal of lower frequency. To be sure that the sampled data in the computer represents the real-world signal, the signal should first be passed through a higher order (e.g., $\geq$ fourth order) low-pass filter to eliminate any high frequency components that are not of interest. Because the low-pass filter has now guaranteed that the filtered signal will have negligible components above the cutoff frequency (f_c) of its pass band, it can be sampled at a rate of at least twice the filter cutoff frequency ($f_s \geq 2f_c$) without danger of aliasing. The sampled data can then be used to accurately and unambiguously represent the analog signal. The original signal can be reconstructed faithfully from data stored in the computer without loss of any information. The minimum frequency to prevent aliasing is called the **Nyquist frequency** and corresponds to twice the highest frequency component of the signal.

ORIGINS OF THE ELECTROMYOGRAM: NEUROPHYSIOLOGICAL BASIS

As muscles undergo a contraction they typically produce a displacement and a force with a concomitant EMG signal. Many biophysical variables impact a given muscle's contractile displacement or force production capability. Each of these variables may or may not have a profound impact upon the EMG signal. To gain insight into these phenomena the origin of the electromyogram will be reviewed.

The outer membrane of a neuron can generate or conduct electrical signals. The initiation of a muscle contraction begins with a volitional or subliminal command: the neural action potential. To increase the speed of electrical conduction the axon may be myelinated—wrapped with Schwaan cells, which function as insulators. Ultimately the nerve and muscle meet at the neuromuscular junction where the neural signals trigger the release of chemical transmitters from the nerve end plates. This triggers a muscular contraction and leads to the depolarization of muscle cells, which results in a measurable EMG signal.

The fluid on the interior of the nerve cell contains different concentrations of charge carrying ions (e.g., sodium: Na^+; potassium: K^+; and chloride: Cl^-). The charge distribution across the membrane establishes a potential difference or voltage. The membrane potential is a function of the ion distributions and concentration gradients and is always expressed as the intracellular charges with respect to the extracellular. Note that very few of the intra- and extracellular ions are involved in the membrane charge distribution that establishes the membrane potential. The neuron is initially at equilibrium, which is known as the resting potential. Upon a suprathreshold stimulation the all-or-none response, or action potential, occurs. The membrane potential first becomes closer to zero (i.e., depolarizes). It then overshoots 0 volts and proceeds to repolarize, (i.e., go away from zero heading back towards resting potential). Because of the significant time the membrane potential undershoots the resting value, a refractory period results during which an action potential cannot be elicited. The ionic distribution gradually returns to the resting potential.

The changing distributions of ions establish a traveling wave in the neuron as if the axon were an electrical cable. Neural action potentials propagate along the axon at speeds as high as 120 m/sec. The fastest speeds of action potential propagation occur in the larger myelinated axons where the action potential jumps from one gap in the myelin (called a *node of Ranvier*) to another. This phenomenon is referred to as saltatory conduction. As a motor neuron approaches the muscle it divides into many branches. The final region of the axon is referred to as the presynaptic terminal or **end plate.**

The neuromuscular junction comprises the motor end plate (axon), post-synaptic membrane (muscle), a 1 to 2 μm cleft, and certain essential biochemicals that complete this electrochemical system. The neural action potential propagates down the axon and leads to **acetylcholine (ACh)** carrying organelles known as vesicles to fuse with the terminal end plate membrane. The neural action potential increases calcium (Ca^{++}) conductance, which in turn enhances vesicle fusion. The ACh is released upon vesicle fusion and interacts with the post-synaptic membrane to elicit muscle action potentials.

The muscle fibers, the fundamental cells within a muscle, have excitable membranes similar to neurons. The key difference is in function. The muscle fiber does not seek to communicate information but to act upon information. Some level of tensile or compressive forces will be generated in accordance with the type of muscle contraction. As long as sufficient amounts of ACh are released from presynaptic terminals and appropriate diffusion into the receptors within the muscle fiber membrane occurs, then the suprathreshold stimuli will elicit a muscle fiber action potential (MAP).

A single functional section of thick and thin filaments arranged in parallel overlapping arrays is referred to as a sarcomere. These filaments can slide past one another to allow for shortening or contraction of a muscle. The amount of force produced within a muscle fiber is proportional to the number of crossbridges formed between the thick and thin filaments.[14] Longitudinally arranged sarcomeres form myofibrils. The parallel organization of myofibrils form a muscle fiber. Each muscle fiber is enclosed in an excitable membrane known as the sarcolemma. The neuromuscular junction (i.e., motor end plate) lies directly on the sarcolemma. Because of the random ACh packet release in the neuromuscular junction and the delays imposed by the slightly different lengths of axonal branches, the muscle fibers within one motor unit are not perfectly synchronized. A time jitter of approximately 20 μs exists in healthy humans.[11] For all intents and purposes this means that the contractions of all the fibers in a single motor unit may be considered to be synchronous.

MAP propagation occurs in both directions along the muscle fiber. As the distribution of ions about the membrane changes, a small electromagnetic field is generated. This electromagnetic field is detected by an indwelling wire or needle electrode that is in close proximity to the excited muscle fiber. In most respects the single MAP has a similar appearance to the neural action potential. The key difference is the requirement of the calcium ion to promote a functional contraction.

The motor unit is comprised of the alpha-motor neuron, the neuromuscular junction, and its associated muscle fibers. This is the most basic functional unit of striated skeletal muscle. The smallest discernible force from a skeletal muscle, known as the twitch tension, will occur in response to one motor unit action potential (MUAP). Morphometrically muscle fibers range from a few millimeters to 30 cm in length and 10 to 200 μm in diameter.[1] The number of muscle fibers within a given motor unit varies from muscle to muscle. For example, the human extraocular muscles have 5 to 6 fibers, and the medial head of the gastrocnemius has 2,000 fibers within a single motor unit.[1] A smaller fiber-to-motor unit ratio appears to correlate to muscles that conduct fine coordinated motions. A muscle fiber can shorten up to 57% of its original length upon excitation.

The spatiotemporal nature of the EMG is illustrated by the manner in which muscle force is modulated in normal motor activities. An increase in the force generated by a muscle is produced by a combination of two mechanisms: (1) an increase in the discharge frequency or firing rate of each alpha-motor neuron and (2) an increase in the number of active motor units. The first mechanism represents a temporal recruitment, and hence muscle action potentials are generated at faster and faster rates. The latter describes a spatial recruitment as more and more motor units contribute to the contraction. For isometric contractions in some muscles, spatial recruitment of motor units distributed throughout the muscle is the principal means of producing forces from 0 to 30% of the maximum voluntary contraction with a secondary role played by modulation of the firing rate. Temporal recruitment becomes increasingly important as force levels approach 70 percent of the maximum. Motor units tend to synchronize at maximum levels of contraction, which is mostly a temporal phenomenon.[3,6]

The recruitment scheme employed to modulate force appears to vary from muscle to muscle. In small muscles, such as those found in the hand, most of the available motor units are recruited below 50% of the maximum voluntary contraction (MVC) possible, whereas in the larger muscles of the extremities, spatial recruitment continues throughout a majority of the range of voluntary contraction.[1] Smaller muscles appear to rely primarily on firing rate, and larger muscles rely primarily on motor unit recruitment to modulate force.

Spatial and temporal recruitment do not operate independently. During contractions of increasing force, the recruitment of new motor units has been observed to decrease the firing rate of previously activated units.[1] The interaction may provide a mechanism for smooth and continuous force output, rather than the jerky output expected if each motor unit generated a discrete quantum of force.

The spatial recruitment of motor units appears to follow a general organizational pattern during isometric contractions. Motor units are recruited and derecruited in an orderly progression, possibly according to their size. Small motor units appear to be activated first, followed by larger and larger units as the developed force increases.[3,23] Derecruitment occurs in the opposite order of recruit-

ment, and modifications in the recruitment order can be induced by the electrical stimulation of sensory nerves.[1] The order of motor unit activation may allow for both the fine control needed to perform intricate tasks and the rapid buildup of force required by movements of a larger scale. Of comparable importance toward accomplishing tasks are the temporal characteristics.

DeLuca and Forrest have described the irregular behavior of the interpulse interval (IPI) as a random variable with characteristic statistical properties.[7] Typically, histograms (i.e., discrete probability distribution functions) are formed. Assuming the IPI ascribes an approximately normal or "bell-shaped distribution" then it may be completely described by two parameters: the mean and standard deviation. Researchers are in disagreement as to the distribution of a muscle's IPI in part because it varies as a function of time (i.e., is nonstationary) and is muscle dependent.

The muscle fibers that comprise a single motor unit need not be isolated or concentrated in an anatomically distinct bundle, but may be distributed throughout the muscle.[28] In effect, recording electrodes sample only a small portion of the total population of active muscle fibers. Signals recorded either from indwelling electrodes or from the surface represent an incomplete picture of the entire activity of the muscle.

Although the muscle fibers constituting a single motor unit are not isolated in an anatomically distinct region, their distribution throughout the muscle is not necessarily uniform. Small, lower threshold units, which are recruited first in a contraction, have been observed in greatest concentration in the deeper layers of the muscle,[4] while larger, high threshold units tended to be superficial.[29] The selective recruitment of the motor units at different distances from a surface electrode may contribute to the nonlinear relationship between surface EMG and muscle force often observed for muscles with a mixture of fiber types and sizes. Larger motor units also generate larger action potentials.[29] The contributions of the small, deep motor units to the surface EMG are attenuated and diffused by the intervening tissue. Large, superficial fibers contribute disproportionately to the EMG due to both their proximity to the recording electrode and their size. At low levels of force, the change in the EMG is often much smaller than the associated change in force because the smaller units in deeper layers of the muscle are recruited first. As force increases, the EMG may grow at a faster rate than the force itself as larger units located closer to the electrode are brought into play.

Action potential trains from a single motor unit can be measured at the surface of the skin during contractions at low levels of force.[5,19] Signals recorded under such conditions often exhibit a strong periodic component due to the firing rate of the alpha-motor neuron associated with the motor unit. Even at these low levels of force when fibers are contracting in response to the regular pulses of the action potential train, mechanical action is smooth due to the filtering action of the tendon-muscle-skeleton complex. The electrical discharges of the nerve are usually asynchronous, except during contractions close to maximal force. All periodic components tend to disappear in the surface EMG for contractions approaching or exceeding 10 percent MVC.[22] With many thousands of motor units active in gross movements and generating action potentials, the activity sensed at the surface appears to be dynamic and almost random.

In a landmark paper by Hill, the thermodynamics of whole muscle contractions were described for active lengthening and shortening.[15] In a manner similar to the length-tension curves of single muscle fibers, there is an optimum length of whole muscle for the production of force. A twitch is the smallest possible mechanical output of the muscle since it reflects only the action of the fibers associated with one motor unit. Hill described the rate-limiting phenomenon of muscle fiber cross-bridge cycling. At the maximum velocity of shortening, no force is produced. Eccentric contractions while the muscle is lengthening can produce forces almost twice as great as during an isometric condition.

The mechanical analog to the Hill model consists of a series elastic element (a spring) connected to the parallel combination of elastic and viscous elements. A variable known as the "active state" was defined to describe the injection of energy into the model. The EMG is sometimes used as a crude estimate of the active state of the Hill model.

Models of the EMG Signal

A mental picture or working theory of how a signal is produced is invaluable to selecting an appropriate processing technique. Several approaches to modeling the EMG have been proposed with varying degrees of accuracy and utility.

The Neurophysiological Approach
DeLuca attempted a mathematical model of the EMG signal based upon the most current knowledge of the neurophysiological mechanisms in-

volved.[6,8] The first building block of this model described the motor unit action potential train (MUAPT) as a combination of impulsive spikes (i.e., the alpha motor neuron action potential train) filtered by transfer functions derived from intervening tissue-electrode effects. A random variable referred to as the generalized firing rate was defined to obviate the precise modeling of jitter within a MUAPT and the difference in firing rates between other motor units. The raw EMG signal was then considered to be a superposition of the individual MUAPTs. DeLuca's model incorporated the number of active motor units (spatial recruitment) and their generalized firing rates (temporal recruitment). In addition, the cancellation due to superposition of MUAPs, the MUAP shape (transfer function) and the synchronization (cross correlation) of motor unit discharges was also included. Much insight into the neurophysiological mechanisms of the EMG has been obtained from this model but its complex solution has delayed its widespread use for various practical applications.

A "top-down" approach toward describing the EMG signal is equally valid and sometimes more useful than building an understanding of the phenomenon from the cellular level upward. The following sections describe how the EMG behaves macroscopically, rather than exhausting the details of the underlying anatomy and electrophysiology associated with its generation.

The Phenomenological Approach
The mechanical output of the muscle is a combination of the activity of all its active motor units. Motor unit output is a combination of the activities of the individual contractile fibers which, in turn, are combinations of the outputs of the individual actin/myosin interactions. Similarly, the electrical activity of the muscle is a combination of many individual events occurring within the muscle. In both mechanical and electrical cases, the macroscopic activity of the muscle is a weighted sum across space and time of a larger number of individual events. Due to the imperfect nature of recording the signal, the attenuation and distortion introduced by the tissue between the muscle cells and the recording electrodes and other physical phenomena, the weighting in the electrical case is fundamentally and radically different from the mechanical case.

Whether or not obtaining a signal directly related to muscle force is possible, spatial and temporal changes in the surface EMG can be observed with changes in muscle force. Even an inexact and gross indication of the state of the underlying muscle can be clinically useful. One way to understand how the EMG signal changes with muscle force is based on a relatively simple, but useful model. In general, the electrical activity at the muscle's surface appears to be almost random. The amplitude of this sequence of noisy spikes grows as muscle force increases. This phenomenon is not surprising, since both temporal and spatial recruitment should increase the electrical activity as more motor units are added or as they contribute more activity in shorter spans of time.

The observation that the surface EMG resembles a sequence of random noise that increases and decreases with muscle force led to the formulation of the Amplitude Modulation (AM) model of the signal. Amplitude modulation means that the amplitude of a higher frequency signal varies with time and carries the information of interest. This process is the same as that used to generate AM radio broadcasts and is illustrated in Figure 20-8. The information of interest (voice or music in the case of AM radio, muscle force in the case of the EMG) is represented in Figure 20-8*A*. If this **modulation** is multiplied by a higher frequency signal called a **carrier** (Figure 20-8*B*), it will form an **envelope** and determine the magnitude of the resulting trace. The modulated carrier is given in Figure 20-8*C*. All the information in the music modulation signal is preserved in the amplitude of the carrier.

The modulation signal can be extracted from the compound signal (the modulated carrier of Figure 20-8*C*) in a number of ways. Since the carrier is of a much higher frequency than the modulation, one of the most straightforward ways to recoup the original information is to rectify the modulated carrier (make all the negative values of the signal positive) and low-pass filter to remove the carrier frequencies and leave the information of interest. This sequence of rectification followed by low-pass filtering is called **envelope detection** and is a simple and useful way of processing the EMG.

The AM model of EMG signal generation is given in Figure 20-9. Instead of a pure sinusoidal carrier as shown in Figure 20-8, the carrier signal in the EMG model appears to be randomly distributed white noise. White noise contains information at all frequencies, just as white light contains all colors. The random noise is band limited by a shaping filter that constrains its spectrum to frequencies to the 10 to 1000 Hz range.

The AM model represents the surface EMG as a zero-mean, white-noise process with a Gaussian distribution, which is passed through a constant filter representing the effects of tissue and electrode system as well as other subcutaneous processes. A static, memory-less function of force modulates this band-limited, random carrier.[19]

In general, this model states:

$$y(t) = c(t)n(t) \tag{5}$$

where $y(t)$ is the raw myoelectric signal, $c(t)$ is the contraction level or force signal, and $n(t)$ is a noise process with unit variance. The AM model dictates that the shape of the spectrum of the EMG remains invariant and force-independent. Variations in force will shift the magnitude of the spectrum defined by the shaping filter while maintaining its shape. These are simplifying assumptions that are extremely useful, even if they are rarely if ever true. In general, the EMG is a nonstationary random process, since muscle force varies continuously with intended motion.

Other phenomena, such as fatigue, also change the EMG signal and muscle output with time. The frequency content of the mechanical output of a muscle is much lower than that of the EMG. With components up to 1 kHz, the EMG has energy at frequencies more than an order of magnitude greater than those of the muscle force associated with it. The difference in frequency content of force and EMG signals justifies the application of smoothing techniques to isolate the slowly varying contraction-level signal and supports the assumption that the signal is stationary with respect to force and the time available for

Figure 20-8 AM Modulation. **A**, A signal that varies with time is modulated or multiplied with a carrier **B**, which is typically a sinusoid. The resulting amplitude modulated signal is shown in **C**.

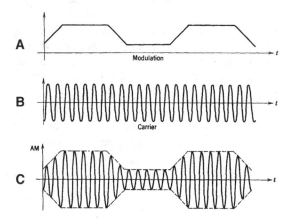

Figure 20-9   AM Model. The amplitude modulation model of the EMG signal states that force or contraction level is multiplied by a zero-mean band-limited Gaussian noise.

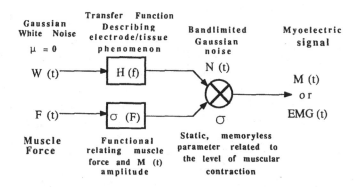

processing.[10,22] The application of low-pass filters to the rectified EMG for envelope detection is a direct result of the AM model. Most processing techniques can be corrupted by low-frequency noises called **motion artifact**, however. As the recording electrode moves slightly on the surface of the skin, a false reading can be generated that can be mistaken for muscle activity. Motion artifact generally manifests itself as a low frequency and transient shift in the baseline of the recording. Because it is usually of much lower frequency than the noisy carrier or the motion of interest, it can be minimized by filtering out all frequencies below 10 Hz with a high pass filter.

Because of the multiplicative nature of the signal model and because the EMG is a zero-mean process, processing is generally nonlinear and consists of rectification followed by smoothing. Many smoothing processors more sophisticated than simple envelope detection have been proposed to relate the EMG to the force generated by a single muscle including integration, averaging, and other smoothing techniques.[4,12,16,17,25] Their relative merits will be discussed in the next section.

Hogan et al. proposed a processing method to relate surface EMG to muscle force that remained faithful to the mathematical characteristics of the raw EMG as measured at the skin's surface.[20] Because the mean and variance completely specify a Gaussian distribution and the EMG has a mean of zero, all of the information pertaining to muscle function and tension must be contained in the signal variance. This is consistent with adopting the amplitude modulation model of Figure 20-9. Computing variance is a nonlinear averaging that also smoothes the signal. Force estimates were obtained by maximum likelihood estimation of the signal variance and inversion of the empirically determined relationship between variance and

force. Hogan extended the processing technique to include multiple channels of myoelectric activity, combining spatial as well as temporal information into the force estimate. A power function, generally found to be quadratic, was used to relate the EMG collected from electrodes over the muscle belly of the biceps brachii to the isometric force developed. The multichannel optimal myoprocessor showed a significant improvement over single-channel processors, which were, themselves, significantly better than traditional rectification and low-pass filtering.

This, and most other processing methods, have excluded the effects of rate of contraction, muscle length, or additive noise. While providing for such considerations may improve performance slightly during the dynamic phase of contraction, it represents a significant increase in system complexity.

EMG Acquisition and Processing

Step 1: Get Yourself a Signal

To acquire the electromyogram involves the appropriate selection of electrodes and instrumentation. The first decision is to select the type of electrodes to record the signal from the body. If one chooses to study a muscle whose fibers are closer to the dermis, or **surface accessible**, then surface electrodes are often an appropriate noninvasive choice. If one chooses to study a deep muscle (e.g., the illiopsoas) then needle or wire electrodes will be required. From the perspective of the patient, surface electrodes are usually preferred due to their pain-free application. From the perspective of the investigator or clinician the choice of electrodes also depends upon the question that is posed.

As illustrated in Figure 20-10*A*, the surface electrode recording system can produce a signal indicative of the overall electrical manifestation of the contracting muscle. Specifically, the spatial and temporal summation of the MUAPTs are smoothed or low-pass filtered via the electrode and tissue electrical properties. The surface EMG is a grand average of the underlying electrical activity. From the surface, the EMG signal is detected with a pair of electrodes typically separated from the epidermis/dermis tissue by an electrolyte. The electrolyte is either a pudding-like or gel-like substance that has a homogeneous dispersion of cations and anions. In this way, the changing distributions of charges occurring about the excitable membranes (muscle fibers) of a muscle may be sensed by the metallic electrodes and transduced for subsequent processing. Stainless steel may be used for surface EMG detection but silver–silver-chloride (Ag-AgC1) is considered to be electrochemically more stable. The raw surface EMG ranges from 10μv to 3 mv in amplitude with a bandwidth between 10 Hz and 1 kHz.[9]

As illustrated in Figure 20-10*B*, the needle electrode recording system produces a signal that is dominated by the motor unit(s) nearest the electrode. Since the tissue electrical properties are less of a factor with indwelling electrodes the amounts of low-pass filtering imposed upon the MUAPT is considerably less than with surface recording. For this reason the bandwidth of needle EMG is typically from 10 Hz to 10 kHz.[9] The amplitude ranges from 10 μv to 1 mv. Once the signal has been sensed by the electrode system it needs to be boosted or amplified to a usable voltage range via an instrumentation amplifier.

The instrumentation amplifier must have several attributes to acquire the EMG signal in a manner that preserves its fidelity. The input impedance should be comprised of a low capacitance ($\leq$ 5 pf) and a high resistance ($\geq$ 1000 MΩ) in parallel. In this way a negligible amount of current is drawn into the instrumentation amplifier so as not to corrupt the EMG signal. Several integrated

FIGURE 20-10   **A,** Surface Electrode Monitoring Problem. Surface electrodes are interfaced to the body via electrolyte to detect EMG. The resulting signal is affected by the time-varying electrical properties of the epidermis, dermis, transcutaneous tissue, and blood, as well as other noise sources. **B,** Needle Electrode Monitoring Problem. A more local view of the nearest motor units contribution to the EMG signal is observed.

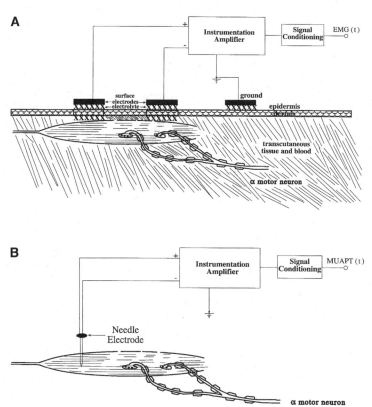

FIGURE 20-11   Typical EMG Instrumentation Amplifier. A differentially configured preamplifier allows for reduction of the noises common to both electrode inputs. A subsequent amplifier with gain is then employed for further noise immunity by increasing the amplitude of the signal.

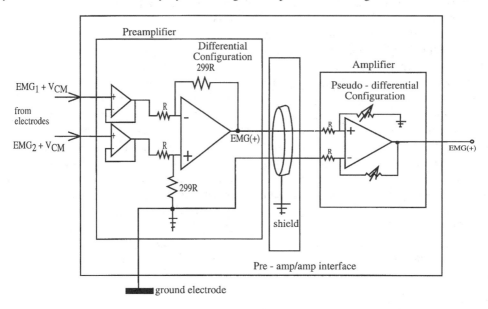

circuits are configured with these attributes but since a minimum noise artifact will result from a minimal lead length between the electrode and first stage of amplification, a separate preamplifier is often employed close to the electrodes themselves. The preamplifier may have the surface electrodes built into it in order to achieve this design goal. To maximize the signal fidelity, or specifically **signal-to-noise ratio (SNR)**, a fixed gain of 300 may also be incorporated within the preamplifier. An additional variable gain spanning 1 to 2000 is required to bring the raw EMG signal to the volt level for recording purposes.

When trying to acquire low-level biophysical signals, noise is always a potential enemy. Figure 20-11 shows the configuration of a typical EMG instrumentation amplifier system. Each electrode transduces a slightly different EMG signal since it takes time for the action potential to move from one electrode to another. However, the same noise voltage often appears on both inputs of the amplifier. The first stage of the preamplifier accurately acquires the EMG signals (EMG1, EMG2) with their respective common mode noise voltages (Vcm). The second stage of the preamplifier subtracts the two input signals yielding a composite representation of the EMG with no common mode noises.

$$EMG = (EMG1 + Vcm) - (EMG2 + Vcm) \quad (6)$$
$$= EMG1 - EMG2.$$

In the real world the complete elimination of common mode noise is not possible. The measure of how well an instrumentation amplifier minimizes this noise is referred to as the **common mode rejection ratio (CMRR)**.

$$CMRR \text{ (dB)} = 20 \log \frac{Vcm}{V_e} \quad (7)$$

V_e is the undesired common mode error voltage at the amplifier output. A differential configuration within the preamplifier is used to achieve the desired level of CMRR ($\geq$ 100 dB). Note that dB or decibels is a unit of gain. A gain of 100 dB implies that Vcm is 100,000 times larger than V_e.

The amplifier section may be some distance from the preamplifier. Such is often the case in a gait laboratory where a long umbilicus of cable may connect the amplifier to the electrode/preamplifier assembly attached to the patient. Even with cable shielding, common mode noises may recorrupt the signal. In such cases it is advisable to implement a pseudodifferential configuration within the amplifier. The pseudodifferential configuration accepts a grounded input on the negative terminal with the assumption that the common mode noise is virtually identical to that appearing on the positive terminal.

The most effective bipolar electrode placement for EMG recording is parallel to the orientation of the muscle fibers within the muscle under study. As shown in Figure 20-12A, if an electrode pair is

Figure 20-12 Traveling Wave **A,** When the electrodes are parallel to the traveling wave (MUAP) then the identical signal appears at the same time instant and when differentially processed yields zero output; **B,** when the electrodes are in series with the traveling wave (MUAP) then the signal that appears at each electrode is different at any given time instant and, when differentially processed, yields the appropriate triphasic signal representative of EMG.

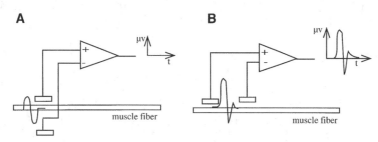

perpendicular to the muscle fiber orientation then each electrode will essentially see the same voltage at the same time. Differential recording of the MUAPT will yield a null signal, even though the electrical activity is significant. The parallel orientation shown in Figure 20-12B, is essential to insure a phasic delay between each electrode's view of the same MUAP, yielding the familiar EMG output. Simply, the MUAP reaches one electrode before the other. For a given MUAP conduction velocity, the signal's arrival time depends upon the interelectrode spacing. Consider Figure 20-13A, where the frequency components of the traveling wave have wavelengths equal to the interelectrode distance (Signal 1) and double the interelectrode distance (Signal 2). Signal 1 actually cancels out and Signal 2 is amplified. Figure 20-13B is a Bode plot (i.e., magnitude versus frequency diagram) of this phenomena. Notice how a cancellation pattern is formed for any frequency component whose wavelength is a multiple of the interelectrode distance or the cancellation frequency. The frequencies canceled and amplified are:

$$f_{cancellation} = nv/d, \text{ for } n = 1,2,3, \ldots \quad (8a)$$

$$f_{pass} = nv/2d, \text{ for } n = 1,3,5, \ldots \quad (8b)$$

where v is the signal's conduction velocity and d is the interelectrode distance.

Notice the dashed line in Figure 20-13 indicates a bipolar electrode. The bandwidth is significantly larger, obviating the frequency "dipping" effect. The signal measured depends upon the electrode geometry, interelectrode distance, electrode/tissue filtering properties, proximity to the active muscle fiber, and its conduction velocity.[1] In short, the closer the electrode spacing, the wider the band-

Figure 20-13 The Frequency Effects of Electrode Spacing. **A,** When the input signal's wavelength is equal to the interelectrode distance the signal cancels; when the input signal's wavelength is double the interelectrode distance the signal is amplified. **B,** In the frequency domain a cancellation pattern is formed. Note that this pattern is modifiable by changing the interelectrode spacing.

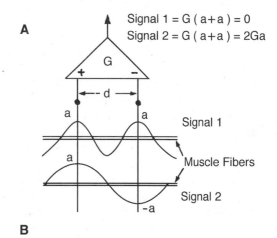

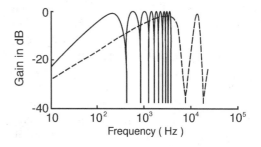

width of frequencies that can be recorded. Electrodes that are farther apart will attenuate higher frequency components and act as low-pass filters.

Step 2: Signal Conditioning

The raw EMG signal is constructed from an infinite number of small triphasic waveforms (MUAPs). As greater levels of contraction are elicited, the spatial and temporal summation of the MUAPT result in the increasing random noise like the signal shown in Figure 20-14. Although the specific time and frequency domain properties are muscle-and task-dependent, the typical raw surface EMG signal contains 95% of its power below 1 kHz. For questions concerning the integrity and distribution of motor units, the raw form of the EMG signal is required. In addition to gaining insight into the underlying physiology, various other uses of the raw EMG include obtaining timing information during dynamic movements. As shown in Figure 20-15, there are numerous other ways to extract information from the EMG. The most common of these techniques are presented first.

The muscle force produced or resulting joint torque is a much lower frequency signal than the raw EMG as shown in Figure 20-14C. As stated previously, the raw EMG resembles a noisy high frequency carrier modulated by the lower frequency force signal. Similar to the $7 handheld AM radio, the goal is to receive the composite signal (modulated radio frequency carrier or raw EMG) and strip away the modulation (music or force signal). Amplitude demodulation, often referred to as linear envelope detection, incorporates an absolute value and low-pass filter. Most of the linear envelope detection techniques require that the absolute value of the EMG signal is first obtained. In analog electronics the circuit that typically performs that function is the full-wave rectifier. As shown in Figure 20-15 this must be followed by some type of smoothing function. The first-order low-pass filter (LPF) is the most common choice and easily implemented in hardware or software. The amount of smoothing is specified by the cutoff frequency, f_c. The lower the cutoff frequency, the smoother the resulting EMG signal will be. The analog hardware implementation of a first-order LPF is of the form depicted in Figure 20-16A. The Bode plot shown in Figure 20-16B, depicts the LPF gain (V_{out}/V_{in}) as a function of frequency. The cutoff frequency is specified by selecting the resistor (R) and capacitor (C) in the feedback path of the operational amplifier circuit .These parameters are related to each other by the following equations:

$$\tau = RC \qquad (9)$$

$$\omega_c = \frac{1}{\tau} \qquad (10)$$

FIGURE 20-14 Raw EMG. **A,** A typical raw EMG is expressed as a function of time. **B,** The power spectral density of this signal contains 95% of its power below 1 kHz. **C,** The force from the muscle that produced the above EMG signal is quite similar to the envelope of the raw signal.

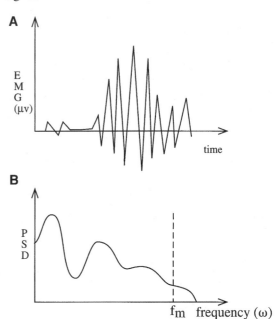

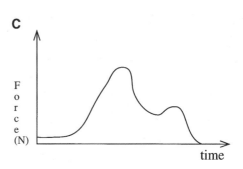

where ω_c is the angular cutoff frequency in radians/second and τ is called the time constant (with units of seconds). But since

$$\omega_c = 2\pi f_c \qquad (11)$$

the cutoff frequency in cycles/second or hertz is expressed as

$$f_c = \frac{1}{(2\pi\tau)} \qquad (12)$$

The cutoff frequency of a first-order LPF is often referred to as the −3 dB point. This is because the frequency components of the signal at that point are attenuated by three decibels when related to the DC value. Recall that the gain in decibels is

FIGURE 20-15   Amplitude Demodulation Type EMG Signal Processing Techniques. Full-wave rectification and low-pass filtering (i.e., linear envelope detection), moving average, integration with time reset, stationary average, and pure integration techniques are depicted.

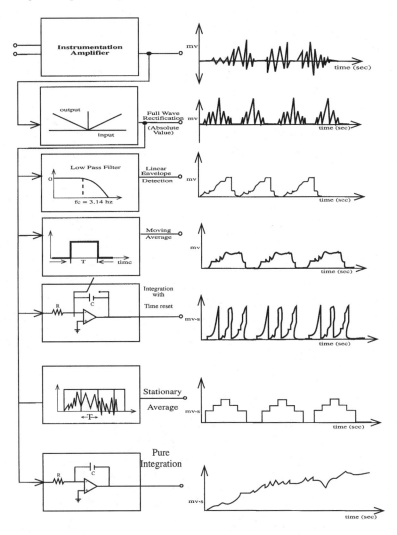

$$\text{Gain (dB)} = 20 \log \left(\frac{V_{out}}{V_{in}}\right) \qquad (13)$$

which implies that the cutoff is that frequency at which the output signal is reduced to 0.707 of the input. The first-order LPF cutoff frequency is also known as the half power point because it is that frequency at which the power in the output signal is half that of the input, or $(0.707)^2 \cong \frac{1}{2}$. Notice that the output signal in a first-order LPF becomes attenuated at a rate of −20 dB/decade of frequencies (see Figure 20-16*B*). If more severe attenuation is required to insure that higher frequencies are eliminated, for example, then a higher-order LPF would be employed. A second-order LPF could be formed by serially cascading two first-order LPFs. The resulting attenuation rate would

be −40 dB/decade. The price paid for increasing the order of an LPF is increased time delay between the input signal and the smoothed signal output. Care should be exercised in choosing a filter order to best match the needs for attenuation and accurate timing or "phase" characteristics.

A time constant often utilized in the linear envelope detection of EMG signals acquired during locomotion is 50 ms. Utilizing Equation 12, this time constant results are a cutoff frequency of approximately 3.2 Hz. There are many other types of low pass filters (e.g., Butterworth, Chebychev, Bessell, Paytner, etc.). Each differs in its attenuation and phase characteristics. Each has special attributes such that, even with identical cutoff frequencies and orders, they may yield different outputs from the same input signal. In general,

FIGURE 20-16   The LPF and the Bode Plot. An analog first-order low-pass filter implementation is shown in **A**. The Bode plot, magnitude versus frequency, is shown in **B**. The effect of increasing the time constant on smoothing the EMG signal is shown in **C**.

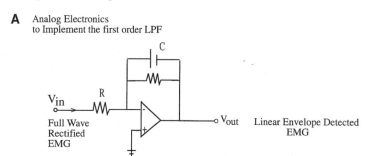

A   Analog Electronics
to Implement the first order LPF

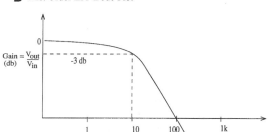

B   First Order LPF Bode Plot

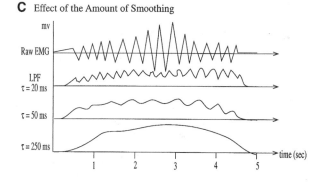

C   Effect of the Amount of Smoothing

selection of a particular LPF implementation or any smoothing function, should be consistent with the model of the signal's origin and hence the investigator's question of interest. For example, if timing is important, a filter that introduces minimal distortion due to phase delays is preferable; if signal fidelity is important, a filter with smooth passbands and rapid attenuation may be more desirable.

The effect of various amounts of smoothing is illustrated in Figure 20-16C. The raw EMG signal is processed using linear envelope detection with a full-wave rectifier and a low-pass filter. The cutoff frequency was varied by adjusting the time constant, τ. Increasing τ yielded decreasing cutoff frequencies and a smoother output signal. The 20 ms time constant LPF lets more high frequencies through, giving a jagged appearance to the output. The 250 ms time constant lets only very low frequencies through, yielding an output with a smoother appearance. Notice that the initial slope of the signal is decreasing. Intuitively one can state that this signal's characteristics are being inappropriately altered due to oversmoothing. The 50 ms time constant LPF yields the most smoothing without compromising significant features of the signal (e.g., slope).

The moving average filter displayed in Figure 20-15 is another smoothing function that is easily implemented on a computer. In this case an average is calculated within a specified window of data points. A new output data point results as the window of fixed width T (ms) moves to the next successive input data point. The output for a particular time, t_1, is

$$\text{Output } (t_1) = \frac{1}{T} \int_{t_1 - \frac{T}{2}}^{t_1 + \frac{T}{2}} |\text{EMG}(t)| \, dt. \qquad (14)$$

To achieve comparable smoothing to the first-order LPF (Siegler et al., 1985),

$$T = \frac{2.7835}{\omega_c} \qquad (15)$$

where ω_c is the angular cutoff frequency in radians per second. Substituting Equation 11 into Equation 15, it follows that the window width of a moving average is equal to

$$T \text{ (ms)} = \frac{2.7835}{2\pi f_c} = 2.7835\tau. \qquad (16)$$

Initially the window must fill, one data point at a time. The output will therefore have a phase lag that is equal to the window width. Because this type of smoothing is generally performed in a computer off-line and not in real time, one may express the output with a phase lag ranging from zero to the number of points within the width of the window. The investigator should describe how the phase lag is handled.

The process of integration generally describes the area under the signal being studied and is expressed in units of millivolt seconds (mv•s). There are many types of integration and they all process the EMG signal in a different way. Integration with time reset (see Figure 20-15) implies that the EMG signal is integrated to a specified time, typically 50 to 200 ms, and the reset to zero (mv•s). The raw EMG signal is converted into a series of spikes. Clearly the width of each spike is dependent upon the reset time as well as the EMG itself.

The stationary average, as shown in Figure 20-15, is similar to the moving average. The main difference concerns the manner in which the data is entered into the window. The moving average progresses through the EMG data one point at a time on a first in/last out basis. The stationary average progresses through the EMG data in blocks of data points equal to the width of the window. For example, the data point at which the first window ends is also where the second window begins. The output signal reflects the arith-metic average of the EMG data within each window. Note that the output of a stationary average is in essence a resampled and smoothed version of the input. The output signal is re-sampled by a factor equal to the number of data points within the chosen window width. Therefore, the effect of resampling is to reduce the number of data points in the output. Care should be taken not to apply too wide a window in a stationary average or the signal may become aliased.

The pure integration function simply integrates indefinitely. Notice, as shown in Figure 20-15, that the pure integral of an absolute value of a signal increases when any significant magnitude of the EMG is present and remains the same when the input signal goes to zero. If a pure integrator were applied to the raw EMG, the output would be zero (mv•s) because raw EMG has zero mean. For these reasons pure integration is of limited value and infrequently utilized. Many investigators have ap-plied some form of integration to their EMG signals and have referred to the output as IEMG.[2, 21,24] The term IEMG rarely refers to pure integration as the name implies. Investigators should clearly state what type of integration is being used in the analy-sis so that others can duplicate and/or interpret the results.

Other signal-processing techniques that have been applied to the EMG signal are illustrated in Figure 20-17. Note that the first two methods operate upon the raw EMG signal and don't require full-wave rectification.

One method of describing EMG activity is to detect the number of times the signal crosses the zero axis. The hardware component that typically performs this function is the comparator. A com-parator compares the input voltage appearing on the positive terminal with that appearing on the negative. If the negative terminal is connected to ground then the comparison is made with respect to zero volts. The comparator's output simply alternates between the positive and negative sup-ply voltages of the circuit depending on whether the EMG signal is above or below zero volts. It is not uncommon to then count the number of zero crossings as a quantification of the EMG activity.

The root mean square (RMS) function is a popular signal-processing technique among engi-neers to quantify errors in various systems. As previously defined, the easiest way to remember the algorithm is to state the name of the function backwards. *Square* is the first step, which refers to squaring the EMG signal. Note that once a signal is squared it will no longer have any negative values. *Mean* is the next step which refers to an

FIGURE 20-17   Other EMG Signal Processing Techniques. The zero-crossing detector, RMS, voltage-to-frequency, integration with voltage reset, and adaptive linear envelope detector techniques are depicted.

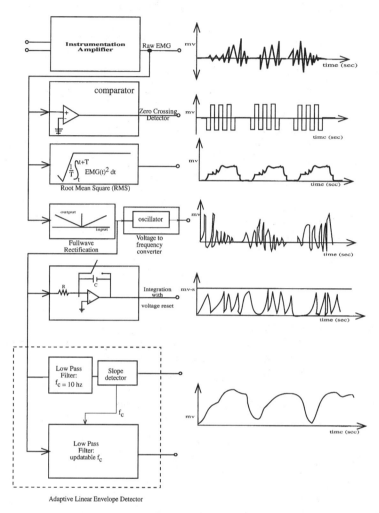

Adaptive Linear Envelope Detector

average calculation of the squared signal. Since the averaging period must be specified, recall the equivalent bandwidth techniques that were established to relate the window width of the moving average to the cutoff frequency of a first-order low-pass filter (see Equation 16). The same principles apply for the RMS function. *Root* is the final operation, which merely implies taking the square root of the entire quantity.

A voltage-to-frequency converter assigns an increasingly higher frequency to increasingly higher magnitudes of the EMG signal. The circuit that typically accomplishes this task is a voltage-controlled oscillator. The output of this circuit is a sine wave whose frequency is proportional to the voltage magnitude of the EMG signal.

A circuit that performs integration with voltage reset will integrate the EMG signal until a preset

voltage level is reached and then reset to 0 (mv·s). When the muscle's activity is low the time until reset will be long. Conversely, when the muscle activity is high the time until reset will be short. In this manner the frequency of integrator resets is an indication of the magnitude of the EMG signal.

The final signal processor to be discussed is the adaptive linear envelope detector. Consider the myoelectric control of a prosthesis. The more spikes from high frequencies within the processed EMG signal, the more jittery the prosthetic limb may respond. If the EMG signal was over-smoothed then the artificial limb may not be able to respond to intentionally rapid motions. Fullmer, Meek, and Jacobsen described an adaptive linear envelope detector consisting of a low-pass filter with an adjustable time constant.[13] This was preceded by a low-pass filter with a fixed time constant, which processed the EMG signal with a bandwidth suffi-cient to preserve the fastest desired limb function. The output of this initial LPF was followed by a differentiator to detect the slope of the EMG signal. If a slow motion was occurring then a gentle slope would be detected and the adaptive low-pass filter would be fed a long time constant (e.g., 500 ms). In this way the extraneous noise within the EMG would be filtered out, yielding a more steady myoelectric control signal. If a fast motion was occurring then a steep slope would be detected and the adaptive low-pass filter would be fed a short time constant (e.g., 50 ms). In this way the prosthesis could respond to a quick, intended motion.

Last-Minute Advice

The International Society for Electrical Kinesiol-ogy (ISEK) has published a must-read report for investigators and clinicians making EMG mea-surements, entitled "Units, Terms, and Standards for Reporting EMG Research" (1980). This docu-ment clearly states the rationale for reporting the instrumentation, gains, bandwidths, sampling rate, signal processing, and associated parameters in-volved in the acquisition and analysis of EMG signals. Standardization in reporting of EMG re-search is essential for accurate interpretation of an investigator's results as well as comparison to the results of other investigators. The National Insti-tute for Occupational Safety and Health (NIOSH) has released a comprehensive text entitled, "Se-lected Topics in Surface Electromyography for Use in the Occupational Setting: Expert Perspec-tives" (1992), which includes the ISEK report. Note that the NIOSH document is available free of charge from the U.S. Department of Health and Human Services by phoning 1-800-35-NIOSH and requesting document 91-100.

Many interesting phenomena concerning the EMG signal are best studied from examining the power spectral density. The fatigue of muscle has received much attention.[9] The median frequency of EMG has been observed to shift downward as the muscle fatigues. The electrode-tissue effects most certainly affect the frequency content of the EMG signal. Kwatny, Thomas, and Kwatny observed that the surface EMG signal is stationary on the time scale. Essentially the signal does not wander within a second's time.[26] Hillstrom et al.[30] concurred with Kwatny et al. on the second scale but found that the surface EMG signal was nonstationary on the minute and hour scales. This implies that for a consistent isometric force signal, the characteristics of surface EMG wander over time. The spectral properties of EMG during various myopathies are not only time varying but different from that of healthy individuals.

Motion artifact and other electrical noise sources should also be given consideration when attempting EMG measurements. The slight disrup-tion of the charge distribution as detected about the epidermis due to even minor motions from the contracting muscle can corrupt the EMG signal. Fortunately the motion artifact is typically below 10 to 20 Hz and can be minimized through appropriate high-pass filtering. It is not unwise to amplify and input the EMG signal into a speaker system. One can often hear a 60-cycle hum or a local radio broadcast, which should signal the investigator that either a ground or related problem exists and is corrupting the EMG signal.

SUMMARY

The surface, wire, and needle EMG signals have received extensive study. Although much knowl-edge has been obtained about the neurophysiologi-cal basis, modeling, and processing of the EMG signal, many questions remain to be answered. In addition to the classic electrodiagnostic study of EMG while sitting (i.e., the open kinetic chain), the study of the agonistic and antagonist EMG activity during posture and locomotion has begun to show value in differential diagnoses, prognoses, and treatment effectiveness demonstration. Still a model that incorporates both firing rate and motor unit recruitment in an accurate and useful manner must emerge. Despite the obvious value of the Hill model, anisometric and multijoint muscles defy the currently employed simplistic amplitude modulation model of the EMG signal. If local sweating and neuromuscular reorganization aid and abet the nonstationary behavior of the surface EMG signal, will it be possible to derive adequate control of artificial limbs? In addition to the obvious valuable timing information that locomo-tion EMG studies can yield, will reliable muscle force and/or velocity estimation become possible?

The investigations that unfold these controver-sial issues will certainly be exciting. All that is needed is the proper attitude.

"Why do they put locks on the Seven-Elevens when they're open twenty-four hours a day?"
Gallager (a contemporary comedian)

REFERENCES

1. Basmajian JV, De Luca CJ: *Muscles alive*, Balti-more, 1989, Williams & Wilkins.
2. Bigland-Ritchie B, Woods JJ: Integrated EMG and oxygen uptake during dynamic contractions of hu-man muscles, *J Appl Physiol* 36:475, 1974.

3. Bouisett S: EMG and muscle force in normal motor activities. In *New development in electromyography and clinical neurophysiology*, New York, 1973, Kager.

4. Crosby PA: Use of surface electromyogram as a measure of dynamic force in human limb muscles, *Med & Comp*: 519, September 1978.

5. De Luca CJ: Physiology and mathematics of myoelectric signals, *IEEE Trans Biomed Eng* 26(6): 1979.

6. DeLuca CJ: A model for a motor unit train recorded during constant force isometric contractions, *Biol Cybern* 19:159, 1975.

7. DeLuca CJ, Forrest WJ: Probability distribution function of the inter-pulse intervals of single motor unit action potentials during isometric contraction. In *New development in electromyography and clinical neurophysiology*, vol 1, Basel, Switzerland, 1973, Karger.

8. DeLuca CJ: Myoelectric analysis of isometric contractions of the human biceps brachii (Master's Thesis), University of New Brunswick, Fredricton, New Brunswick, Canada, 1968.

9. DeLuca CJ, Sabbahi MA, Stulen FB et al: Some properties of the median frequency of the myoelectric signal during localized fatigue. In Knuttgen HK et al: *Biochemistry of exercise*, vol 13, 1983.

10. Doerschuk PC, Gustafson DE, Wilsky AS: Upper extremity limb function discrimination using EMG signal analysis, *IEEE Trans Biomed Eng* 30(1):18, 1983.

11. Ekstedt J: Human single muscle fiber action potentials, *Acta Physiol Scand* 61(suppl 226): 1964.

12. Evans H, Pan F, Parker P et al: Signal processing for proportional myoelectric control, *IEEE Trans Biomed Eng* 31:207, February 1984.

13. Fullmer RR, Meek SG, Jacobsen SC: Optimization of an adaptive myoelectric filter, *Proc. 6th Annual Conference IEEE EMBS*, Los Angeles, September 1984.

14. Gans C: *Biomechanics: approach to vertebrate biology*, Ann Arbor, 1980, University of Michigan Press.

15. Hill AV: Production and absorption of work by muscle, *Science* 131:897, 1960.

16. Hoff AL, van der Berg JW: EMG to force processing (Parts I-IV), *J Biomech* 14(11):747, 1981.

17. Hoff AL, van der Berg JW: Linearity between weighted sum of the EMGs of the human triceps surae and the total torque, *J Biomech* 10:529, 1977.

18. Hogan N: A review of the methods of processing EMG for use as a proportional control signal, *Biomed Eng* 10:81, March 1976.

19. Hogan N, Mann R: Myoelectric signal processing: optimal estimation applied to electromyography. Part I: Derivation of the optimal myoprocessor, *IEEE Trans Biomed Eng* 27(7):382, 1980.

20. Hogan N, Mann R: Myoelectric signal processing: optimal estimation applied to electromyography. Part II: Experimental demonstration of optimal myoprocessor performance, *IEEE Trans Biomed Eng* 27(7):396, 1980.

21. Inman VT, Ralston HJ, Saunders J et al: Relation of human electromyogram to muscular tension: electroencephalogram, *Clin Neurophysiol* 4:187, 1952.

22. Kadefors R: Myoelectric signal processing as an estimation problem. In *New developments in electromyography and clinical neurophysiology*, New York, 1973, Karger.

23. Kandel ER, Schwartz JH: Motor systems of the brain: reflex and voluntary control of movement. In *Principles of neural science*, New York, 1985, Elsevier.

24. Kouri PV: Relationship between muscle tension, EMG and velocity of contraction under concentric and eccentric work. In Desmedt JE: *New Development in electromyography and clinical neurophysiology*, Basel, Switzerland, 1973, Karger.

25. Kriefeldt JG: Signal versus noise characteristics of filtered EMG used as a control source, *IEEE Trans Biomed Eng* 18(1):1971.

26. Kwanty E, Thomas DH, Kwanty HE: An application of signal processing techniques to the study of myoelectric signals, *IEEE Trans Biomed Eng* 17(4): 303, 1970.

27. Loeb GE, Gans C: *Electromyography for experimentalists*, Chicago, 1986, University of Chicago Press.

28. Stein RB: *Nerve and muscle*, New York, 1980, Plenum Press.

29. Woods JJ, Bigland-Ritchie B: Linear and non-linear surface EMG/force relationships in human muscles, *Am J Phys Med* 62(6):287, 1983.

30. Hillstrom HJ, Moskowitz GD: Robust intent recognition for prosthetic control. Proceedings of 14th Annual International Conference IEEE. *Engineering in Medicine and Biology Society* 1448-1449, 1992.

CHAPTER 21

EMG METHODOLOGY

Gary L. Soderberg
Loretta M. Knutson

KEY TERMS

Artifact

Crosstalk

Data average

EMG amplitude

EMG timing

Filtering

Preamplification

Rectification

Reliability

Sampling rate

Telemetry

This chapter presents methodologic considerations and recording techniques for the electromyogram (EMG) derived during gait. A section on data presentation and interpretation follows. Examples and citations are included to facilitate understanding of how various factors influence the data collection and interpretation. For more detailed discussion of the theoretical basis for the systems described in this chapter, refer to the preceding chapter by Hillstrom and Triolo.

METHODOLOGICAL CONSIDERATIONS

The EMG during gait can be derived for a number of purposes and with a wide variety of methods. Several factors of general nature should be considered prior to the actual collection of the data of interest. These considerations are the purpose and intent of the work, whether to use a cabled system or telemetry, and what system is to be used for the collection of the data. The following sections address each of these considerations.

Purpose and Intent

Gait has been the focus of a wide variety of studies. The EMG, as the electrical record of the activation of muscle, has been used during many investigations and reported in reviews[3] and texts.[42] Questions of central nervous system (CNS) control are addressed by evaluating the temporal sequencing of the recorded activity.[21,29,36,41] Association of the EMG data with biomechanical parameters of interest, such as muscle force, has also been attempted.[34,48,49] Normalcy of gait pattern for different age groups has also been described with EMG data.[35,45] Furthermore, differentiation of normal from pathological motion has been attempted.[9,19] However, few studies have been published regarding the efficacy of treatments designed to alter functions such as human gait.[18] In each case EMG data have served a useful purpose within the constraints associated with the technique.

The assessment of the appropriateness of the EMG should be focused on the intention of the application. Such a decision will at least, if not directly, determine whether a surface or an indwelling technique is used. Criteria associated with each electrode type will be discussed in later sections of this chapter.

Cabling versus Telemetry

Another factor to consider in assessing completed studies or when considering completing a study using gait in which the EMG is included is whether to use telemetry or a system using cabling. When purchasing equipment to initiate recording of the EMG, a thorough analysis of the available systems is necessary. The primary advantage associated with telemetry is the freedom from encumbrance. There are, however, disadvantages, including the ability to modify the number of channels, the gain of the instrumentation, and the transmitting range. These are discussed in the volume by Loeb and Gans[30] and in a NIOSH manual.[44] Note that these techniques have successfully been used in evaluating activities such as locomotion.[4,5]

Should cabling be chosen, the use of preamplifying electrodes is highly recommended for purposes of controlling or eliminating the artifacts discussed in later sections of this chapter.[43,44] The key factor for anyone analyzing and interpreting the gait literature, regardless of which of these techniques are used, is to ascertain that the work includes EMG collected by appropriate procedures and results in high-quality data.

Data Collection Technique

Previous studies of gait inclusive of EMG have primarily used hardware systems including graphic, FM, and digital recorders. The classic form of recorder is considered inadequate for the recording of EMG data because the response frequency is rarely greater than 60 Hz. Demodulated data, such as the root mean square (RMS), can be adequately recorded but the user needs to be sure that the raw information is free of artifacts. Other graphic systems such as light beam and thermal recorders have appropriate response rates but there are potential limitations on control of paper speed. For all these graphic forms, interpretation is limited to the visual examination of the data from the record produced.

Other recording systems, such as the FM and digital recorders are considered more desirable because of the improved response rate and the ability to reevaluate unmarked data on any occasion. Signal-to-noise ratios can be problematic, as can overall size of storage capability.[44] More recently, sophisticated software has become available, allowing for online collection and subsequent analysis of data without the superimposition of other devices. Online collection may be limited in ability to record large quantities of data sampled over relatively large intervals at high sampling rates, but there are a number of techniques that can be used effectively for recording multiple-channel data from multiple muscles over numerous gait cycles. Examples of data presentation from each of these techniques will be given throughout this chapter. The key factor in determining the quality of the data is whether the collection and analysis techniques produce an accurate record. The standards specified in the previous chapter should be upheld.

RECORDING TECHNIQUE

Surface

The surface electrode is the most common type of electrode used in gait studies. These electrodes are of various configurations but usually comprise a disk composed of silver-silver chloride. The size of these circular-shaped disks varies from 1 mm to about 5 mm in diameter. Selection of the size of the electrode will depend on the muscle or muscles to be studied. The usual rule is that the smaller the muscle the smaller the electrode diameter, but there are no stringent requirements or published rules. The disks are usually encircled by Teflon or similar material that serves as a mechanism to affix the electrode to the skin surface by means of a doubled-sided washer or adhesive collar. In some cases, the electrodes have been mounted into a lightweight housing containing instrumentation that will amplify the signal close to the site of the electrode pickup. These electrodes, commercially available, are often referred to as preamplifiers because the EMG is amplified prior to being cabled to the main amplifier.

Applications and Limitations   Surface electrodes, generally easy to obtain, apply, and use, provide a more general representation of muscle activity. Their ability to record the performance of small muscles or muscles located deep in the body—such as the tibialis posterior, vastus intermedius, the brachialis and the intrinsic muscles of the hand—is limited. Often, surface EMG is most appropriate because information about specific muscles or deep muscles is not required. However, in many circumstances the issue of cross talk is not adequately considered.[31] Cross talk occurs when signals from muscles other than those being investigated are recorded at the electrode site through volume conduction.[28] Such instances can lead to inaccurate data and subsequent erroneous interpretations. Thus, because most EMG applications in gait use surface electrodes, both the user and the consumer need to consider the possibility of contaminated records as a result of cross talk.

Use of preamplifying electrodes has become more popular with the onset of better technology and methods of electrode fabrication. While the size of the electrode increases the mass of the on-site electrode, a major advantage of preamplification is that the signal will likely be free of the unwanted artifacts. In addition, preparation of the electrode site only requires a wiping with denatured alcohol as compared with a sanding or abrading of the skin and the alcohol wipe usually required by the more conventional surface electrode.

The assessment of any literature dealing with this topic should ascertain that the authors have taken adequate steps to assure the quality of the data by maintaining the necessary instrumentation standards while at the same time avoiding artifacts.

Indwelling

Recording the EMG during gait with indwelling electrodes has been performed only in limited situations. Primary applications include basic and clinical studies assessing preoperative function of muscle during gait and for those cases when the muscles of interest are only accessible by indwelling electrode. An example of the latter would be a study of the function of the posterior tibialis muscle during gait.[37]

Applications and Limitations   Use of the indwelling electrode has the advantage of minimizing or eliminating issues associated with cross talk, but raises the question of whether the sampling area is representative of the whole muscle function. Discussion of this issue will probably continue into the foreseeable future, with little immediate resolution. Given the correct equipment—primarily preamplifying electrodes—and a suitable connection technique for the fine wires once inserted into muscle, the method is very manageable. Artifacts may be more likely to develop with indwelling electrodes. The connectors between the electrodes and the amplifiers often expose the conducting wire to the environment. This poor connection increases susceptibility to noise and artifact in comparison to surface electrode and preamplifier connections.

Site Selection

Despite the relatively long-term use of EMG by clinicians and investigators in a wide variety of disciplines, little information is available in the literature as to the preferred location for electrodes. When fine wire insertions are desired or necessary the electrode can be placed directly in the belly of the muscle of interest for diagnostic EMG.[14] For the surface EMG, however, the decision as to where to put the electrode is less clear.

Some have advocated the use of the site where the muscle can be the most easily stimulated (motor point) on the basis that the maximum amplitude of potentials will be located there. Basmajian and DeLuca, however, state that this location will not yield the greatest signal amplitude.[6] Rather, they suggest an interelectrode-surface spacing of 1 cm for surface electrodes because this spacing is "compatible with the architecture of most muscles in the human body."[6]

Some electromyographers have suggested specific anatomic locations for electrodes. Davis did so in a now antiquated government document.[13] More recently selected locations have been specified by Zipp.[56] Most of the figures from this latter work include a mechanism for body dimension normalization, a technique judged to be desirable. With consideration given to issues of signal-to-noise ratio, stability (reliability and cross talk), and a presentation of selected data relative to EMG output, Basmajian and DeLuca state that the preferred location of an electrode is approximately halfway between the center of the innervation zone and the further tendon.[6] More specific guidelines have been provided by Loeb and Gans, but their experience is more with animal studies than with human locomotion.[30]

In fact, few studies using the EMG in gait have attended to any specific selection criteria for either surface or indwelling electrode recording sites. Regardless, numerous techniques are available to validate or verify the electrode location. This process is often overlooked on the basis that the surface electrode will record from the area beneath the electrode. For the indwelling electrode if the technique is accurate there should be no need for verification because there would be no other possibility of signal generation from other than the muscle impaled. Most investigators, however, space individual surface electrodes at distances they have determined—using clinical, surface, and applied anatomy—will record from the volume of muscle of interest. Thus, interelectrode distances will vary between studies. In cases where electrodes are permanently mounted in a preamplifying electrode, the interelectrode distance is fixed and the recording area is assumed to be suitable. In summary no standards are available. Both the user and consumer need to make judgments to assess the validity of the signals generated.

Artifacts

To have ideal valid recording, the data must contain no artifacts. There are several major types of artifacts. Mechanically induced artifacts are common and occur when cables are handled or allowed to move when the subject is active. Changes may also be seen with electrode movement occurring between the skin and electrode interface. These artifacts are usually of low frequency (see Figure 21-1A). Another artifact that can be a major problem is 60-cycle (Hz) interference (Figure 21-1B). This occurs when a reference electrode is not applied appropriately on the subject, when a wire is loose, or when electrical fields persist. The latter can come from improper shielding of wires. If 60-cycle interference (50 cycle in some countries) continues to be a problem in recording, attention should be paid to the environment, including grounding of all outlets and evaluation of equipment in use in adjacent areas. Another important artifact the electromyographer needs to be aware of is that produced through the electrocardiogram, which is particularly noticeable over the lumbar portion of the erector spinae muscles and in certain other muscles such as the gluteus medius (Figure 21-1C).

To eliminate artifacts an optimal design that will minimize electrode impedance is advised. In addition, high-quality instrumentation is essential—including a differential amplifier with a high common-mode rejection ratio. Further, an adequate reference electrode and the minimization of the number of devices concurrently collecting data help to avoid ground loops. The use of battery-driven equipment is also recommended,[30] as is the continuous monitoring of the raw signal, usually by means of an oscilloscope.

Reliability and Validity

Considering the number of factors influencing the information content of the EMG during gait, one needs to prudently question the reliability of information obtained. The principles, as cited in the chapter by Strube and DeLitto, apply to the EMG measurements made during gait as well. Fortunately, many of the studies are performed only once on a given day, minimizing the impact of issues of reliability. Many factors can be controlled, particularly if surface electrodes are used. The size and type of the electrode, the preparation of the recording site, the interelectrode spacing, and the standardized location of electrodes relative to anatomical landmarks are all factors that may be controlled to improve the reliability of the measure. Anatomical variation within and between sexes and inconsistencies due to motivation are more difficult to assess and control.

The reliability of each available method is an important factor in investigating muscle function

FIGURE 21-1 Common artifacts encountered during EMG recordings: **A,** Low frequency shift caused by cable or electrode movement; **B,** 60 Hz; **C,** EKG.

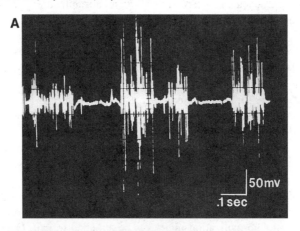

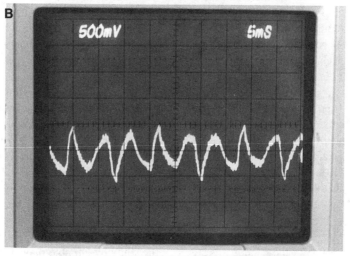

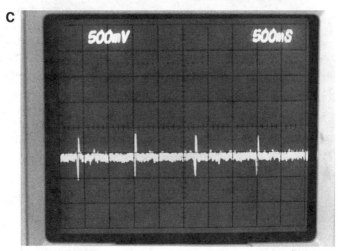

during gait. In general, across-channel (muscle) comparisons are precluded because of differences in instrumentation and constituencies of body tissues from one recording area to another. Between-subject comparisons are also precluded on the basis of individual differences and subcutaneous fat, muscle geometry, and other variances. In many instances, therefore, a normalization process should be completed to allow for comparisons. Frequently, both clinicians and investigators have used the recording of EMG during a maximum voluntary contraction and conversion of the values recorded during the test or procedure to a percentage of the EMG produced during the maximum voluntary contraction. Individual variations that preclude direct comparisons, thus, can be taken into account. The criterion for normalization may need to be reconsidered in some cases—for example, when the patient with cerebral palsy cannot effectively generate maximum voluntary efforts. The chapter by Knutson and Soderberg in this volume contains a more complete discussion of this issue.

Despite the early application of EMG in the study of normal patterns[17,23] and extensive use of EMG for the last several decades, little work has been completed that examines reliability. Kadaba et al. have shown that the variance ratio can be used to demonstrate that surface electrode recordings produce higher reliability than those from fine wire electrodes for cycle-to-cycle, run-to-run, and day-to-day comparisons.[25] In a follow-up study on other normal subjects, some of these same investigators found that repeatability within a day, as measured by a "coefficient of multiple correlation," was slightly better than between test days.[24] Two studies of relevance were reported by Arsenault in the same year. One addressed the issue of the number of strides required for the analysis of EMG data in gait. Normal subjects were used for the study of five lower extremity muscles. Results of the within-day reliability analysis produced intraclass correlation coefficients (ICCs) of .96 to .99 for three strides for three subjects and .99 and above for ten strides for eight subjects.[5] The second of the studies assessed the existence of the normal profile of EMG activity during gait. This work also reported within-day reliability for eight healthy subjects, noting ICCs of .84 to .99, depending on which of the five muscles is considered. The authors did note that statistically significant differences existed in amplitude of activity across subjects for all muscles.[4] Winter and Yack followed with a 1987 report on EMG patterns for 16 muscles, providing a detailed report of the

variability between subjects.[50] Results indicated, through use of the coefficient of variation (CV), that normalization reduces variability and that some muscles are more variable than others. Use of the CV and other measures to report repeatability have added some confusion to data interpretation, and users of EMG as a measure during gait should be cognizant of the meaning of the various statistics that can be applied. (Review of Chapter 22 by Knutsson and Soderberg is advised relative to these issues.)

Often, numerous assumptions are made regarding such issues as selectivity of recording, artifacts, and cross talk, and frequently the lack of these considerations brings some doubts to the credibility of the work and the meaning that may be attached to gait. One study that can be used as an example did not use gait as the activity performed. However, the issue of reliability in determining the onset of muscle activity via surface EMG was evaluated by means of perturbing the standing posture. In this paper DiFabio demonstrated differences in determinations of times of onset of muscle activity when examiner's visual judgments are compared to a computerized analysis system.[15] The author makes the point about the need for visual determinations for purposes of validity and indicates the utility of the computerized system for the reliability component of the EMG analysis. Because EMG data from studies or trials involving gait are most frequently judged in terms of onset and amplitude, implications from the study by DiFabio may apply to EMG measurements derived during gait.

In some instances studies have compared results from data collected simultaneously with surface and fine wire electrodes.[20,25,55] Only the study by Kadaba was performed during gait, indicating that cycle-to-cycle and run-to-run reproducibility were better for the surface electrodes than for the fine wire electrodes. Day-to-day measures were considered good only for surface electrodes and poor for the fine wire electrodes.

DATA PRESENTATION AND INTERPRETATION: FACTORS INFLUENCING EMG DATA

Hardware Considerations and Instrumentation Characteristics

Standards for instrumentation characteristics have been suggested by the International Society of Electrophysiologic Kinesiology.[47] Despite existence of standards, a variety of hardware and software systems are employed by investigators. This situation, in addition to varied processing methods, have made comparisons across studies difficult. Furthermore, the time is right for reviewing and embellishing the standards in light of the changes that have occurred in computers and software programs in recent years.

Selection of a method for managing data requires that the electromyographer consider alternatives relative to the hardware used to manage the data. Decisions will relate to the type of filter, the number of poles to be used in a filter, the time constants in the smoothing element, and the data sampling frequency. Each of these have an effect on the data and can lead to data distortions and subsequently alter interpretations applied to either temporal or amplitude features.[22,26] Any article reporting EMG methodology should adequately specify the hardware characteristics so the reader can determine suitability of the chosen instruments. Texts such as those by Basmajian and DeLuca,[6] Loeb and Gans,[30] and the NIOSH manual[44] are all helpful resources in elucidating the characteristics associated with each component.

Sampling Rate

The sampling rate is the frequency with which data is accepted by the analog-to-digital converter, the A-to-D board, which is usually housed within the computer. Sampling an analog EMG signal collected using surface electrodes is probably satisfactory between 500 to 1000 Hz. Sampling the analog EMG signal collected using fine wire electrodes should employ a higher rate of 1000 to 2000 Hz. These guidelines are influenced by the work of Winter whose published plot of the frequency spectrum of EMG signals is reprinted in Figure 21-2. The frequency spectral density for surface electrodes is lower than that for fine wire electrodes. In general, researchers follow these guidelines to select the sampling rate employed.

Data sampled at 1000 Hz (samples per second) for a gait cycle that was 1 second in duration would provide 1000 data points—that is, 1000 voltage values. For a 1.2 second gait cycle, 1200 data points would be collected. If the sampling rate is doubled, 2000 Hz, the number of data points doubles (2000 for a 1 second gait cycle and 2400 for a 1.2 second gait cycle.)

Averaging Data

Because of the large number of values collected, it is frequently desirable to select points in the cycle and retain values at these points for the analysis, (e.g., averaging several gait cycles). The fewer the points used (e.g., every 10% of the gait cycle), the smoother the EMG signal over the course of the

FIGURE 21-2 Frequency spectrum of EMG as recorded via surface and indwelling electrodes. Higher frequency content of indwelling electrodes is due to closer spacing between electrodes. From Winter DA: *Biomechanics and motor control of human movement,* New York, 1979. J. Wiley and Sons.

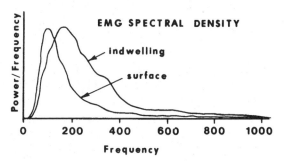

gait cycle. On the other hand, many points fail to smooth the curve and the original appearance of the signal is retained. Selecting values at each 5% increment results in 20 data points across the 100% gait cycle. If the data were sampled at 1000 Hz this approximates the 6 Hz analog filter (managed within the hardware), which creates the linear envelope of the signal as recommended by Winter.[51] A signal smoothed with a 50 msec time constant creates a similar effect. In a digital format the ideal situation is not to select points at each 5% increment of the gait cycle but rather to apply a moving window averager that averages all values within the interval rather than averaging an absolute time period. With data that is time normalized, the number of values in this interval will obviously vary as a function of the varying gait cycle durations.

Number of Repetitions

When EMG signals were first gathered and analyzed, researchers focused on the raw record for one trial that contained three to eight gait cycles. Variations from cycle to cycle were described, if observed. With the introduction of computers, procedures emerged that allowed the cycles to be averaged. While averaging removes individual cycle traits that may be of interest, the average is favored as being a more valid representation of performance than random or arbitrary selection of one gait cycle. The question arises, however, as to how many cycles are needed to form the average. Arsenault et al. found in adult normal subjects an average of three gait cycles was as satisfactory as 12 cycles.[5]

Data Management Considerations

Management of EMG data can be done using either an unprocessed (raw form) or a processed version of the signal. "Scoring" of the contraction intensity or quantification of the raw signal has limited utility, which is probably a primary reason why many electromyographers decline to use this form. Some software programs are now available that allow the computer screen to simulate the oscilloscope function of immediate monitoring.

Most often, EMG users will select some form of signal processing. Rectification is frequently selected because this procedure will allow the data to be numerically manipulated. While half-wave rectification has been done, literature citations that document this procedure are uncommon. Its use is extremely limited because this process would essentially eliminate one half of the usable data available for analysis. The literature much more commonly includes full-wave rectified data. Examples of this technique can be found in a number of works.* Whether data processing in addition to full-wave rectification is completed depends on the study purpose and the intent of the electromyographer. An important aspect is the effect of the smoothing process because if the smoothing or integration is too great, some characteristics of the muscle's activity during gait may be lost. In spite of this effect, rectification followed by smoothing are the most common forms of processing.[52]

Software Programs for Data Analysis

Software programs were written on large minicomputers in the early to mid-1970s for use in analyzing biological signals. A majority of these programs were lab specific; however, by the early 1980s software programs were available on the PDP 11 and the Apple II. With the advent of more powerful computers in the mid-1980s—specifically the IBM XT, and later other IBM personal computers and IBM clones—more powerful and research-specific commercial software systems became more widely available. Some programs are written to accompany specific hardware systems whereas others are configured to manage a variety of biological signals, including the flexibility to work with most EMG hardware systems.

Methods of Data Analysis

Variations in the technique of analyzing EMG data abound. Use of EMG data collected and evaluated in the clinical setting is relatively unusual but several systems purport to be applicable to the clinical environment. The simplest and probably the most common is the biofeedback form, where the signal can be directed back to the client either visually or via an audio amplifier. The latter is the most appropriate during gait but the limitation is that only one channel can be "fed back" at one time. Usually complicating the clinical situation is that the patient is also concentrating on other issues, such as balance, degree of load bearing, and equality of swing and stance times and distances. Thus, clients are most frequently evaluated in a specialized laboratory facility with the capability for multichannel EMG data collection and the more complex analyses desired.

The two parameters of interest from the EMG data are the timing and amplitude of the muscle activity. Timing is judged by the onset and cessation of activity as discussed in this chapter. Changes in these times relative to normal are considered to be alterations or errors in the timing of the contraction. Perry has described these deviations as follows:

> **Premature.** Action begins before the normal onset
> **Prolonged.** Action continues beyond the normal cessation
> **Continuous.** EMG uninterrupted for 90% or more of gait cycle
> **Curtailed.** Early termination of the EMG
> **Delayed.** Onset later than normal
> **Absent.** EMG of insufficient amplitude or duration
> **Out of phase.** Swing or stance time reversed.[37]

These descriptors help distinguish the deviation from normal and provide the clinician with information that may suggest how the client is treated.

Difficulty arises with the judgment surrounding the onset and termination of the EMG. Essentially two choices—visual (subjective) and quantitative (objective)—are available. The visual approach requires only the EMG record of interest, displayed either in hard copy or via an instrument such as an oscilloscope or video display terminal (VDT). An example of a hard copy record is shown in Figure 21-3. Such records are used in some centers for determining onset for muscles in a more gross sense, (i.e., without a precise time of onset and termination of EMG activity). For making clinical decisions this form of analysis is likely sufficient; however, these decisions are somewhat dependent on the gain of the amplification system.

---

* Refer to the following sources: 10, 39, 40, 52, 53, 54.

FIGURE 21-3   Example of raw EMG collected during gait. Tibialis anterior muscle activity, the top trace, and gastrocnemius muscle activity, the middle trace, were recorded with surface electrodes. The posterior tibialis muscle activity, the lowest trace, was recorded via a fine wire electrode. Footswitch showing stance (downward deflection) and swing is also shown. Voltage units are shown for each channel and vary to accommodate for appropriate scaling.

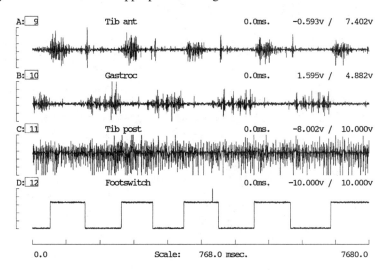

More quantitative approaches are reported in the literature, but even when quantitative techniques are used operational definitions of the EMG must be established. Perry has indicated that the EMG from 5% of the maximal contractile effort registered on a manual muscle test was an appropriate threshold.[37] DiFabio, in a balance study, used a sliding window that searched for the first set of 25 data points that exceeded three standard deviations of the current mean baseline values.[15] Another possibility is to use some value of the raw or processed EMG signal in order to make a determination of onset and termination of activity. One option is to use plus or minus 2 or 3 standard deviations above the quietest portion of the EMG record obtained during a dynamic activity. This situation may be problematic, however, when subjects display consistently high levels of EMG during the activity under study. Winter has been among those who have shown differences in onsets and durations of EMG due to the selection of differing threshold values of the raw signal.[53] Ten, 20, and 30 microvolt levels were used for six different subjects to show how phasic patterns would differ for the rectus femoris muscle.

Numerous reports in the literature, while addressing the normal pattern of activity (Figure 21-4), do not assist the reader with making interpretations associated with temporal events.[16,50] While these authors provide averages of the EMG profiles, no information is given about when the muscle should be considered as active or inactive.

Figure 21-5 also provides an example of potential difficulties associated with on-off determinations during gait. In this case the raw signal has been full-wave rectified and passed through a 50 millisecond time constant. Selecting the time for the onset and cessation of EMG activity would be difficult. Indeed, this figure suggests that these three muscles are active throughout the gait cycle. Numerous works have identified the influence of the technique for signal processing.[26,44]

Objective criteria for determining activation time have been used under more static test conditions when response to a stimulus is the focus of study. For example, Nashner describes the use of a baseline derived from the 100 millisecond time period prior to the introduction of a postural perturbation as a criterion of muscle activation.[32] An increase in EMG amplitude of more than 1½ standard deviations from the baseline is called "on." One alternative for the dynamic condition of gait has been used whereby the EMG taken during resting serves as a baseline, and signals 2 or 3 standard deviations above resting level were considered "on."[46] This reportedly compared well against another criterion of 5% of peak.

Chong and investigators reported summary EMG data on gait at each year of age in ten children 4 to 16 years old with hip internal rotation associated with cerebral palsy.[11] No designation of criteria to determine onset or offset of myoelectric events recorded from the surface electrodes on four muscles in normal or cerebral palsy

Figure 21-4   EMG of rectus femorii and hamstrings. An EMG record for right rectus femoris, right hamstrings, left rectus femoris, and left hamstrings (top to bottom). Raw signal has been full-wave rectified and subjected to smoothing by a 50 millisecond time constant.

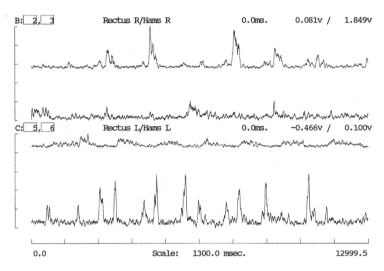

subjects was given, and reports were limited to temporal representations of typical cases. The normal medial hamstring activity shown and described for a 9-year-old was active towards the end of swing and during the initial one third of stance. The apparent use by Chong et al. of visual analysis to judge EMG phasic activity in muscles during gait is typical of a majority of reports in the literature.

In 1979, Csongradi et al. reported temporal EMG data from surface recordings of rectus femoris, vastus medialis, and medial hamstrings in normal and spasticity children.[12] They reported two patterns of medial hamstring activity in their 26 normal subjects. A majority showed a single burst of activity beginning in late swing and ending in mid-stance. From the authors' report, activity was seen for a continuous time period from about 84 to 100% and 0 to 24% of the gait cycle. Five of the normal subjects had a second burst of EMG. In these children, the figure suggested the first burst of activity occurred between 90 to 100% and 0 to 12%, and the second burst at 46 to 56%. Again, these researchers apparently used visual inspection to judge on and off.

At this point there is no collective agreement as to the criterion for determination of initiation or termination of muscle activity. Perry, however, indicates that the timing of normal is 1 standard deviation from the mean.[37] No rationale or statistics are applied to support this statement. Factors taken into consideration include signal processing/instrumentation characteristics, intent of the study,

and application for the data collected. The fact that the decisions made will continue to vary compounds the interpretation of the reports and limits comparisons between the investigators or clinicians completing the work.

Similar difficulties exist in the analysis of amplitude data. Comparisons within and between muscles are of data normalized to some magnitude of reference contraction or standard as discussed earlier in this chapter. The significance of the differences in the amplitudes are frequently left for reader interpretation. Winter has published profiles of muscular activity for selected muscles during gait (see Figure 21-6) showing mean EMG signals in microvolts along with ± 1 standard deviation.[50] The suggestion is made that these data can be used in the diagnostic process.

Little utility can be gained in considering the on/off information without consideration for the amplitude and differences in the patterns of EMG evoked during an activity such as gait. Note in Figure 21-7 that the initiation and termination of muscle activity is precisely the same according to the selected threshold. However, the level of activity varies greatly over the interval in which the muscle would be labeled as active. Even though the timing of the activity is the same for all three examples, the amplitudes vary significantly over the duration of this same interval. Consideration of both the duration and amplitude are therefore important to the understanding of the information derived by EMG. In fact, DiFabio cites the need to use visual verification for purposes of validating

FIGURE 21-5 EMG data of rectus femoris. Processed EMG data averaged over several cycles for three different groups of patients for the rectus femoris muscle. From Sojka A: Variations in the kinematic, temporal-distance and electromyographic characteristics of children with cerebral palsy who exhibit genu recurvatum (Master's thesis), University of Nebraska, Lincoln 1993, 52.

FIGURE 21-6 EMG profiles. Ensemble average of EMG profiles from 15 strides for a typical normal subject. Solid line is the average EMG at each 5% of the stride period, the dotted line indicates ± 1 SD. The coefficient of variation (CV) is indicated for each muscle. The mean cadence for the 15 strides was 114, ± 2. From Winter DA, Yack HJ: *Electroencephalogr Clin Neurophysiol* 67:402, 1987.

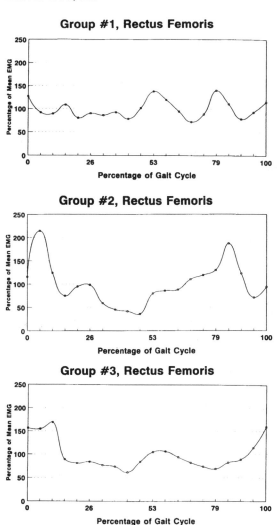

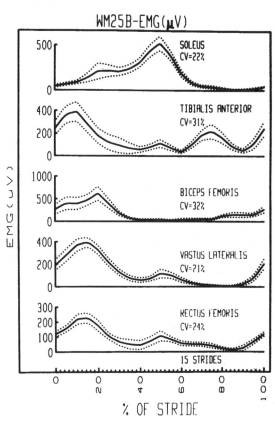

muscle onsets determined by objectified methods.[15] In two studies, Bogey et al., have used both temporal and amplitude factors.[7,8]

Regardless of whether temporal, amplitude, or both determinations are made from the EMG data there will often be a need to normalize these data to account for discrepancies in cycle times. Figure 21-8 shows results from a gait trial of a patient with knee pathology. The footswitch, indicating the difference between stance and swing phases, shows the variability in the cycle time, i.e., from one heel strike to the next. To accommodate for this variation a procedure should be used to normalize the time from one heel strike to the next (or other corollary points in the gait cycle) to 100%. Then, EMG data can be considered representative, assuming that a number of trials are averaged for reasons of producing a more representative data set. With systems available for computerized collection of EMG data, this process of normalization is rather simple when compared to the limitations of the visual analysis.

EMG signals derived during gait are evaluated in either a raw or processed form. Maintaining the file of the raw data is advantageous because of the opportunity for retrieval. Assessment of this record is limited to visual analysis, about which judgments of onset, termination, and amplitude can be

FIGURE 21-7   EMG vs. percentage of gait cycle time. EMG, in arbitrary units, plotted versus the percent of gait cycle time. Threshold level for determining the onset and termination of muscle activity is shown for three patterns of muscle activity that occurred during the gait cycle.

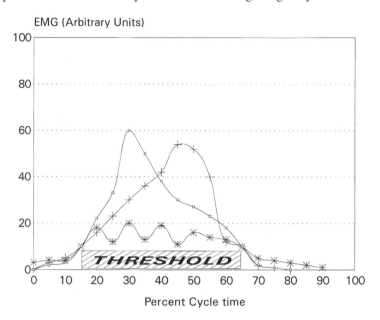

FIGURE 21-8   EMG data and footswitch. Record showing footswitch that designates stance (downward deflection) and swing phases of gait. Raw EMG records are for muscles right rectus femoris, right hamstrings, right gluteus medius, left rectus femoris, left hamstrings, and left gluteus medius muscles from top to bottom. Voltage units shown for each channel vary to accommodate for appropriate scaling.

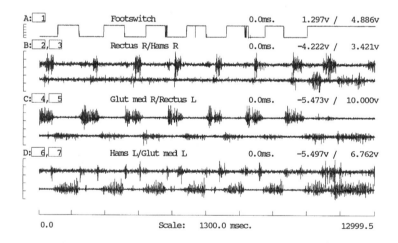

made. Adler et al. and Rose, Oonpuu, and DeLuca provide examples of this type of analysis.[1,38] Clinically this method has some advantages, particularly in that expense for software and the time for personnel to reduce data is minimized, and decisions can be made immediately as to the recommended course of treatment. The potential for incorrect decisions is higher, however, without completing more objective analyses over a number of gait cycles.

The most common data analysis technique yields a processed form of the EMG data. Of the processing techniques available for EMG data the ensemble average has been used to describe the pattern of EMG for subjects considered normal. This method includes full-wave rectification and low-pass filtering of the signal before the averaging of multiple trials is completed.* Output is

*See references 2,4,5,33,45,50,53.

typically an analog curve for the specified number of gait cycles, with some indication of the variability such as the standard error (Figure 21-6). Other forms of signal analysis are also available, including full-wave rectification followed by smoothing by a time constant.[25,27] An example of a full-wave rectified signal followed by a 50 millisecond time constant was shown in Figure 21-4. Any of these forms are acceptable for determining timing and amplitude variations of the EMG signal during gait. Decisions associated with the selection of instrumentation characteristics are most frequently a function of the purpose of the work and availability of equipment within the facility.

SUMMARY

This chapter has presented information about how EMG assists our understanding of gait. Many factors influence the collection and interpretation of the information, but none of these factors negate our ability to use this information for patient assessment and treatment. While presently underutilized in practice, the EMG can enrich our knowledge of muscle function and may, in fact, guide the clinician to even more effective patient care.

REFERENCES

1. Adler N, Bleck EE, Rinsky LA: Gait electromyograms and surgical decisions for paralytic deformities of the foot, *Dev Med Child Neurol* 31:287, 1989.
2. Arendt-Nielsen L et al: Electromyographic patterns and knee joint kinematics during walking at various speeds, *J Electromyogr Kinesiol* 1:89, 1991.
3. Arsenault AB, Winter DA, Marteniuk RG: Characteristics of muscular function and adaptation in gait: a literature review, *Physiother Canada* 39:5, 1987.
4. Arsenault AB, Winter DA, Marteniuk RG: Is there a "normal" profile of EMG activity in gait? *Med Biol Eng Comput* 24:337, 1986.
5. Arsenault AB et al: How many strides are required for the analysis of electromyographic data in gait? *Scand J Rehabil Med* 18:133, 1986.
6. Basmajian JV, DeLuca CJ: *Muscles alive: their function revealed by electromyography,* ed 5, Baltimore, 1985, Williams & Wilkins.
7. Bogey RA, Barnes LA, Perry J: Computer algorithms to characterize individual subject EMG profiles during gait, *Arch Phys Med Rehabil* 73:835, 1992.
8. Bogey RA, Barnes LA, Perry J: A computer algorithm for defing the group electromyographic profile from individual gait profiles, *Arch Phys Med Rehabil* 74:286, 1993.
9. Cahan LD et al: Instrumented gait analysis after selective dorsal rhizotomy, *Dev Med Child Neurol* 32:1037, 1990.
10. Chen, JJ, Shiavi R: Temporal feature extraction and clustering analysis of electromyographic linear envelopes in gait studies, *IEEE Trans Biomed Eng* 37:295, 1990.
11. Chong KC et al: The assessment of the internal rotation gait in cerebral palsy, *Clin Orthol Rel Res* 132:145, 1978.
12. Csongradi J, Bleck E, Ford FW: Gait electromyography in normal and spastic children, with special reference to quadriceps femoris and hamstring muscles, *Dev Med Child Neurol* 21:738, 1979.
13. Davis JF: *Manual of surface electromyography,* WADC Technical Report No. 59-184, 1959.
14. Delagi EF et al: *Anatomic guide for the electromyographer,* Springfield, Ill, 1975, C. C. Thomas.
15. DiFabio RP: Reliability of computerized surface electromyography for determining the onset of muscle activity, *Phys Ther* 67:43, 1987.
16. Dubo HI et al: Electromyographic temporal analysis of gait: normal human locomotion, *Arch Phys Med Rehabil* 57:415, 1976.
17. Eberhart HD, Inman VT, Bresler B: The principal elements in human locomotion. In Klopsteg PR, Wilson PD, editors: *Human limbs and their substitutes,* New York, 1954, Hafner Publishing Co.
18. Etnyre B et al: Preoperative and postoperative assessment of surgical intervention for equinus gait in children with cerebral palsy, *J Pediatr Orthop* 13:24, 1993.
19. Fung J, Barbeau H: A dynamic EMG profile index to quantify muscular activation disorder in spastic paretic gait, *Electroencephalogr Clin Neurophysiol* 73:233, 1989.
20. Giroux B, Lamontagne M: Comparisons between surface electrodes and intramuscular wire electrodes in isometric and dynamic conditions, *Electromyogr Clin Neurophysiol* 30:397, 1990.
21. Grillner S: Neurobiological bases of rhythmic motor acts in vertebrates, *Science* 228:143, 1985.
22. Herschler C, Milner M: An optimality criterion for processing electromyographic signals relating to human locomotion, *IEEE Trans Biomed Eng* 25:413, 1978.
23. Hirschberg GG, Nathanson M: Electromyographic recording of muscular activity in normal and spastic gaits, *Arch Phys Med Rehabil* 33:217, 1952.
24. Kadaba MP et al: Repeatability of kinematic, kinetic, and electromyographic data in normal adult gait, *J Orthop Res* 7:849, 1989.
25. Kadaba MP et al: Repeatability of phasic muscle activity: performance of surface and intramuscular wire electrodes in gait analysis, *J Orthop Res* 3:330, 1985.
26. Kleissen RFM: Effects of electromyographic processing methods on computer-averaged surface electromyographic profiles for the gluteus medius muscle, *Phys Ther* 70:716, 1990.
27. Knutsson E, Richards C: Different types of disturbed motor control in gait of hemiparetic patients, *Brain* 102:405, 1979.
28. Koh TJ, Grabiner MD: Evaluation of methods to minimize cross talk in surface electromyography, *J Biomech* 26 (Suppl 1):151, 1993.
29. Lass P et al: Muscle coordination following rupture of the anterior cruciate ligament, *Acta Orthop Scand* 62:9, 1991.

30. Loeb GE, Gans C: *Electromyography for experimentalists,* Chicago, 1986, University of Chicago Press.

31. Morrenhof JW, Abbink HJ: Cross-correlation and cross-talk in surface electromyography, *Electromyogr Clin Neurophysiol* 25:73, 1985.

32. Nashner LM, Shumway-Cook A, Marin O: Stance posture control in select groups of children with cerebral palsy: deficits in sensory organization and muscular coordination, *Exp Brain Res* 49:393, 1983.

33. Neumann DA, Cook TM: Effect of load and carry position on the electromyographic activity of the gluteus medius muscle during walking, *Phys Ther* 65:305, 1985.

34. Olney SJ, Winter DA: Predictions of knee and ankle moments of force in walking from EMG and kinematic data, *J Biomech* 18:9, 1985.

35. Õunpuu S, Winter DA: Bilateral electromyographical analysis of the lower limbs during walking in normal adults, *Electroencephalogr Clin Neurophysiol* 72:429, 1989.

36. Patla AE: Some characteristics of EMG patterns during locomotion: implications for the locomotor control processes *J Mot Behav* 17:443, 1985.

37. Perry J: *Gait analysis: normal and pathological function,* Thorofare, N.J., 1992, Slack Inc.

38. Rose SA, Oonpuu S, DeLuca PA: Strategies for the assessment of pediatric gait in the clinical setting, *Phys Ther* 71:961, 1991.

39. Shiavi R et al: Variability of electromyographic patterns for level-surface walking through a range of self-selected speeds, *Bull Prosthet Res* 18:5, 1981.

40. Shiavi R et al: Pattern analysis of electromyographic linear envelopes exhibited by subjects with uninjured and injured knees during free and fast speed walking, *J Orthop Res* 10:226, 1992.

41. Sinkhaer T, Arendt-Nielsen L: Knee stability and muscle coordination in patients with anterior cruciate ligament injuries: an electromyographic approach, *J Electromyogr Kinesiol* 1:209, 1991.

42. Smidt, GL, editor: *Gait in rehabilitation,* New York, 1990, Churchill Livingstone.

43. Soderberg GL, Cook TM: Electromyography in biomechanics, *Phys Ther* 64:1813, 1984.

44. Soderberg GL, editor: *Recording techniques in selected topics in surface electromyography for use in the occupational setting: expert perspectives* (Pub No. 91-100), Washington, D.C., 1992, U.S. Department of Health and Human Services, National Institute for Occupational Safety and Health

45. Tata EG, Peat M: Electromyographic characteristics of locomotion in normal children, *Physiotherapy Canada* 39:161, 1987.

46. Threlkeld AJ: Personal communication. Combined Sections Meeting of the American Physical Therapy Association, New Orleans, La., 1990.

47. *Units, terms and standards in the reporting of EMG research city,* 1980, International Society of Electrophysiological Kinesiology.

48. White SC, Winter DA: Predicting muscle forces in gait from EMG signals and musculotendon kinematics, *J Electromyogr Kinesiol* 2:217, 1992.

49. Winter DA, Scott SH: Technique for interpretation of electromyography for concentric and eccentric contractions in gait, *J Electromyogr Kinesiol* 1:263, 1991.

50. Winter DA, Yack HJ: EMG profiles during normal human walking: stride-to-stride and intersubject variability, *Electroencephalogr Clin Neurophysiol* 67:402, 1987.

51. Winter DA: *Biomechanics of human movement,* ed 2, New York, 1979, John Wiley & Sons.

52. Winter DA: Electromyogram recording, processing, and normalization: procedures and considerations, *J Hum Muscle Perform* 1:5, 1991.

53. Winter DA: Pathologic gait diagnosis with computer-averaged electromyographic profiles, *Arch Phys Med Rehabil* 65:393, 1984.

54. Yang JF, Winter DA: Surface EMG profiles during different walking cadences in human, *Electroencephalogr Clin Neurophysiol* 60:485, 1985.

55. Young CC et al: The effect of surface and internal electrodes on the gait of children with cerebral palsy, spastic diplegic type, *J Orthop Res* 7:732, 1989.

56. Zipp P: Recommendations for the standardization of lead positions in surface electromyography, *Eur J Appl Physiol* 50:41, 1982.

CHAPTER 22

EMG: Use and Interpretation in Gait

Loretta M. Knutson
Gary L. Soderberg

KEY TERMS

Amplitude referenced norms

Concentric contraction

Duration reference norms

Eccentric contraction

Maxium voluntary isometric contraction

Muscle profiles

Normalization

The focus of this chapter is on the use and interpretation of the electromyogram as derived during gait. The chapter begins with a review of the ways electromyographic (EMG) gait data have been used to help clinicians understand human walking behavior and improve patient function. Normal profiles, the relationship of EMG data to other variables, and the methods of presenting EMG data in normal and pathological states are then discussed. The chapter concludes by detailing the importance of normalizing data to time and amplitude when creating normal templates and comparing data within and across studies of pathologic gait performance.

EMG APPLIED TO THE STUDY OF GAIT

The application of electromyography in gait is well documented. Review articles have been published on the subject of EMG gait analysis.[2,69,80] EMG data has been used to describe non-disabled adult gait,[*] non-disabled and maturing childhood gait,[†] and the emergence of walking behavior in infants.[‡] Gait studies including EMG data have addressed persons with neuromotor pathology.[§]

A primary application in pathologic gait has been for pre- and postoperative evaluations of patients with paralytic disorders or with cerebral palsy. Traditionally this application addressed the effects of orthopaedic procedures,[¶] however, reintroduction of neurosurgical rhizotomy has led to pre- and postoperative EMG evaluation of that procedure as well.[13] Clinicians and researchers have employed dynamic EMG to guide decisions about the type of orthopaedic surgery to be performed[5,7,63] and to evaluate if the surgical decision was improved by using electromyography.[1,47] The general consensus holds preoperative EMG evaluation is helpful. Unlike orthopaedic surgery, decisions regarding selective posterior rhizotomy surgery are not guided by preoperative EMG study but rather by intraoperative EMG recordings of muscle responses to spinal cord nerve rootlet stimulation. Preoperative EMG study for guiding rhizotomy decisions may warrant further attention. Besides the applications noted, EMG analysis has also been used to evaluate orthotic devices.[*]

A sample of a preoperative recording is shown in Figures 22-1*A* and 22-1*B*. This evaluation was completed on a 12-year-old child with right hemiplegia who demonstrated dynamic and postural cavovarus foot deformity. The primary concern was foot control and posture during gait. To determine which muscle was the most likely culprit in causing cavovarus in gait, the EMG was recorded first from surface electrodes placed over the gastrocnemius and tibialis anterior muscles (Figure 22-1*A*) to examine phase of activity for the tibialis anterior muscle. Recordings suggested normal phase but prolonged gastrocnemius muscle activity was accompanied by tibialis anterior activity that was almost constant, except perhaps for brief quiescence in mid-to-later swing. Also, a higher burst or peak of tibialis anterior muscle activity occurred appropriately at early swing. These recordings suggested that the likely source of cavovarus was the tibialis anterior muscle due to its sustained activity throughout the stance phase. To be assured the tibialis posterior was not a more serious source of the cavovarus, an EMG was recorded from a fine wire electrode inserted into that muscle and a surface electrode placed over the peroneal muscles (Figure 22-1*B*). Tibialis posterior muscle activity was considered acceptable despite a tendency for premature stance activity. Peroneal muscles were active appropriately in stance but apparently were not able to counter the inversion pull of the tibialis anterior muscle. Timing and level of activity in the muscles studied suggested orthopaedic surgery would be most effective if treatment involved transfer anteriorly of the tibialis anterior.

Figure 22-2 shows a record from a postoperative study of a 7-year-old child who had undergone heel cord release. Note the co-contraction of the tibialis anterior and gastrocnemius muscles during stance as well as the additional phase of contraction of the tibialis anterior muscle during mid-to-late swing phase. While co-contraction of these muscles may be seen in infants beginning to walk, by 7 years of age the profile for the tibialis anterior muscle should look like the normal adult profile having biphasic bursts, at heel strike and at toe off. Even the mid-to-late swing phase tibialis anterior activity is deviant; early swing activity is more normal. Unlike the child described in Figure 22-1, surgery to alter tibialis anterior muscle activity may not be wise for this child. Clinical findings of "crouched gait"—walking with hips, knees, and ankles flexed—and evidence from the postoperative EMG record that the vastus lateralis and medial hamstring muscles are also inappropriately active

---

* Refer to the following sources: 6, 14, 23, 36, 40, 53, 59, 70, 79, 82, 97, 100.

† Refer to the following sources: 9, 74, 83, 84, 86.

‡ Refer to the following sources: 8, 25, 41, 57, 58, 88.

§ Refer to the following sources: 10, 11, 19, 20, 32, 39, 42, 45, 46, 49, 50, 54, 60, 61, 65, 68, 71, 76, 78, 81, 98.

¶ Refer to the following sources: 24, 26, 29, 30, 62, 85, 87.

* Refer to the following sources: 10, 12, 15, 34, 43, 48.

FIGURE 22-1   EMG data of subject with cavovarus foot. EMG raw recordings from the right leg of a 12-year-old child with right hemiplegia and cavovarus foot deformity. Avoiding discomfort at onset of testing, surface recordings were made first of the gastrocnemius and tibialis anterior muscles (**A**). Thereafter recordings were made with a fine wire electrode inserted into the tibialis posterior muscle and surface electrodes on the gastrocnemius and peroneal muscles (**B**). Stance phase is represented on the footswitch record by the lowest level, swing by the highest level. Findings confirmed inappropriate tibialis anterior activity throughout gait plus appropriate bursts at early swing. The tibialis posterior muscle seemed a less likely culprit for the cavovarus because its activity occurred normally in stance, despite occasional premature onset in swing.

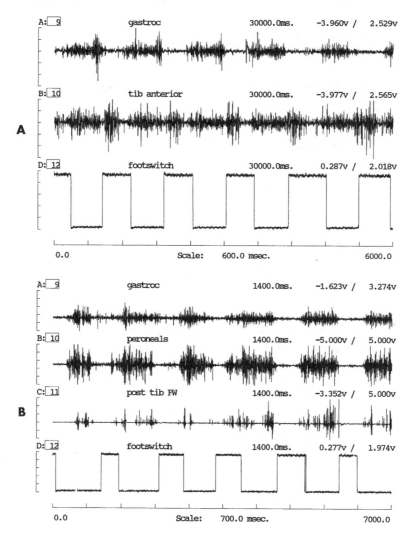

in stance suggests excess muscle activity may be needed for stability. Alteration of the tibialis anterior muscle, which may be providing stability in stance, could be detrimental for this child. In fact, overall effectiveness of the original heel cord release might be questioned even with the gastrocnemius muscle looking appropriately active in stance. To address this question adequately, comparison with a preoperative record is needed.

Without the preoperative record no statements can be made about whether the out-of-phase (stance) activity in the tibialis anterior, vastus lateralis, and medial hamstring muscles was always present or resulted from surgery. Complementary documentation of joint angles from kinematic plots would also aide interpretation.

Holt was perhaps the first person to report on the use of EMG data to analyze the movement of

FIGURE 22-2   EMG data of subject with cerebral palsy. Raw EMG record from the right lower extremity of a 7-year-old child with moderate spastic quadriplegic type cerebral palsy. Stance phase, represented by the lowest level on the footswitch, demands activity from all muscles. Only the gastrocnemius muscle activity compares to activity that would be seen in a person without neuromotor dysfunction. vl = vastus lateralis muscle; mh = medial hamstring muscles; ta = tibialis anterior muscle; gastroc = gastrocnemius muscle.

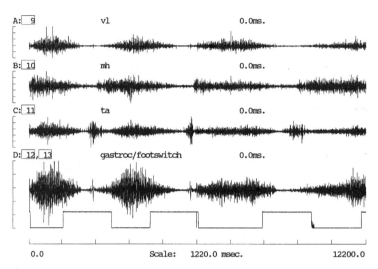

children with cerebral palsy.[33] He stated, on the basis of EMG evidence, that locomotion cannot be judged by visual inspection alone. On the other hand, some degree of caution is needed in interpreting EMG data obtained from patients with pathology. Young et al., studying 36 children with cerebral palsy, found that temporal-distance characteristics of unencumbered gait were effected by wearing electrodes.[103] The greatest change occurred with fine wire electrodes, but even wearing surface electrodes resulted in a significant reduction in cadence. Furthermore, while the presentation of raw data (Figures 22-1 and 22-2) may serve many situations well, increased objectivity is important for evaluating groups and making broad statements regarding treatment. For example, to even make comparisons between muscles, particularly amplitude contrasts, data should be referenced to another contraction specific to each patient. This will be discussed in greater detail later in this chapter.

Investigations on patients in the 1950s and 1960s were primarily descriptive based on visual inspection of the EMG record. Most studies addressed only the temporal characteristics of the muscle, i.e., when is the muscle active versus quiescent.[6,17,18,62] In these patient studies, the criterion or selection of threshold for calling the muscle "on" was not specified. Other investigators provided amplitude information referenced to a full gait cycle.[23,35,45,53,94] Early representations of amplitude were schematic. As technology improved, raw EMG signals were processed and averaged to create a mean linear envelope or ensemble average. The advantage of amplitude information is the indication of the muscle's relative contraction intensity level, a factor Winter suggests is of more interest and significance in gait analysis than temporal on/off data.[94,95] In later sections of this chapter, methods for presenting EMG gait data will be discussed in greater detail. First, however, the normal profile important for comparison in the presence of pathology will be reviewed.

THE NON-DISABLED PROFILE

The benefit of having a template based on non-disabled subject EMG gait patterns can be seen when drawing distinctions between normal and abnormal patterns or elucidating the need for or effectiveness of treatment. Overlaying the pathologic gait profile on a normal profile is a simple way to allow visual inspection so judgements can be made relative to the nature of the deviance. This was done by Winter when he superimposed plots of EMG patterns for a patient with cerebral palsy over normal patterns.[94] Using more objective statistical approaches is also possible. Measures that could be used to explain deviations from "normal" include variations in onset times and signal amplitude. Unfortunately universal agreement on what comprises the normal data base does not exist.

The very notion of a non-disabled pattern of EMG activity has been questioned by Arsenault et al.[3] Studying the soleus, rectus femoris, vastus medialis, and tibialis anterior muscles in eight normal subjects, these authors noted highly repeatable EMG outcomes within individuals but differences for a given muscle between subjects. The differences in profiles were particularly significant for the rectus femoris muscle. Therefore, there may be limits associated with the use of the non-disabled profile.

The EMG signal is known to be influenced by a host of factors including instrumentation and the form of data analysis used. Unless standards across facilities are uniformly agreed upon, development of non-disabled profiles will tend to be facility dependent. In view of the lack of a common standard, the consumer tends to be limited to interpreting each study independently. Winter's 1984 call for increased effort in developing a data bank of non-disabled EMG profiles could be repeated today.[94]

Duration-Referenced Norms

In the late 1950s Sutherland initiated gait analysis efforts at Shriner's Hospital of San Francisco. This work was supported by others in the 1960s and early 1970s, and in 1973 led to the creation of a chart defining active periods based on fine wire electrode studies of lower extremity muscles in 12 normal adults (Figure 22-3). These data or other similar temporal summaries generated for laboratory-specific applications continue to be used today. A review of EMG patterns in adult locomotion as reported across various laboratories and including studies with a temporal focus has been published by Shiavi.[69]

Recently, Sutherland and colleagues also provided an excellent summary of temporal data for children.[83] Using surface electrodes on seven lower extremity muscles, Sutherland et al. gathered EMG data as part of a comprehensive study of more than 300 children between ages 1 and 7 years. Stance and swing phase data are separately

referenced from 0 to 100%. The investigators chose this method of plotting because stance phase was longer in the younger children. Normalizing each of the two main phases of gait to 100% facilitated comparison between the children at different ages. However, comparison to adult norms or joint rotation data (generally plotted as 100% for the full gait cycle) is difficult. Converting Sutherland's data to a 100% base would be possible for those interested.

Temporal data described in existing normal templates for both children and adults have generally been based on visual appraisal of EMG data. While this method may be valid, it is of concern from a reliability perspective. DiFabio found that while making valid decisions about EMG onset may require visual appraisal, reliability using computerized selection of muscle onset was clearly superior to experienced appraiser judgment.[21] Winter also demonstrated how setting different arbitrary signal amplitude thresholds changed interpretation of the on/off data.[94]

Peak Activity-Referenced Norms

In 1972, Carlsöö published a book in which a schematic plot of lower extremity muscle activity showed rising and declining EMG signals suggestive of when peak activity in the muscle occurs. This plot presumably based on normal adult gait is reproduced in Figure 22-4. The mechanism for creating amplitude plots in the 1950s involved hand marking along the top border of raw, rectified, and sometimes filtered EMG records. Later, computer sequences to create linear envelopes were introduced.[53] As the desire for objectivity grew, the ensemble average, a mean of two or more linear envelopes, emerged using various mathematical manipulations.[31,73] Today, software programs written for personal computers are standard additions to hardware systems used in motion analysis laboratories. They operate quickly and readily to create and plot linear envelopes and ensemble averages. The ensemble average is probably most important to supporting objective, statistical analysis of the data gathered.

Plots of linear envelopes or ensemble averages created from computerized techniques have been published for normal adults[96,102] and normal children[86] for select muscle groups. Synthesis of this information into a chart or template has not occurred in the same way as has the data from visual appraisal of duration by Sutherland et al.[83] or schematic representation of amplitude by Carlsöö.[14]

Figure 22-3   Non-disabled temporal EMG patterns for adult lower extremity muscles. Graph created in 1973 by research efforts of Sutherland, Hagy, and Mann (personal communication, John Hagy and Larry Lamoreux). Reprinted with permission of San Francisco Shriners Hospital for Crippled Children.

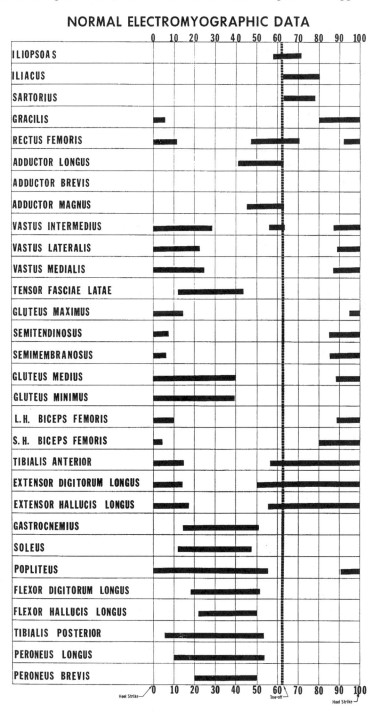

Obviously, with computer software systems available this creation of templates should be an easy next step for the ambitious student of EMG gait analysis. Publishing both a printout and a computer-stored version of a normal amplitude template is needed for different ages and most lower extremity muscles.

Profiles for Specific Muscles

Non-disabled profiles of muscle action in gait have been studied using a variety of techniques. Variations in the results may be influenced by this fact. For example, some investigators favored fine wire electrodes for all muscles, while others reserved

FIGURE 22-4 Schematic representation of normal lower extremity muscle activity based on EMG recordings. Reprinted with permission of Sven Carlsöö, professor emeritus, former professor of anatomy, Karolinska Institute, Stockholm, Sweden. Figure published previously in *How Man Moves*.[14]

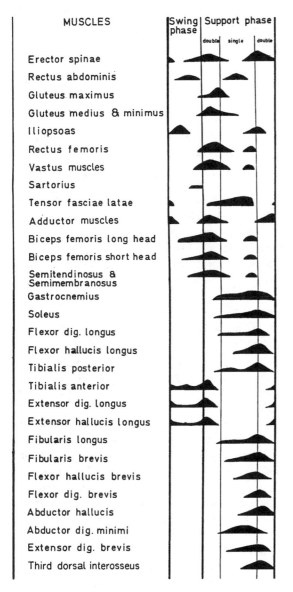

bursts, one in stance and one in swing.[91] Similar profiles were seen for the paraspinal muscles although the time of onset may be slightly shifted to encompass the stance and swing phase transitions or the burst duration may be prolonged.[91] The erector spinae may not show the swing-stance transition burst but instead have a small burst on either side of heel contact.[91] Vink and Karssemeijer studied low back muscles in 11 subjects looking for correlation to pelvic rotation in gait.[90] Bilateral activity was found during double support with ipsilateral activity often greater than contralateral activity at heel strike. A relationship to pelvic rotation was not confirmed. Based on frequent and bilateral activity, and low back muscle activity not associated with pelvic motion, trunk muscles may simply have general utility for creating stable walking behavior.

Because persons with upper limb amelia can normally walk, clinical evidence exists that upper extremity muscle action is not required for gait. On the other hand, observation and several kinematic studies confirm that normal unencumbered gait involves arm swinging reciprocal to forward progression of the opposite lower limb. The value of this pattern is unclear when the movement is not obligatory. One study addressed the relationship of upper and lower extremity EMG activity looking for evidence of intersegmental interactions.[92] If synchronous phasing had been found, support would be given for using upper extremity activity to trigger lower extremity functional electrical stimulation in persons with paralysis. Eight women were studied while walking and wearing surface electrodes on several upper extremity muscles and the contralateral tibialis anterior. Using objective criteria to identify from a smoothed EMG record when the muscles were on or off, the investigators failed to confirm intersegmental coupling consistently present between one upper limb muscle and the tibialis anterior.

Studies of upper extremity and trunk muscle EMG activity during gait are not common and appear limited to adults. No studies were found in the literature regarding children.

Lower Extremities   The majority of studies have focused on the lower extremities. Proximal muscles show more variability than distal muscles as do two-joint muscles versus single-joint muscles.[97] Foot intrinsic muscles are normally active in mid-stance or late mid-stance until toe off,[51] however flat-footed individuals show earlier onset of activity in some muscles.[28] Foot intrinsic muscle activity is considered helpful for stabilizing the foot.

their use for deep muscles not accessible by surface electrodes. Despite variations in the description of the "normal profile," sufficient agreement exists to make the following points about maturing and non-disabled adult gait EMG profiles.

The Trunk and Upper Extremities   Waters and Morris reported abdominal muscles may remain active throughout the gait cycle or show biphasic

The gastrocnemius and soleus muscles are active from approximately 10 to 50% of the gait cycle.[22,53,82] Because the foot is dorsiflexing until late mid-stance, 40% of the cycle, the contraction is accepted as being primarily eccentric to control forward rotation of the tibia over the foot.[79,82] Late in stance, the foot begins to plantarflex continuing through toe off. As Sutherland points out, however, EMG activity in the plantarflexors has ceased or begun to cease.[83] Even with plantarflexor muscle activity lasting until 50% of the gait cycle; the last 10 to 12% of stance phase, during which the foot continues to plantarflex, occurs without corresponding electrical activity in the plantarflexors. Thus, plantarflexion at late mid-stance must either be a passive phenomenon or the result of residual tension that remains in the muscle after electrical activity ceases. Sutherland has also suggested that the gastrocnemius muscle assists knee extension during stance although some kinesiologists consider knee extension in the latter half of stance to be a function of momentum.[79,82] Shiavi et al. report the gastrocnemius and soleus muscles show earlier onset of activity as walking speed increases and at fast walking begin during the swing-stance transition.[72]

The tibialis anterior muscle shows biphasic activity in non-disabled gait, first from toe off through mid-swing then at heel strike (loading).[6,22,53] The swing phase activity helps foot clearance with concentric contraction bringing the foot out of plantarflexion at toe off and towards dorsiflexion. The level of muscle activity during swing phase varies but the inversion and dorsiflexion action common to the muscle may also prepare the foot for loading onset in the normally supinated position. Loading phase activity is eccentric to decelerate the plantarflexor moment created at impact. This period of activity is brief, ending early in stance. However, Shiavi et al. have described mid-stance tibialis anterior muscle activity in normal subjects.[72] Similarly prolonged activity was reported by Gray and Basmajian in flat-footed subjects[28] and in new walkers.[57,58] Differing from the more common description of a biphasic pattern for adult normal subjects, Shiavi et al. suggested the tibialis anterior muscle is monophasic at slow speeds and multiphasic at fast speeds. In another study, the tibialis anterior was the only lower extremity muscle that Milner et al. found did not respond in a linear fashion to increasing walking velocity.[53] In this study, the muscle showed a parabolic-like curve where the point of lowest activity occurred at the person's comfortable walking velocity.

The peroneal muscles and the tibialis posterior muscle, which act antagonistically, are both active during stance phase but the peroneal muscles may begin and end slightly later than the tibialis posterior muscle.[79] EMG study shows the tibialis posterior muscle activity ending in late stance whereas the peroneal muscles may remain active into early swing. The activity in these two muscles corresponds to the normal motion seen in the coronal plane as the foot moves from supination at heel strike to pronation at mid-stance and back to supination at late stance and toe off. Activity of the peroneal muscles after mid-stance probably fails to keep the foot pronated (everted), even though tibialis posterior muscle activity is decreasing, because onset of the tibialis anterior muscle counters pronation and facilitates supination (inversion).

Unlike the antagonistic dorsiflexors and plantarflexors, which work in opposite periods of gait, the antagonistic peroneal and tibialis posterior muscles work in approximately the same period of gait. The antagonistic quadriceps and hamstring muscles also work at approximately the same time.[22,23,72] They both show their primary function in the swing-to-stance phase transition but may show additional activity at stance-to-swing transition, particularly as walking speed increases.[23] Hamstring muscle activity is eccentric with onset in late swing to decelerate the passively extending knee. Active knee extension in late swing is unlikely because quadriceps muscle onset occurs after the knee is already extending and typically lags behind hamstring muscle onset. Quadriceps muscle activity is important for knee stability at initial loading. The external moments at this time would otherwise flex the knee. The quadriceps muscles remain active slightly longer than the hamstring muscles. Their action in early stance is eccentric given kinematic evidence that knee flexion is occurring. Thereafter, as mid-stance is approached, kinematic plots show the knee beginning to extend despite reducing quadriceps muscle activity. Thus knee extension at mid-stance, like plantarflexion at toe off, may be a passive phenomenon or influenced by residual muscle tension.

The gluteus maximus muscle contributes to hip extension and stability in the swing-to-stance phase transition.[6,23] Hamstring muscle activity in early stance also assists hip extension. Inconsistently, the gluteal muscles may be active in the stance-to-swing transition possibly to stabilize against iliopsoas hip flexion activity, which began in mid-stance and will continue through mid-swing.[6,23] The hip abductors are well known for their frontal plane action, which prevents a positive Trendelenburg during stance. The gluteus medius, likely along with other hip abductor muscles, gluteus minimus and tensor fasciae latae, is active from heel strike through mid-stance, ceasing as the opposite extremity begins to bear weight.[72] With increased walking speed, activity in these muscles may begin earlier, in late swing. Some normal subjects have shown gluteus medius activity during the stance-to-swing phase transition evidently to gain slight limb abduction which will help clear the foot from the floor.[72] Hip adductors are active in both transitions of gait.[23]

RELATIONSHIP OF EMG TO OTHER VARIABLES

Joint Motion

Kinematic plots of joint angular motion are often compared to EMG plots to determine if the muscle activity can explain joint motion or if the joint motion can explain muscle activity. Addition of moment data from kinetic plots further clarifies the complex picture of our biological system in motion. One example of joint motion occurring without concurrent muscle activity is seen when the knee flexes from 45% (heel off) to 62% (toe off) of the gait cycle, a motion that increases farther from toe off to 70% (early swing) of the gait cycle when the knee begins to extend. This knee flexion is not created by hamstring muscle activity because hamstring muscle activity does not begin until late swing when its onset slows the extending knee. Such examples of joint motion without EMG activity in the muscles that ordinarily create movement in a given direction are common in gait. Muscle function in gait is often one of control, with onset of eccentric activity for protection against motion occurring in the opposite direction. Electromyographic study also reveals that a muscle's role during gait is often different from that described as its primary muscle action in anatomy texts. With the foot progressing from heel strike to flat foot, the knee flexes slightly but the hip extends more notably. Hamstring muscle activity during this early stance period is considered more important for creating hip extension proximally than knee flexion distally despite the muscle's primary action listed as a knee flexor in anatomy texts. The hip extension is crucial to forward propulsion.

Because the majority of motion in gait occurs in the sagittal plane, the muscles responsible for stability and action in this plane are the most commonly studied. The iliopsoas, gluteus maximus, quadriceps, hamstrings, tibialis anterior, gastrocnemius, and soleus muscles are primarily associated with sagittal plane motion. Nonetheless, stability is vital to normal joint motion in frontal and coronal planes as well. Hip abductor, hip adductor, peroneal, tibialis posterior, and tibialis anterior muscles provide control in these planes.

Age and Gender

The EMG characteristics associated with gait have also been studied in children of varying ages, partly to describe maturation of motor control systems and partly with the intention of developing profiles against which children with motor problems could be compared.* Sutherland and co-authors have shown maturational affects studying temporal EMG data on seven muscles in a large number of children between 1 and 7 years of age.[83] Although 369 EMG studies were completed and 309 normal children participated in some phase of comprehensive gait analysis, the number of children included at each age group and for each muscle varied from four to 44. Based on differences across some of the ages, results were plotted on bar graphs showing mean times of onset and cessation of EMG activity for the 10 age groups studied—at each year and half-year to age 3, then each year thereafter. Comparison of results across the ages revealed the majority of changes took place by 2 years of age. Specifically, the tibialis anterior, medial hamstring, and lateral hamstring muscles had a mature pattern by 2 years of age. The major changes in the vastus medialis muscle occurred by 2 years of age but earlier swing phase onset persisted until age 4 years. Gluteus medius and gluteus maximus muscle activity periods were similar across all age groups. The gastrocnemius muscle findings were most discrepant from descriptions of adult normal profiles and this held for all age groups with less frequency in older children. Discrepancy was influenced by the presence of two patterns: the "immature" pattern consisting of late swing phase onset and the "mature" pattern following adult norms of activity limited to stance phase. Although frequency of the immature pattern decreased after age 2, 25% of the children at 2 years and older continued to exhibit this pattern.

Findings by Tata and Peat employing an EMG amplitude perspective failed to find any significant

---

*Refer to the following sources: 8, 9, 25, 41, 57, 58, 74, 83, 84, 86, 88.

differences across the ages in children of 1 to 7 years.[86] Studying four muscles in 70 children did, however, suggest a trend toward changing recruitment patterns with development. More prolonged levels of activity were seen in the 1-year-old children, with the gastrocnemius muscle most unlike the adult pattern. The authors concluded that an adult pattern of lower extremity muscle activity during walking occurs by the third year of life. This finding agrees with that of early investigators.[41,57,58,88] Due to the confounding effect of maturation, normal profiles for each age between 1 and 3 years would facilitate comparison when evaluating very young children with pathology. Thereafter, normal adult standards could be used.

Öberg et al. have provided temporal-distance data on normal subjects between 10 and 79 years of age.[56] This study is valuable for its focus inclusion of older persons. Similar data on EMG changes in the normal elderly do not appear available. Gender differences have also received little attention relative to EMG data, despite studies reported in this area on other gait parameters.

Force

Amplitude of EMG signals derived during gait may also be interpreted as a measure of relative muscle tension. In effect, data seem to support that the linear envelope of the EMG signal reflects the relative amount of muscle tension. Whether that relationship is linear or nonlinear has been the subject of many studies, which have concluded that the relationship is influenced by technique and physiological factors. Woods and Bigland-Ritchie, however, found in their 20 subjects that the relationship was determined by anatomical and physiological factors and not recording technique.[99] Reviews on the variety of factors influencing the EMG-force relationship have been published.[64,77,93] An important conclusion may be that to understand the meaning of EMG signal amplitude, factors such as energy generation and absorption, length-tension, and tension-velocity must simultaneously be addressed. That is, during study and interpretation of data, attention should be given to factors such as muscle length, velocity of contraction, type of contraction, and muscle fiber types.

Contraction Type and Fiber Type

Studies suggest that the relationship between tension and EMG activity, whether linear or nonlin-

ear, is influenced by the type of contraction. To determine contraction type, kinematic data must be merged with EMG data. A technique for interpretation of EMG for concentric and eccentric contractions in gait has been suggested by Winter and Scott.[96] Using a biomechanical model based on average kinematic data of hip, knee, and ankle joint angles from 30 adult subjects, muscle length for six commonly examined lower extremity muscles was determined. Subsequently calculations were made of muscle fiber shortening and lengthening velocity. Then, employing computer graphics, overlays of the contraction type were projected onto EMG linear envelopes normalized to the mean gait cycle EMG for the same six muscles. This technique contributes to the clinical interpretation of EMG data by providing information about the type of contraction undertaken by the muscle at different points in the gait cycle. As analytical techniques become increasingly available through computer software programs and as applicability is defined, use by clinicians will become more prevalent and treatment efficacy can more actively be studied.

Velocity

Investigators agree that increased velocity elongates the period of muscle activity by leading to activity that starts earlier or lasts longer.[53,70] Milner et al. found that values recorded from indwelling electrodes in six subjects were dependent on walking speed for the vastus lateralis, biceps femoris, and lateral gastrocnemius muscles, but not the tibialis anterior muscle.[53] The general trend was for increasing EMG amplitude with increasing walking speed, but the tibialis anterior muscle produced a somewhat curvilinear profile. In general, subjects showed a minimum of EMG activity in the muscles studied while walking at their comfortable speed. Milner et al. suggested that without a pace constraint, subjects naturally selected a walking velocity associated with a minimum of muscular activity. This is similar to the finding that energy expenditure per meter traveled increases with walking speeds that are slower or faster than free speed.[66] Despite this finding, concern about the effect of velocity on the EMG signal leads some researchers to control velocity during gait testing whereas others favor allowing subjects to walk at their comfortable walking speed.[38,45] In fact, the imposition of an unnatural velocity has been shown to decrease the repeatability of the EMG signal.[31,38]

Methods for Presenting EMG Gait Profiles in Non-Disabled and Pathological States

EMG data obtained during gait have most often been plotted against a time base on the X axis in one of several ways. Examples of such plots are shown in Figures 22-3 and 22-4. Creation of these plots requires knowledge of when the gait cycle begins and ends. This information can readily be obtained from a footswitch or from camera recordings of joint kinematics. The first step in viewing plots of this sort is to consider the X axis. Both Figure 22-3 and 22-4 begin with 0% and go to 100%, but Figure 22-3 references heel strike as 0% and progresses from stance to swing, whereas Figure 22-4 begins with swing phase. Temporal plots by some investigators may add a short period of EMG activity before stance begins at 0%.[23] Sutherland's data on children are presented with stance and swing phase separately representing 0 to 100%.[83] In any event, interpretations and comparisons require attention to the time base of the plot. Rather than use a time base, EMG amplitude of one muscle can be plotted against that of another muscle (Figure 22-5). This alternative plot method is much less common in the literature. A further alternative is to report numbers corresponding to EMG voltage output (Table 22-1) or indices without graphical plots.[70,89]

Duration and Time-Referenced Presentation

One of the most common approaches to plotting EMG data demonstrates when the muscle is on or active during the gait cycle and when it is off or quiet. A simple bar graph such as shown in Figure 22-3 provides this on/off information. Traditionally, muscle active periods were judged according to the examiner's visual inspection of the raw or processed EMG signal. As Winter demonstrated, the labeling of on/off can vary noticeably depending on the criteria employed.[94] Thus, a key limitation to this approach is agreement between examiners in the absence of criteria for making visual judgments. Even with computer programs available to introduce objectivity, another limitation remains. Amplitude information is ignored in a duration approach and, as Winter has stated, "more than passing concern should be made concerning the problems and errors associated with the use of 'phasic' EMG patterns as diagnostic tools."[94] Nonetheless, descriptions of temporal aspects of muscle activity can be valuable in motor

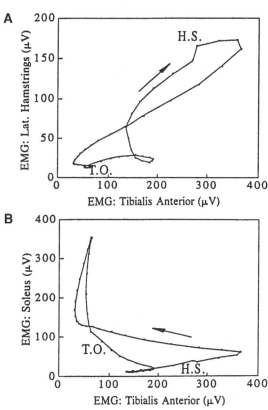

Figure 22-5 EMG muscle amplitude. EMG amplitude of one muscle plotted against the amplitude of another. (**A**) Positive slope; (**B**) negative slope. Reprinted with permission from Butterworth-Heinemann Ltd. Source: Davis BL, Vaughan CL: Phasic behavior of EMG signals during gait: Use of multivariate statistics. *J Electromyogr Kinesiol* 3:51-60, 1993.

control studies. Applications in motor control literature may present normal data in terms of latency for muscle activation from some point in the gait cycle (e.g., heel strike or toe off) or refer to a muscle's activation latency relative to another muscle becoming active or quiet. In these studies, objective criteria for determining on and off periods and latency are important.

Amplitude and Time-Referenced Presentation

A different and often more comprehensive approach than temporal representations of the EMG signal attends to signal amplitude. The raw signal is processed, and recognizable periods of rising and declining activity are retained. This approach has the advantage of considering not only when the muscle is active but how active. Amplitude

TABLE 22-1 *Vastus Lateralis Muscle EMG Voltage.* Voltage values based on the average within each 5% increment of six gait cycles. Values were preamplified 35× at the surface electrode and amplified 5000× at the main amplifier.

Percent of gait cycle	Cycle 1	Cycle 2	Cycle 3	Cycle 4	Cycle 5	Cycle 6
5%	0.442	0.346	0.425	0.371	0.325	0.333
10	0.138	0.225	0.433	0.230	0.157	0.489
15	0.142	0.111	0.259	0.111	0.121	0.079
20	0.175	0.149	0.289	0.054	0.038	0.106
25	0.169	0.151	0.284	0.086	0.064	0.136
30	0.171	0.176	0.142	0.067	0.071	0.120
35	0.194	0.072	0.125	0.087	0.061	0.077
40	0.130	0.079	0.173	0.089	0.017	0.078
45	0.238	0.117	0.080	0.062	0.014	0.013
50	0.039	0.080	0.026	0.071	0.013	0.015
55	0.030	0.063	0.041	0.096	0.014	0.022
60	0.019	0.032	0.011	0.042	0.030	0.015
65	0.035	0.022	0.045	0.030	0.041	0.018
70	0.034	0.036	0.029	0.026	0.042	0.023
75	0.043	0.037	0.025	0.036	0.039	0.022
80	0.033	0.053	0.032	0.033	0.028	0.034
85	0.036	0.036	0.044	0.083	0.041	0.054
90	0.068	0.026	0.035	0.075	0.056	0.036
95	0.106	0.044	0.090	0.111	0.123	0.092
100	0.300	0.090	0.203	0.153	0.102	0.211

interpretation may be based on visual appraisal or computerized summation. For example, in Figures 22-4 and 22-6 *A* and *B* the suggestion could be made that the muscle *appears to have a peak* at some point, has a *low level of activity* at another point, and is *quiescent* at yet another time. However, using computerized summation from Figures 22-6 *A* and *B* as shown in Table 22-1, voltage levels can clearly be identified at each 5% increment of the gait cycle. In this case, the investigators' considerations do not need to be confined to amplitude of the signal but can extend to temporal considerations if criteria for calling the muscle "on" or "off" are set. These criteria might best be referenced to 2 or 3 standard deviations above some resting level or as a percent of maximum. Use of the lowest point in the gait cycle as "resting level" is not ideal—particularly for subjects with known pathology—because the muscle may be active constantly, just to varying degrees. The resting level should be defined as resting in recumbent, sitting, or standing positions, not during the lowest point of EMG activity during gait.

Alternative Presentations

Although plotting the EMG data on a time base provides an immediate reference for what is occurring between 0 and 100% of the gait cycle, alternative presentations can direct the attention to the relationship between muscles during gait. Figure 22-5 presents amplitudes of pairs of muscles plotted against each other. In Figure 22-5*A* the relationship between two muscles acting in synchrony shows a positive slope. By contrast, the tibialis anterior and soleus muscles shown in Figure 22-5*B* have a negative slope and are somewhat curvilinear because they act at different phases of the gait cycle. The X and Y axes represent a percentage of some contraction level (amplitude normalized EMG data) and the focus is on the contraction relationship between muscles. Muscle relationships that deviate from the normal profile would then be the subject of focus. For example, the children with spastic cerebral palsy described in Figures 22-1 and 22-2 and new walkers who show excessive co-contraction of calf muscles might demonstrate a profile more like that of the

FIGURE 22-6   EMG data of subject with mild spastic diplegic cerebral palsy. (**A**) Rectified and (**B**) linear envelope processed EMG gait records from a 4½-year-old child with mild spastic diplegic cerebral palsy. Processing entailed smoothing rectified signals with a 50 millisecond time constant, which acted like a moving average. Stance phase from the footswitch record is represented by the lowest level, swing by the highest level. vl = vastus lateralis muscle; mh = medial hamstring muscles; ta = tibialis anterior muscle; gastroc = gastrocnemius muscle. Corresponding average voltage values for each 5% increment of six gait cycles for the vastus lateralis muscle only are found in Table 22-1, based on an amplifier gain of 5000.

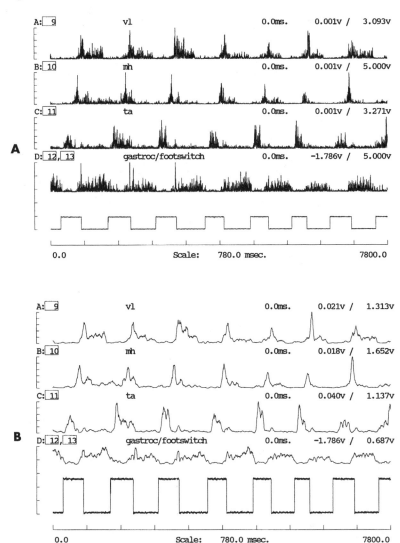

tibialis anterior and lateral hamstrings in Figure 22-5A.

Rather than plot EMG data, values can be used to draw attention to the findings of interest. For example, persons with neuromotor pathology often show abnormal co-contraction of muscles. Vaughan et al. have described a "co-contraction index" (CCI) for this purpose.[89] A value of 1.0 indicated both muscles were firing at the same relative levels, and a value of 0.0 meant that one muscle was firing at a maximum while the other muscle was at a minimum. In other situations, the variation-to-signal ratio (V/S) described by Shiavi et al. may be useful.[70] Similar to the coefficient of variation, the V/S is a measure of variability defined by the ratio of signal variation over the stride to average EMG value over the stride. Shiavi used the V/S to demonstrate how signal variability decreased at faster walking velocities for several lower extremity muscles. Yet a further alternative is to present all the EMG values across a linear envelope, such as shown in Table 22-1 for 5% increments of six gait cycles. Conversion of the analog EMG signal to a digital signal, which is typically managed by an A-to-D board in the computer, creates a list of voltage values associated with the sampling or data conversion rate. Signals converted at 1000 Hz would provide digital voltage values every millisecond. Because dealing with 1000 values every second is cumbersome, signal processing often reduces the number of digital values available. Presenting EMG voltage values as in Table 22-1 is uncommon; however the information is basic to data analysis.

Time Normalized Data

Whenever EMG data from gait are averaged over several cycles, a first consideration must be the differing duration of the gait cycles. The normal adult subject walking at free velocity has a gait cycle of about 1 second duration, although the likelihood of every cycle being exactly that duration is small. Thus, every cycle considered in an averaging equation must first be normalized to 100%. This time-normalization step is particularly critical when studying patients who show wide disparity in their gait cycle duration. An example of such a situation is shown in Figure 22-7. The 5-year-old child with cerebral palsy demonstrated gait cycle durations between 3 and 6 seconds. If signals were averaged every 1 or 2 seconds, the results would be invalid relative to the gait cycle. By first normalizing the cycle to 100% and then averaging at perhaps every 5% increment, results remain relative to the gait cycle.

Amplitude Normalized Data

Basis

Amplitude normalization is important because EMG signal quality and quantity can be influenced by such factors as instrumentation, signal gain at the amplifier, electrode placement, and the subject's subcutaneous fat. Referencing the EMG amplitude to a common level for each individual is needed to validate amplitude comparisons, which otherwise might be erroneous. The procedure of referencing the EMG data from a contraction to the EMG from some other contraction is called "normalizing." This might better be labeled "amplitude normalizing," because it is the signal amplitude that is being divided by the reference value and then multiplied by 100%. Addition of the adjective "amplitude" distinguishes the procedure from "time normalization," which was described in the previous section.

Figure 22-7 EMG data of subject with cerebral palsy. Raw EMG record of a 5-year-old child with spastic diplegic type cerebral palsy who showed mild involvement except when judging from walking behavior clinically and as seen from laboratory study. Gait cycle durations varied from 3 to 6 seconds compared to normal, which is closer to 1 second.

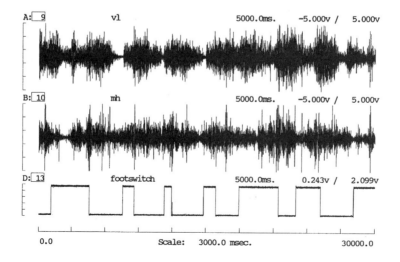

Conditions Requiring and Not Requiring Amplitude Normalization

The most compelling reason for using amplitude normalization is to allow for between-subject, between-day, and between-muscle comparisons. When subjects within a study serve as their own control, normalizing the signal is not required. However, if the electrodes are removed and replaced between sessions, data should be amplitude normalized. A further consideration of a repeated measures design study that does not normalize the amplitude of the EMG signal is that comparisons to other studies are problematic. Thus, a good general rule is to normalize data.

Selection of the Reference Contraction and Limitations

Many methods of amplitude normalization have been described in the literature but the most common has been comparison of the task-related EMG to one reference contraction, usually a maximum voluntary isometric contraction (MVIC).[4,27,55,99,101] The EMG subsequently obtained is expressed as a percentage of MVIC. Although the most common reference contraction has been the MVIC, a number of investigators in the past decade or two have used submaximal MVIC contractions[101,102] or a value taken from the dynamic event under study.[16,45,75,102] During isometric contractions, submaximal efforts have been found to be more reproducible than maximal efforts.[101] Suggestions for taking a value from the dynamic event have included using (1) the peak EMG during a dynamic activity[37,45,102] or (2) the mean EMG during a dynamic activity.[97,102] Knutsson and Richards selected the peak dynamic integrated EMG as the criteria for normalization in their study aimed at describing variations in the gait pattern of subjects with hemiplegia and differences between the subjects with hemiplegia and those with normal motor control.[45] Use of the dynamic contraction, however, can be confounding because of the change in muscle volume under the electrode site, thus affecting the magnitude of the detected EMG.

The rationale for what reference value to choose when amplitude-normalizing EMG data has not been well established. In a study using 11 normal subjects aimed at improving the sensitivity of electromyography as a diagnostic tool in gait analysis, Yang and Winter advocated either the peak or the mean of the subject ensemble average, because the dynamic values produced lower inter-subject coefficient of variations (CVs) than data normalized to 50% MVIC or to a mean EMG per

unit of isometric moment of force calibration method.[102] A weakness of this focus is that low variability between subjects is descriptive and not necessarily of value, even when developing diagnostic criteria.[44] Data must be described as they exist; manipulation to lower the variability does not make the findings more powerful diagnostically. Further, data are more likely to be reproducible if some variability exists. In the extreme case, data without variability makes consideration of reproducibility a mute point. If the ultimate goal is to generalize findings to a population, approaching the matter from a reliability perspective is most logical; findings must be reproducible.

Because we considered the reliability focus to be most appropriate for selecting the reference contraction and we noted an increasing trend to use the mean EMG from the dynamic event as the reference contraction, we undertook an investigation to identify which of three EMG values provided the best amplitude normalization value from a reproducibility perspective. The gastrocnemius muscle EMG results from 20 normal persons and 20 individuals with anterior cruciate deficiency were normalized to EMG values obtained from MVIC, peak dynamic, and mean dynamic contractions. Values were then subjected to evaluation using four statistical measures; inter- and intra-subject coefficients of variation (CV), variance ratio (VR), and intraclass correlation coefficient (ICC). Measures of group variability and precision provided respectively by the inter- and intrasubject CVs were lower for the dynamic conditions. However, use of the MVIC as the reference contraction for normalization was supported based on the VR and ICC, which related to reproducibility.[44] Future study should address reliability of gait data using the EMG from a submaximal versus a maximal voluntary contraction for the normalization value.

Maximal and Submaximal Voluntary Contraction When MVIC or submaximal MVIC are used, the electromyographer must also make the decision about what sampling period of the reference contraction is most appropriate. Probably the most common is a 3 to 5 second period, often with a 1 or 2 second interval at the beginning to assure the record is stable. A primary concern is to avoid fatigue during the MVIC, which could negatively influence performance of the task of interest. The number of repetitions to secure the reference EMG level has also varied across studies; investigators have used the greatest EMG value produced or the mean of a number of trials to arrive at the criterion for normalization.

None of these techniques appears to have a singularly stronger theoretical basis. In a study that may be applicable, nine subjects performing isometric contractions showed increased reliability in their data as the number of trials increased for both maximal and submaximal contractions.[101] Thus, a satisfactory approach may be to complete more than one reference contraction and perhaps use the mean of three contractions.

Dynamic Contraction Levels   When either the mean or the peak of the dynamic contraction is employed as the amplitude normalization reference value, the value is taken from the gait cycle. In most cases, a gait cycle is denoted by a footswitch or kinematic data, and the step to obtain the value from the mean or peak EMG signal across any gait cycle is a simple subroutine within a computer software program. As with other reference contractions decisions must be made about using the values from one gait cycle or averaging over several gait cycles. The value from the mean EMG signal should inherently be more stable than the peak value. Caution, for example, is needed to assure that the peak value does not reflect an error in the data collection or storage or artifact interfering with the EMG signal. Usually, the electromyographer can detect spurious signals by viewing raw or unprocessed data first.

Resting Level Activity   The resting level EMG signal can also be used for amplitude normalization. The disadvantage is that the EMG user may not be able to ascertain if the subject's muscle is truly in a resting state or if some level of effort is being exerted. The primary application appears to be for testing patients who have impairments that preclude maximum or other grades of maximum voluntary effort. Examples include persons with cerebral palsy and hemiplegia. Other potential applications exist for testing the elderly and those with osteoporosis, but examples in the literature are difficult to find. The advantage over using a reference from the dynamic event may be that the resting level reference provides an indication of how much muscle activity is needed above a resting level. The reliability and validity of using resting level EMG over other values of EMG for use in the normalization equation is currently being evaluated by Knutson and Soderberg.

Summary

Electromyography has been employed by numerous investigators to evaluate gait. Examples were reviewed in the introduction and throughout this chapter. Existence of a normal template of EMG during gait can aid clinical and research investigations of pathology and treatment interventions aimed at restoring normal function. Although some consensus on the normal profile of EMG activity in gait has emerged, descriptions still vary. Universal agreement may be missing because human behavior is as variant in gait as in other life situations. However, differences can also be attributed to variant technology and methodology across laboratories.

Electromyographic data is influenced by other variables. Accordingly, the relationship of the EMG to other variables was discussed. Ways investigators present normal and pathological EMG data were reviewed. New presentation formats appear to be emerging although common standards across laboratories are lacking. If diagnostic value of kinesiological EMG data is to be achieved, more efforts should be dedicated to selecting standards or guidelines in methodology. Because data normalization is necessary for averaging data, and averaged data are needed to create normal templates and establish treatment efficacy, the methods of normalizing EMG data to time and amplitude must receive attention. Methods of data normalization were discussed in this chapter.

Acknowledgment
Figures 22-1, 22-2, 22-6, and 22-7 were created using DATA-PACII Software from RUN Technologies, Laguna Hills, California.

References

1. Adler N, Bleck EE, Rinsky LA: Gait electromyograms and surgical decisions for paralytic deformities of the foot, *Dev Med Child Neurol* 31:287, 1989.
2. Arsenault AB, Winter DA, Marteniuk RG: Characteristics of muscular function and adaptation in gait: a literature review, *Physiotherapy Canada* 39(1):5, 1987.
3. Arsenault AB, Winter DA, Marteniuk RG: Is there a "normal" profile of EMG activity in gait? *Med Biol Eng Comput* 24:337, 1986.
4. Arsenault AB, Winter DA, Marteniuk RG et al: How many strides are required for the analysis of electromyographic data in gait? *Scand J Rehabil Med* 18:133, 1986.
5. Barto PS, Supinski RS, Skinner SR: Dynamic EMG findings in varus hindfoot deformity and spastic cerebral palsy, *Dev Med Child Neurol* 26:88, 1984.
6. Battye CK, Joseph J: An investigation by telemetering of the activity of some muscles in walking, *Med Biol Eng* 4:125, 1966.
7. Bennet GC, Rang M, Jones D: Varus and valgus deformities of the foot in cerebral palsy, *Dev Med Child Neurol* 24:499, 1982.

8. Berger W, Altenmueller E, Dietz V: Normal and impaired development of children's gait, *Hum Neurobiol* 3:163, 1984.

9. Berger W, Quintern J, Dietz V: Afferent and efferent control of stance and gait: developmental changes in children, *Electroencephalogr Clin Neurophysiol* 66(3):244, 1987.

10. Branch TP, Hunter R, Donath M: Dynamic EMG analysis of anterior cruciate deficient legs with and without bracing during cutting, *Am J Sports Med* 17(1):35, 1989.

11. Brunt D, Scarborough N: Ankle muscle activity during gait in children with cerebral palsy and equinovarus deformity, *Arch Phys Med Rehabil* 69(2):115, 1988.

12. Brodke DS, Skinner SR, Lamoreux LW et al: Effects of ankle-foot orthoses on the gait of children, *J Pediatr Orthop* 9(6):702, 1989.

13. Cahan L, Adams J, Perry J et al: Instrumented gait analysis after selective posterior rhizotomy, *Dev Med Child Neurol* 32(12):1037, 1990.

14. Carlsöö S: *How man moves: kinesiological methods and studies,* New York, 1972, Crane, Russak & Company.

15. Cerny K, Perry J, Walker JM: Effect of an unrestricted knee-ankle-foot orthosis on the stance phase of gait in healthy persons, *Orthopedics* 13(10):1121, 1990.

16. Chen JJ, Shiavi R: Temporal feature extraction and clustering analysis of electromyographic linear envelopes in gait studies, *IEEE Trans Biomed Eng* 37:295, 1990.

17. Chong KC, Vojnic B, Quanbury AO et al: The assessment of the internal rotation gait in cerebral palsy, *Clin Orthop Rel Res* 132:145, May 1978.

18. Close JR, Todd FN: Phasic activity of muscles of lower extremity and effect of tendon transfer, *J Bone Joint Surg* 41:189, 1959.

19. Csongradi J, Bleck E, Ford FW: Gait electromyography in normal and spastic children, with special reference to quadriceps femoris and hamstring muscles, *Dev Med Child Neurol* 21:738, 1979.

20. Dietz V, Quintern J, Berger W: Electrophysiological studies of gait in spasticity and rigidity, *Brain* 104:431, 1981.

21. De Fabio RP: Reliability of computerized surface electromyography for determining the onset of muscle activity, *Phys Ther* 67:43, 1987.

22. Dubo HIC, Peat M, Winter DA et al: Electromyographic temporal analysis of gait: normal human locomotion, *Arch Phys Med Rehabil* 57:415, 1976.

23. Eberhart HD, Inman VT, Bresler B: The principal elements in human locomotion. In Klopsteg PE, Wilson PD, editors: *Human limbs and their substitutes,* New York, 1954, McGraw Hill.

24. Entyre B, Chambers CS, Scarborough NH et al: Preoperative and postoperative assessment of surgical intervention for equinus gait in children with cerebral palsy, *J Pediatr Orthop* 13(1):24, 1993.

25. Forrsberg H: Ontogeny of human locomotor control. I. Infant stepping, supported locomotion and transition to independent locomotion, *Exp Brain Res* 57:480, 1985.

26. Gage JR, Perry J, Hicks RR et al: Rectus femoris transfer to improve knee function of children with cerebral palsy, *Dev Med Child Neurol* 29(2):159, 1987.

27. Giroux B, Lamontagne M: Comparisons between surface electrodes and intramuscular wire electrodes in isometric and dynamic conditions, *Electroencephalogr Clin Neurophysiol* 30:397, 1990.

28. Gray ER, Basmajian: Electromyography and cinematography of leg and foot (normal and flat) during walking, *Anat Rec* 161:1, 1968.

29. Griffin PP, Wheelhouse WW, Shiavi R: Adductor transfer for adductor spasticity: clinical and electromyographic gait analysis, *Dev Med Child Neurol* 19:783, 1977.

30. Gueth V, Abbink F, Reuken R: Comparison of pre- and postoperative electromyograms in children with cerebral palsy, *Electromyogr Clin Neurophysiol* 25:233, 1985.

31. Herschler C, Milner M: An optimality criterion for processing electromyographic (EMG) signals relating to human locomotion, *IEEE Trans Biomed Eng* 25:413, 1978.

32. Hirschberg GG, Nathanson M: Electromyographic recording of muscular activity in normal and spastic gaits, *Arch Phys Med Rehabil* 33:217, 1952.

33. Holt KS: Facts and fallacies about neuromuscular function in cerebral palsy as revealed by electromyography, *Dev Med Child Neurol* 8:255, 1966.

34. Hunt KG: *The effects of fixed and hinged ankle foot orthoses on gait myoelectric activity in children with myelomeningocele.* Published thesis, University of Iowa, Iowa City, 1993.

35. Inman VT, Ralston HJ, Saunders JB et al: Relation of human electromyogram to muscular tension, *Electroencephalogr Clin Neurophysiol* 4:187, 1952.

36. Inman VT, Ralston HJ, Todd F: *Human walking,* Baltimore, 1981, Williams & Wilkins.

37. Kadaba MP, Ramakrishnan HK, Wootten ME et al: Repeatability of kinematic, kinetic, and electromyographic data in normal adult gait, *J Orthop Res* 7:849, 1989.

38. Kadaba MP, Wootten ME, Gainey J et al: Repeatability of phasic muscle activity: performance of surface and intramuscular wire electrodes in gait analysis, *J Orthop Res* 3(3):350, 1985.

39. Kalen V, Adler N, Bleck EE: Electromyography of idiopathic toe walking, *J Pediatr Orthop* 6:31, 1986.

40. Kameyama O, Ogawa R, Okamoto T et al: Electric discharge patterns of ankle muscles during the normal gait cycle, *Arch Phys Med Rehabil* 71(12):969, 1990.

41. Kazai N, Okamoto T, Kumamoto M: Electromyographic study of supported walking of infants in the initial period of learning to walk, *Biomechanics V,* Baltimore, 1976, University Park Press.

42. Kerrigan DC, Gronley J, Perry J: Stiff-legged gait in spastic paresis: a study of quadriceps and hamstrings muscle activity, *Am J Phys Med Rehabil* 70(6):294, 1991.

43. Knutson LM, Soderberg GL: The effects of ankle foot orthotics on gait myoelectric activity in children with cerebral palsy: part I. (In preparation for publication 1994)

44. Knutson LM, Soderberg GL, Ballantyne BT et al: A study of various normalization procedures for within day electromyographic data, *J Electromyogr Kinesiol* 4(1):47, 1994.

45. Knutsson E, Richards C: Different types of disturbed motor control in gait of hemiparetic patients, *Brain* 102:405, 1979.

46. Lass P, Kaalund S, leFevre S et al: Muscle coordination following rupture of the anterior cruciate ligament. Electromyographic studies of 14 patients, *Acta Orthop Scand* 62(1):9, 1991.

47. Lee EH, Goh JC, Bose K: Value of gait analysis in the assessment of surgery in cerebral palsy, *Arch Phys Med Rehabil* 73(7):642, 1992.

48. Lehmann JF, Condon SM, Price R et al: Gait abnormalities in hemiplegia: their correction by ankle-foot orthoses, *Arch Phys Med Rehabil* 68:763, 1987.

49. Leonard CT, Hirschfeld H, Forssberg H: The development of independent walking in children with cerebral palsy, *Dev Med Child Neurol* 33(7):567, 1991.

50. Limbird TJ, Shiavi R, Frazer M et al: EMG profiles of knee joint musculature during walking: changes induced by anterior cruciate ligament deficiency, *J Orthop Res* 6(5):630, 1988.

51. Mann R, Inman V: Phasic activity of intrinsic muscles of the foot, *J Bone Joint Surg* 406-A:469, 1964.

52. Middleton EA, Hurley GRB, McIlwain JS: The role of rigid and hinged polypropylene ankle-foot-orthoses in the management of cerebral palsy: a case study, *Prosthet Orthot Int* 12:129, 1988.

53. Milner M, Basmajian JV, Quanbury AO: Multifactorial analysis of walking by electromyography and computer, *Am J Phys Med* 50(5):235, 1971.

54. Møller BN, Jurik AG: Tidemand-Dal C et al: The quadriceps function in patellofemoral disorders: a radiographic and electromyographic study, *Arch Orthop Trauma Surg* 106:195, 1987.

55. Neumann DA, Cook TA: Effect of load and carry position on the electromyographic activity of the gluteus medius muscle during walking, *Phys Ther* 65:305, 1985.

56. Öberg T, Karsznia A, Öberg K: Basic gait parameters: reference data for normal subjects, 10–79 years of age, *J Rehabil Res Dev* 30(2):210, 1993.

57. Okamoto T: Electromyographic study of the learning process of walking in 1- and 2-year-old infants, *Medicine and Sport* 8:328, 1973.

58. Okamoto T, Kumamoto M: Electromyographic study of the learning process of walking in infants, *Electromyography* 12(2):149, 1972.

59. Õunpuu S, Winter DA: Bilateral electromyographical analysis of the lower limbs during walking in normal adults, *Electroencephalogr Clin Neurophysiol* 72(5):429, 1989.

60. Peat M, Dubo HI, Winter DA et al: Electromyographic temporal analysis of gait: hemiplegic locomotion, *Arch of Phys Med Rehabil* 57:421, 1976.

61. Peat M, Woodbury MG, Ferkul D: Electromyographic analysis of gait following total knee arthroplasty, *Physiotherapy Canada* 36:68, 1984.

62. Perry J, Hoffer MM: Preoperative and postoperative dynamic electromyography as an aid in planning tendon transfers in children with cerebral palsy, *J Bone Joint Surg* 59-A(4):531, 1977.

63. Perry J, Hoffer MM, Giovan P et al: Gait analysis of triceps surae in cerebral palsy: a preoperative and postoperative clinical and electromyographic study, *J Bone Joint Surg* 56-A:511, 1974.

64. Perry J, Bekey GA: EMG-force relationships in skeletal muscle, *CRC Crit Rev Biomed Eng* 7(1):1, 1981.

65. Pinzur MS, Asselmeier JM, Smith D: Dynamic electromyography in active and limited walking below-knee amputees, *Orthopedics* 14(5):535, 1991.

66. Ralston HJ: Energy speed relation and optimal speed during level walking, *Int Zeitschrift für Angewandte Physiologie* 17:277, 1958.

67. Richards CL, Knutsson E: Evaluation of abnormal gait patterns by intermittent-light photography and electromyography, *Scand J Rehabil Med* Suppl 3:61, 1974.

68. Richards CL, Wessel J, Malouin F: Muscle activation patterns in gait of rheumatoid arthritic patients, *Physiotherapy Canada* 37(4):220, 1985.

69. Shiavi R: Electromyographic patterns in adult locomotion: a comprehensive review, *J Rehabil Res Dev* 22(3):85, 1985.

70. Shiavi R, Bugle HJ, Limbird T: Electromyographic gait assessment. Part 1: Adult EMG profiles and walking speed, *J Rehabil Res Dev* 24(2):13, 1987.

71. Shiavi R, Bugle HJ, Limbird T: Electromyographic gait assessment. Part 2: Preliminary assessment of hemiparetic synergy patterns, *J Rehabil Res Dev* 24(2):24, 1987.

72. Shiavi R, Champion S, Freeman F et al: Variability of electromyographic patterns for level-surface walking through a range of self-selected speeds, *Bull Prosthet Res*, 18(1):5, 1981.

73. Shiavi R, Green N: Ensemble averaging of locomotor electromyographic patterns using interpolation, *Med Biol Eng Comput* 21:573, 1983.

74. Shiavi R, Green N, McFadyen B et al: Normative childhood EMG gait patterns, *J Orthop Res* 5(2):283, 1987.

75. Shiavi R, Limbird T, Borra H et al: Electromyographic profiles of knee joint musculature during pivoting: changes induced by anterior cruciate ligament deficiency, *J Electromyogr Kinesiol* 1:48, 1991.

76. Shiavi R, Zhang LQ, Limbird T et al: Pattern analysis of electromyographic linear envelopes exhibited by subjects with uninjured and injured knees during free and fast speed walking, *J Orthop Res* 10(2):226, 1992.

77. Soderberg GL, Cook TM: Electromyography in biomechanics, *Phys Ther* 64:1813, 1984.

78. Sudarsky L, Simon S: Gait disorder in late-life hydrocephalus, *Arch Neurol* 44(3):263, 1987.

79. Sutherland DH: An electromyographic study of the plantar flexors of the ankle in normal walking on the level, *J Bone Joint Surg* 48-A(1):66, 1966.

80. Sutherland DH: Gait analysis in cerebral palsy, *Dev Med Neurol* 20:807, 1978.

81. Sutherland DH, Cooper L: The pathomechanics of progressive crouch gait in spastic diplegia, *Orthop Clin North Am* 9(1):143, 1978.

82. Sutherland DH, Cooper L, Daniel D: The role of the ankle plantar flexors in normal walking, *J Bone Joint Surg* 62-A(3):354, 1980.

83. Sutherland DH, Olshen R, Biden EN et al: *The development of mature walking,* London, 1988, Mac Kieth Press.

84. Sutherland DH, Olshen RA, Cooper L et al: The development of mature gait, *J Bone Joint Surg* 62-A(3):336, 1980.

85. Sutherland DH, Schottstaadt ER, Larsen LJ et al: Clinical and electromyographic study of seven spastic children with internal rotation gait, *J Bone Joint Surg* 51-A:1070, 1969.

86. Tata EG, Peat M: Electromyographic characteristics of locomotion in normal children, *Physiotherapy Canada* 39(3):167, 1987.

87. Thometz J, Simon S, Rosenthal R: The effect on gait of lengthening of the medial hamstrings in cerebral palsy, *J Bone Joint Surg* 71(3):345, 1989.

88. Tsurumi N: An electromyographic study on the gait of children, *J Jpn Orthop Assoc* 43(8):611, 1969.

89. Vaughan CL, Bowsher KA, Sussman MD: Spasticity and gait: knee torques and muscle cocontraction. In Sussman MD, editor: *The diplegic child: evaluation and management,* Rosement, Ill, 1992, American Academy of Orthopaedic Surgeons.

90. Vink P, Karssemeijer N: Low back muscle activity and pelvic rotation during walking, *Anat Embryol (Berl)* 178(5):455, 1988.

91. Waters R, Morris J: Electrical activity of muscles of the trunk during walking, *J Anat* 111:191, 1972.

92. Weiss PL, St. Pierre D: Upper and lower extremity EMG correlations during normal human gait, *Arch Phys Med Rehabil* 64:11, 1983.

93. White SC, Winter DA: Predicting muscle forces in gait from EMG signals and musculotendon kinematics, *J Electromyogr Kinesiol* 2:217, 1993.

94. Winter DA: Pathologic gait diagnosis with computer-averaged electromyographic profiles, *Arch Phys Med Rehabil* 65:393, 1984.

95. Winter DA: Personal communication. International Society of Electrophysiological Kinesiology Meeting, Baltimore, 1990.

96. Winter DA, Scott SH: Technique for interpretation of electromyography for concentric and eccentric contraction in gait, *J Electromyogr Kinesiol* 1(4):263, 1991.

97. Winter DA, Yack HJ: EMG profiles during normal human walking: stride-to-stride and inter-subject variability, *Electroencephalogr Clin Neurophysiol* 67(5):402, 1987.

98. Winters TF, Gage JR, Hicks R: Gait patterns in spastic hemiplegia in children and young adults, *J Bone Joint Surg* 69(3):437, 1987.

99. Woods JJ, Bigland-Ritchie B: Linear and non-linear surface EMG/force relationships in human muscles, *Am J Phys Med* 62(6):287, 1983.

100. Wooten ME, Kadaba MP, Cochran GV: Dynamic electromyography. II. Normal patterns during gait, *J Orthop Res* 8(2):259, 1990.

101. Yang JF, Winter DA: Electromyography reliability in maximal and submaximal isometric contractions, *Arch Phys Med Rehabil* 64:417, September 1983.

102. Yang JF, Winter DA: Electromyographic amplitude normalization methods: improving their sensitivity as diagnostic tools in gait analysis, *Arch Phys Med Rehabil* 65:517, 1984.

103. Young CC, Rose SE, Biden EN et al: The effect of surface and internal electrodes on the gait of children with cerebral palsy, spastic diplegic type, *J Orthop Res* 7:732, 1989.

PART IV

APPLICATIONS

♦ This section applies gait analysis methods and theory to human examples of locomotion. Variables described in previous sections are used to discuss the information necessary to evaluate performance. The stage is set in Chapter 23, which reviews goals of assessment and introduces the concept of selecting the appropriate "gold" standard. Each of the subsequent chapters serves as an example to illustrate the use of gait analysis to meet a particular goal. The advantages and disadvantages of using gait analysis to compare individual performance to optimal non-disabled performance or to classify disability are exemplified in this section. Knowledge gained from gait studies is used to form a conceptual framework for gait problems in disabled persons. Common laboratory findings are presented to demonstrate how variables lead to clinical diagnosis. Several chapters use gait analysis methods to describe gait as an outcome measure rather than to examine mechanisms which produce gait disorders. Gait data collected on a patient population are used to classify the severity of functional disability. The efficacy of interventions used to optimize walking is examined in several chapters. Gait is used in one chapter as a treatment tool rather than as an assessment or diagnostic tool. Chapter 32 demonstrates how data from gait studies can be used to pose hypotheses about the effect of aging on motor performance.

CHAPTER 23

GOALS OF GAIT ASSESSMENT

Carol A. Oatis

KEY TERMS

Disability

Disease

Handicap

Impairment

Treatment efficacy

The first parts of this book have presented the tools used to analyze gait, including the theories and technologies available to perform the analysis. Representative normative data in each area of analysis have also been presented. The clinician, however, may rightfully be asking, "So what?" Will all of these complicated theories and sophisticated technologies yield any more useful information than is obtained by a standard physical assessment? The next portion of this book presents applications of these technologies in clinical and athletic settings. The following chapters will serve as examples of how gait analysis can be used to ask specific questions. The reader will see that the questions to be answered will influence the depth of theory and complexity of technology required.

The goals of gait analysis appear to fall into five large categories:

1. To describe the difference between a patient's performance and a nondisabled subject's performance.
2. To classify the severity of a disability.
3. To determine the efficacy of intervention.
4. To enhance performance.
5. To identify the mechanisms causing the gait dysfunction.[8]

The chapters that follow are demonstrations of gait analysis directed to each of these categories. The reader is challenged to consider the goals carefully as gait analysis is undertaken. Before reading the application chapters, however, we must consider the goals themselves and the implications each has for the investigation.

COMPARISONS OF DISABLED AND NONDISABLED

Judging by the quantity of normative data reported in the first portion of this book (see Craik and Dutterer, Wu, Winter et al., and Knutson and Soderberg), considerable information is known about the walking patterns of nondisabled subjects. Comparisons between the performance of disabled and nondisabled performance are common—perhaps the most common use of gait analysis. The detailed description of normal locomotion was expected to provide an understanding of the mechanisms of locomotion. Thus variation from normal could be expected to lead to a similar understanding.[3] The usefulness of such comparisons, however, is limited. As Craik and Dutterer noted earlier in this volume, the gait pattern is the outcome of a multiplicity of factors, including gender, age, and walking velocity. The complexity

of the factors that influence gait reduces the meaningfulness of the simple bimodal descriptor, normal/abnormal.

Krebs, in Chapter 24 of this book, directly addresses the issue of the standards chosen for comparison in gait analysis. He suggests that there are occasions in which an external standard such as a nondisabled standard is useful. It seems particularly useful when the expectation is for a "normal" performance. However, many studies comparing the performance of disabled subjects to that of nondisabled standards had no such expectations.[18,25] The reader in these circumstances could justifiably wonder if the comparisons yielded any information that an experienced clinician would not have obtained from a clinical evaluation.

Most comparisons to normal kinematic parameters use data collected by Murray et al.[24] or by Eberhart et al.[12] These studies, however, were not designed to provide normative data bases. Instead, they are characterized by small, homogeneous samples and generally lack statistical descriptive data such as confidence intervals. Thus the comparison of subjects who are older or younger or are walking at a different velocity from the "standards" will yield information of limited application.

Several factors are of particular importance when choosing a standard for comparison. These include gender, age, and walking velocity. Many studies have supported the view that women walk differently from men of similar height and weight.[15,26] Differences include a faster cadence and a shorter single support time in women. Similarly, numerous data suggest that age and level of maturation effect the walking pattern.* Debate continues about the exact effects of age on the gait pattern and the ages at which these changes emerge; however, comparisons between subjects of significantly varied ages will be difficult to explain because of inherent differences among the subjects.

Walking velocity has similarly intrinsic effects on gait. Walking speed has dramatic effects on the walking patterns of nondisabled subjects including changes in step length, swing stance ratios, and the EMG activity of the muscles of the lower extremity. Since the majority of normative data were collected at "free speed,"[12,24] and gait disabilities frequently lead to abnormally slow gait patterns,[25,31,35] comparisons between disabled and nondisabled subjects may lead to erroneous con-

---

* Refer to the following sources: 1, 2, 17, 23, 32, 33.

clusions regarding the impact of the disability on the movement pattern. The effect of speed may explain some or all of the differences between the two populations. Thus in order to characterize the effects of pathology on the gait pattern, the intrinsic factors of gender, age, and walking velocity must be considered or controlled.

Krebs notes in his chapter that on occasions the disabled subject serves as a more meaningful standard than the nondisabled standard. This is particularly true when the goal of assessment is to classify the level of disability. The implications of this assessment goal follow.

Disability Levels

The sociologist Saad Nagi proposed a classification scheme to help explain the relationship between health and functional status.[27] Nagi uses the term *disease* to describe the organic alteration. *Impairment* identifies the alteration in the bodily processes resulting from the disease. *Disability* is the resulting functional loss, and *handicap* is the resulting ability or inability to function within society. For example, rheumatoid arthritis is the disease; decreased knee joint range of motion is the impairment; gait dysfunction is the disability; and the ability of the patient to continue his or her job is a measure of handicap.

As healthcare reimbursement becomes more and more tied to alleviating disability and handicap, gait assessment may become particularly well suited to measure the severity of disability. Measures of disability have been used successfully in the evaluation of chronic disorders such as arthritis[16] and low back pain[29] and are gathering appeal in clinical settings.[7,14] A recent study of the use of diagnoses to drive treatment among physical therapists in the Netherlands reported that the therapists studied used measures of impairment most frequently to plan and implement treatments.[9] However the importance of establishing a relationship between impairment and disability was discussed.

Knutsson and Richards demonstrated the use of EMG patterns during locomotion to classify patients with hemiplegia.[19] These authors reported three distinct patterns of muscle activity during locomotion in patients with spastic hemiplegia. By identifying such distinctions the authors suggested that treatment might be directed more specifically to the functional limitation. Delitto et al. have also described a classification scheme for patients with low back pain.[10] These authors, too, note that a classification scheme based on functional ability

may lead to more direct and thus more successful interventions.

Similarly Richards et al. in this volume used walking velocity to classify patients during the recovery stage of stroke. The authors then investigated the relationships between velocity and other standard clinical measures of function. They noted that walking velocity seemed to discriminate better among the different functional levels and may be more sensitive to physiological changes during recovery.

In all of these examples the authors use functional abilities as outcome measures to classify patients within a single diagnostic category. Such classification may yield a more specific and efficient application of treatment to improve recovery. Treatment efficacy is a critical concern for clinicians and the use of gait assessment to evaluate treatment efficacy is the next goal to be discussed. While comparisons with normal may be the most common application of gait analysis, assessment of treatment efficacy is probably the most common *clinical* application of gait assessment.

Efficacy of Intervention

Implicit in the comparison of disabled performance to nondisabled performance is the goal of "normalizing" performance or at least improving function. Classification of disability also implies a more directed treatment regimen to optimize results. Two factors are primary forces in healthcare today: the need to shorten hospital stays[13] and the need to maximize function.[21] These two apparently opposite forces compel the healthcare provider to search for and utilize the most effective treatment regimens.

Thus another common goal of gait assessment is evaluation of treatment efficacy. Here again, a judicious choice of measurement standard is important. If the expectation is the return to "normal" behavior, normal standards of comparison are logical, indeed essential. In a subsequent chapter in this volume, Snyder-Mackler and Eastlack discuss the effects of disruption and repair of the anterior cruciate ligament on functions including walking. Information regarding preinjury status is rarely available; however, most patients have unilateral injuries only. The opposite knee, an apparently normal knee, then serves as a common and useful measure of performance. Achieving the functional capacity of the uninvolved knee provides a measurable goal. Thus locomotion performance provides a useful outcome measure to assess the effectiveness of intervention.

In many studies, however, the subjects demonstrate disabilities not expected to be normalized by intervention.[20,22] The investigators use preintervention status or the functional abilities of comparable subjects to assess the effects of a treatment approach. Rodgers and Selby-Silverstein, in later chapters in this section, also use gait analysis to provide outcome measures following intervention. Treatment is provided to improve functional performance, not to restore normal function. These chapters utilize the pretreatment status of the subjects as the basis for comparison. As healthcare dollars are guarded more carefully, studies such as these may be essential to justify continued intervention. Clinicians who have been accustomed to measuring *impairment* may look to gait analysis to provide a measurement of *disability*.

Clinicians who intervene to improve *normal* performance also find gait analysis a useful outcome measure, which leads us to the next goal of gait assessment.

TO ENHANCE PERFORMANCE

Athletes, along with their coaches, have followed the advancement of motion analysis with anticipation and have utilized the technological advances in order to enhance their performance. Such application may take the form of recommending alterations in swimming stroke or the position of the lift in a ski jump. Cavanagh and colleagues have examined the running form of runners, in part to identify differences between average runners and elite runners.[4-6] Williams et al. reported differences in some kinematic variables when elite female runners were compared to elite male runners measured at the same running velocity.[39] Williams and Cavanagh noted that certain biomechanical variables appeared to be related to running efficiency as measured by VO2.[38] However they cautioned that the relationship appeared complex and was likely to incorporate a set of variables rather than a single parameter. In fact, Williams suggested that thus far gait analysis has proven to be more useful in understanding the source of injuries in runners than providing information to improve running efficiency.[37]

Implicit in the goal of improving performance is the belief that gait analysis can provide information to explain the mechanism of performance. Similarly, the treatment of gait pathologies is based on hypotheses regarding the mechanisms of the movement pathology. Understanding the mechanisms of the movement pathology is the last and perhaps most compelling goal of gait analysis.

TO DETERMINE THE MECHANISMS OF THE GAIT ABNORMALITY

The first goal of gait analysis reviewed in this chapter was the comparison of normal gait patterns with abnormal patterns. However, such a comparison may not yield sufficiently meaningful information to explain the abnormal performance. This critique implies that there is usefulness in understanding *why* a patient walks in a particular manner. Such a belief suggests that understanding the mechanisms of the movement will result in a more specific and thus more successful intervention.

The mechanisms responsible for normal gait have been studied intensively during the twentieth century and have been considered for hundreds of years. The extension of this interest in the mechanics of gait to abnormal gait appears to have accelerated in the second half of this century; Ducroquet wrote a classic clinical text describing the apparent cause of numerous gait deviations.[11] The more recent interest seems to have paralleled the expansion of technical capabilities and the concomitant increase in survival rate of individuals with disabilities.

Countless studies have attempted to explain the abnormal phenomena in pathological gait patterns.[28,34] A difficult part in the task of understanding the mechanisms of gait disorders is the discrimination of primary mechanisms from compensatory mechanisms. Simon et al. used mathematical analysis to separate the primary from the compensatory mechanisms in children with cerebral palsy.[30] Weintraub et al. have presented a computerized diagnostic system for gait analysis that attempts to consider the multiple movement faults and their interactions to determine the "best" explanation of the pathology, including primary and compensatory mechanisms.[36] The ability to make this distinction could certainly have implications for treatment. One could hypothesize that the compensatory changes would be eradicated if the primary problems could be treated effectively.

A similarly difficult task is to identify the essential tasks of gait and the mechanisms utilized to accomplish these tasks in the presence of other pathology. Winter has suggested that the two primary tasks of locomotion are support and propulsion.[40] The author reported variability among healthy subjects in the ways support was provided but a constancy among these subjects in the total support moment generated. (For a more complete discussion see Winter in this volume.) However the author reported less variability in the generation of the support moment in subjects with gait pathologies suggesting that, while the task of support remains the same, the ways of accomplishing the task may vary according to the capacity of the subject.[41] It is conceivable that the mechanisms used to maintain normal locomotion are different from those used to maintain locomotion under abnormal conditions. Thus it is not surprising that a number of diverse approaches are used to try to explain the mechanisms of pathological gait patterns.

The following chapters by Esquenazi and Hirai, McClay, Basille and Bock, and Patla provide a variety of perspectives on the way mechanistic information can be obtained and utilized. The chapter by Esquenazi and Hirai demonstrates an approach that focuses on the individual elements of the gait cycle and the effects of pathology in the neuromusculoskeletal system in order to identify the causes of gait pathologies on patients following brain injuries. They offer solutions, that substitute for lost or inadequate movement. McClay uses an analysis of the structural abnormalities of the musculoskeletal system to evaluate the sources of injuries in runners. Basille and Bock propose a model of intervention based on a combined biomechanical, neurophysiological, and dynamical systems approach. Their chapter focuses more on treatment rather than on assessment as in the other chapters. However the treatment is based on underlying assumptions regarding the mechanisms for the deviations. Patla, on the other hand, takes a more global approach and considers the effect of the other special sensory systems on the altered behavior reported in aging. Such diversity emphasizes the spectrum of approaches being brought to the vexing task of explaining the mechanisms controlling abnormal motor behavior such as gait. It is hoped that this variety will ultimately yield a better understanding and thus more directed, efficient, and successful methods of reducing the pathologies.

Summary

This chapter identifies the five central goals of gait assessment found in the literature. It provides examples of these goals already in the literature and introduces the following chapters in light of these goals. The five goals,

1. to distinguish between normal and abnormal,
2. to classify severity of disability,
3. to assess treatment efficacy,
4. to enhance performance, and
5. to identify underlying mechanisms,

influence the kinds of technologies and controls needed in the assessment. The specific goal of gait analysis should be identified prior to the onset of the assessment.

References

1. Barron RC: Disorders of gait related to the aging nervous system, *Geriatrics* 22:113, 1967.
2. Beck RJ, Andriacchi TP, Kuo KN et al: Changes in the gait patterns of growing children, *J Bone Joint Surg* 63-A:1452, 1981.
3. Cappozzo A: The mechanics of human walking. In Patla AE, editor: *Adaptability of human gait: implications for the control of locomotion,* Amsterdam, 1991.
4. Cavanagh PR, Kram R: Stride length in distance running: velocity, body dimensions, and added mass effects, *Med Sci Sports Exerc* 21:467, 1989.
5. Cavanagh PR, Lafortune MA: Ground reaction forces in distance running, *J Biomech* 13:397, 1980.
6. Cavanagh PR, Pollock ML, Landa J: A biomechanical comparison of elite and good distance runners, *Ann NY Acad Sci* 301:328, 1977.
7. Chiodo LK, Gerety MB, Mulrow CD et al: The impact of physical therapy on nursing home patient outcomes, *Phys Ther* 72:168, 1992.
8. Craik RL, Oatis CA: Gait assessment in the clinic: issues and approaches. In Rothstein JM, editor: *Measurements in physical therapy,* New York, 1985, Churchill Livingstone.
9. Dekker J, van Baar ME, Curfs EC et al: Diagnosis and treatment in physical therapy: an investigation of their relationship, *Phys Ther* 73:568, 1993.
10. Delitto A, Cibulka MT, Erhard RE et al: Evidence for use of an extensor-mobilization category in acute low back pain syndrome, *Phys Ther* 73:216, 1993.
11. Ducroquet R, Ducroquet J, Ducroquet P: *Walking and limping: a study of normal and pathological walking,* Philadelphia, 1968, J.B. Lippincott.
12. Eberhart HD, Inman VT, Saunders JB et al: *Fundamental studies of human locomotion and other information relating to design of artificial limbs.* A Report to the National Research Council, Committee on Artificial Limbs, University of California, Berkeley, 1947.
13. Emery MJ: The impact of the prospective payment system: Perceived changes in the nature of practice and clinical education, *Phys Ther* 73:18, 1993.
14. Fairbank JCT, Couper J, Davies JB et al: The Oswestry Low Back Pain Disability Questionaire, *Physiotherapy* 66:271, 1980.
15. Finley FR, Cody KA, Finizie RV: Locomotion patterns in elderly women, *Arch Phys Med* 50:140, 1969.
16. Fries JF, Spitz PW, Young DY: Dimensions of health outcomes: the health assessment questionaire, *J Rheumatol* 9:789, 1982.
17. Imms FJ, Edholm OG: Studies of gait and mobility in the elderly, *Aging* 10:147, 1981.
18. Jevsevar DS, Riley PO, Hodge WA et al: Knee kinematics and kinetics during locomotor activities

of daily living in subjects with knee arthroplasty and in healthy control subjects, *Phys Ther* 73:229, 1993.

19. Knutsson E, Richards C: Different types of disturbed motor control in gait of hemiparetic patients, *Brain* 102:405, 1979.

20. Kroll MA, Otis JC, Sculco TP et al: The relationship of stride characteristics to pain before and after total knee arthroplasty, *Clin Orthop Rel Res* 239:191, 1989.

21. Kuhn KE, Fried LP: Functional implications of chronic disease and physiological changes with aging: the imperative of geriatric rehabilitation, *Phys Ther Pract* 1:7, 1992.

22. Lee EH, Goh JCH, Bose K: Value of gait analysis in the assessment of surgery in cerebral palsy, *Arch Phys Med Rehabil* 73:642, 1992.

23. Murray MP, Kory RC, Clarkson BH: Walking patterns in healthy old men, *J Bone Joint Surg* 53-A:259, 1971.

24. Murray MP: Gait as a total pattern of movement, *Am J Phys Med* 48:290, 1967.

25. Murray MP, Gore DR, Clarkson BH: Walking patterns of patients with unilateral hip pain due to osteo-arthritis and avascular necrosis, *J Bone Joint Surg* 53-A:259, 1971.

26. Murray MP, Kory RC, Sepic SB: Walking patterns of normal women, *Arch Phys Med* 51:637, 1979.

27. Nagi SZ: An epidemiology of disability among adults in the United States, *Milbank Q* 54:439, 1976.

28. Olgiatti R, Burgunder JM, Mumenthaler M: Increased energy cost of walking in multiple sclerosis: effect of spasticity, ataxia, and weakness, *Arch Phys Med Rehabil* 69:846, 1988.

29. Roland M, Morris R: A study of the natural history of back pain. Part 1: Development of a reliable and sensitive measure of disability in low back pain, *Spine* 8:141, 1983.

30. Simon SR, Deutsch SD, Nuzzo RM et al: Genu recurvatum in spastic cerebral palsy: report on findings by gait analysis, *J Bone Joint Surg* 60-A:882, 1978.

31. Smidt GL, Wadsworth JB: Floor reaction forces during gait: comparison of patients with hip disease and normal subjects, *Phys Ther* 53:1056, 1973.

32. Steinberg FV: Gait disorders in old age, *Geriatrics* 21:134, 1966.

33. Sutherland DH, Olshen R, Cooper L et al: The development of mature gait, *J Bone Joint Surg* 62-A:236, 1980.

34. Tardieu C, Lespargot A, Tabary C et al: Toe-walking in children with cerebral palsy: contributions of contracture and excessive contraction of triceps surae, *Phys Ther* 69:656, 1989.

35. Waters RL, Frazier J, Garland DE et al: Electromyographic gait analysis before and after treatment for hemiplegic equinus and equinovarus deformity, *J Bone Joint Surg* 64-A:284, 1982.

36. Weintraub MA, Bylander T, Simon SR: QUAWDS: a composite diagnostic system for gait analysis, *Comput Methods Programs Biomed* 32:91, 1990.

37. Williams KR: *Optimization of movement,* Denver, 1992, American Physical Therapy Association.

38. Williams KR, Cavanagh PR: Relationship between distance running mechanics, running economy, and performance, *J Appl Physiol* 63:1236, 1987.

39. Williams KR, Cavanagh PR, Ziff, JL: Biomechanical studies of elite female distance runners, *Int J Sports Med* 8 (Suppl 2):107, 1987.

40. Winter DA: Overall principle of lower limb support during stance phase of gait, *J Biomech* 13:923, 1980.

41. Winter DA: Biomechanics of normal and pathological gait: implications for understanding human locomotor control, *J Motor Behav* 21:337, 1989.

CHAPTER 24

INTERPRETATION STANDARDS IN LOCOMOTOR STUDIES

David E. Krebs

KEY TERMS

Accuracy

Functional standards

Individual standards

Normative standards

Precision

Reliability

Validity

Currently, no widely recognized standards exist for interpreting locomotor studies. Since the University of California at Berkley studies[13] in the 1940s, top computer scientists, engineers and clinicians have worked to enhance locomotor data collection, analysis, and viewing. Locomotor analysis—including assessment of gait, stair ascent and descent, chair rise, jumping, gait initiation and termination, and standing posture's EMG, kinematics, and kinetics—has benefitted from an explosion of technical improvements in the past decade. Why, then, are there no accepted means of *interpreting* locomotor studies? Two competent clinicians can examine the same data and yet not arrive at the same clinical decision or treatment recommendation. The usual explanation for this dilemma in health-related fields is that the test interpreters differ their clinical experience and weight the relative risks and benefits of treatment differently, leading them to make different recommendations.

This chapter argues that, in locomotor analysis, hardware and software limitations and the extremely complex technology used in locomotor analysis are, in part, at fault. Indeed, a few years ago the National Institute of Health (NIH) funded a major research project (#R01 AM38297) chiefly to enable several U.S. pediatric gait labs that use similar equipment to pool and compare their results.[7] Besides these very real technical differences among clinicians and among laboratories, another, perhaps more important consideration is that few standards exist to guide any clinical decision.* In locomotor analysis, some initial attempts have been made in generating standards for personnel, technical (equipment), and laboratory procedures, but interpretation standards have to date not been addressed.

Locomotor Analysis Standards

Since the time humans first found social contracts and explicit rules to be useful in maintaining order, standards have found a place in law, measurement, and pedantry. Indeed, Hermes' mission was to translate the Olympic gods' messages to humans, and therefore hermeneutics is the name given to the science and method of interpretation. When the instructor states that at least 92% of test answers must be correct for you to be awarded an "A," he/she is setting 92% as the standard. The instructor also determines a standard for what constitutes a correct

answer. In short, a standard is a level of performance or of quality that is established by custom, authority, or by general acclaim as an example or model.

Standards are set in part because no knowledge is certain. Neither empirical data nor theory are ultimate sources of knowledge.[35] Thus, in any field, standards are set somewhat artificially. Hence, some *rules of evidence* (as the term is used in litigation) and *decision rules*—that call for standards if the decisions are to be replicated or critically examined—are required for any clinical decision. In this chapter and in clinical discussions in general, standards are typically developed by consensus panels convened nationally to determine optimal therapies for costly and controversial diseases,[15] or locally by the expert opinions of community practitioners. Peer review standard organizations (PR-SOs) of the 1970s exemplified the latter approach, while NIH consensus conferences are examples of the former. Locomotor analysis standards, then, should be widely accepted levels of **quality of locomotor performance** against which pathological gait, stair, chair rise, and other locomotor activities of daily living (ADL) are judged.

In certifying a locomotor laboratory, standards **could** be set to specify the number of engineers, therapists, physicians, and technicians; the precision and accuracy of the kinematic, kinetic, and EMG data; the repeatability of the test results and their false-positive and false-negative rates; as well as many procedural details, such as how frequently the system should be calibrated and how electrodes are cleaned.[9] In addition to the standards for the technical aspects of the equipment used to gather the data and the professional aptitude of the clinicians generating the interpretations of that data, interpretation standards that guide the determination of "normal" values against which a given patient's test results are compared have a critical impact on locomotor analysis. These interpretation standards and their inherent difficulties are considered in some depth below.

The Need for Explicit Standards

Explicit standards are guideposts. Unwritten— especially unstated—standards, like assumptions, have a habit of changing when they should be steadfast, and stubbornly resisting examination when they should be changed.[1] If clinical knowledge and clinical decisions could be exact, infallible, and made equally well by all practitioners, then explicit standards might be unnecessary. Gait analysis and the clinical decisions made from gait data, however, are rife with unstated assumptions, such as the system's accuracy in all six degrees of freedom (three translations and three rotations for

---

*As of this writing one of President Clinton's "new" national health proposals is rumored to be the formation of panels to recommend standards for treatment of common problems such as otitis media; having read the foregoing chapters in this book, the reader can begin to appreciate the formidable task inherent in setting standards for gait interpretation.

each body segment and joint, respectively). As Woltring[44,45] and others have pointed out, joint angles computed using the 3-1-2 Cardan angles method[40] may be different by a factor of two or three from another approach, such as a 2-1-3 Cardan angle method. The gait analyst wishing to communicate to the surgeon about degrees of knee valgus or hip external rotation present in a patient prior to knee arthroplasty faces a lack of clinical standards as well as a lack of technical and engineering standards in gait analysis measurement and reporting conventions.

Given all this uncertainty, the sophisticated clinician is led to inquire about the nature of the uncertainty. Is my system as certain (accurate) in the sagittal as it is in the frontal and transverse planes? Are some motion and force representations more trustworthy than others? For instance, the obvious and most-cited uncertainty in clinical gait analysis systems is skin movement artifact. There is some evidence that clusters of markers (arrays)[2,3] such as used in the Massachusetts General Hospital MGH Biomotion Lab minimize this problem[2]; however, no system in current clinical use tracks bone motions—unless bone pins have been inserted! Uncertainties in calculating joint moments may be due in part to errors in defining the putative joint centers—many systems place a reflective marker on "the joint axis."[17,20] A small error in estimating the joint center can turn a "flexion moment" into an "extension moment."[20] Indeed, changes in the excursion, range, and variability of the ground reaction vector can be observed in ostensibly static stacks of weight merely by increasing the weight's mass![43] And these are only a small sample of the many uncertainties subject to as many interpretations as there are interpreters.

Clinicians are not alone in this imperfect world of decision making. Other professions, notably the law, have grappled with this epistemological problem by requiring explicit standards of increasing rigor, proportionate to the hazard inherent in the decision.

Examples of Standards from Other Medical/-Legal Realms Civil law uses less stringent decision standards than criminal law, in part because the penalty for an erroneous judgement is greater in criminal law. Misdemeanors are judged according to the standard that the charges are "most likely true" whereas in murder cases, the defendant must be found guilty "beyond a shadow of doubt." Thus, we as a society have decided we would rather allow incorrect "not guilty" judg-

ments in misdemeanors than in murder cases. The same logic should, I propose, be applied to gait analysis. Depending on the hazard, the interpretation of the gait data should be more or less conservative. For example, if my system is good in sagittal knee kinematics, and the risk from an incorrect brace prescription is small (inconvenience, cost of travel to the fitting, device fabrications costs, etc.), then asserting that a "Saltiel" ground reaction orthosis should be attempted to control the initial contact to mid-stance crouching in this child with cerebral palsy would be prudent. But to recommend to a surgeon, with any current system, to change the patient's genu valgum via a tibial osteotomy 7.23° toward varus, or that the muscle powers (angular velocity times torque, both of which are fallible) in the cervical spine are greater than normal, would probably be judged reckless by most experienced gait analysts.

Standards from other medical decisions should be used when analogies are apt. Hypertension and its treatment is an example of an important public health problem in which normal values and normative values may be different. In the United States, normative 120/80 mm Hg values are accepted, but in primitive cultures, these same values represent hypertension. Optimal (or healthy) normal blood pressure (BP) is probably lower than 120/80, but the data are scant at present. We know that BP can be too low, but the precision and accuracy of the measured BP values depend on the home, "lab," or office in which the measurements are made, and the lab-specific standards for interpreting the Korotkoff sounds. No one would argue that a BP of 121/80 denotes hypertension, but some would argue that a 1 mm Hg difference in systolic BP is not a clinically measurable, acceptable level of precision. Hence, a standard of, say, 20 mm HG is often the accepted deviation required to initiate treatment. To follow on the analogies just presented, suggesting that a varus osteotomy of 7° (not 7.23°) might be considered, or that ankle (not neck) sagittal joint powers are excessive, would be within the accuracy and precision of many state-of-the-art gait laboratories. Whether such recommendations would withstand the scrutiny of a consensus conference of experts is a question that has yet to be addressed in the literature.

Limitations to Interpretation: Signals and Noise

My colleagues and I have shown that the "real life event"[18] (gait) is virtually impossible to measure through observational gait analysis (OGA) techniques.[21] Restricting the number of ratings made and rating less disabled subjects may improve OGA,[12] but the results remain very "noisy," making discrimination of even very different brace systems difficult.[22] If the gait of a child walking is the 0-order (or life event) data, then instrumented gait analysis (IGA) kinematics, kinetics, and EMG are first- or second-order data.[18] The statistical and engineering models whose assumptions form the basis of the data the IGA lab team interprets are often unknown to the clinicians consuming the data. Worse, the "purveyors" (the IGA team) of these data are often unaware of their system's sampling rate, smoothing or filtering routines, system accuracy and precision, interpolation routines invoked when markers are covered or data are otherwise missing, and other limitations imposed by their systems. For example, placing a reflective marker at the putative "knee joint axis" and another at the hip and ankle served Sutherland and colleagues admirably for simple kinematic questions, but test-retest (marker placement variability and system precision) was limited, as was the system's ability to determine joint moments.[39] The remainder of this section explores some of the more important determinants of IGA signal limitations, which in turn limit the scope of its data interpretation.

Sampling Frequency   The Nyquist sampling theorem states that an event must be sampled at least twice as fast as its fastest component. Hence, a 3 Hz sine wave must be sampled at no less than 6 Hz to obtain a usable signal; sampling at least 4 times the "fundamental" frequency is required to maintain high fidelity. Some gait analysis systems use 30 Hz sampling rates, which provide interpretable data from some aspects of slow walking,[22] but are useless for analysis of running or jumping. Faster events alias ("fold over") to higher or lower amplitude signals and add to or subtract from those measured real signals. We have evidence that normal gait has some kinematic components with frequencies of 10 to 30 Hz.[3,4,5] In my laboratory normal gait kinematics are sampled at over 150 Hz; higher sampling rates for kinetics and surface EMG (up to thousands of Hz) may be necessary to prevent signal aliasing.

Filtering and Smoothing Effects   Various smoothing and filtering routines exist to reduce noise in the signal and to hide data acquisition blemishes. In any system of even the highest quality, the signal-to-noise ratio cannot be infinite, so judicious use of noise-reduction techniques can

enhance the interpretability and information content of any data acquired. But to what standard should signal conditioning be held, given that we cannot obviate filtering and smoothing altogether, and given that over-conditioning removes telltale signs that the data are bad and *should* be ignored? In our laboratory, we currently acquire and usually present unfiltered force place data. EMGs are usually unfiltered for fine wire electrodes but surface EMG data are hardware rectified and low-pass filtered at 18 Hz (Figure 24-1) or RMS conditioned in hardware. We low-pass filter the kinematic data in software at 6 Hz, despite recognizing that 6 Hz is probably too high for the head and too low for the foot segments.[3] We use three types of the many digital smoothing techniques: digital median (especially useful for reducing occasional "spikes" in the data), mean ("moving average" boxcar filters, useful for rounding overly square corners), and *n*-order splines (time-consuming but useful in fitting functions of a given order to data of a known order); in each case the "window" over which the data are smoothed can be user-set.[6] Figures 24-1 through 24-5 summarize the effects of various "linear envelope" display routines, as well as the appearance of our unfiltered force plate and filtered kinematic data.

Precision and Accuracy, Reliability and Validity   Data precision refers to the number of bits or digits used to describe the signal; accuracy, however, refers to the meaningfulness of these numerical representations. Hence, a digital watch may display the time in seconds or milliseconds. Although the latter would be more precise, both or neither may have sufficient accuracy: both may be incorrect by several hours or even days. Overprecision can be especially misleading to clinicians interpreting gait lab results. For example, our system has 12-bit resolution, and our computer routines display some numeric output to 6 decimal places. Thus, although our system precision is high, in fact, our kinematic system accuracy is at best 0.25° and <1 mm orientation and position, respectively.[27] The term *at best* is used because the most troubling inaccuracies in motion analysis arise from marker-on-skin artifact as described earlier,[2,30] whereas our system accuracy numbers stem from tests of rigid objects with markers tightly attached. Again, just because the computer displays knee angles to .000001 degrees does not mean that the results are accurate to that level of precision.

Finally, no discussion of standards would be complete without consideration of reliability and

Figure 24-1   EMG data low-pass filtered at 18 Hz. Same data as in Figure 24-2, but digitally low-pass filtered at 18 Hz. Note the amplitude attenuation. In addition to appearing rounder and smoother, the height of each peak is lower than in the "raw" data.

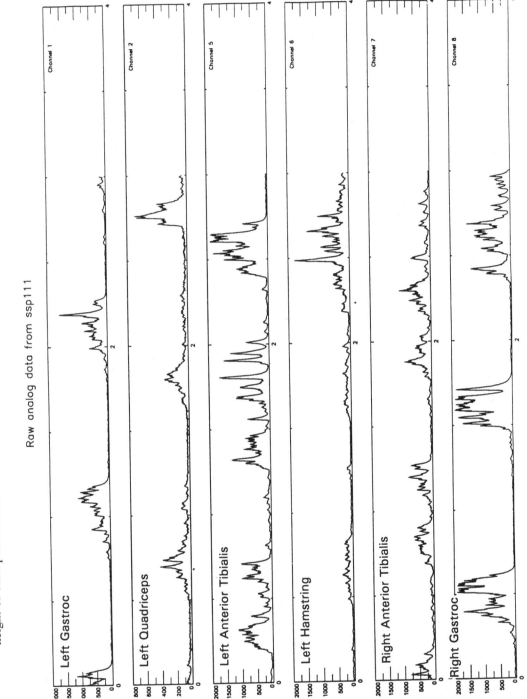

Raw analog data from ssp111

FIGURE 24-2 EMG data of lower limb. Lower limb EMG data from a gait trial of a 25-year-old healthy male graduate student in our lab. Muscles over which the surface electrodes were placed appear to the left and above each graphic strip. Abscissa is time in seconds, ordinate is arbitrary computer A-D units. "Raw data" in fact refers to rectified and filtered EMG from surface electrodes (manufactured by Cyberthetics Inc, 130 Pond Circle, Mashpee, MA 02649), whose integrated silver-silver chloride electrodes and preamplifiers have a system gain of 3750, bandpass of 3 dB points at 45 and 500 Hz, Common Mode Rejection Ratio of 95 dB, noise of <1 u V, and input impedance of 10^{12} ohms (The importance of these terms and the associated values are more fully explained in Krebs DE: Biofeedback in neuromuscular re-education and gait training. In Schwartz, MS (editor): *Biofeedback: a practitioner's guide,* New York, 1987, Guilford Press.) The EMG signals are full-wave rectified and low-pass filtered in hardware at 18 Hz and then sampled at 1000 Hz. The further filtering illustrated in the subsequent figures is performed in software using digital filter routines. *(See figure on page 340).*

FIGURE 24-3 EMG data low-pass filtered at 6 Hz. Same data as in Figure 24-2, but digitally low-pass filtered at 6 Hz. Note the amplitude attenuation is yet greater than in Figure 24-1, and there are more abrupt artifacts at the beginning and end of the sampling period, especially when as in the left gastroc/soleus site, a substantial EMG signal appears at those times. The serene smooth appearances of these data are fairly trustworthy, since we've seen the "raw" signals and they appear to be valid. Compare the phasic patterns of the top and bottom strips, for example; these mid-stance left and right gastroc bursts are exactly as expected. The tibialis anterior (TA) patterns at .5 and 1.75 sec on the left and 1.0 and 2.0 sec on the right show bimodal firing patterns during these swing phases. This unusual pattern is apparently not abnormal for this robust youngster—at least by individual (his left and right sides are symmetric) and functional (his gait is otherwise unimpaired) standards. However, by normative standards this pattern is clearly abnormal. The bimodal firing pattern effect is seen more clearly on this highly smoothed data than on the "raw" data in Figure 24-2. Which is the more representative and informative figure is left to the reader's judgment. *(See figure on page 342)*

FIGURE 24-2 EMG data of lower limb. *(See legend on page 339)*

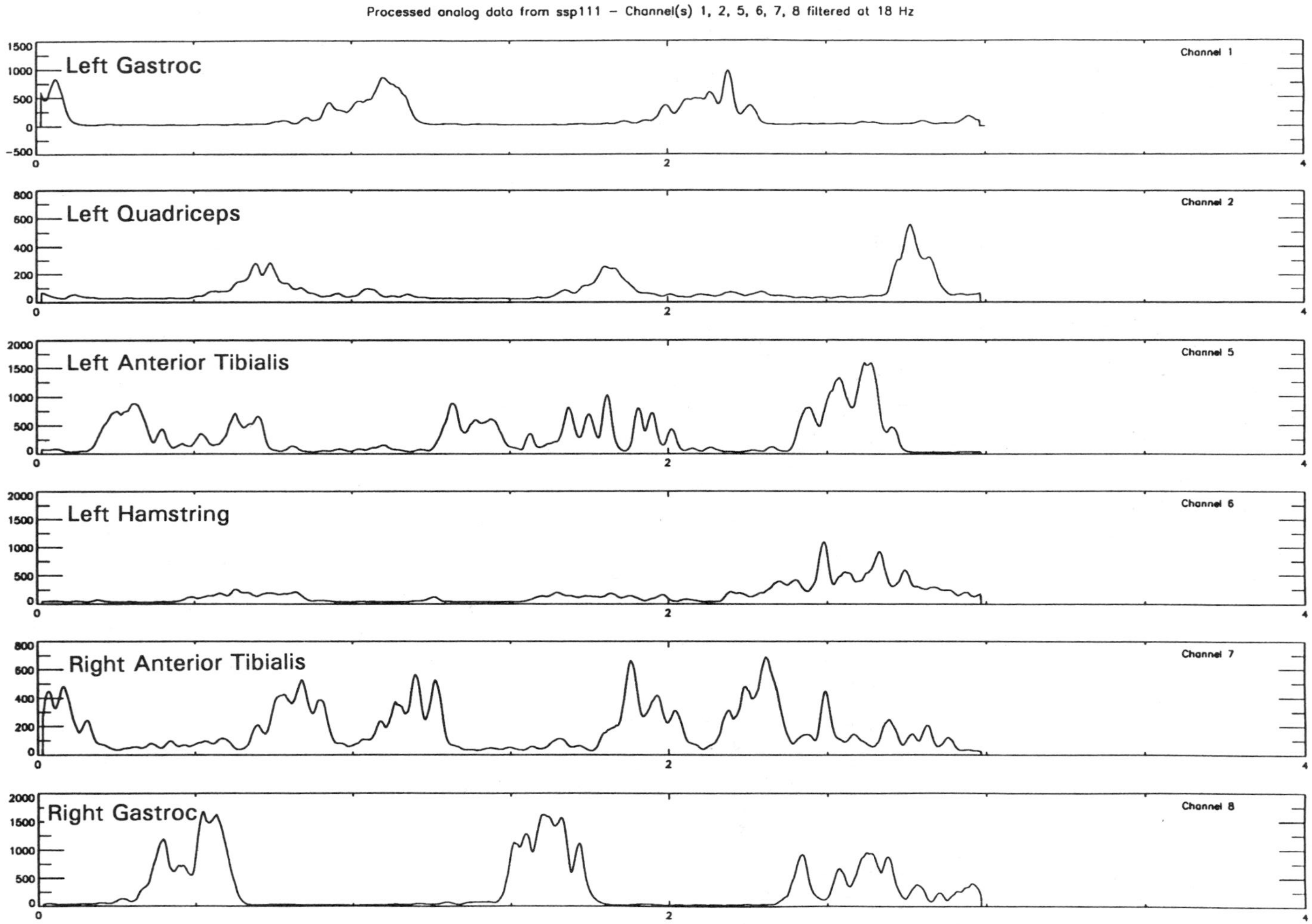

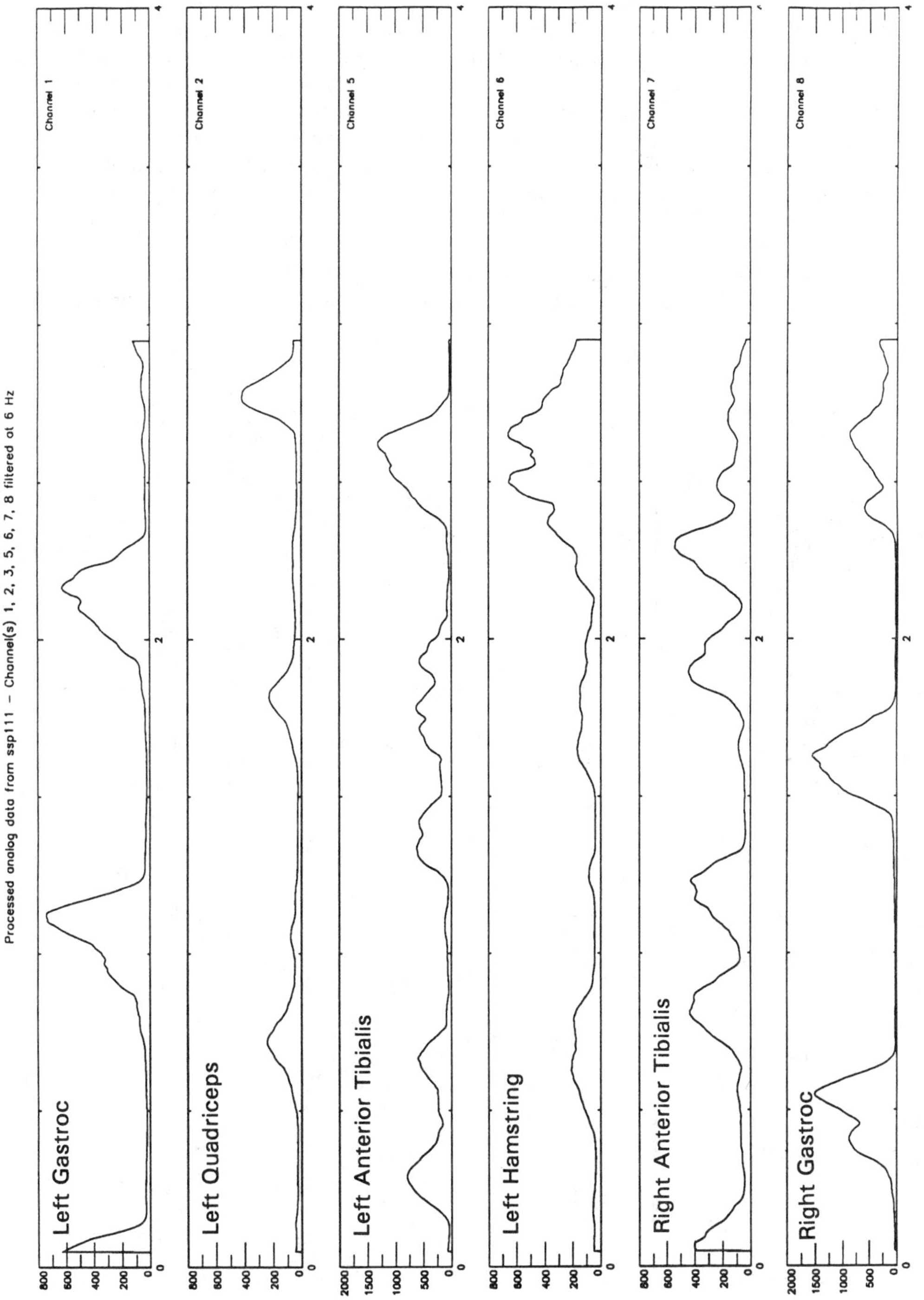

Figure 24-3 EMG data low-pass filtered at 6 Hz. (*See legend on page 339*)

FIGURE 24-4 Kinematic data during stair descent. Kinematic data from the same subject during stair descent are relatively smooth, in part because they are sampled very rapidly (153 Hz) compared to the fundamental frequency of stair climbing.[4] However, the force plate patterns (2nd row down, extreme left) are essentially identical to those reported in the literature except for some baseline "noise." We do not routinely filter the force plate data, in part to prevent amplitude attenuation and in part because the exact initial contact and toe off times are critically important to understanding the phase relationships of the other (kinematic and EMG) data. In addition, the small "notch" about half-way up the first "leg" of each vertical ground reaction trace is a "heel strike impulse," which is quite informative concerning the vigor with which a subject walks or negotiates stairs. Filtering (or too low a sampling rate) obviates this information. Abscissa of all these summary graphs is time in sec; from top left to lower right the nine plots show: (1) instantaneous center of gravity COG antero-posterior velocity; (2) antero-posterior CG (dark line) and Center of Pressure (light line) displacement; (3) whole-body moment arm (light trace: RMS distance between CP and CG in both pitch and roll planes); (4) vertical ground reaction force (shown for right limb during right stance) in percent body weight; (5) base of support (interfoot distance, top trace) and vertical CG displacement (dark trace); (6) left (dark trace) and right (light) knee flexion/extension; (7) left (dark trace) and right (light) foot heights; (8) lateral CG displacement (dark or bottom trace) and CP (top or light trace) displacement; and (9) left (dark trace) and right (light trace) hip flexion/extension. Curve reversals on hip and knee curves can be used to determine cycle durations.

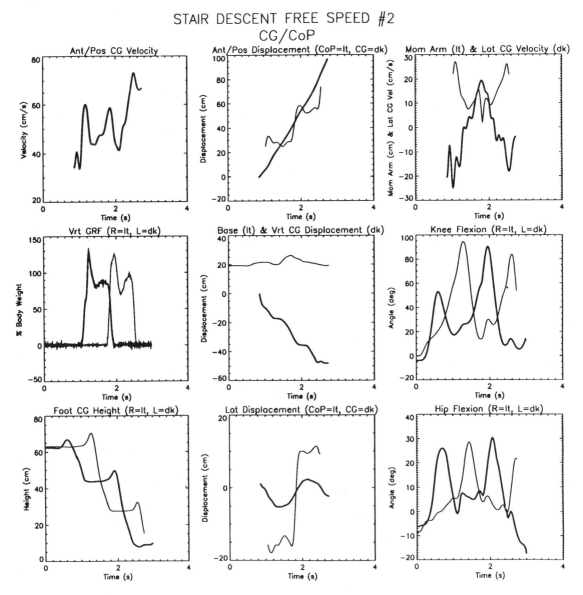

Figure 24-5   EMG data from stair descent. "Raw" EMG data from the same trial as Figure 24-4. Note that the minimally filtered appearance of the EMG data permits the interpreter to establish temporal relationships among gait events by estimating on/off times and comparing these to the kinematic data.

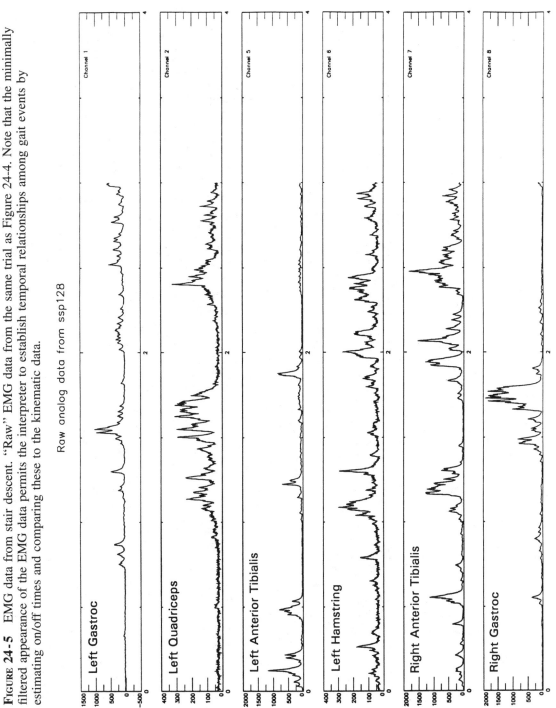

Raw analog data from ssp128

validity, as discussed more fully by Strube and Delitto in the present book. Precision and accuracy refer to the *instrumentation's* numeric output; reliability and validity refer more generally to the test results. Reliability is the extent to which repeated tests yield consistent results. Validity is the extent to which a test actually measures what it is purported to measure.[18] Hence the overall credibility of the locomotor tests rests upon both the stability of the behavior being measured and the fidelity of the signals emanating from the instrumentation.

Valid measurements in locomotor analysis carry an additional burden: one cannot simply ask a subject to walk in the lab and expect the results to be meaningfully interpretable. One of the most common errors in clinical gait analysis is to collect only free, preferred speed gait. For normal subjects who select a normal cadence and stride length (and thus velocity), preferred gait differs little from paced cadence, or velocity-controlled gait.[16,25] Subjects with pathology, however, often walk significantly slower than normal. When their gait is measured before and after some therapeutic intervention the expensive gait lab degenerates into a fancy stopwatch unless some constant velocity comparisons are available. That is, most gait lab variables (EMG, kinematics, and kinetics) are highly velocity-dependant.[29,31,32] If one claims that surgery, braces, or other therapies improve the knee flexion amplitude, EMG amplitude, or ground reaction force magnitude, then one needs velocity-controlled trials to make such a claim—or at least to show that the "improvements" exceed those expected from changing walking speed alone. With a stop watch I can measure gait velocity: if the patient walks faster following surgery, then it would be expected that joint motion and muscle EMG amplitudes would increase, as would ground reaction forces.

Moreover, gait is often not the best locomotor task to analyze. Many knee pathologies are better analyzed during stair ascent or descent,[16,41] and we have shown that rising from a chair can stress the hip substantially more than gait.[38] Some authorities argue no presurgical analysis is complete until the child is anesthetized.[14] Standards in locomotor task selection, as well as data analysis and interpretation, should be developed more fully in the coming decade as current hardware limitations are overcome by technological improvements that permit more than gait alone to be analyzed.

THREE INTERPRETATION STANDARDS IN LOCOMOTION

Clinicians use at least three standards to interpret locomotor test results: individual, functional, and normative. Each has its advantages and disadvantages, and in certain cases, all three may be employed. Most previous discussions of gait analysis and clinical decision making based on these data apparently assume normative standards, but none explicitly address the standard by which a given patient's data are to be interpreted.[14,34,42]

Individual standards are referenced solely to the subject being tested. The most common example in rehabilitation is to compare the subject's range of motion (ROM) or manual muscle testing (MMT) on the impaired side to the "good" side. This individual standard has been implicitly accepted for years in isokinetic testing.[19] In gait analysis, one might compare the right and left side kinematics of a subject with hemiplegia, or the pre- and postoperative kinetics of that same subject.[41] Individual standards are by definition less dependable than normative standards; but where normative data are not available, individual standards are often the only reasonable choice. The aesthetics or appearance of the subject's locomotion may be the most important outcome of analyses employing individual standards.

Functional standards are task oriented; they require that a criterion movement or locomotor activities of daily living (ADL) be accomplished. The key question is, "*Can* the patient perform the task sufficiently to satisfy his/her ADL needs?" Secondary questions are, "Does the locomotion observed increase energy/oxygen consumption in subjects with limited cardiovascular reserves; affect other determinants of gait, such as shock absorption in patients with degenerative joint disease; or preserve stability in patients, such as those with vestibulopathy?"[24] The major limitation of functional standards is their dichotomous (can/cannot perform the function) outcomes. Determining if a patient with low back pain can lift a 50 kg weight from the floor to a waist-height shelf is often less informative than determining *how* the subject performs the lift. Hence, comparisons of back kinematics, torques, and EMG during successful and unsuccessful lifts might provide diagnostic insight into the impaired tissue structure or into inappropriate postures assumed by various body segments during lifting.

Normative standards are used in comparing a given aspect of patient performance to normal values. Hence, normative standards require that a normative data base exists for the variable being interpreted. Such population parameters as walking speed, double support time, and even knee flexion/extension patterns (although not absolute magnitudes in anatomical coordinates) have been widely reported and can probably be considered to have normative databases available. Hence, if a child with cerebral palsy does not have a "double flexion" wave form in sagittal knee ROM during gait, one could assert an abnormality on normative standards; however, because some labs measure "knee" motion in camera, lab, or marker coordinates (rather than anatomical coordinates the way a clinician would use a goniometer), some labs report 5° and others 25° as the normal magnitude for the peak knee flexion in stance. Similarly, if a gait trail had a velocity of <.9 m/min, or double support times of > 25% of a gait cycle, we could, on the basis of population (parametric) normative values judge these gaits to be abnormal. As another example, some researchers report a moment (torque) tending to extend the knee in the first 100 msec of stance; others report the initial stance moment to be flexor.[20] Unfortunately, no comprehensive (magnitude and pattern) normative data exist for EMG, kinetics, or most kinematics.

Indeed, even where averaged data exist for sample populations, authors have been a bit lax in supporting their particular choice of "normative" standards. Winter's excellent anthology on gait suggests that we use 1 standard deviation (SD) to "arrive at a 'differential' diagnosis" of a given subject's EMG as compared with a small sample of incompletely described "normals" from the text.[42] One wonders why only 1 SD is the correct standard, when only 68% of even the "normal" population would then be judged normal? Why not the (statistically) more common 2 SDs to define normal? However, Winter must be credited for advancing at least some defensible and explicit criteria; it is at worst a criticizable, publically expressed beginning.

Moreover, the units in which these EMG, kinetic, and power variables should be expressed remain a matter of controversy: should they be in microvolts, newtons, and joules, respectively, or in percent maximum for the trial, percent of body weight, or some other normalized form? In fact, there is little agreement on a convention for determining positive and negative joint moments. Some labs describe moments tending to extend the knee as extensor moments, while others call them flexor moments reasoning that the knee flexor muscles must be employed to resist these torques. Nonetheless, general agreement exists on the *timing* of lower limb firing during gait, sagittal kinematic patterns, and peak magnitudes of sagittal joint moments.[17]

Several books have recently been published, which provide practical guidance to gait lab workers. However, to date none have explicitly defined interpretation standards against which to judge

pathological locomotor data. Soderberg even suggests that "[w]ithout such [standards] the clinician cannot be sure that the data are meaningful. . . ."[37] Frequently, each lab is exhorted to determine its own "normal" values. Doing so, however, merely proliferates small-sample, idiosyncratic data bases. Because each lab defines, for example, knee frontal plane rotation differently, no amount of "normal values" from lab A will help lab B make normative decisions on excessive genu valgum/varum. Such values could, of course, assist in deciding on the basis of individual or functional standards.

In short, although it might be preferable to have large, representative samples of normal subjects included in normative data bases on all conceivable locomotor analysis variables, it is unlikely such an ambitious undertaking will ever occur. In our lab, we use an 11 segment, 66 degree-of-freedom (dof) kinematic model; it would require tabulation of 198 values (66 dof times displacement, velocity, and acceleration for each dof). Torques and forces for each rotation and translation, the various combination variables (e.g., moment arm, double support, stride length, and other temporodistance values), and EMG for each muscle would similarly need to be tabulated to generate a fully specified normative database. For now, at least, clinical locomotor analysis measures are judged against a veritable pantheon of standards: some individual, some functional, some normative, and some none of the above. The last category, of course, is employed by many motion analysis labs currently providing "gait analysis" services, not from sloth or ignorance but at least somewhat because no federal (or even state) standards have been promulgated, as they have for other clinical testing labs in the United States.[10] Indeed, at present, no U.S. society or association speaks for gait analysis (or locomotor analysis) laboratories or certifies their competence, in part because few explicit standards exist by which a lab's test data—much less interpretation thereof—could be evaluated.[28] The Computer Aided Motion Analysis in a Rehabilitation Context (CAMARC) society in Europe has several subcommittees attempting to set equipment and technical minimum standards, but is not addressing interpretation standards.[26] The United States has no comparable committees at present.

EXAMPLES OF STANDARDS-BASED CLINICAL DECISIONS

Individual, functional, and normative standards provide a basis for the clinical community to begin exchanging ideas on how locomotor analysis influences clinical decisions. For example, Perry stresses the importance of first, second, and third rocker in stance (shank vs. ground rotation occurring about the heel at heel strike, about the talocrural joint during foot flat, and about the metatarsophalangeal joint during late stance, respectively) to normal gait.[34] Normal knee and shank muscle activity is critical to attaining heel strike (e.g., spastic hamstring muscles preventing full knee extension in terminal swing obviates first rocker); but Dr. Perry does not tell us what EMG amplitude or phasic pattern is required to permit normal foot rocker kinematics. When many persons analyze, for example, a child with cerebral palsy and determine that only toe (and not heel) strike occurs during the initial contact phase, we now know to look for hamstring and triceps surae spasticity, thanks to Dr. Perry's work. But according to her, unless we use fine wire EMG, we can only guess at which muscles are in fact at fault. Hence, as indicated at the outset of this chapter, interpretation standards are impeded not only by conceptual difficulties but by lack of equipment and technical standards shared by labs in this field. In addition, these same concepts do *not* apply to stair ascent or descent foot motions.[46] It would be helpful if, in clinical reports, the interpretation standards used were explicitly identified, if only by indicating, for example, "We compared the left (normal) side to the right (impaired) side and found. . . ." Further work is clearly required in this area.

The following interpretations of a patient studied in our lab is intended to be an illustrative case only. The report as mailed to the referring clinician is presented *en toto* but the subject's identification is protected. This example looks at individual and normative standards and attempts to answer the question of whether physical therapy (PT) helped to improve this patient's locomotor ADL? This patient (see Appendix for her case analysis), according to normative standards, had a slow gait with excessively long double support durations, both pre- and post-therapy. However, she did improve both velocity and double support duration following PT. In addition, the locomotor analysis was able to determine through comparison of variables for which there are no normative data which aspects of her locomotor ADL improved. For example, Figure 24-6 of the Appendix provide phase-plane analysis results of the whole body center of gravity displacement and velocity during (from left to right, top to bottom): two trials of eyes open, feet together (Romberg position); two trials of eyes closed, feet together (Sharpened Romberg); two trials of semitandem (feet in heel-

toe but mediolaterally same width as the prior four tests); and finally, standing with feet 30 cm (12 in) apart. Note the latter condition shows least dynamics (velocity changes) on both test dates, while the semitandem condition shows less dynamics (lower center of gravity (COG) displacements and velocities) post- than pretreatment.[36] Similarly, the maximum whole-body moment arm measure of stability[24] during locomotor ADL improved by 20% post PT (see cover letter, Appendix). As indicated by the prior two references, both these measurements have been featured in publications, and we are fairly confident in their utility, but neither measurement has representative sample, population-based normative data available; hence individual comparison of this patient before and after treatment was as rigorous as we could be with the phase plane and moment arm measures. The gait velocity and double support durations, of course, were compared to normative data bases.

Summary

Even by standards of the most ardent critics,[8] instrumented analysis is useful for detecting and recording locomotor events that can not be observed in the clinic, including forces, and motions too small or rapid to detect by eye, so long as the results are reliable and can be presented to clinicians in an understandable form.[33] Humans' acute pattern recognition capabilities, even without other clinical information, is sufficient to allow total novices to discriminate familiar from unfamiliar gaits only from retroreflective markers[11]; hence, experts no doubt glean more insights from patterns of joint displacements and forces than merely judging obtained curves against "normal" values using an arbitrary statistical decision rule. Whether the precision offered by instrumented analysis is warranted by the demands of the clinical decision is the subsequent, but no less important, question. By a more stringent standard, that of expert clinical observation and patient interrogation, instrumented locomotor analysis is demonstrably better. Even among patients judged by clinical examination to be fully rehabilitated and scoring "excellent" on interrogative questionnaires, quantitative locomotor analysis could detect knee angular velocity, range of motion, and extensor moment deficiencies.[16] However, in all cases, individual clinicians need clear standards for interpretation of test results. For most locomotor pathologies, such standards are not now available, so this chapter proposes a tentative framework from which such discussions can begin. For example, even if one were to apply "individual" standards to patients following unilateral knee arthroplasty, what constitutes "full recovery?" Must the operated and unoperated knees perform exactly identically? Must they perform within, say, 5% of one another? Or is operated knee performance within 15% of the contralateral knee acceptable? At present, no clear answers to these questions exist.

Would your personal physician proclaim you cured following treatment for a bout of pneumonia or osteomyelitis without insisting that you undergo laboratory tests? Probably not, but he/she probably would use such a lax standard if you only had a mild cold. Similarly, few clinicians would insist that patients with uncomplicated ankle sprains have a normal locomotion test result before returning to recreational sports, but many pediatric orthopaedists correctly insist on simultaneous EMG and kinematic findings before performing muscle transfers or lengthening procedures on children with cerebral palsy. With society's current emphasis on cost-effective medical care, it seems likely that more physical therapy procedures will be investigated to determine if in fact patients do perform gait, stair, and chair locomotor ADL better following therapy. Such questions beg definition of standards to enable a set of decision rules that can be fairly applied to all cases, and test results interpreted according to those consistent, fairly applied standards.

REFERENCES

1. American Educational Research Association, American Psychological, National Council on Measurement in Education: *Standards for education and psychological testing,* Washington, D.C., 1985, American Psychological Association.
2. Angeloni C, Cappozzo A, Catani F et al: *Quantification of relative displacement between bones and skin- and plate-mounted markers,* Proceedings of the VIII Meeting of the European Society of Biomechanics, Rome, Italy, June 21-24, 1992.
3. Angeloni C, Riley PO, Krebs DE: Frequency content of whole body gait kinematic data. *IEEETrans Rehab Eng* 2:40, 1994.
4. Antonsson EK, Mann RW: The frequency content of gait, *J Biomech* 18:39, 1985.
5. Antonsson EK, Mann RW: Automatic 6-DOF kinematic trajectory acquisition and analysis, *J Dynamic Systems Measure Control, Trans ASME* 111:31, 1989.
6. Benda BJ, Riley PO, Tucker CA: *Use of a computerized 3-D wire model to display and analyze kinematic gait lab data,* Proceedings of the IEEE Conference on Gait Analysis, Newport, Rhode Island, 1989.
7. Biden E, Olshen R, Simon S et al: Comparison of gait data from multiple labs, *Trans Orthop Res Soc:* January 1987.
8. Brand RA, Crowninshield RD: Comment on criteria for patient evaluation tools, *J Biomech* 14:655, 1981.
9. Centers for Disease Control: Regulations for implementing the clinical laboratory improvement amendments of 1988: a summary, *MMWR* RR-2:1, 1993.
10. Centers for Disease Control: Regulations for implementing the clinical laboratory improvement amendments of 1988: a summary, *MMWR* RR-2:1, 1992.
11. Cutting JE, Koxlowski LT: Recognizing friends by their walk: gait perception without familiarity cues, *Bull Psychonomic Soc* 9:353, 1977.
12. Eastlack MF, Arvidson J, Snyder-Macker L et al: Interrater reliability of videotaped observational gait analysis assessments, *Phys Ther* 71:465, 1988.
13. Eberhart HD, Inman VT, Saunders JB et al: *Fundamental studies of human locomotion and other information relating to the design of artificial limbs,* Report to the National Research Council, Committee on Artificial Limbs, University of California, Berkeley, 1947.
14. Gage JR: *Gait analysis in cerebral palsy,* New York, 1991, Cambridge University Press.
15. Healy B: Does vasectomy cause prostate cancer? *JAMA* 269:2620, 1993.
16. Jevesvar DS, Krebs DE, Riley PO et al: Knee kinematics and kinetics during locomotor of activities of daily living, *Phys Ther* 73:229, 1993.
17. Kadaba MP, Ramakrishnan HK, Wootten ME et al: Repeatability of kinematic, kinetic, and electromyographic data in normal adult gait, *J Orthop Res* 7:849, 1989.
18. Krebs DE: Measurement theory, *Phys Ther* 67:1834, 1987.
19. Krebs DE: Isokinetic, electrophysiologic and clinical function relationship following tourniquet-aided arthrotomy, *Phys Ther* 69:803, 1989.
20. Krebs DE: *Seize the moment: dynamics and estimated moments of force in locomotion analysis.* Paper presented at the 12th Annual Eugene Michels Research Forum, Alexandria, Va, 1992.
21. Krebs DE, Edelstein JE, Fishman S: Reliability of observational gait analysis, *Phys Ther* 65:1027, 1985.
22. Krebs DE, Edelstein J, Fishman S: Plastic/metal and leather/metal knee-ankle-foot orthoses for disabled children: prescription considerations, *Am J Phys Med Rehabil* 67:175, 1988.
23. Krebs DE, Elbaum L, Riley PO et al: Exercise and gait effects on in vivo hip contact pressures, *Phys Ther* 71:301, 1991.
24. Krebs DE, Gill-Body KM, Riley PO et al: Double-blind placebo-controlled trial of rehabilitation for bilateral vistibular hypofunction: preliminary report. *Otolaryngol Head Neck Surg* 109:735, 1993.
25. Krebs ED Wong DK, Jevsevar DS et al: Trunk kinematics during locomotor activities, *Phys Ther* 72:505, 1992.
26. Leo T, Cappozzo A, Fioretti S: *CAMARC-II: a European project for clinical application movement analysis: methods and techniques.* Paper presented at the VIII Meeting of the European Society of Biomechanics, Rome, Italy, June 21-24, 1992.
27. Mann RW, Antonsson EK: Gait analysis: precise, rapid, automatic, 3-D position and orientation kinematics and dynamics, *Bull Hosp Jt Dis Orthop Inst* XLKII:137, 1983.

28. Miller F: *Accreditation for diagnostic gait laboratories: is it necessary?* Proceedings of the 8th East Coast Clinical Gait Laboratory Conference, Rochester, May 5-8, 1993.

29. Milner M, Basmajian JV, Quanbury AO: Multifactorial analysis of walking by electromyography and computer, *Am J Phys Med* 50:235, 1971.

30. Murphy MC et al: In vivo measurement of the three-dimensional skeletal motion of the normal knee. In *Advances in bioengineering,* New York, 1984, American Society of Mechanical Engineers.

31. Murray MP, Kory RC, Clarkson BH et al: Comparison of free and fast walking patterns of normal men, *Am J Phys Med* 45:8, 1966.

32. Murray MP, Mollinger LA, Sepic SB et al: Gait patterns in above knee amputee patients: hydraulic swing control vs. constant-friction knee components, *Arch Phys Med Rehabil* 64:339, 1983.

33. Olsson E: Gait analysis in orthopaedics, *Semin Orthop* 4:111, 1989.

34. Perry J: *Gait analysis: normal and pathological function,* Thorofare, N.J., 1992, Slack Inc.

35. Popper KR: *Conjectures and refutations: the growth of scientific knowledge,* New York, 1968, Harper & Row.

36. Riley PO, Benda BJ, Krebs DE: Phase plane analysis of stability in quiet standing. *J Rehabil Res Develop,* in press, 1994.

37. Soderberg GL: Gait and gait retraining. In Basmajian JV, Wolf SL: *Therapeutic exercise,* ed 5, Baltimore, 1990, Williams & Wilkins.

38. Strickland EM, Fares M, Krebs DE et al: In vivo acetabular contact pressures during rehabilitation. Part I. acute phase, *Phys Ther* 72:691, 1992.

39. Sutherland DH, Hagy JL: Measurement of gait movements from motion picture film *J Bone Joint Surg* 54:787, 1972.

40. Tupling SJ, Pierrynowski MR: Use of cardan angles to locate rigid bodies in three-dimensional space, *Med Biol Eng Comput* 25:527, 1987.

41. Weinstein JN, Andriacchi TP, Galante J: Factors influencing walking and stair climbing following unilateral knee arthroplasty, *J Arthroplasty* 1:109, 1986.

42. Winter DA: *The biomechanics and motor control of human gait: normal, elderly and pathological,* ed 2, Waterloo, Ontario, 1991, University of Waterloo Press.

43. Wisleder D, Mclean B: Movement artifact in force plate measurement of posturalsway, *J Biomech* 26:340, 1993.

44. Woltring HJ: Estimation of the trajectory of the instantaneous centre of rotation in planar kinematics, *J Biomech* 23:1273, 1990.

45. Woltring HJ: Representation and calculation of 3-D joint movement, *Hum Movement Science* 10:603, 1991.

46. Zachazewske JE, Riley PO, Krebs DE: Biomechanical analysis of body mass transfer during stair ascent and descent in normal subjects. *J Rehab Res Develop* 30:412, 1993.

APPENDIX TO CHAPTER 24
Dear Dr. S:

Summary
Ms. TKW underwent two tests at the MGH Biomotion Lab, on April 21 and July 1, 1992, before and after physical therapy at MGH for her gait and balance disorders. Major changes between the two tests include a more rapid and stable gait and significantly improved ability to arise from a chair following PT. She reports she now walks alone in her "lumpy" yard and for greater distances on the street without using a cane, as compared to her abilities prior to PT treatment.

History and Complaints
Ms. TKW is a 78-year-old female with vestibulopathy and multiple sensory deficits who first experienced persistent dizziness in 1989, following a single episode in 1985. In 1989 she underwent physical therapy at Braintree Hospital including "positional challenge" exercises (BPPV exercises). Her dizziness stopped thereafter but she continued having balance and gait problems, treatment for which she is now referred to MGH. In addition, Ms. TKW reports left knee osteoarthritis and right foot metatarsalgia.

Balance and stability control is assessed in our laboratory while performing: (1) quiet standing, (2) free speed and paced gait, (3) walking in place, (4) stair ascent, and (5) rising from a chair. Ms. TKW did not perform stair ascent, because she required a handrail or other support during the April 21 visit.

Standing Balance
Quiet standing balance in Romberg position differed little between eyes open and eyes closed conditions. The attached phase-plot diagrams reveal slightly decreased sway during all standing activities in the July visit, particularly in semitandem stance (second row, last two plots of phase-plot diagrams, see Figure 24-6). Greatest instability was seen in the first visits' second trail of semitandem stance with eyes open, but Ms. TKW was able to perform this comparatively difficult task with eyes closed (not shown) as well

Figure 24-6 Phase plot diagram before (April 21) and after (July 21) physical therapy. Note increased stability (less plot dispersion) after therapy.

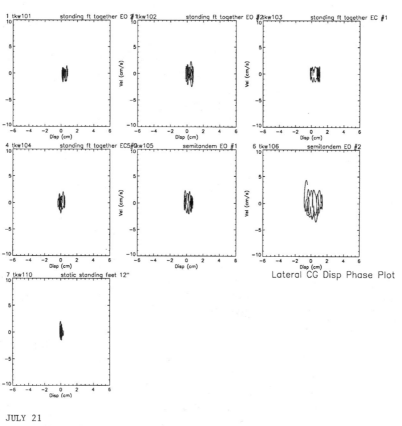

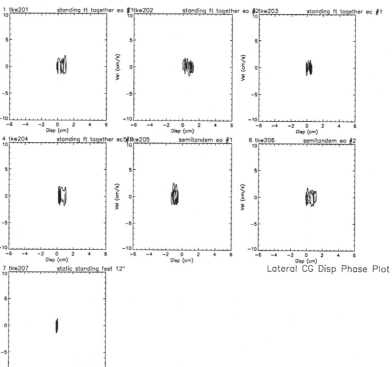

Figure 24-7 Standing positive.

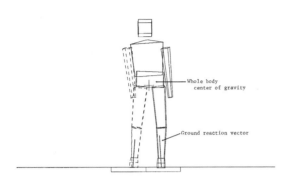
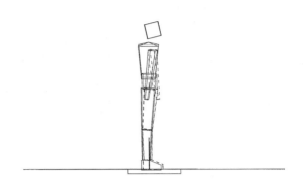

as eyes open at each visit. Standing with a wide (30 cm) base of support was most stable. Posture was normal and weight distribution was relatively symmetric during both visits (see attached "box-person," Figure 24-7).

Gait During the April 21 visit, Ms. TKW's preferred pace gait was slow with reduced arm-swing, broad base of support (≈ 20 cm, compared with our lab's normal 13.3 cm), and slight left leg limping. During the July 1 visit, Ms. TKW significantly increased her gait velocity, armswing, and her kinematics (particularly the maximum moment arm, an indicator of how far she would allow her center of gravity to be from her center of pressure/support), which improved commensurately.

During paced (1 cycle per second) gait trials, she walked more rapidly than her preferred pace, and her kinematics improved substantially as a result. At the imposed pace, there was improvement in double support duration, moment arm, and lateral velocity between visit 1 and 2. The following table and attached graphics summarize Ms. TKW's gait findings. Solid vertical lines on the graphics represent left heel strike and toe off (Figure 24-8).

Visit Date	GCGAVX	HDSTIM	HMOMAX	HCGLVA
Apr-21	64.91	44%	10.17	30.63
Jul-01	83.45	28%	12.22	40.59

GCGAVX = Average antero-posterior velocity in cm/sec, during preferred pace.
HSDTIM = Double support duration, in % cycle, during paced (120 beats/min) gait.

HMOMAX = Maximum moment arm, in cm, during paced gait
HCGLVA = Center of gravity medio-lateral maximum velocity, in cm/sec, paced gait

Walking in place differed little between visit 1 and 2. Stair ascent tests were not performed because during her first visit she was fearful of ascending.

Chair Rise During the first visit, Ms. TKW required several initial rocking motions of her trunk before she was able to rise. On July 1, she rose more smoothly in less time (2.37 compared with 2.59 sec on April 1) and without the rocking motions (note top left graph during visit 1 [TKW127] has 2 antero-posterior [A/P] center of gravity [CG] velocity peaks whereas only the normally required 1 peak is present during visit 2 [TKW227] (Figure 24-9).

Conclusion

Ms. TKW clearly improved her standing and locomotor stability both in preferred and paced activities. She reports she still lacks confidence in her abilities and expresses fear of falling, to which she attributes her slow preferred pace. However, when required to walk more rapidly she appears more stable than during preferred pace gait.

Recommendations

We recommend that Ms. TKW continue home exercises to enhance her confidence in her now-improved capabilities. She should probably continue to walk, at least while practicing at home, at a near normal pace and speed, perhaps using a

FIGURE 24-8. **A,** Gait kinematics and kinetics prior to physical therapy.

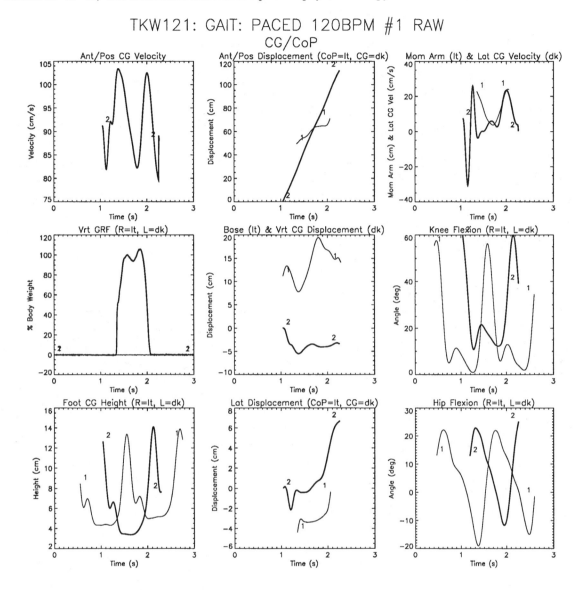

metronome set at 120 beats per minute. Her confidence may be boosted further by encouragement from you and her other health care providers for whom she expresses great admiration and whose opinions she holds in high esteem.

Thank you for referring this patient. Please contact us if you have any questions about these test results or if we can be of further assistance.

Very truly yours,

David E. Krebs, PhD, PT
Professor and Director, MGH Biomotion Lab

FIGURE 24-8   **B,** Gait kinematics and kinetics after physical therapy.

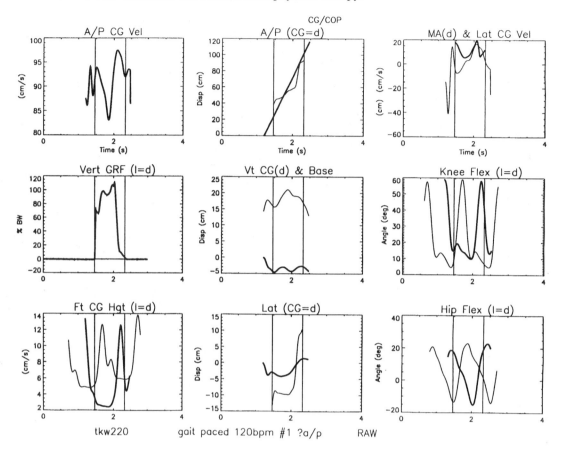

FIGURE 24-9   A, Chair rise kinematics prior to therapy.

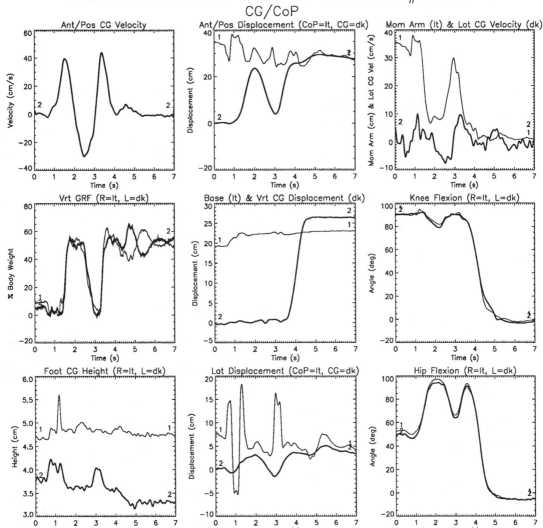

FIGURE 24-9 **B,** Chair rise kinematics after therapy.

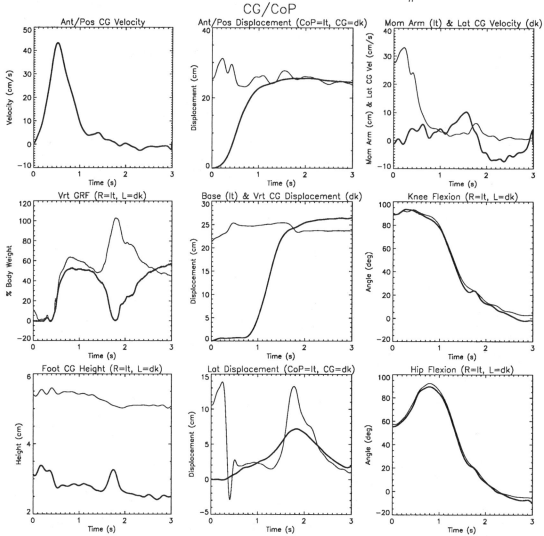

FIGURE 24-9 **C,** Chair rise "box person" kinematics after therapy.

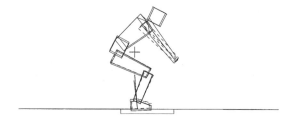

CHAPTER 25

GAIT VELOCITY AS AN OUTCOME MEASURE OF LOCOMOTOR RECOVERY AFTER STROKE

Carol L. Richards
Francine Malouin
Francine Dumas
Daniel Tardif

KEY TERMS

Barthel index

Berg Balance test

Cerebrovascular accident (CVA)

Fugl-Meyer test

Gait velocity

Hemiplegia

The use of meaningful but easy to obtain outcome measures is critical to study therapy effectiveness, especially in clinical trials with a large sample size. Outcome measures should be sensitive enough to reflect physiological and functional changes taking place over the whole range of the recovery process and be reliable whether obtained by the same or different evaluators. Gait velocity is potentially a good outcome measure for studying locomotor recovery, because it is simple to measure and has been shown to be a reliable measure under both clinical and laboratory testing conditions.[5,21,32] Moreover, results from transversal studies have shown gait velocity to be sensitive to the stage of recovery[3] and positively correlated to strength[2] and the propulsive power produced by the ankle plantarflexors[22] but not to spasticity of the thigh muscles[20] in hemiplegic patients. Furthermore, gait velocity is positively correlated to scores obtained in clinical tests of function such as the Fugl-Meyer, Barthel, and Berg tests.[4,18,24,31] Gait velocity has also been shown to be a sensitive primary outcome measure in a recent clinical trial designed to compare three physical therapy approaches to promote gait recovery in acute stroke.[16,25] These results thus suggest that gait velocity may be a measure of choice to reflect physiological and functional changes taking place during locomotor recovery. Systematic comparisons, however, of gait velocity to clinical and laboratory measures of locomotor recovery in acute stroke subjects have not been reported.

The aims of this chapter are to:

1. Describe locomotor recovery in a group of subjects six weeks poststroke using laboratory measures from a walking test (kinematics and EMG) and gait-related clinical scales.
2. Compare the sensitivity of clinical and laboratory measures of gait recovery.
3. Study the relationship between gait velocity and other measures (clinical and laboratory) of gait recovery.
4. Discuss the use of gait velocity as an outcome measure of gait recovery poststroke.

SUBJECTS AND METHODS

Eighteen patients, nine men and nine women (nine with left-sided paresis), with a first episode of hemiplegia due to a thromboembolic infarct of the middle cerebral artery (confirmed by CAT scan) were included in a study. All were able to complete a walking task under laboratory conditions with or without external support provided by caregivers. Values of gait parameters obtained for the patients were compared to those obtained in a group of healthy elderly (58 ± 7.6 yrs; mean ± 1 SD) subjects walking at metronome-induced cadences equal to 75% of their respective free cadences to represent slow normal gait.

Patients were evaluated 6 weeks poststroke after receiving 5 weeks of physical therapy administered within the confines of a randomized clinical pilot trial. (For details of the physical therapy approaches see Malouin et al.[16,17] and Richards et al.[25]) Clinical tests of function, made by a trained physical therapist, included the Fugl-Meyer[9] test of sensorimotor function, the Barthel Index,[15] and the Berg balance test.[1] Both the Fugl-Meyer and Barthel tests have been used in a number of clinical trials and have been shown to be valid and reliable,* while the recently developed Berg balance test[1] has shown much promise. Since the focus of this chapter is on gait-related clinical measures, emphasis will be placed on two subscores of the Fugl-Meyer and Barthel tests that are particularly related to gait performance—the Fugl-Meyer leg subscore (FM-L) and the Barthel ambulation subscore (BAMB)—rather than the total test scores.

The gait capacity of the patients was estimated from an analysis of the walking performance of the patients over a distance of 4 m, repeated at least twice. When possible, 10 gait cycles were averaged. The gait analysis included records of the gait movements in the sagittal plane by means of an electrogoniometer system (modified TRIAX system, Isacson et al.[12]), activation patterns of four muscle groups (Quad = quadriceps; Hamst = hamstrings; TS = triceps surae; TA = tibialis anterior) of the affected leg, and spatiotemporal parameters. The EMG activity was picked up by surface electrodes placed over the muscles' bellies. The myosignals were then fed to miniature preamplifiers close to the electrodes—to limit the recording of movement artifacts—and then to an electrode selector box attached to the patient's waist. They were amplified and recorded to test for the quality of the signals prior to being rectified and time averaged (time constant 20 ms) and recorded on polygraphic paper as well as being fed to an IBM compatible computer for recording and further analysis. The foot fall pattern was recorded by means of footswitches taped to both shoes. Mean gait velocity over a 4 m distance, delineated by photocells broken by the patients as they walked across the walkway, was calculated by the computer.[7,24,26,27]

---

*Refer to the following sources: 6, 8, 9, 10, 11, 14.

Data Analysis

Correlations among the gait parameters were made using simple correlations (Pearson correlation coefficients) and regressions calculated by the GB statistical package and the Stanford graphics software program. Gait movement and muscle activation profiles for the patients are illustrated in comparison to mean normal values (with confidence limits of ± 2 SE). For the statistical analyses, the muscle activation profiles are represented by variables defined as the area under a specific segment of the muscle activation profile as shown for the TA in Figure 25-1. These segments were chosen because of the functional importance of the activation bursts.[7,24,26,27]

Results

Gait Velocity and Clinical Gait-Related Performance Level Six Weeks Poststroke

The gait velocity (n = 18) achieved 6 weeks poststroke ranged from 12 to 65 cm/s. A frequency distribution analysis clearly demonstrated the existence of three clusters of gait velocities. Nine patients were found to walk very slowly (group I) with gait velocities ranging from 12 to 20 cm/s; six others (group II) walked at intermediate veloci-

ties at a range of 28 to 37 cm/s; whereas, the last three patients were fast walkers (group III) with gait velocities ranging from 55 to 65 cm/s (Table 25-1). In fact, the mean gait velocities for groups I, II, and III represented 23%, 48%, and 88% (see Figure 25-3) of the mean gait velocity (68.3 ± 6.7 cm/s; mean ± 2 SE, n = 8) of healthy elderly subjects walking at 75% free cadence (see previous section on Methods).

While patients in groups II and III were able to walk independently, all patients in group I needed some assistance to manage the walking test. The amount of assistance, however, varied markedly among the patients of group I. Six of them needed only minimal support of one upper extremity, largely for security. The three other patients, however, required bilateral upper extremity support for both balance and weight support. If we compare the gait velocity of the slow walkers of group I who needed maximal support (group Ia) to those who only needed minimal help (group Ib), there is less than 1.5 cm/s difference or about 2.2%, as illustrated in Figure 25-2.

The main difference, however, between the two subgroups of slow walkers was found in the Berg balance scores. As shown in Figure 25-2, which plots clinical scores in percent of the maximum value and gait velocity in percent of the mean velocity obtained in the normal controls, for subgroups Ia and Ib, the slow walkers requiring only minimal support (group Ib) had a Berg score of 70 ± 15% (mean ± 1 SD, n = 6), as compared to 23.8 ± 12.5% (mean ± 1 SD, n = 3) for the others needing help for both balance and weight support (group Ia). Similar observations can be made for the FM-L and BAMB scores, which are all above 50% in the Ib group and below 50% in the Ia group (Figure 25-2). These results suggest that for very slow walkers gait velocity is not as discriminative as the Berg balance test, and to a lesser extent as other gait-related clinical scores, to monitor gait recovery.

Figure 25-3 compares the clinical scores and gait velocities (in percent of maximal or reference values) for the three groups. First, note how the gait velocity is low in groups I and II in comparison to respective clinical scores, suggesting that a higher level of performance must be reached in the gait-related tests to attain higher gait velocities. This figure also shows that for subjects achieving gait velocities over 50% of normal values, clinical scores become less discriminative. In fact, there is no difference in the clinical scores between groups II and III, whereas the gait velocity of group III is almost twice that of group II. These results

Figure 25-1   Muscle activation profiles. Illustration of the activation parameters used in the statistical analyses to represent the tibialis anterior muscle. The shaded areas outline the area under specific segments of the activation profile during the gait cycle: 0-16% (TA1), 60-80% (TA2) and 84-100% (TA3).

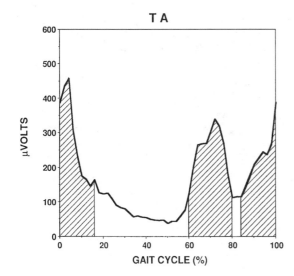

TABLE 25-1   Characteristics of the patients with hemiplagia determined by gait velocity 6 weeks poststroke

Group Paretic side		I ($n = 9$) 4L, 5R			II ($n = 6$) 2L, 4R			III ($n = 3$) 3L		
	(Max.)	X	(SD)	range	X	(SD)	range	X	(SD)	range
Gait vel.	(68.3)	15.7	(2.9)	12–20	32.8	(3.1)	28–37	60.0	(5.0)	55–65
Berg	(56)	30.6	(15.0)	6–43	47.7	(7.7)	36–54	50.3	(2.9)	47–52
FM-L	(34)	20.2	(6.5)	10–30	29.2	(3.9)	22–33	29.7	(1.5)	28–31
BAMB	(47)	21.7	(14.5)	7–41	37.2	(7.7)	28–47	42.0	(4.0)	38–46
Age (yrs)		67.3	(11.3)	48–85	66.2	(5.4)	60–74	70.0	(10.6)	62–82

L: left-sided paresis; R: right-sided paresis; Max.: maximum of respective reference value.

FIGURE 25-2   Clinical scores of function. [Barthel ambulation subscore (BAMB), Fugl-Meyer leg subscore (FM-L), and Berg balance test] in percent of respective maximum score and gait velocity (in percent of the mean velocity of normal controls walking at 75% of free cadence) for patients with hemiplegia in subgroups Ia and Ib.

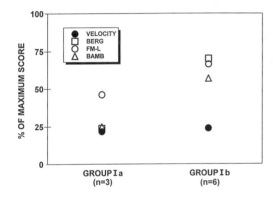

FIGURE 25-3   Comparison of clinical scores and gait velocities. Clinical scores of function [Barthel ambulation subscore (BAMB), Fugl-Meyer leg subscore (FM-L), and Berg balance test] and gait velocity in percent of respective maximum values (Y-axis) for each of the three subgroups (I–III) of patients with hemiplegia (X-axis).

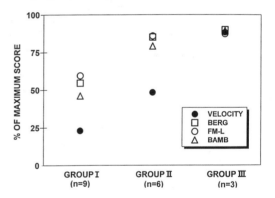

indicate that the clinical scores saturate well before maximal locomotor recovery. This saturation and lower sensitivity of the clinical tests to higher levels of gait performance are likely associated with the nominal and ordinal scales of measurement. Similar limitations of these scales in comparison to ratio scales have been well documented for muscle testing.[28]

These findings thus suggest that for very slow walkers, the Berg balance test may better reflect locomotor capacity than gait velocity; as gait velocity increases up to about 50% of normal values, the clinical tests become less discriminative than gait velocity. Therefore, gait velocity should be more appropriate as an outcome measure to detect improvement from about 50% of normal values up to maximal locomotor recovery.

On the other hand, the Berg balance test appears to be more sensitive than gait velocity to monitor locomotor capacity (balance and strength) of subjects in the early stage of recovery.

When the 18 subjects from all three groups were pooled (Figure 25-4A), the correlation coefficients for BAMB, FM-L, and Berg scores with gait velocity were $r = 0.58$, $r = 0.62$ and $r = 0.60$, indicating a relationship of similar strength. This graph also clearly illustrates how the scores from the fast walkers of group III are clustered away from the subjects of groups I and II suggesting that for gait velocity above 37 cm/s (or 54% of normal values), the clinical scores are not as meaningful. As expected, when recalculating the correlation coefficients (r) without subjects from group III, the coefficients between gait velocity and both FM-L and Berg scales increased to $r = 0.73$ and $r = 0.64$ respectively (Figure 25-4*B*). Removal of the fast walkers (group III), from the analysis had little effect on the coefficient between gait velocity and the BAMB score. Moreover, the Y intercept of the BAMB linear regression lines (Figure 25-4) are always higher than those of the Berg and FM-L indicating that the BAMB score has a higher gait velocity threshold. The latter finding and the fact that in contrast to the Berg and FM-L scales, the BAMB relationship with gait velocity was not strengthened by taking out the fast walkers, may indicate that the BAMB scale is a less sensitive measure of locomotor recovery than the FM-L and Berg scales, especially for slower walkers at an early stage of gait recovery.

FIGURE 25-4 Score correlations with gait velocities. Correlations between three clinical scores [Barthel ambulation subscore (BAMB), Fugl-Meyer leg subscore (FM-L), and Berg balance test] given in percent of respective maximum scores on the X-axis, and gait velocity given in percent of the mean velocity of normal controls walking at 75% of free cadence on the Y-axis. Pearson correlation coefficients (r) calculated for total sample ($n = 18$) in (**A**) and in (**B**) for groups I and II ($n = 15$).

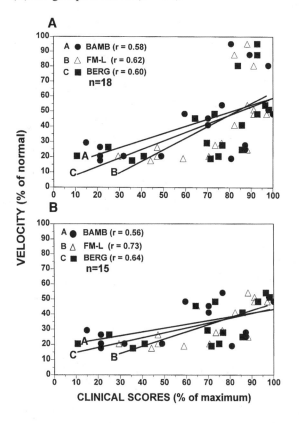

Relationship of Gait Velocity to Kinematic and EMG Measures at Six Weeks Poststroke

Since both kinematic and EMG measures are known to be sensitive to gait velocity,[19,29,30,36] specific patterns of gait recovery should be discernible in the movement and muscle activation profiles of the three velocity-determined groups of patients. As expected, there were marked differences in the movement and muscle activation profiles that could be related to the level of gait velocity at 6 weeks poststroke. This is illustrated in Figure 25-5, which gives individual ankle movement and activation patterns for the TS and TA for subjects of groups I through III (Figures 25-5*A*, *B*, *C*). The ankle movement patterns are perhaps the feature that best distinguishes the fast (Figure 25-5*C*) from the slower walkers (Figures 25-5*A* and *B*). Both the total excursion and the timing of the ankle movements are much closer to normal values for the fast walkers. Surprisingly, in group II marked dorsiflexion (>20 degrees) is still present in four of six subjects, but the timing seems essentially preserved. In contrast, both the timing of the movements and the dorsiflexion excursion are disturbed in most subjects of group I.

The amplitude and timing of the TS and TA activation also differ among the groups (Figure 25-5). It is interesting to note that only one subject of group III (Figure 25-5*C*) had a peak TS activation burst within normal limits. Moreover, despite near normal gait velocities, two subjects from group III have very low levels of activation in the TS, and only one subject of group II had a TS activation burst above 20% (about 45%) of normal values. On the other hand, the timing and the level of the TA2 (60 to 80% of the gait cycle) activation bursts are near normal in most subjects of groups II and III. This TA2 activation burst may represent a compensatory mechanism for the lack of push off power normally provided by the TS.[13,22] The TA2 activation burst at the stance-swing transition most likely contributes to swing phase initiation by lifting the foot, thus compensating for the lack of propulsion force due to weak plantarflexors.[22] Other compensatory mechanisms implicating proximal segments that can explain, for instance, how subjects with excessive ankle dorsiflexion and weak plantarflexors can develop the necessary support moment to stand and walk were also observed.[13,23,34] Figure 25-6 illustrates such compensatory mechanisms by comparing the movements and muscle activations of four patients of group II that walked with excessive stance phase dorsiflexion.

FIGURE 25-5 Kinematic and EMG measures. Comparison of ankle movement and activation profiles of the triceps surae (TS) and tibialis anterior (TA) muscles during the gait cycle for the three groups of patients with hemiplegia with normal values (mean ± 2 SE, *n* = 8). Thin lines represent each patient. Ankle movements not measured for two patients in group I.

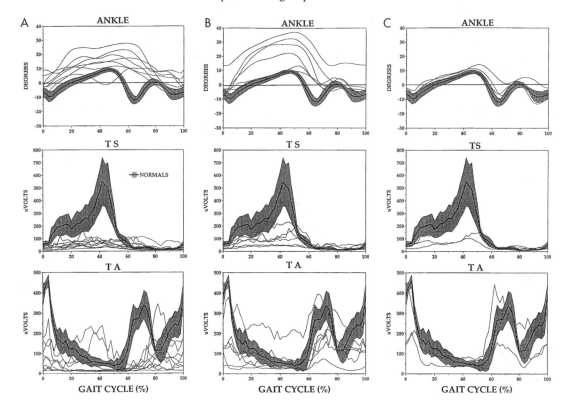

For example, case P 212, who walked at a velocity of 31 cm/s, had excessive flexion of all three lower extremity joints during the stance phase. Given the very low TS activation, it is reasonable to assume that the delayed but prolonged stance phase activation burst of high amplitude of the quadriceps combined with a lower but in-phase activation burst of the hamstrings, acting as hip extensors, produce the necessary support moment.[23,34] Moreover, the genesis of the quadriceps and hamstrings activation bursts may be related to the stretch imposed on the respective muscles by the joint flexions,[13] except for the TS that does not respond due most likely to profound paresis.[13] The excessive ankle dorsiflexion of case P 108 may be related to the lack of adequate compensation by the quadriceps and hamstrings muscles for the weak TS. Is it possible that in the other two cases the contribution of the TS to the control of stance phase ankle dorsiflexion and subsequent push off power negated the need for proximal compensations? Interestingly, the activation profiles of the TA show a preservation of the phasic activation bursts in three of the four cases.

Because we are looking at transversal data, it is difficult to determine if these patterns reflect mainly the degree of impairment or a continuum related to the stage of recovery. Longitudinal studies are needed to determine the relative contributions of impairment and compensatory strategies developed in the course of recovery in the locomotor pattern adopted by the patients.

Relationships Between Gait Spatiotemporal Parameters and Muscle Activations

Table 25-2 summarizes the correlations between selected variables representative of the main muscle activation bursts (see Figure 25-1) and gait velocity, stride length, and cadence. First, note that the strongest correlations were found between gait velocity and the distal muscles and that these were stronger than respective correlations with stride length and cadence. The TA2 had the highest correlation ($r = 0.71$) with spatiotemporal parameters, suggesting that the level of activation of the TA2 may contribute more to gait velocity than the TS or the proximal muscles. These findings are in

FIGURE 25-6 Compensatory mechanism measures. Comparison of the movement and activation profiles of the quadriceps (QUAD), hamstrings (HAMST), triceps surae (TS), and tibialis anterior (TA) muscles of four hemiplegic patients with normal values (represented as mean ± 2 SE, *n* = 8). All four patients belonged to group II; velocity range: 31–37 cm/s.

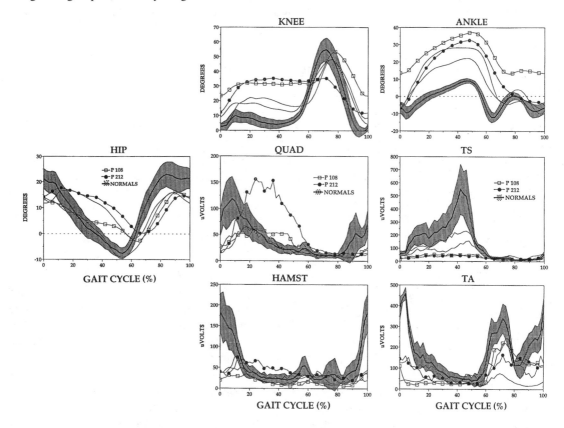

accordance with the low activation levels found in the TS (even in subjects from groups II and III) as compared to the TA, and further support the role of the TA2 burst for lifting the foot at swing phase initiation to compensate for the low TS activation burst. The proximal muscles were not significantly correlated with the spatiotemporal parameters, and only weak correlations (about *r* = 0.50) were obtained between the proximal muscles and the distal muscles. Stronger correlations were found between the TS and TA, suggesting concomitant recovery and perhaps a proximal-distal distinction in the sequence of recovery. One must keep in mind, however, that compensatory strategies implicating the proximal muscles (see Figure 25-6) may confound the direction of the changes related to recovery in the proximal muscles and affect the strength of the correlations. These results indicate that gait velocity, dependent on both stride length and cadence, is more sensitive than stride length or cadence alone to gait recovery. Moreover, gait velocity is more significantly related to distal than to proximal muscles, and in particular, the TA2 activation burst.

Relationships Between Muscle Activations and Clinical Gait-Related Measures

Table 25-3 gives Pearson correlation coefficients (*r*) computed between the BAMB, FM-L, and Berg scores and activation bursts in proximal and distal muscles. Here again, the strongest correlations are found for the distal muscles. Note also that only the Berg and FM-L scores are significantly related with TA and TS activations. In contrast to gait velocity, the clinical gait-related scores show relationships of similar strengths for both the TS and TA activation bursts, suggesting that gait velocity may be more sensitive than clinical scores to physiological changes associated with locomotor recovery.

DISCUSSION

This chapter analyzed the relationships between gait velocity and gait-related clinical measures of function as well as other measures obtained from gait analysis in a group of patients with hemiplegia in the acute poststroke rehabilitation phase. The re-

TABLE 25-2   Pearson correlation coefficients (r) between recovery in muscle activation bursts and gait spatiotemporal parameters at 6 weeks poststroke

Muscle	Quad (0–40%)	Hamst (0–40%)	TS (20–50%)	TA1 (0–16%)	TA2 (60–80%)	TA3 (84–100%)
Quad	1	.70**	.46	.24	.22	.50*
Hamst	.70**	1	.49*	.33	.32	.48*
TS	.46	.49*	1	.57*	.63**	.59**
TA1	.24	.34	.57*	1	.86**	.85**
TA2	.22	.32	.63**	.86**	1	.81**
TA3	.50*	.48*	.59**	.85**	.81**	1
Vel	.19	.20	.64**	.53*	.71**	.47*
Str L	.22	.10	.58*	.46	.58*	.47*
Cad	.06	.25	.47*	.48*	.69**	.35

Vel: velocity; Str L: stride length; Cad: cadence; Quad: quadriceps; Hamst: hamstrings; TS: triceps surae; TA1–TA3: tibialis anterior.
*$p < .05$ **$p < .01$

TABLE 25-3   Correlations (r) between recovery in muscle activation bursts and clinical measures of function 6 weeks poststroke in the total group of patients with hemiplegia ($n = 18$)

	BAMB	FM-L	BERG
Quad (0–40%)	−.06	.06	.16
Hamst (0–40%)	.31	.21	.26
TS (20–50%)	.45	.49*	.54*
TA1 (0–16%)	.42	.53*	.55*
TA2 (60–80%)	.44	.57*	.56*
TA3 (84–100%)	.27	.49*	.46

BAMB: Barthel ambulation subscore; FM-L: Fugl-Meyer leg subscore; BERG: Berg balance score; Quad: quadriceps; Hamst: hamstrings; TS: triceps surae; TA: tibialis anterior
*$p < .05$ **$p < .01$

sults showed that patients with lesions of the same cerebral territory sustained 6 weeks earlier presented very different levels of gait recovery thus confirming the multifactorial nature of disability creation in stroke patients (for a review, see Wood-Dauphinee[35]). Scrutiny of the gait velocity distribution led to the distinction of three groups of patients: near normal (group III), intermediate (group II), and slow (group I) walkers. This finding supports the use of gait velocity to measure the level of gait recovery even in the very acute phase.[4,18,25,30]

Patients in group I could further be divided into groups Ia and Ib on the basis of the need for support. Those in group Ia, required maximal bilateral support to walk whereas those in Ib could

walk with minimal support. In the very slow walkers of group I, gait velocity did not discriminate between the patients of groups Ia and Ib. On the other hand, of the clinical scores used, the Berg balance score appeared to best distinguish the need for support among the patients. This is not surprising because the Berg balance test evaluates elements of posture and balance that are necessary prerequisites of independent walking.[1,33] These results thus suggest that for very slow walkers (range: 12–20 cm/s), the Berg balance test is more sensitive than gait velocity to measure the level of locomotor recovery.

Further analysis indicated that clinical scores, including the Berg balance score, plateaued when patients achieved a gait velocity equal to about 50% of the velocity of elderly normal controls walking at 75% of free cadence. This corresponds to a velocity of about 33 cm/s or about 30% of the velocity of normal controls at 100% free cadence.[24] In fact, except for the Barthel ambulation subscore, the strength of the relationships between the gait-related clinical scores and gait velocity was weakened when results of the patients in group III were included in the analysis. Such a saturation of the clinical scores has important implications because it means that clinical scales such as the Barthel ambulation subscore, the Berg balance test, and the Fugl-Meyer leg subscore are not sensitive enough to monitor small changes in locomotor recovery even for patients in mid-range (50%) of locomotor recovery. This lack of sensitivity, due in part to the limitations associated with gait-related motor behaviors to infer gait recovery and in part to the ordinal scales of measurement used to score the behaviors,[28] argues for the selection of gait velocity rather than clinical measures as an outcome measure once patients have attained about 50% of normal gait velocity or as in the present case are able to walk independently at a velocity of about 33 cm/s.

This chapter also presented new information on the movement and muscle activation profiles during gait of a relatively homogeneous group of patients in terms of lesion location and time poststroke. As expected, patients in group I, who walked very slowly, had the most disturbed profiles while those in group III had the least disturbed. A most important finding was the possibility of relating characteristic movement and activation profiles to one of the three levels of locomotor recovery defined on the basis of gait velocity. This is critical because it suggests that gait velocity reflects aspects of the underlying physiological change. Interestingly, it was found that the most frequent type of disturbed motor control was the lack of adequate muscle activations or type 2 as described by Knutsson and Richards.[13] Whether the predominance of type 2 disturbances in this cohort of patients can be associated to the type and severity of the lesion, the time poststroke, or to early physical therapy is at present unknown.

Consistent findings were also reported between clinical tests and muscle activations on the one hand and between gait velocity and muscle activations on the other hand. Both sets of relationships pointed out that distal muscles contributed more than proximal muscles to the level of locomotor recovery. Moreover, while the contribution of the TS to recovery was expected,[22] it was surprising to see how the TA at the stance-swing transition could be important for locomotor recovery. The weak correlations between gait velocity and the proximal muscles may in part be due to biomechanical compensations[13,23,34] such as illustrated in Figure 25-6. Finally, as expected, gait velocity is more strongly related to the muscle activations or gait-related clinical scores than either stride length or cadence alone.[24]

In summary, the results of the present chapter support gait velocity as an outcome measure of choice to monitor locomotor recovery over the whole range of velocities, and even more so when patients with hemiplegia are capable of independent gait. Gait velocity reflects both functional and physiological changes and remains sensitive to change even in the upper levels of recovery.

Acknowledgment: *This work was supported by the Canadian National Health Research and De-velopment Program and the Hôpital de l'Enfant-Jésus Foundation.*

REFERENCES

1. Berg K et al: Measuring balance in the elderly: preliminary development of an instrument, *Physiother Can* 41:304, 1989.
2. Bohannon RW: Strength of lower limb related to gait velocity and cadence in stroke patients, *Physiother Can* 38:204, 1986.
3. Brandstater ME et al: Hemiplegic gait: analysis of temporal variables, *Arch Phys Med Rehabil* 64:583, 1983.
4. Dettmann MA, Linder MT, Sepic SB: Relationships among walking performance, postural stability, and functional assessments of the hemiplegic patient, *Am J Phys Med* 66:77, 1987.
5. Drouin LM et al: Correlation between gross motor function measure scores and gait spatiotemporal measures in children with neurological impairments. (submitted to *Dev Med Child Neurol*)
6. Duncan PW, Propst M, Nelson SG: Reliability of the Fugl-Meyer assessment on sensorimotor recovery following cerebrovascular lesion, *Phys Ther* 63:1606, 1983.
7. Durand A, Richards CL, Malouin F et al: Motor recovery after arthroscopic partial meniscectomy: analysis of gait and the ascent and descent of stairs, *J Bone Joint Surg* 75A:202, 1993.
8. Eggert GM et al: Caring for patients with long-term disability, *Geriatrics* 32:102, 1977.
9. Fugl-Meyer AR et al: Post-stroke hemiplegic patient. I. Method for evaluation of physical performance, *Scand J Rehab Med* 7:13, 1975.
10. Granger CV et al: Stroke rehabilitation: analysis of repeated Barthel Index measures, *Arch Phys Med Rehabil* 60:14, 1979.
11. Gresham GE et al: Residual disability in survivors of stroke: the Framingham study, *N Eng J Med* 293:954, 1975.
12. Isacson J, Gransberg L, Knutsson E: Three-dimensional electrogoniometric gait recording, *J Biomech* 19:627, 1986.
13. Knutsson E, Richards C: Different types of disturbed motor control in gait of hemiplegic patients, *Brain* 102:405, 1979.
14. Kusoffsky A et al: The relationship between sensory impairment and motor recovery in patients with hemiplegia, *Scand J Rehab Med* 14:27, 1982.
15. Mahoney FD, Barthel DW: Rehabilitation of the hemiplegic patient: a clinical evaluation, *Arch Phys Med Rehabil* 35:359, 1954.
16. Malouin F et al: Effects of an intense task-oriented gait training program in acute stroke patients: a pilot study. In Woollacott M, Horak F, editors: *Posture and gait: control mechanisms,* Eugene, Ore, 1992, University of Oregon Books.
17. Malouin F et al: Use of an intensive task-oriented gait training program in a series of patients with acute cerebrovascular accident, *Phys Ther* 72:781, 1992.
18. Mizrahi J et al: Variation of time-distance parameters of the stride as related to clinical gait improvement in hemiplegics, *Scand J Rehab Med* 14:133, 1982.

19. Murray MP et al: A comparison of free and fast speed walking patterns of normal men, *Am J Phys Med* 45:8, 1966.
20. Norton B et al: Correlation between gait speed and spasticity at the knee, *Phys Ther* 55:355, 1975.
21. Olney SJ et al: An ambulation profile for clinical gait evaluation, *Physiother Can* 31:85, 1979.
22. Olney SJ et al: Work and power in gait of stroke patients, *Arch Phys Med Rehabil* 72:309, 1991.
23. Perry J: Kinesiology of lower extremity bracing, *Clin Orthop* 102:18, 1974.
24. Richards CL, Malouin F, Dumas F et al: The relationship of gait speed to clinical measures of function and muscle activations during recovery post-stroke, *Proceedings NACOB II*:299, 1992.
25. Richards CL et al: Task-specific physical therapy for optimization of gait recovery in acute stroke patients, *Arch Phys Med Rehabil* 74:612, 1993.
26. Richards CL et al: Muscle activation level comparisons for determining functional demands of locomotor tasks, *Sem Orthop* 4:120, 1989.
27. Richards CL, Malouin F, Dumas F: Effects of a single session of prolonged plantarflexor stretch on muscle activations during gait, *Scand J Rehab Med* 23:103, 1991.
28. Rothstein JM: Measurement and clinical practice, In Rothstein JM, editor: *Measurement in physical therapy,* New York, 1985, Churchill Livingstone.
29. Shiavi R, Bugle HJ, Limbird T: Electromyographic gait assessment. Part 1: Adult EMG profiles and walking speed, *J Rehabil Res Dev* 24:13, 1987.
30. Shiavi R, Bugle HJ, Limbird T: Electromyographic gait assessment. Part 2: Preliminary assessment of hemiplegic synergy patterns, *J Rehabil Res Dev* 24:24, 1987.
31. Skilbeck CE et al: Recovery after stroke, *J Neurol Neurosurg Psychiatry* 46:5, 1983.
32. Wall JC: Measurement of the temporal gait parameters from a videorecording, In Woollacott M, Horak F, editors: *Posture and gait: control mechanisms,* Eugene, Ore, 1992, University of Oregon Books.
33. Winstein CJ et al: Standing balance training: effects on balance and locomotion in hemiparetic adults, *Arch Phys Med Rehabil* 70:755, 1989.
34. Winter DA: Overall principle of lower limb support during stance phase of gait, *J Biomech* 13:923, 1980.
35. Wood-Dauphinee S: The epidemiology of stroke: relevance for physical therapists, *Physiother Can* 37:377, 1985.
36. Yang JF, Winter DA: Surface EMG profiles during different walking cadences in humans, *Electroencephalogr Clin Neurophysiol* 60:485, 1985.

EFFECT OF FUNCTIONAL ELECTRICAL STIMULATION

Mary M. Rodgers

KEY TERMS

Biomechanical model

Cutaneous electrodes

Hybrid systems

Implanted electrodes

Multichannel implanted FES system

Reciprocating gait orthosis (RGO)

Spinal cord injury (SCI)

The purpose of this chapter is to review how gait analysis has been used to evaluate functional electrical stimulation (FES) applications for walking. Two main patient populations with different types of paralysis have been targeted for FES-assisted walking applications: stroke and spinal cord injury (SCI).[3,9,13,31,40] Although a variety of definitions have been assigned to FES, this chapter will focus on FES used to produce muscle contractions for joint stability and/or limb movement during walking.

The underlying model used in FES applications is the normal biomechanical model. Since those patients who can benefit from FES-assisted walking have compromised neurological systems (paralysis), FES is utilized to produce normal—or at least functional—movement patterns. In this model, the individual's nervous system is not part of the movement system. FES works peripherally to produce normal movement patterns. The biomechanical measurements incorporated in gait analysis can provide the objective means of assessing the efficacy of FES-assisted walking.

Historical Perspective and Background of FES

From a historical perspective, the use of electrical stimulation for treatment of a variety of disorders has been used for centuries.[3,9,13,31,40] The application of FES to improve walking is a more recent innovation that began with the 1961 work of Liberson and colleagues.[19] These researchers used FES of the peroneal nerve to activate dorsiflexion for preventing foot drop during the swing phase of gait following stroke. From 1968 to 1975, numerous clinical locations in the United States and Europe trained several hundred patients with stroke to use FES.[15] The large-scale multicenter functional evaluation determined that foot drop FES systems in general did not prove satisfactory in terms of clinical usefulness, adequate functionality, cost effectiveness, and practicality. These findings led to a diminished interest in FES for a few years. After 1980, FES again started to be of interest as research continued, particularly in the field of gait restoration in patients with SCI.

FES was first applied to a patient with paraplegia to assist in standing in the 1960s.[40] Methodology for FES restrengthening of paralyzed muscles following SCI and for FES-assisted standing was developed by a research group in Ljubljana, Slovenia, in the seventies.[18] This group presented results of FES with implanted electrodes to assist in standing and swing-to and swing-through crutch supported gait. They also reported prolonged as-

sisted standing and reciprocal biped gait using FES in patients with SCI in the late seventies.[15,16] The FES application methodology using surface electrodes was adapted and utilized after 1981 by different research groups and centers around the world, including locations in the United States (Chicago), Scotland, Germany, Yugoslavia, and Israel.[15] FES-assisted walking for patients with SCI was adopted by other centers using significantly modified or different approaches, such as hybrid systems that combine FES with orthotic devices and systems using implanted electrodes.[23,32]

Most FES-assisted ambulation has been confined to laboratory settings. Of the few studies that include gait analysis, most are based on data for single subjects or small sample sizes. A variety of parameters have been measured in those studies. FES has been reported to improve walking velocity, stride length, and stride time. Energy expenditure, center of gravity trajectory, cadence, step length, physiologic cost index, temporal measures (stance and swing times), heart rate, and oxygen consumption are all measurements that have been incorporated in the analysis of FES walking done by different researchers. However, few studies are reported in the literature that support the efficacy of FES treatment for walking. Although this lack of research may be due to the difficulty of well-controlled efficacy research, such research is essential to justify the use of FES in rehabilitation.

Applications with Patients with Hemiplegia

Description of Systems

The first successful applications of FES for walking were in patients with hemiplegia following cerebrovascular accident (CVA) whose primary deficit was inadequate foot clearance for walking or inadequate ankle control.[3] Cutaneous electrodes over the peroneal nerve distribution have been used to dorsiflex the foot or to elicit hip, knee, and ankle flexion for limb advancement.[19,38] Single-channel implanted electrode systems were first used over 20 years ago, and surviving patients are still using their walking systems. Multichannel implanted FES systems, which offer greater selectivity of muscle action and reduce the potential need for tendon transfer to balance the foot during dorsiflexion, are now in clinical trial.[3]

Gait Evaluation Results

Gait analysis reports of FES-assisted gait of patients with hemiplegia have come primarily from three research group locations: Rancho Los Ami-

TABLE 26-1 Summary of studies reporting gait analysis evaluation of FES-assisted walking systems for patients following cerebrovascular accident (CVA) or traumatic brain injury (TBI).

Research	Subjects	FES System Type	Results
Waters et al. (1988)	3 CVA, 1 TBI	Epimysial electrodes in thigh and hip muscles	Increased hip and knee flexion, household or limited community walking for three out of four subjects
Meadows et al. (1991)	1 CVA	Same; nine epimysial electrodes, eight-channel stimulator	Increased walking velocity (> 30 m/min), cadence, stride length, knee extension at heel strike
Bogataj et al. (1989)	20 CVA	Six-channel microprocessor stimulator, surface electrodes over muscles and peroneal nerve	Decreased stride time and loading on assistive device; increased velocity, stride length, ground reaction force, and loading time for uninvolved leg, and increased endurance
Malezic et al. (1990)	10 CVA	Adaptive dual-channel stimulator, surface electrodes	Decreased stride time, increased velocity, and increased stride length
	10 TBI	Same	Decreased stride time; increased stride length and velocity
Marsolais et al. (1990)	6 CVA	Implanted electrodes, varied numbers of muscles	Varied results

gos Rehabilitation Engineering Center in Downey, California; Israel Institute of Technology and Loewenstein Rehabilitation Hospital in Israel; and Case Western Reserve University and Cleveland Veterans Administration Medical Center, Cleveland, Ohio. Table 26-1 summarizes the techniques used and general results reported by each group. Figure 26-1 shows a comparison of those researchers who reported numerical values for velocity and stride length changes with FES in patients with stroke.

The group of researchers at Rancho Rehabilitation Engineering (Los Amigos Research and Education Institute, Downey, California) have used epimysial electrodes to stimulate the deep muscles of the thigh and hip in six subjects with hemiplegia during walking.[38] They report safe walking in these patients at velocities greater than 30 m/min (0.5 m/s). The subjects, some of whom had not walked in the 10 to 15 years since their stroke, have become comfortable in walking about their community with the aid of their percutaneous FES system.[3,38] Subjects who could not stand or walk have become independent in their home or household environment, reducing the need for attendant care and offering new vocational rehabilitation opportunities. Waters et al. evaluated the success of their system in one subject by walking speed

FIGURE 26-1 Stride length and walking velocity percentage increases from no FES to FES-assisted walking from three studies: Malezic et al.[20] (n = 10), Bogataj et al.[2] (n = 20) and Meadows et al.[27] (n = 1).

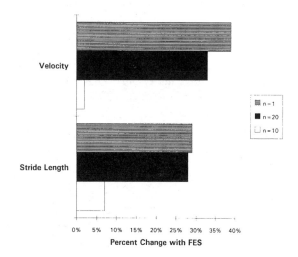

achieved and walking comfort.[38] This subject showed increased stride length and a more extended knee angle at heel strike for more stable limb support with FES. The subject could walk faster and farther with the stimulation system.

More specific gait analysis measurements with a larger sample size were reported by the Israeli research group.[2,20] These researchers applied multichannel FES to 20 patients with hemiplegia secondary to stroke or head injury using a six-channel microprocessor stimulator–stride analyzer. Bogataj and associates utilized this system to restore independent gait and to reestablish a normal gait pattern in a 2- to 3-week therapy period.[2] Twenty-one combinations of stimulation sites for the peroneals, hamstrings, quadriceps, gluteus maximus, and triceps brachii (for reciprocal arm swing) muscles were utilized.[20] Corrections of equinovarus, knee extension and hyperextension, elbow flexion, and hip extension were recorded during gait. Ground reaction forces (from instrumented shoes) were measured at the beginning and end of each therapy session. Heel switches were used to determine stride length and velocity. Mean stride length was calculated as the ratio of the distance to number of steps, and mean velocity was calculated as ratio of mean stride length to mean stride time. A three-dimensional electrogoniometric system was utilized to measure joint angles. The authors claim that gait improved significantly in all subjects during the therapy period, resulting in partly or completely independent gait. Mean stride time decreased 20% by the end of the therapy period for all subjects except one subject for whom increased stride time was an improvement. Mean gait velocity increased 62.6% and mean stride length 46.3%. Changes also occurred in gait without FES after the therapy sessions. Mean stride time was shorter, and gait was more regular. The load on the impaired leg was greater and lasted longer; the load on a crutch, if used, was decreased. The center of gravity trajectory was closer to normal, and endurance increased. Figure 26-2 shows the variables that were significantly different following the therapy period.

The Cleveland research group reported improvements in gait for a sample of six stroke patients using implanted electrodes for FES.[25] Marsolais et al. cite gait improvements with FES in this sample as evidenced by less scissoring, increased walking endurance, increased walking speed, and improved symmetry.

APPLICATIONS TO PATIENTS FOLLOWING SPINAL CORD INJURY

Description of Systems

FES walking for individuals following SCI has been demonstrated primarily in research settings and has not had the more widespread clinical

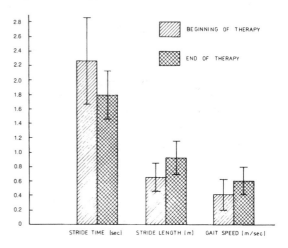

FIGURE 26-2 Diagram of mean stride time, mean stride length, and mean velocity with their standard deviations at beginning and at end of an FES therapy period for 20 subjects. (From Bogataj U et al: *Phys Ther* 69:319, 1989. Reprinted with the permission of the American Physical Therapy Association.)

testing that FES walking for patients with stroke has received. Two major approaches to FES-aided gait have been utilized by different research groups: (1) to stimulate many lower extremity muscles directly to provide the necessary movements or (2) to stimulate the necessary movement by both reflex action and direct stimulation.[13,22,23,28] A third approach uses a constant stimulation of the quadriceps to stabilize the knee combined with a swing-to or swing-through gait similar to that achieved with long-leg braces.[9] Presently, the energy costs of walking with FES are reported to be comparable to those of walking using long-leg braces.[21,39]

A commercially available system called "Parastep" (Sigmedics, One Northfield Plaza, Northfield, Illinois) is similar to the four-channel surface electrode system first proposed by Kralj in 1973 and subsequently refined by the research group in Ljubljana.[13] Bilateral stimulation of the quadriceps provides stabilization of the knee for quiet standing and during the stance phase of gait. Push buttons near the handgrips of the walker are used to trigger swing phases of gait by turning off quadriceps and stimulating the peroneal nerve near the head of the fibula to elicit a flexor withdrawal response to initiate a step. Although surface electrodes enable the user to try the system easily in a physical therapy setting, the flexor withdrawal reflex is not present bilaterally in all patients with SCI. In addition, the flexor withdrawal reflex is often variable and may accommodate to the FES over time so that a step cannot be taken. Because of the importance of this response, the intensity of the flexion withdrawal reflex stimulation is also adjustable from the walker. However, the quality of gait with the system is reportedly inferior to that with percutaneous or implanted electrode systems.[9,22]

Hybrid systems, which combine FES with orthotic devices in order to maximize advantages and minimize disadvantages of a single approach to SCI gait, have been developed. The hybrid assistive system combines FES with an externally powered modular orthosis in which the orthotic joints can move freely, be fixed, or provide torque to assist limb movement. Hybrid systems that utilize the reciprocating gait orthosis (RGO) involve the most bracing.[6,33] Although this hybrid system may have the widest application for patients with either quadriplegia or paraplegia since the brace provides most of the antigravity support and allows stabilization of trunk, it is costly and presents some practical difficulties in controlling movement.

Gait Evaluation Results

Early FES-assisted walking was often subjectively evaluated by the ability of the individual to walk regularly at home or outside of the home with FES and assistive devices. However, a number of different research groups have reported more objective gait analysis results using various FES-assisted walking systems. Table 26-2 provides a summary of these studies.

Researchers in the United Kingdom evaluated gait in three paraplegic subjects using the Oswestry Para Walker orthosis system with and without FES.[26,30] Gluteal muscle FES produced abduction and extending moments about hip at the appropriate phases of gait cycle. Patient-controlled switches in the crutch handles initiated stimulation of the gluteal muscle of the stance leg to supplement the mechanical action of the orthosis in resisting adduction and to reduce the force required from the latissimus dorsi muscle acting through the crutch to bring about extension of the stance leg. Nene and associates reported on five patients using ORLAU ParaWalker with FES of gluteal muscles as part of the hybrid system.[29,36,37] The addition of gluteal FES produced a further reduction in energy cost of 6 to 9%, with the fifth showing no change. Still, energy cost was up to five times that for a normal subject, so the clinical relevance of a 6 to 9% reduction in energy cost is questionable. Stallard showed that crutch-loading

force was reduced by between 10 and 50% for these patients, who all reported that the action of reciprocal walking became much easier.[37] Figure 26-3 shows a sample comparison of crutch loading for a patient using the ParaWalker with and without gluteal FES. Increases in gait velocity were also reported. Despite the gait improvements, the researchers also encountered a number of problems with FES. These included associated abdominal wall muscle contractions, difficulty in applying electrodes accurately, unreliable adherence of electrodes, and inconvenience of cables connecting the crutch control switch to the stimulator.

Israeli researchers compared gait analysis results for an individual with T4 complete paraplegia walking with three different systems: RGO, hybrid (RGO and FES), and FES alone.[7,8] Table 26-3 summarizes the results reported by Isakov and associates. Although the hybrid system had a minimal effect on walking speed, the reduction in patient effort demand was greater as evidenced by the heart rate increase—which was half that of the RGO (61 bpm increase for the RGO vs. 39 bpm increase with the hybrid). The researchers defined a physiologic cost index (PCI) as resting heart rate subtracted from walking heart rate and divided by walking speed (in m/min). This PCI during walking with RGO was 2.55 bts/m, and decreased to 1.54 bts/m with the hybrid system. The efficacy of using the proposed hybrid system was more evident with the PCI values than with other gait analysis measurements.

Mizrahi and associates evaluated FES-assisted walking in four patients with paraplegia.[8,28] Quadriceps and gluteal muscles were stimulated simultaneously in the supporting extremity, while the flexor reflex was triggered to obtain swinging of the contralateral limb. Time and distance parameters of gait were measured using an electrical contact system. Low walking speed and short stride length, accompanied by long stance and swing times, were recorded at the onset of training. Significant increases of stride length and gait velocity, along with decreased stance phase and stride time were observed in all subjects following a training program of 10 to 30 days. Heart rate and oxygen consumption during FES-induced walking increased 150% from rest. Oxygen uptake was five times higher during walking compared to resting values. These results demonstrate the high level of effort required during FES-induced walking and the dependence on anaerobic sources of energy.

Marsolais and associates have reported gait analysis results from their implanted FES walking system.[11,12,22,25] The FES system consists of fine

TABLE 26-2 Summary of studies reporting gait analysis results with FES-assisted walking in subjects with SCI.

Research	Subjects	FES System Type	Results
Kobetic et al. (1991, 1993) and Marsolais et al. (1988, 1990)	$n = 11$	Implanted electrodes, varied numbers of muscles	Improved velocity to .8 m/s in 2 subjects, 4 subjects standing, 4 subjects walking, 5 subjects able to ascend/descend stairs
McClelland et al. (1987)	$n = 3$	Gluteal FES and Para Walker Orthosis using surface electrodes	Increased velocity, decreased crutch loading
Nene et al. (1989)	$n = 5$	Same system	Decreased energy cost and crutch loading; increased speed in 3 subjects, decreased speed in 2 subjects
Isakov et al. (1986, 1992) and Mizrahi et al. (1985)	$n = 4$	Hybrid plus FES	Increased speed, stride length, HR, and VO_2; decreased stance and stride time; maximum distance 400 m, velocity 0.9 m/s, VO_2 two to three times normal—less than with lower leg braces, less energy costs at faster speeds
Kralj et al. (1979)	$n = 3$	Four channels FES to thigh muscles and peroneal nerve	Walking speed .2-.45 m/s, stance 82%, swing 18% of stride time
Heller et al. (1990)	$7 = 2$	Same FES system compared to braces	Increased stride length, cadence, speed with crutches, increased stride length, decreased cadence and speed with walker
Hirokawa et al. (1990) and Solomonow et al. (1989)	$n = 6$	RGO with FES for thigh muscles	With FES: increased distance walked, velocity, cadence, hip range; decreased energy cost, HR
Phillips et al. (1989)	$n = 1$	RGO with FES	Increased distance walked, velocity; decreased energy cost
Petrofsky et al. (1990)	$n = 4$	Modified RGO with FES	Increased velocity; decreased energy costs and loading on assistive device

FIGURE 26-3 A representative graph of impulse (force-time integral) of vertical crutch–ground reaction forces with and without FES of gluteal muscles. (From Pedotti A, Ferrarin M, editors: *Restoration of walking for paraplegics: recent advancements and trends,* Milan, Italy, 1992, IOS Press.)

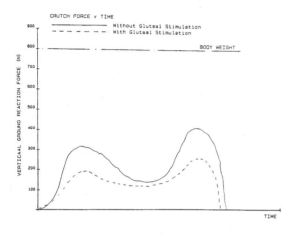

TABLE 26-3 Gait analysis results for four individuals with SCI.

	RGO	Hybrid + FES
Cadence (steps/min)	39	42
Step length (m)	0.61	0.59
Speed (m/min)	23.9	25.2
Heart rate (b/min)	61	39
PCI (bts/m)	2.55	1.54

Source: Isakov et al: Ambulation using the reciprocating gait orthosis and functional electrical stimulation, *Paraplegia* 30:239–245, 1992.

wire electrodes implanted in knee extensors, hip flexors, hip extensors, hip abductors, ankle dorsiflexors, and ankle plantarflexors to synthesize a stimulation pattern individually—as close as possible to the normal activity of muscles during gait—for each subject. Each step is started by a hand switch, while the pattern of particular muscle action is generated and stored by a microcomputer program. Gait evaluation was performed by assessing foot-floor contacts, walking speed, foot reaction forces, and joint goniograms (electrogoniometer measurement of joint angles). A walking speed of 0.8 m/s was measured with two subjects using the FES system. Gait improvements with FES were demonstrated by less scissoring, increased walking endurance, increased walking

speed, and improved symmetry. Criteria used by the researchers for "practical ambulation" include a walking rate of 1.0 m/s, energy use for walking less than 50% of individual's maximum aerobic capacity, donning and doffing time of a few minutes, component failure rate of only a few times per year, and safety.

This group compared two different patterns of FES-assisted gait using their implanted system.[22,24,25] The first pattern included FES of hip flexors, knee extensors, and ankle dorsiflexors. The second pattern added hip extensors and abductors and ankle plantarflexors. With the second pattern, stride length and speed of walking were significantly increased, double stance time was decreased, and weight transfer to the walker was decreased. Force plate studies showed that FES of the gluteus medius muscle was most effective in assisting mediolateral body weight shift during walking, while gluteus maximus and semimembranosus FES helped in the forward progression of the center of pressure.

Marsolais and associates also compared FES-assisted walking to walking with long leg braces.[22,24,25] The energy cost of FES walking in complete paraplegic subjects was similar to that of long leg brace ambulation. However, the energy cost increased as the speed of walking in long leg braces increased. During FES-assisted walking, no significant variation of energy cost was seen with increasing speed. The researchers assert that FES has, therefore, the potential to use less energy than long leg braces at speeds approaching those of normal walking. For a walking speed of 0.18 m/s, energy expenditure was 4.2 times greater than normal; for 0.35 m/s, 2.5 times normal; and for 0.56 m/s, 2.2 times normal. (Energy expenditure of normal walking is about 40 cal/min/kg at low walking speed of .33 m/s). A sample of eight subjects with paraplegia walked a maximum distance of 400 m, at a maximum velocity of 0.9 m/s. Oxygen uptake was two to three times normal, but less than with long leg braces. The major deviations of gait kinematics were exaggerated hip flexion during swing, early knee extension during swing, absent knee flexion in early stance, and early dorsiflexion following toe off.

The research group of Kralj and associates, based in Ljubljana, Yugoslavia, has reported gait analysis results for their FES-assisted gait system.[17] The system used four channels of surface FES for stimulation of the quadriceps and the peroneal nerve to elicit a flexor withdrawal response. Kralj and associates observed a low walking speed in three patients with paraplegia using this

FES system (0.2 to 0.45 m/s). Stance phase lasted 82% and swing phase 18% of stride time in these subjects as compared to a 60 to 40% stride time ratio seen in able bodied subjects. The double stance phase was 27 to 32% of stride time for these subjects.

Heller and associates, researchers from the United Kingdom, compared the use of FES for knee flexion in swing-through gait to fixed knee bracing.[5] These researchers showed in two patients that swing-through gait with knee flexion during swinging phase increased stride length (in both subjects) and speed (in one subject) compared to conventional fixed knee caliper bracing. Subject A, using crutches, had a 26% increase in stride length and cadence leading to a 58% increase in speed. Subject B, using a rolling walker, had a 51% increase in stride length with a reduction in cadence, which led to a speed reduction of 21%.

Several research groups in the United States have used gait analysis to evaluate the use of the hybrid system consisting of the RGO in combination with FES. Hirokawa and associates reported gait analysis data on six subjects using a modified RGO with surface FES to the quadriceps and hamstring muscles.[6] The orthosis consists of an ankle-foot plastic splint (AFO), a lockable knee joint, and a free hip joint. Lateral aluminum uprights connect the AFO with the knee and hip and extend upward to the mid-thoracic level. The two hip joints are connected with cables so that hip flexion of one leg will produce hip extension of the opposite leg. The authors compared energy costs of walking in the RGO with and without FES and compared their findings to energy costs of walking in long leg braces, the ParaWalker, and the implanted FES system from the literature. Figure 26-4 shows energy expenditure and heart rate findings of the study. The researchers also reported walking distances of 0.27 to 1.24 miles (0.43 to 1.99 km), maximum velocities of 31.1 to 68.68 ft/min (0.16 to 0.35 m/s), cadence of 41 to 50 steps/min, and hip range of motion of 32 to 50 degrees with the RGO-FES system. The authors conclude that the FES-powered RGO provided substantial improvements in energy cost over other currently available options.

Phillips et al. evaluated a system that uses surface FES of the quadriceps femoris and hamstring muscles in combination with the RGO in one quadriplegic subject.[33,34] They reported walking distance of 0.8 km and walking velocity of 1.2 to 2 km/hr (0.33 to 0.56 m/s). The group also compared walking with and without FES and found a reduction in blood pressure, oxygen con-

Figure 26-4A Comparison of energy expenditure in KCAL/kg-min (top) and KCAL/kg-M (bottom) during walking in long leg braces (LLB), the hip guidance orthosis (ORLAU), reciprocating gait orthosis (RGO), RGO+FES, and implanted FES (Marsolais[21]). (From Hirokawa S et al: *Arch Phys Med Rehabil* 71:687, 1990.)

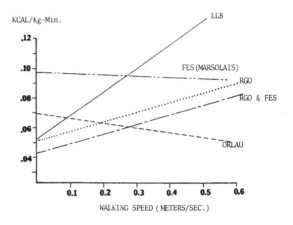

sumption, and task cost with FES. They concluded that for this subject, cardiopulmonary stresses were less when walking in the RGO with FES than with the RGO alone.

Petrofsky et al. reported on a modified RGO system with FES of the gluteus maximus and hamstring muscles.[32] The RGO was constructed of plastic and graphite, weighing approximately 10 pounds. Four able-bodied (control) subjects walking in the modified RGOs were compared to four SCI patients using the RGO with and without FES. Metabolic efficiency (calculated from the external work performed and the oxygen uptake) was best at 2.0 mph (54 m/min) for the control subjects, 1.5

FIGURE 26-4B Comparison of pooled heart rate at the beginning (shown in the bottom graph) and end (top) of a 30 m walk using long leg braces (LLB), reciprocating gait orthosis (RGO), RGO+FES, and implanted FES (Marsolais[21]). (From Hirokawa S et al: *Arch Phys Med Rehabil* 71:687, 1990.)

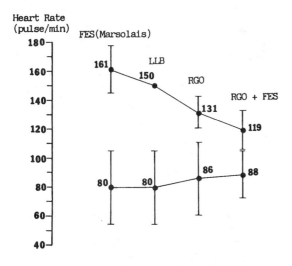

mph (40 m/min) for the SCI subjects using the RGO and FES, and 1.0 mph (27 m/min) for the SCI subjects walking in the RGO without FES. The difference in VO_2 between the control and SCI subjects using FES was statistically different at speeds more than 1.5 mph. VO_2 and cardiac output were lower in subjects who walked with FES compared to RGO alone, but higher than the control subjects. Average weight exerted on the walker through the hands was 4.9% of body weight during walking with FES. Walking without FES increased the hand loading to 27% of body weight.

USEFULNESS OF GAIT ANALYSIS TO EVALUATE FES EFFICACY

Limitations of Current Findings

As evidenced by the research findings available, the ability of FES-aided walking systems to restore real, functional walking generally has had more anecdotal than scientific documentation.[9] The problems of restoration of walking in SCI and stroke patients are compounded by individual variations in residual muscle function at particular levels of injury. A number of different protocols—with a broad spectrum of complexity, from relatively simple (single channel of FES) for individuals with a mild unilateral deficit, to complex, multichannel devices that stimulate most of

the lower extremity muscles for those with more involved injuries—may be required. For many patients, assistive technologies other than FES may be more appropriate for achieving gait.

Limited FES ambulation has been accomplished in patients with both hemiplegia and SCI. More severely involved hemiplegic patients have achieved this goal with fewer channels of stimulation and minimal orthotic requirements when compared to SCI patients who require more extensive bracing and stimulation.[3,14,38] Although the extensive bracing afforded by the RGO in combination with surface FES permits the SCI individual to stand and walk at a slow velocity, navigating stairs and other basic community maneuvers are not possible. For some SCI individuals, this is a worthwhile addition to their wheelchair mobility. For others, surface FES walking systems are discarded because of the time required for donning and operating the system and the marginal benefit to their daily routine.[14] Percutaneous systems utilizing up to 48 channels of stimulation permit joint movement and limited walking as well as stair climbing and ramp negotiation.[23] These systems, however, require an excessive energy demand that is similar to the use of knee-ankle-foot orthoses and crutches.[21,39] Energy consumption during FES walking continues to decrease as the experience in synthesizing movement improves. However, the energy required to walk is still more than twice that of able bodied individuals and greater than that of propelling a wheelchair.[31]

At this point, there are no clinically available, fully functional FES systems for the individual with complete SCI.[3] Creating FES walking in such a patient is an extremely difficult undertaking. Most of the existing work in FES has been for the incompletely paralyzed patient groups, who comprise the majority of potential FES users in the United States. Each improvement in FES technology and clinical application in this population is a step toward the future realization of FES walking in the completely paralyzed.

Suggested Evaluation Procedures

One problem evident in the research work, which includes gait analysis of FES-assisted walking, is the lack of a consistent approach to analysis. Katakis has recommended an assessment program that could be utilized by those who evaluate the performance of synthesized gait of SCI patients using FES.[10] In this program, gait performance is evaluated using a subjective questionnaire and objective measurement of kinematic and kinetic parameters of gait. The individual is subjectively classified as a physiological walker, limited household, unlimited household, limited community, or unlimited community walker. Kinematic parameters (those which describe the motion) can be collected using electrogoniometers or camera systems (for joint angles), foot-mounted switches, and foot-mounted inked markers. The base of support (and mediolateral stability) can be measured using step width or step angle or both. Right and left sides can be examined for symmetry (a basic characteristic of normal gait). Weakness and lack of control in flexing and extending the leg at knee, hip, and ankle joints may be indicated by stride and step lengths. Temporal parameters (the time taken to perform the phases of gait such as swing through, single support, transfer or body support, contact time, etc.) can be examined. Time from heel contact to toe contact can be measured, and joint movements during the gait cycle can be compared with normal values.

Ground reaction forces (the forces produced when the foot or walking aid is in contact with the ground) are collected from force plates. Impulse from the GRF indicates a change in linear momentum of the body as it is reflected in the lower limb during its stance phase (expressed as % of total). Other information provided by GRF includes loading and unloading rate of each foot (vertical component), mid-stance period (vertical component), magnitude of braking force and duration of braking phase (A-P component), magnitude of propulsive force and duration of propulsive phase (A-P component). The same information can be provided for patients with crutches or other assistive devices.

Gait evaluation is necessary in order to detect, describe, measure, and assess the errors (deviations from normal) of synthesized walking using FES. These gait errors may be classified as pathological (from neuromuscular deficiencies of patient), functional (from artificial stimulation of muscles), or control (from applied artificial control strategies of gait). Using detailed knowledge of normal function, appropriate corrective measures can be taken to minimize these errors and improve the stability, symmetry, and propulsion of synthesized gait.

Summary

A review of how gait analysis has been utilized to evaluate FES applications for walking has been presented in this chapter. Patients with paralysis from stroke and SCI have been the primary populations targeted for FES-assisted applications. In both cases, the normal biomechanical model is applied, with the FES working peripherally to produce normal movement patterns. The biomechanical measurements incorporated by different research groups have varied, making comparisons difficult. Although limited FES ambulation has been accomplished in patients with both stroke and SCI, more functional results have been achieved in patients with stroke. Currently, there are no clinically available FES walking systems for individuals with SCI, which allow standing, walking, and basic maneuvers required for activities of daily living. However, as research continues, future realization of functional walking using FES in individuals with complete lower limb paralysis may be accomplished.

References

1. Bajd T et al: Restoration of walking in incomplete spinal cord injured patients by use of surface electrical stimulation, preliminary results, *Prosthet Orthot Int* 9:109, 1985.
2. Bogataj U et al: Restoration of gait during two to three weeks of therapy with multichannel electrical stimulation, *Phys Ther* 69:319, 1989.
3. Campbell JM, Meadows PM: Therapeutic FES: from rehabilitation to neural prosthetics, *Assist Technol* 4:4, 1992.
4. Graupe D et al: Patient-controlled electrical stimulation via EMG signature discrimination for providing certain paraplegics with primitive walking functions, *J Biomed Eng* 5:220, 1983.
5. Heller B et al: Preliminary studies of swing-through gait using FES. In DB Popovic, editor: *Advances in external control of human extremities X,* Belgrade, Yugoslavia, 1990, Nauka.
6. Hirokawa S et al: Energy consumption in paraplegic ambulation using the reciprocating gait orthosis and electric stimulation of the thigh muscles, *Arch Phys Med Rehabil* 71:687, 1990.
7. Isakov E, Douglas R, Berns P: Ambulation using the reciprocating gait orthosis and functional electrical stimulation, *Paraplegia* 30:239, 1992.
8. Isakov E, Mizrahi J, Najenson T: Biomechanical and physiological evaluation of FES-activated paraplegic patients, *J Rehabil Res Dev* 23:9, 1986.
9. Jaeger RJ: Lower extremity applications of functional neuromuscular stimulation, *Assist Technol* 4:19, 1992.
10. Katakis JN: A program to evaluate the synthesized gait of SCI patients using FNS. In Pedotti A, Ferrarin M, editors: *Restoration of walking for paraplegics: recent advancements and trends,* Milan, Italy, 1992, IOS Press.
11. Kobetic R et al: Analysis of paraplegic gait induced by functional neuromuscular stimulation, *Proc Ann Int Conf IEEE Eng Med Biol Soc* 13:200, 1991.
12. Kobetic R et al: The next step: artificial walking. In Inman, editor: *Human walking,* Baltimore, 1993, Williams & Wilkins.

13. Kralj A, Bajd T: *Functional electrical stimulation: standing and walking after spinal cord injury,* Boca Raton, Fla, 1989, CRC Press.

14. Kralj A, Bajd T, Turk R: Enhancement of gait restoration in spinal injured patients by functional electrical stimulation, *Clin Orthop* 233:34, 1988.

15. Kralj A, Bajd T, Turk R: FES for gait restoration: a practicality and clinical issues discussion. In Pedotti A, Ferrarin M, editors: *Restoration of walking for paraplegics: recent advancements and trends,* Milan, Italy, 1992, IOS Press.

16. Kralj A et al: Paraplegic patients standing by functional electrical stimulation, *Digest 12th Int Conf Med Biol Eng:* 59, 1979.

17. Kralj A et al: Gait restoration in paraplegic patients: a feasibility demonstration using multichannel surface electrode FES, *J Rehabil Res Dev* 20:3, 1983.

18. Kralj A, Grobelnik S, Vodovnik L: *Electrical stimulation of paraplegic patients—feasibility study,* Proceedings of the International Symposium on External Control Human Extremities, Dubrovnik, Yugoslavia, 1973.

19. Liberson WT et al: Functional electrotherapy: stimulation of the peroneal nerve synchronized with the swing phase of the gait in hemiplegic patients, *Arch Phys Med Rehabil* 42:101, 1961.

20. Malezic M et al: Evaluation of adaptive dual channel electrical stimulator for gait. In Popovic DB, editor: *Advances in external control of human extremities X,* Belgrade, Yugoslavia, 1990, Nauka.

21. Marsolais EB, Edwards BG: Energy costs of walking and standing with functional neuromuscular stimulation and long leg braces, *Arch Phys Med Rehabil* 69:243, 1988.

22. Marsolais EB, Kobetic R: Development of a practical electrical stimulation system for restoring gait in the paralyzed patient, *Clin Orthop* 233:64, 1988.

23. Marsolais EB, Kobetic R: Functional electrical stimulation for walking in paraplegics, *J Bone Joint Surg* 69A:728, 1987.

24. Marsolais EB et al: Orthoses and electrical stimulation for walking in complete paraplegia, *J Neurolog Rehabil* 5:13, 1991.

25. Marsolais EB, Kobetic R, Jacobs JL: Comparison of FES treatment in the stroke and spinal cord injury patient. In Popovic DB, editor: *Advances in external control of human extremities X,* Belgrade, Yugoslavia, 1990, Nauka.

26. McClelland M et al: Augmentation of the oswestry parawalker orthosis by means of surface electrical stimulation: gait analysis of three patients, *Paraplegia* 25:32, 1987.

27. Meadows P et al: *Multichannel electrical stimulation system for gait assist and cyclical stimulation,* Proceedings of the 14th Annual RESNA Conference, Kansas City, Mo, 1991.

28. Mizrahi J et al: Quantitative weightbearing and gait evaluation of paraplegics using functional electrical stimulation, *Med Biol Eng Comput* 23:101, 1985.

29. Nene AV, Jennings SJ: Hybrid paraplegic locomotion with the parawalker using intramuscular stimulation: a single subject study, *Paraplegia* 27:125, 1989.

30. Nene AV, Patrick JH: Energy cost of paraplegic locomotion using the paraWalker: electrical stimulation "Hybrid" orthosis, *Arch Phys Med Rehabil* 71:116, 1990.

31. Peckham PH, Creasey GH: Neural prostheses: clinical applications of functional electrical stimulation in spinal cord injury, *Paraplegia* 30:96, 1992.

32. Petrofsky JS, Smith JB: Physiologic costs of computer-controlled walking in persons with paraplegia using a reciprocating-gait orthosis, *Arch Phys Med Rehabil* 72:890, 1991.

33. Phillips CA: Functional electrical stimulation and lower extremity bracing for ambulation exercise of the spinal cord injured individual: a medically prescribed system, *Phys Ther* 69:842, 1989.

34. Phillips CA, Hendershot DM: Functional electrical stimulation and reciprocating gait orthosis for ambulation exercise in a tetraplegic patient: a case study, *Paraplegia* 29:268, 1991.

35. Solomonow M et al: Muscle stimulation powered orthosis: a practical walking system for paraplegics, *Proc XIII Int Con Biomech:* 7, 1989.

36. Stallard J: The relative energy cost of paraplegic ambulation. In Pedotti A, Ferrarin M, editors: *Restoration of walking for paraplegics: recent advancements and trends,* Milan, Italy, 1992, IOS Press.

37. Stallard J: Hybrid systems: results and performance monitoring. In Pedotti A, Ferrarin M, editors: *Restoration of walking for paraplegics: recent advancements and trends,* Milan, Italy, 1992, IOS Press.

38. Waters RL, Campbell JM, Nakai R: Therapeutic electrical stimulation of the lower limb by epimysial electrodes, *Clin Orthop:* 44, 1988.

39. Waters RL, Lunsford B: Energy cost of paraplegic locomotion, *J Bone Joint Surg* 67:1245, 1985.

40. Yarkony GM et al: Neuromuscular stimulation in spinal cord injury. I. Restoration of functional movement of the extremities, *Arch Phys Med Rehabil* 73:78, 1992.

Gait Analysis as an Outcome Measure After Anterior Cruciate Ligament Injury

Lynn Snyder-Mackler
Marty Eastlack

Key Terms

Anterior cruciate ligament

Clinical decision making

Cocontraction

Disability

Flexed-knee gait patterns

Impairment

Quadriceps avoidance gait

Anterior cruciate ligament (ACL) rupture is among the most frequent traumatic knee injuries.[8,9,39] Approximately 100,000 surgical reconstructions of the ACL are performed each year. Historically, outcome following ACL rupture and reconstruction has been evaluated based on joint laxity measurements: presence of excessive anterior tibial displacement on the femur, positive pivot shift test, and more recently, anterior tibial displacement as measured by an arthrometer.[8,9,27] Measurements of thigh muscle strength and range of motion have also been used to quantify recovery.[*] Questionnaires have been developed that attempt to assess function after knee injury in an effort to describe more accurately the disability associated with ACL injury.[†] In some cases (e.g., quadriceps femoris muscle strength), the measured impairment has correlated well with self-reports of knee functional status.[26,32,33,36] In other cases (e.g., joint laxity), the relationship is less clear.[12,28] In an attempt to quantify dysfunction during locomotion that occurs after ACL injury, gait analysis has been used.[5,33,38,41] We will describe how gait analysis has been used to (1) describe the disability associated with ACL rupture, (2) describe changes after reconstruction and/or rehabilitation, and (3) also discuss what systems can be used to analyze gait in this population.

DESCRIBING PATIENT POPULATIONS

Patients Who Are ACL Deficient

Most of the studies of gait after ACL injury examine patients who have anterior cruciate ligament deficiency (ACLD). Some investigators have described kinematics;[‡] some have described kinetics;[§] and others have described patterns of muscle activity using electromyography.[||] Patients have been studied during level walking, fast walking, running, and ascending and descending stairs.[#] The only consensus among these studies is that there is great variation in the kinetics, kinematics, and muscle activity patterns of patients who have ACLD during gait. We suggest that although the picture is not complete, some common patterns can be extracted from this literature.

The fact that level walking is rarely difficult for patients with anterior cruciate ligament deficiency is supported by the relative similarity between the kinematics of the cruciate deficient and normal knees in most studies.[15,30,31,37] However, the studies of knee joint kinetics suggest that this normalcy belies alterations in gait that may either protect the joint from or, in some instances, accelerate joint destruction.[5,22] Shiavi et al.[18,30,31] and Sinkjaer, Arendt-Nielsen, and co-workers[3,32] in a series of studies have described patterns of knee joint muscle activity in patients who are cruciate deficient, which are not tremendously different from the muscle activity of nondisabled individuals during level walking. Studies of knee joint kinematics during free-speed, level walking have also not demonstrated large differences from those of healthy subjects[15,30,31,37] (Figure 27-1).

Berchuck and colleagues, however, have described a drastic change in knee joint kinetics during level walking, in the absence of serious kinematic differences[2,5,41] (Figure 27-2).

In the majority of the patients with ACLD, there was a total absence of the external knee flexion moment during stance phase of the involved lower extremity.[5,41] Berchuck and colleagues maintain that this strategy removes any need for the quadriceps (providing an internal extension moment) to contract and have termed this gait pattern "quadriceps avoidance."[5,41] Kadaba and colleagues have described several alterations in knee joint kinetics during gait, the most predominant of which was **not** "quadriceps avoidance," but rather a pattern of increased stance phase knee flexion and external knee flexion

---

FIGURE 27-1 Muscle activity of ACLD knees versus controls during level walking (0% incline) and at various inclines. (From Sinkjaer T, Arendt-Nielsen L: Knee stability and muscle coordination in patients with anterior cruciate ligament injuries: an electromyographic approach, *J Electromyograph Kinesiol* 1:209, 1991. Used with permission.)

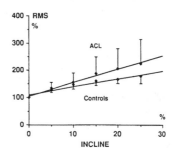

---

* Refer to the following sources: 1,10,11,16,33,37,40.

† Refer to the following sources: 6,14,17,19,23,24,29.

‡ Refer to the following sources: 3,5,15,26,30,31,36.

§ Refer to the following sources: 5,13,15,23,24,30,31,37.

|| Refer to the following sources: 3,7,15,18,26,30,31,32,37.

Refer to the following sources: 3,5,7,13,15,18,20,22,26, 30,31,32,37.

Figure 27-2   Knee external moment data and kinematic data from nondisabled and ACLD knees during level walking. (From Berchuck M, Andriacchi TP, Bach BR et al: Gait adaptations by patients who have a deficient anterior cruciate ligament, *J Bone Joint Surg* 72-A:871, 1990. Used with permission.)

Figure 27-3   Kinematic and moment data of ACLD knees, Groups 2 and 3 (which comprised 78%) showed increased stance phase knee flexion and external knee flexion moments balanced by increased quadriceps femoris muscle activity. (From Kadaba MP, Ramakrishnan HK, Gainey JC et al: Gait adaptation patterns in patients with ACL deficiency, *Trans Orthop Res Soc* 18(2):361, 1993. Used with permission.)

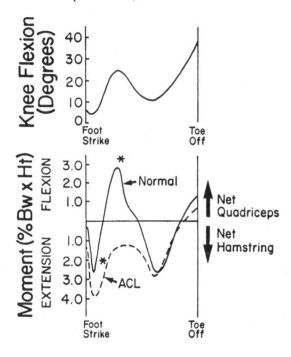

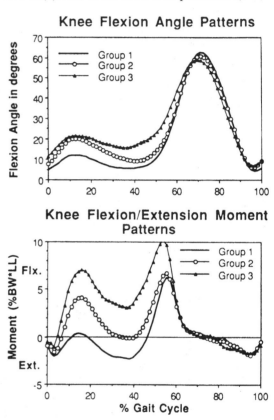

moments balanced by increased quadriceps femoris muscle activity[15] (Figure 27-3). They hypothesize that the patients use a flexed knee gait to minimize anterior shear forces at the knee.

The flexed-knee gait pattern is similar to the pattern we have observed in patients with weak quadriceps femoris muscles after ACL reconstruction.[33]

Sinkjaer and colleagues, in a recent study of gait in patients who are ACL deficient, have identified a relationship between perceived stability (as measured by a Lysholm scale, a knee stability scale) and abnormal muscle activation patterns.[19,32] Patients who activated their medial gastrocnemius muscles for a longer period of time than nondisabled subjects were more stable than those patients whose activation patterns were more like those of the nondisabled subjects (Figure 27-4).

In addition, training a small subpopulation of the unstable patients to walk more like the stable patients with ACLD improved their Lysholm scores. This study suggests that an "abnormal" gait pattern may actually represent a positive

adaptation (reprogramming) due to the absence of the ACL. This notion is underscored by a study of the effect of ACL transection (ACLT) on osteoarthritis (OA) in dogs by O'Conner and colleagues.[25] Dogs who underwent ipsilateral dorsal root ganglionectomy (DRG) and ACLT had higher vertical ground reaction forces during gait and developed much more severe OA than dogs with ACLT and intact sensation. This suggests a protective function of altered gait patterns mediated by muscular reflexes. Dogs who received a DRG 52 weeks after ACLT showed altered vertical ground reaction forces for a short time, but rapidly returned to pre-DRG levels.[25] Timoney stated that "successful surgery should predictably restore a normal gait pattern."[38] This expectation may be overly optimistic. In addition, a normal gait pat-

Figure 27-4   Electromyographic data of medial gastrocnemius muscle of controls and ACLD knees. Those with poor stability and excellent stability have been separated. (From Sinkjaer T, Arendt-Nielsen L: Knee stability and muscle coordination in patients with anterior cruciate ligament injuries: an electromyographic approach, *J Electromyograph Kinesiol* 1:209, 1991. Used with permission.)

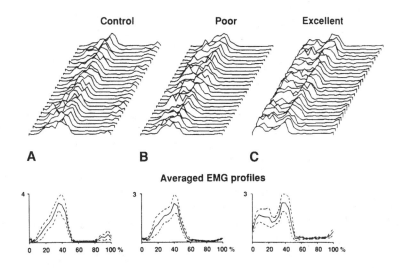

tern may not really be desirable. An adaptation or "reprogramming" of gait to stabilize the knee when the patient is ACLD may persist after anterior cruciate ligament reconstruction (ACLR) and may or may not be advantageous.

There is consensus that, during stressful activities, there are measurable disturbances in kinetics, kinematics, and patterns of muscle activation after ACL rupture. However, there is no consensus about typical responses. We believe that two characteristic strategies emerge from a careful reading of the literature: (1) a strategy where the hamstrings act dynamically to stabilize the knee and (2) a strategy where overall muscle activity increases (co-contraction) to quasi-statically stabilize the knee. Sinkjaer and Arendt-Nielsen found that as the grade of an incline increased, all five muscles tested acting at the knee joint (medial hamstrings, lateral hamstrings, medial gastrocnemius, vastus medialis, and vastus lateralis muscles) had earlier onset times and longer duration of EMG activity in persons with ACLD knees when compared to persons with nondisabled knees[3] (Figure 27-5).

This tendency was greatest in the lateral hamstrings and medial gastrocnemius presumably owing to their synergistic actions with the ACL. In another study, Sinkjaer and Arendt-Nielsen noted that the biceps femoris and semitendinosus were activated earlier in stance in the patients who were

Figure 27-5   Mean onset, offset, and duration of electromyographic activity in ACLD and nondisabled knees. Recorded at varying increased inclines with respect to heel strike. (From Sinkjaer T, Arendt-Nielsen L: Knee stability and muscle coordination in patients with anterior cruciate ligament injuries: an electromyographic approach, *J Electromyograph Kinesiol* 1:209, 1991. Used with permission.)

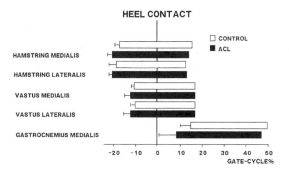

ACLD compared to nondisabled subjects.[32] Shiavi and co-workers, in a study of patients with ACLD during pivoting found that all muscles tested had periods of abnormal activity and that muscles which were ACL synergists were active during the points in the gait cycle when the ACL would normally be providing a passive restraint to anterior tibial translation and/or internal tibial rotation.[13]

Berchuck et al.[5] and Wu et al.[41] have also demonstrated gait alterations in patients who are ACLD with more strenuous testing (stair climbing, jogging, and running to a sidestep cut), including increased hamstring (extension) moments during weight bearing, presumably to compensate for the absent ACL. McNair et al. found quadriceps and hamstring activity were both increased in early stance in jogging.[20] Tibone found increased medial hamstring firing and earlier onset of firing in the involved vastus medialis muscle during running.[36] Surprisingly, Berchuck et al. found that the "quadriceps avoidance" gait persisted to some degree during jogging; the external knee flexion moment was diminished but not absent.[5]

In stair climbing, Tibone et al. found earlier cessation of vastus medialis oblique muscle firing as the contralateral limb leaves the step below and increased biceps femoris activity at initial contact in the ACLD limb during ascent of stairs[36] (Figure 27-6).

The authors attributed these findings to the limb's attempt to stabilize the knee and avoid anterior translation of the tibia as the limb approaches full extension. They found no difference in descending stairs. The authors, however, did not specify which limb led in ascending or descending stairs. Both ascending and descending stairs should be stressful to the ACLD limb.[2] This activity should be a good marker of function if the ACLD limb has to support the body weight as the uninvolved limb descends first and if in ascending

FIGURE 27-6 Vastus medialis oblique muscle activity during ascent of stairs. (From Tibone JE, Antich TJ, Fanton JS et al: Functional analysis of anterior cruciate ligament instability, *Am J Sports Med* 14(4):276, 1986. Used with permission.)

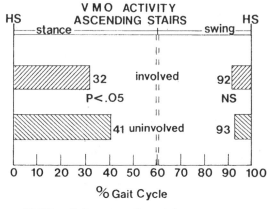

VMO activity ascending stairs.

stairs the involved limb has to propel the body weight forward as it leads. Andriacchi has emphasized the importance of assessing the kinematics and kinetics of stair ascent and descent to evaluate the knee in a more intensive functional activity than level walking.[2]

The kinematics, kinetics and EMG findings after ACLD are not tremendously different from the nondisabled during level walking. However, during stressful activities (eg stairclimbing, fast walking) kinetic, kinematic and EMG abnormalities occur in the ACLD knees. Typically, the subject will either co-contract the muscles around the knee to stabilize the knee statically and decrease anterior tibial translation or increase hamstring muscle activity to decrease anterior tibial translation. In either case the subject can display a flexed knee gait and an increased extension moment during stance.

Patients Who Have Undergone ACL Reconstruction

The literature regarding gait *after* anterior cruciate ligament reconstruction is limited. In our laboratory, we have demonstrated that patients in the early postoperative phase after ACLR have significant alterations in knee flexion during the stance phase of gait.[33] We have further defined the postoperative kinematic abnormalities by dividing the abnormalities into two separate categories, one strongly correlated to quadriceps femoris muscle strength and one apparently unrelated. The first is a tendency for the patients who have undergone ACLR with weak quadriceps femoris muscle to flex slightly at heel strike and then fix the knee in slight flexion throughout the period of single support (Figure 27-7). Weakness of the thigh musculature could lead to a decreased ability for the knee to counter the increased external flexion moment associated with flexed knee stance. Co-contraction or co-activation of antagonistic muscles, in this case the quadriceps femoris and hamstring muscles, has a role in maintaining joint stability[4,34,35] (Figure 27-8). Solomonow and colleagues have suggested that the thigh muscles and anterior cruciate ligament act synergistically to maintain joint stability.[34,35] Co-contraction tends to stabilize a joint in a single position. Therefore, in an effort to counter the external flexion moment that occurs during flexed knee stance, a fixed knee angle during stance or decreased stance time might be noted in patients who have weak quadriceps femoris musculature.

The second postoperative kinematic problem is the lack of full extension of the involved knee

FIGURE 27-7   Quadriceps femoris muscle weakness after ACLR. Subject with quadriceps femoris muscle weakness after ACLR displays a gait pattern in which the knee is fixed in slight flexion throughout stance as compared to nondisabled side. (From Snyder-Mackler L, Delitto A, Bailey S et al: Quadriceps femoris muscle strength and functional recovery after anterior cruciate ligament reconstruction: a prospective randomized clinical trial of electrical stimulation, *J Bone Joint Surg* (in press). Used with permission.)

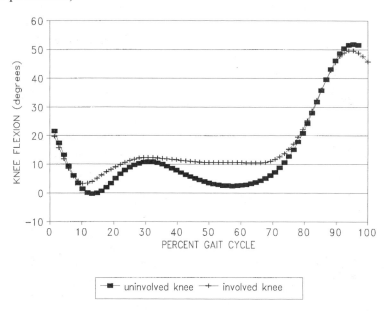

during the stance phase of gait even when full active range of motion (ROM) is attainable in nonfunctional situations and regardless of the quadriceps strength of the involved extremity (Figure 27-9). Findings of Snyder-Mackler and colleagues' study of ten patients in the early postoperative phase after ACL reconstruction suggest that kinematic alterations consistent with a co-contraction strategy continue after surgery when the quadriceps are weak.[33] A recent report by Timoney et al. demonstrated a significant reduction in the mid-stance knee flexion moment in ACLR patients even 8 to 12 months after surgery, although they failed to demonstrate a full "quadriceps avoidance" pattern[38] (Table 27-1). The lack of full extension in ACLR patients after surgery may represent an adaptation that was learned before surgery when the knee was unstable. Berchuck et al. rationalized that the quadriceps avoidance gait pattern is learned in an effort to minimize the anterior tibial translation that can be caused by quadriceps contraction when the ACL is ruptured.[5] Patients rarely undergo acute ACL reconstruction because acute reconstruction is associated with an increased risk of arthrofibrosis.[21] Therefore, most patients walk for some time before surgery without an intact ACL. Perhaps persistence of altered gait patterns early after ACL reconstruction represents a learned pattern from before surgery. A comprehensive analysis of gait (kinetics and kinematics), however, in patients who are ACLD and ACLR where the same patients are followed longitudinally has not been reported in the literature.

In a follow-up study done by Tibone and Antich on subjects who had undergone a ACLR (patellar tendon autografts), six of the 11 subjects had difficulty with the functional tests performed (i.e., single limb jumping, half squat, stair climbing, straight cutting, and cross cutting). The authors did not elaborate on what difficulties the subjects had or how the performance was graded (e.g., observation of kinematics, etc.), therefore it is difficult to interpret the findings. However, Tibone et al. do report that nine of their 11 subjects lacked at least 5 degrees of knee extension, and all subjects had at least a 15% quadriceps femoris muscle strength deficit in their involved knees as compared to their other limb. Perhaps the subjects who demonstrated deficits in strength and range of motion also display more abnormal kinematics and kinetics in all activities; however, the authors did not look at this relationship.[36]

Perry et al. recorded electromyographic activity from the sartorius, semitendinosus, gracilis, and the vastus lateralis muscles and revealed greater EMG activity in the involved limbs for all patients

FIGURE 27-8 Coactivation of antagonistic muscles in an ACLD knee in an attempt to maintain joint stability. (From Solomonow M, Baratta R, Zhou BH et al: The synergistic action of the anterior cruciate ligament and thigh muscles in maintaining joint stability, *Am J Sports Med* 15:207, 1987. Used with permission.)

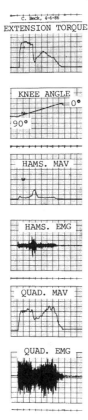

for the same activities as in the normal subjects.[26] Also, the muscles of the involved side were more active than those of the uninvolved side in the subjects who had undergone surgery. Although the surgical technique, advancement of the pes anserinus group, is not currently done, we believe that these subjects might have been employing a co-contraction strategy that we have hypothesized is commonly demonstrated in subjects with ACLD to stabilize their knees during functional activities. Perry et al.'s subjects also demonstrated decreased velocities and stride lengths during fast walking and running. The subjects that subjectively reported that they had a "good result" after surgery had significantly stronger quadriceps than the subjects who reported they had a "poor result." We feel that this finding reaffirms that quadriceps femoris muscle strength is a good predictor of functional outcome.

The electromyographic data in patients who have had an ACLR is scarce. Ciccotti et al. collected EMG data on the vastus medialis oblique, vastus lateralis, rectus femoris, semimembranosus, biceps femoris, tibialis anterior, gastrocnemius, and the soleus muscles of healthy ACLD and ACLR subjects (bone-patellar tendon-bone autografts) during several functional activities (e.g., walking, ascending and descending stairs, ascending and descending ramps, running, and cross cutting). They found increased activity in the vastus lateralis, biceps femoris, and tibialis anterior muscles in the patients with ACLD across all functional activities (Figure 27-10).

The patients who were ACLR had muscle activity patterns much like those of the healthy, control subjects. Ciccotti et al. attributed this increased muscle activity in the patients with ACLD to a protective mechanism to avoid pivoting of the knee joint. In the ACLD group, the quadriceps activity was statistically similar to or increased from those of healthy subjects. This finding also suggests that the quadriceps avoidance gait proposed by Berchuck as an explanation for the altered moments in his study *may not* occur. Ciccotti and colleagues also identified a coordinated hamstring/quadriceps activation pattern *in all three groups* that seems to suggest that ACL transection has no effect on the neurophysiological control of these activation patterns.[7]

In the ACLR population there is minimal literature available, but it appears that kinematic and kinetic changes are largely dependent on quadriceps femoris muscle strength. In the subjects who have fully recovered quadriceps femoris muscle strength (maximal voluntary isometric contraction close to the nondisabled side), the kinetics and kinematics appear similar to normals. If quadriceps femoris muscle weakness persists, the kinematic and kinetic data continue to appear as they did prior to surgery. Electromyographic findings appear to be similar to the nondisabled population in all activities after ACLR.

GAIT ANALYSIS AND CLINICAL DECISION MAKING

An examination of the existing research invokes some interesting questions about how gait analysis can be used to aid clinical decision making in patients after ACL injury. The literature suggests that gait analysis might be able to help us to determine whether a patient is a candidate for a brace and rehabilitation or for surgery and whether a patient needs to be braced after surgery. Some studies report that gait training with a template

FIGURE 27-9   Subject after ACLR. This patient does not display full extension during stance phase despite adequate quadriceps femoris muscle strength and no active range of motion limitations. (From Snyder-Mackler L, Delitto A, Bailey S et al: Quadriceps femoris muscle strength and functional recovery after anterior cruciate ligament reconstruction: a prospective randomized clinical trial of electrical stimulation, *J Bone Joint Surg* (in press). Used with permission.)

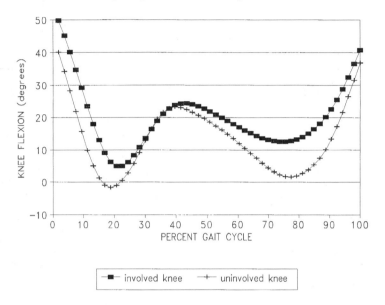

TABLE 27-1   Reduction in mid-stance knee flexion moments (MKFM) in ACLR knees as compared to nondisabled knees during level walking. (From Timoney JM, Inman WS, Queseda PM et al: Return of normal gait patterns after anterior cruciate ligament reconstruction, *Am J Sports Med* 21:887-889, 1993; with permission.)

Group	PVV (m/min)	FWV (m/min)	VDLR (BW/sec)	TDLR (BW/sec)	HKEM (%BW × H)	MKFM[a] (%BW × H[b])
Injured	21.0	70.1	51.9	50.3	2.69	2.02
Injured[c]			44.3	43.2	2.17	
Uninjured	22.3	69.5	52.4	50.3	2.70	3.10
Uninjured[c]			48.2	46.5	2.60	
Controls	24.7	73.6	66.6	64.1	2.83	3.74

[a]PVV, pre–heel strike vertical foot velocity; FWV, average free-walking velocity; VDLR, maximum vertically directed loading rate; TDLR, maximum tibially directed loading rate; HKEM, heel strike external knee extension moment; MKFM, midstance external knee flexion moment. $P > 0.05$ for all measurements; H, height.
[b]$P < 0.01$.
[c]Data calculated excluding subject with inconsistent heel strike.

derived from analysis of patients who compensate well for the absence of an ACL might improve functional performance of patients who are ACLD without surgery.[32] At the very least, gait analysis should be able to provide information about whether a patient requires an assistive device for ADL. The clinical usefulness of gait analysis as an outcome measure in this population is largely related to the level of sophistication of equipment used to answer these questions.

In most of the papers we have reviewed, gait analysis involves the use of rather sophisticated instrumentation.[5,33,38,41] An assessment of gait analysis as an outcome measure should certainly involve an analysis of the clinical usefulness of these measures. Clinical gait analysis has traditionally been observational: the therapist watches the patient walk. Videotaping has also been used to allow the examiner to view the tape repeatedly and stop or slow the tape for more careful analysis.

FIGURE 27-10 EMG data of knees. Electromyographic data of vastus lateralis (VL), biceps femoris (BF) and anterior tibialis muscles of ACLD (rehab), ACLR (recon), and nondisabled (control) knees during level walking. (From Ciccotti MG, Kerlan RK, Perry J et al: An electromyographic analysis of the knee during functional activities: the normal, ACL deficient and reconstructed profiles, *Am J Sports Med* (in press). Used with permission.)

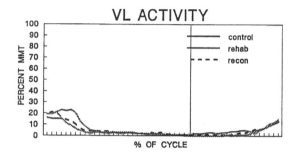

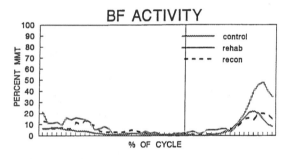

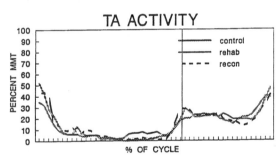

Two- and three-dimensional link-segment analysis as well as 6-degree-of-freedom rigid body analysis have been used for kinematics in combination with EMG analysis and/or analysis of kinetics (moment and/or forces). Given that this equipment is not readily available to every clinician, when is it necessary to use these instruments? When is it appropriate to use other means of gait analysis, and what types of information can they give the clinician?[*]

As with all measurement, which system is appropriate to use for making assessments of outcome after ACL injury depends on the kinds of judgments one intends to base on the data. Suppose the clinician is trying to decide whether to allow the patient to walk without crutches. If the decision only requires discerning whether the patient has an observable limp, then observational gait analysis (OGA) may be sensitive enough to allow for an accurate judgment. If however, the clinician is interested in comparing the knee joint flexion and extension excursions among patients, OGA or even videotaped OGA is probably not sensitive or reliable enough to detect subtle changes that may be clinically meaningful.[†]

If the clinician or researcher is interested in obtaining information on motion occurring in a single plane, two-dimensional kinematic analysis can provide accurate data with relatively low errors. In a recently completed study of rehabilitation after ACLR, we studied the gait of 131 patients at 6 to 8 weeks post-surgery after 4 weeks of rehabilitation. Once again, we found that the quadriceps femoris muscle strength has a profound effect on the knee flexion and extension excursions of the patients during the subphases of stance as measured by two-dimensional motion analysis. Four centers in four different parts of the country participated in this study. Gait analysis was performed at each site, while the computerized analysis of the videotapes was all performed at a single site. Since we were examining motion in a single-plane (sagittal) where the amount of excursion is typically large (flexion/extension) during walking, two-dimensional analysis was sufficient. Using a more rigorous setup would have prevented clinics from becoming involved in the project as cost and the need for dedicated space for the equipment would have been prohibitive.

If the clinician is interested in motion occurring in more than one plane, (e.g., in knee flexion/extension and internal/external rotation), then the error associated with use of a two-dimensional system will probably be too great to give an accurate assessment. In the situation where the clinician is either trying to measure rotational instability at the knee or assessing whether the patient is dynamically preventing the tibia from translating forward on the femur—in order to determine whether the patient is a bracing or surgical candidate—a more sophisticated system may be required. In these cases, detection of

---

[*]   See also Chapter 14.

[†]   See also Chapter 10 and 11.

the small translations (millimeters of motion) would likely be impossible with a two-dimensional or even a three-dimensional link-segment model. In this case, 6-degrees-of-freedom (3 rotations, 3 translations) rigid body analysis provides the most accurate assessment of movement. This type of system is sensitive enough to analyze movement of even a few degrees with little error. However, the patient will need to be referred to a center where this kind of analysis is performed, since it is impractical for most clinical settings.[*]

Perhaps we can determine which muscles fire during gait in the patient who demonstrates a good compensatory strategy via electromyography (EMG) and kinematic analysis. We may then be able to teach "poor compensators" (patients who are ACLD and are unstable) to stabilize the knee dynamically during activities by activating the muscles of the lower extremity in a similar way to those patients who compensate well for the injury.[32] We may eventually predict a gait pattern for patients who are poor compensators for ACLD and will likely progress to further ligamentous damage or meniscal tear. In order to ascertain which muscles are firing at a given point in the gait cycle, some form of EMG must be used. Most often, surface electrodes are used for analysis of dynamic motion. EMG can be used in a stand-alone format or can be interfaced with most motion analysis systems to give an accurate picture of the muscles that are firing during each phase of gait. The use of EMG to infer muscle force from muscle activity patterns is problematic. However, relative timing of muscle activity during gait can be accurately determined from even the most basic system. If research scientists are able to identify patterns in a few key muscles that then can be used to categorize and potentially train patients to walk in a more "stable" manner, then clinical settings with a simple EMG system may be able to translate the research into practice.[†]

The simplest way to assess the temporal components of gait accurately is to use footswitches with OGA. In a setting where force plates are unavailable, footswitches can give an accurate measure of step time, stance time, and velocity if the test is performed over a known distance. Since many kinematic and kinetic gait variables are velocity dependent, precise measures of velocity are often necessary to interpret results accurately.

The use of photoelectric cells allows easy and accurate calculation of velocity.[‡]

Evaluation of ground reaction forces requires the use of a force platform. If calculation of joint moments or center of pressure measurements are required, it is necessary to have a system that can measure both kinetics and kinematics. Several investigators have used the examination of external joint moments to predict muscle forces. Noyes and co-workers, in a study of patients who are ACLD and also have varus deformities, have identified the presence of an increased adduction moment at the knee in these patients.[22] The data were interpreted to indicate that the knee abductor torques (internal moments) must be high in these patients. Similarly, Berchuck and colleagues interpreted the absent external knee flexion moment in their subjects to suggest that the quadriceps femoris muscles (internal extension moment) are not active during the stance phase of gait.[5] The EMG data in this population, however, underscores the danger of inferring muscle activity patterns from measures of external moments. External moments are net moments. Many combinations of muscle activity patterns can combine to produce a given external moment. Identification of muscle activity patterns and their responsibility for alteration in "normal" or even "desirable" moments about the knee in different subphases of stance can only be determined by combining moment, EMG, and precise velocity measurements. This requires a sophisticated motion analysis setup and gait laboratory.[§]

SUMMARY

Gait analysis has been used to describe the disability resulting from rupture and reconstruction of the ACL. We have reviewed the pertinent literature and identified areas where investigation is incomplete. The clinical usefulness of various gait analysis methods for evaluation of different aspects of the disability have been presented. We believe that gait analysis provides an invaluable compliment to measurements of impairment and self-report in capturing the total disability and recovery after ACL injury. The effects of ACL rupture on function are enigmatic and gait analysis gives us insight into the mechanisms that affect an individual's ability to compensate for its loss during functional activity. Unfortunately, very little of

---

what has been uncovered experimentally is transferable to clinical measures that can be applied easily in the clinic.

REFERENCES

1. Arvidsson I, Eriksson E, Haggmark T et al: Isokinetic thigh muscle strength after ligament reconstruction in the knee joint: results from a 5–10 year follow-up after reconstruction of the anterior cruciate ligament in the knee joint, *Int J Sports Med* 2:7, 1981.

2. Andriacchi TP, Andersson GBJ, Fermier RW et al: A study of lower limb mechanics during stair climbing, *J Bone Joint Surg* 62A:749, 1980.

3. Arendt-Nielsen L, Sinkjaer T, Nielsen J et al: Electromyographic patterns and knee joint kinematics during walking at various speeds, *J Electromyograph Kinesiol* 1(2):89, 1991.

4. Baratta R, Solomonow M, Zhou BH et al: Muscular coactivation: the role of the antagonist musculature in maintaining knee stability, *Am J Sports Med* 16(2):113, 1988.

5. Berchuck M, Andriacchi TP, Bach BR et al: Gait adaptations by patients who have a deficient anterior cruciate ligament, *J Bone Joint Surg,* 72-A:871, 1990.

6. Bollem S, Seedhom BB: A comparison of the Lysholm and Cincinnati knee scoring questionnaires, *Am J Sports Med* 19:189, 1991.

7. Ciccotti MG, Kerlan RK, Perry J et al: *An electromyographic analysis of the knee during functional activities: the normal, ACL deficient and reconstructed profiles.* Unpublished manuscript.

8. Daniel DM, Stone ML, Sachs R et al: Instrumented measurement of anterior cruciate ligament disruption, *Am J Sports Med* 13:401, 1985.

9. Daniel DM: *Current concepts: ACL Injury: who is at risk?* Paper presented at the 59th Annual Meeting of the AAOS, Washington, D.C., February 1991.

10. Delitto A, Rose SJ, McKowen JM et al: Electrical stimulation versus voluntary exercise in strengthening thigh musculature after anterior cruciate ligament surgery, *Phys Ther* 68:660, 1988.

11. Elmqvist LG, Lorentzon R, Johansson C et al: Does a torn anterior cruciate ligament lead to changes in the central nervous drive of the knee extensors? *Eur J Appl Physiol* 58:203, 1988.

12. Harter RA, Osternig LR, Singer KM et al: Long-term evaluation of knee stability and function following surgical reconstruction for anterior cruciate ligament insufficiency, *Am J Sports Med* 16(5):434, 1988.

13. Hasan SS, Edmondstone MA, Limbard TJ et al: Reaction force patterns of injured and uninjured knees during walking and pivoting, *J Electromyograph Kinesiol* 1(3):218, 1991.

14. Jensen JE, Slocum DB, Larson RL: Reconstruction procedures for anterior cruciate ligament insufficiency: a computer analysis of clinical results, *Am J Sports Med* 11:240, 1983.

15. Kadaba MP, Ramakrishnan HK, Gainey JC et al: Gait adaptation patterns in patients with ACL deficiency, *Trans Orthop Res Soc* 18(2):361, 1993.

16. Kannus P, Latvala K, Jarvinen M: Thigh muscle strengths in the anterior cruciate ligament deficient: isokinetic and isometric long-term results, *J Orthop Sports Phys Ther* 9(5):223, 1987.

17. Larson R: Rating sheet for knee function. In Smillie I, editor: *Diseases of the knee joint,* New York, 1974, Churchill Livingstone.

18. Limbard TJ, Shiavi R, Frazer M et al: EMG profiles of knee joint musculature during walking: changes induced by anterior cruciate ligament deficiency, *J Orthop Res Soc* 6:630, 1988.

19. Lysholm J, Gillquist J: Evaluation of knee ligament surgery results with emphasis on use of a scoring scale, *Am J Sports Med* 10:150, 1982.

20. McNair PJ, Marshall RN, Matheson JA: Gait of subjects with anterior cruciate ligament deficiency, *Clin Biomech* 4(4):243, 1989.

21. Mohtadi NGH, Webster-Bogaert S, Fowler PJ: Limitation of motion following anterior cruciate ligament reconstruction: a case control study, *Am J Sports Med* 19:620, 1991.

22. Noyes FR, Schipplein OD, Andriacchi TP et al: The anterior cruciate ligament-deficient knee with varus alignment: an analysis of gait adaptations and dynamic joint loadings, *Am J Sports Med* 20(6):707, 1992.

23. Noyes FR, McGinniss GH, Mooar PA: Functional disability in the anterior cruciate insufficient knee syndrome: review of knee rating systems and projected risk factors in determining treatment, *Sports Med* 1:278, 1984.

24. Noyes FR, Mooar PA, Matthews DS et al: The symptomatic anterior cruciate-deficient knee. Part 1: The long-term functional disability in athletically active individuals, *J Bone Joint Surg* 65A:154, 1983.

25. O'Connor BL, Visco DM, Brandt KD: Gait alterations in dogs with unstable knee joints: evidence that the central nervous system is reprogrammed to protect unstable joints, *Trans Orthop Res Soc* 17:478, 1992.

26. Perry J, Fox JM, Boitano MA et al: Functional evaluation of the pes anserinus transfer by electromyography and gait analysis, *J Bone Joint Surg* 62A:973, 1980.

27. Queale WS, Snyder-Mackler, Handing KA et al: *Instrumented examination of knee laxity in patients with anterior cruciate deficiency.* Unpublished manuscript.

28. Seto JL, Orofino AS, Morrissey MC et al: Assessment of quadriceps/hamstring strength, knee ligament stability, functional and sports activity levels five years after anterior cruciate ligament reconstruction, *Am J Sports Med* 16(2):170, 1988.

29. Sgaglione NA: *Interpretation of ACL surgery data: critical analysis of outcome comparing knee ligament rating systems.* Paper presented at the 59th Annual Meeting of the AAOS, Washington D.C., February 1992.

30. Shiavi R, Zhang LQ, Limbard T et al: Pattern analysis of electromyographic linear envelopes exhibited by subjects with uninjured and injured knees during free and fast speed walking, *J Orthop Res Soc* 10:226, 1992.

31. Shiavi R, Limbard T, Borra H et al: Electromyography profiles of knee joint musculature during pivoting: changes induced by anterior cruciate

ligament deficiency, *J Electromyograph Kinesiol* 1(1):49, 1991.

32. Sinkjaer T, Arendt-Nielsen L: Knee stability and muscle coordination in patients with anterior cruciate ligament injuries: an electromyographic approach, *J Electromyograph Kinesiol* 1:209, 1991.

33. Snyder-Mackler L, Ladin Z, Schepsis AA et al: Electrical stimulation of the thigh muscles after reconstruction of the anterior cruciate ligament, *J Bone Joint Surg* 73A:1025, 1991.

34. Solomonow M, Baratta R, Zhou BH et al: The synergistic action of the anterior cruciate ligament and thigh muscles in maintaining joint stability, *Am J Sports Med* 15:207, 1987.

35. Solomonow M, Zhou BH, Baratta R: Coactivation patterns of the knees antagonist muscles, *Proc IEEE-Engineering Med Biol,* 1987.

36. Tibone JE, Antich TJ: A biomechanical analysis of anterior cruciate ligament reconstruction with the patellar tendon, *Am J Sports Med* 16(4):332, 1988.

37. Tibone JE, Antich TJ, Fanton JS et al: Functional analysis of anterior cruciate ligament instability, *Am J Sports Med* 14(4):276, 1986.

38. Timoney JM, Inman WS, Quesada PM et al: Return of normal gait patterns after anterior cruciate ligament reconstruction, *Am J Sports Med* 21:887, 1993.

39. Torg JS, Wayne C, Kalen V: Clinical diagnosis of anterior cruciate ligament instability in the athlete, *Am J Sports Med* 4:84, 1976.

40. Wigerstad-Lossing I, Grimby G, Jonsson T et al: Effects of electrical muscle stimulation combined with voluntary contractions after knee ligament surgery, *Med Sci Sports Exer* 20:93, 1988.

41. Wu CD, Birac D, Andriacchi TP et al: A study of compensatory function in ACL deficient knees in walking and more stressful activities, *Trans Orthop Res Soc* 17:659, 1992.

Gait Assessment of Children to Enhance Evaluation of Foot and Ankle Function and Treatment Efficacy

Lisa Selby-Silverstein

Key Terms

Coefficient of variation
Down syndrome
Foot angle
Foot and ankle function

Foot contact index
Pronation-supination index
Protocol

The objective of this chapter is to discuss how gait assessment can be used with children to enhance understanding of foot and ankle function and the effects of foot orthoses. Logistical recommendations will be made to assist the clinician in obtaining gait data from young children. In addition, parameters that might provide useful information about foot and ankle dysfunction and its remediation will be discussed. Finally, specific examples of differences seen in parameters between a child without disability and a child with Down Syndrome (DS) and the changes documented when the child with Down Syndrome wore foot orthoses will be presented.

An important step towards using gait data obtained from young children is collecting that data in a valid manner. There are a few things a clinician can do, in addition to the standard playing and cajoling used when working with children, to facilitate a useful data collection session. The walkway should be well delineated and no wider than necessary. Everything should be ready for the data collection to start when the child arrives. The data collection session should follow a regimented procedure with which all data collectors are familiar. Everything needed during data collection should be readily available. The investigator should have a data collection sheet on which to record any anecdotal information about the trials collected, such as what the child was doing with the arms during the trial or if the child did or did not appear to be using a typical gait pattern. A consistent data collection staff with consistent jobs should decrease the chance of staff error during data collection. The protocol should be rehearsed with adults first. Once the method is perfected with adults, data should be collected from some children without disabilities. Besides assisting in building a normative data base, this procedure helps to identify problems with the protocol before data from the children to be studied are collected.

From a research design perspective, as much as possible should be done to maximize the number of valid trials obtained during data collection. Toward this end, both the type of data being collected and the number of conditions should be minimized. Investigators should not expect to collect data from a child for more than a 2-hour time span. The child probably will not be cooperative for more time and even if he/she is, the data probably will be more representative of fatigued rather than typical performance. In addition, the child and the parents are more likely to be willing to return for future analyses if data are not collected for the entire time during which the child is cooperative. In order to have a minimum of three usable trials, a minimum of five to ten trials that are believed to be usable will need to be collected.

From a protocol perspective, particular methods are suggested to insure valid data collection and analysis. The investigator should have a way of naming data files, which consistently names all data collected from each trial and documents the number of trials attempted before the data were recorded. The marker placement should be documented such that it could be repeated for follow-up assessment. For force plate data to be useful in calculating joint torques or powers, the child must step on the plate with one foot *only* as data from force plates are affected by any force exerted on them at any instant in time. Nyquist's sampling theorem should be observed so that, minimally, the gait pattern is sampled at two times the frequency of the movement of interest.[2] The investigator or clinician should decide whether it is important to evaluate kinematic data within the context of the laboratory coordinate system or a local coordinate system, as this has bearing on how the data are interpreted. For example, when assessing pelvic sway as an indicator of standing balance, measuring pelvic movement relative to the laboratory would be better than measuring pelvic movement relative to the trunk. However, when assessing knee motion during gait, measuring lower leg movement relative to the laboratory would not be as informative as measuring lower leg movement relative to the femur. Toward this end, the marker sytem used during data collection should provide the data necessary to calculate kinematics using an appropriate mathematical model.

When evaluating corrective footwear, use of new shoe gear is important because shoes take on the shape of the foot as it has been functioning. In addition, it is usually assumed that the child will not exhibit a representative gait the first time the child walks in corrective footwear. Ideally, data should be collected in barefeet and in standard footwear (shoes or sneakers) as well as in the corrective footwear being evaluated. One of these conditions may need to be neglected to collect enough trials to assure a valid representation of the child's behavior under the remaining conditions. If this is necessary, collecting data in barefeet may be neglected since barefoot walking is not a critical functional condition; that is, the child will not be able to walk outside regularly in barefeet. Finally, it is important to recognize that foot and ankle function are dependent on multiple factors, particularly how the body moves over the foot. Hence, movement of the body proximal to the ankles should be considered when evaluating foot and ankle function or the efficacy of any treatment aimed at modifying foot and ankle function.

A number of parameters may provide useful information about foot and ankle dysfunction and its remediation. The following are brief descriptions of various parameters and what each tells us. Preceding chapters have described these variables and their collection processes in greater detail. What follows serves as a basis for demonstrating their usefulness in clinical applications.

Foot angle describes the degree of intoeing or outtoeing of the foot relative to the forward line of progression. This method for measuring foot angle from a Musgrave Footprint™* was adapted from Shores[4] (Figure 28-1). Draw a line along the medial (AB) border of the footprint between the most medial activated sensor in the bottom half and top halves of the print. Then draw lines at the end of the toes (AC) and at the back of the heel (BD) perpendicular to the line AB. The length of the foot along AB can then be divided by three, and lines (EF and GH) can be drawn across the foot to trisect it (also with lines perpendicular to AB). A line can then be drawn along the lateral (DH) border of the footprint. The lowest two "across foot" lines (BD and EF) can then be bisected and a line (IJ) connecting these two bisection points can be drawn to extend so that it crosses the line of forward progression (KL). The angle in degrees that line IJ forms with regard to the forward line of progression (KL) can be called the foot angle. A zero degree foot angle indicates that the foot angle line is parallel to the line of progression. Internal (or medial) rotation is represented by negative numbers and external (or lateral) rotation by positive numbers.

The **pronation-supination index** was developed as an indirect method of measuring the relative amount of pronation or supination the foot was in when the distal third of the foot was in contact with the ground. This may be an important parameter to assess since it is thought that foot supination is what provides a rigid lever for push off. The value is computed by dividing the distance, center of pressure to medial footprint border, by the distance from the medial to the lateral

*Musgrave Footprint™ Preston Communications, Ltd., New Ross, Dinbren Rd, Llangollen, Clwyd, N. Wales, United Kingdom.

FIGURE 28-1   Musgrave Footprint.™ The lines are drawn to measure foot angle (the angle between lines IJ and KL), pronation-supination index (the ratio of GM/GH), and foot contact index (IN/ length of actual sneaker). Note: The gray scale indicates the amount of pressure between the ground and the sole of the foot in kg/unit area.

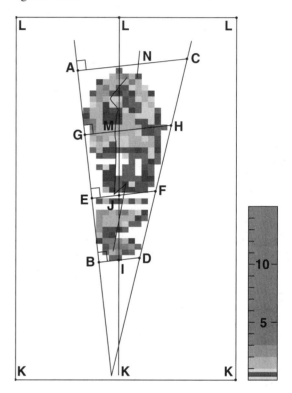

footprint borders at the distal third of the footprint. This value can be obtained by using the Musgrave Footprint,™ (Figure 28-1) and the same medial border line (AB) drawn to measure foot angle. The perpendicular distance between the medial border of the foot (AB) and the furthest point of the center of pressure (M) can be measured across line GH. As a normalization procedure, this distance can be divided by the length of GH, the width of the footprint at the distal third of the print. This is approximately the widest point of the footprint and is presumed to be close to the location of the metatarsal heads. A decrease in the value of this ratio indicates foot pronation and an increase in the value indicates foot supination.

The **foot contact index** also can be calculated using data from the Musgrave Footprint™. First, the length of the footprint is measured along the foot angle line (IN) (Figure 28-1). Then as a normalization procedure, this distance is divided by the actual length of the child's sneaker at its longest point. A decrease in the value of this ratio indicates that less of the length of the foot was in contact with the ground, and an increase indicates that more of the length of the foot was in contact with the ground.

Joint torques for each step analyzed can be calculated using kinematic and ground reaction force data (Figure 28-2). These values are usually graphically depicted and normalized to 100% of stance phase or 100% of the gait cycle using linear interpolation. Torque values (in newton meters) are usually normalized by dividing the values by the child's weight (in newtons). This allows group data comparison. Specific aspects of joint torque curves, which may prove interesting, include the phase of the peaks, the value of the highest peak(s), and the smoothness of the curves.

Electromyography, joint kinematics, joint powers, and full body center of mass displacement data could also yield interesting information with regard to aspects of a child's overall gait that might influence or be influenced by foot and ankle function. It is important to recognize, however, that many gait variables vary with velocity, so it is important to measure average velocity and consider it when gait data is being assessed.[1]

In addition to actual parameter values, coefficients of variation for the parameters over a number of trials indicate the stability or instability of a behavior. That is, if there is a high coefficient of variation, then there is a high degree of variability and the behavior might be more easily influenced than if the variability is low and hence the behavior is stable.

The following were data collected from a 4-year-old child without disability walking while wearing sneakers, and a 4-year-old child with Trisomy 21 type Down syndrome, first walking while wearing sneakers and then while wearing sneakers and foot orthoses. The child without disability had no history of medical, orthopaedic, or neurological dysfunction. The child with Down syndrome exhibited hypotonia and overall joint hyperextensibility. She also had a history of a ventricular septal defect, severe intestinal dysfunction, and hiatal hernia surgery. She was enrolled in an early intervention program and was receiving physical therapy at home twice per month. She also was involved in a swimming program. None of her medical problems appeared to be issues at the time of data collection.

In standing, the child with Down syndrome exhibited 4 degrees of heel eversion as measured through a Plexiglas grid. The foot orthoses realigned her feet so that lines drawn to bisect her calcanei moved from a position of 4 degrees of eversion to vertical. The following data reflect differences detected between gait of the child without disability, and gait of the child with Down syndrome, and the change in gait when the child with Down syndrome wore foot orthoses (Figure 28-3A through 28-4C).

Figures 3A and 3B are sample Musgrave right sneaker prints during gait of a child with DS in sneakers alone (Figure 28-3A) and while wearing sneakers and foot orthoses (Figure 28-3B). Figure 28-3C is a sample right Musgrave sneaker print during gait of a child without disability. Note the foot angles in relation to the forward line of progression (line next to sneaker print), the location of the center of pressure throughout stance phase (black line) and the medial arch areas (left side) of all three prints depicting the amount of pressure in that area (see gray scale to right of sneaker prints).

From these data it is evident that the child with DS exhibited more outtoeing than the child without disability and that the foot orthoses decreased the child's outtoeing problem. The pronation-supination index indicates that the foot moved from a more pronated to a more supinated position when the center of pressure was near the distal third of the footprint. This could be interpreted as a desirable effect since the pronation-supination index for the child without disability showed more supination at the same footprint location. The change in pressure distribution in the arch area

---

FIGURE 28-2 Torque about the transmalleolar axis.

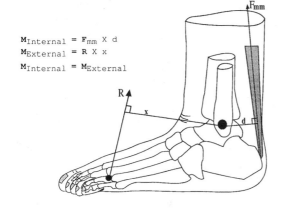

$$M_{Internal} = F_{mm} \times d$$
$$M_{External} = R \times x$$
$$M_{Internal} = M_{External}$$

F_{mm} = force from muscles.
 d = lever arm for muscles.
 x = lever arm for ground reaction force.
 R = ground reaction force.

FIGURE 28-3 **A**, Sneaker print from child with DS wearing sneakers alone. **B**, Sneaker print from child with DS wearing sneakers and NPFOs. **C**, Sneaker print from child without disabilities wearing sneakers. *Note:* The forward line of progression is the line next to the sneaker print, the center of pressure is represented by the black line through each sneaker print, the gray scale to right of sneaker prints represents the amount of pressure being detected in kg/unit area.

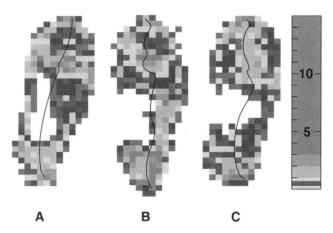

A   **B**   **C**

further supports the interpretation of improvement in that wearing sneakers alone, the child with DS exerted more medial arch pressure on the ground than the child without disability and orthoses decreased the pressure. The jaggedness of the center of pressure line when the child with DS was wearing foot orthoses reflects a more unstable foot performance compared to either child's foot movement in sneakers alone. This "instability" could be a lasting consequence of the changed foot alignment or it could be an effect that will stabilize over time. Determining the permanence of the foot instability would require collecting this type of gait data over time. The child's performance during function tasks would also need to be assessed to see if the foot instability has a negative effect on the child's function.

Figures 28-4*A* and 28-4*B* are sample three-dimensional ankle torque curves about the transmalleolar axis during gait of a child with DS in sneakers alone (Figure 28-4*A*) and while wearing sneakers and foot orthoses (Figure 28-4*B*). Figure 28-4*C* is a sample three-dimensional ankle torque about the transmalleolar axis of a child without disability. They are all normalized to 100 percent of the stance phase of gait. Note the heights and phases of the peaks, the jaggedness of the curve in Figure 4*A,* the phase at which the curve crosses zero (when center of pressure is beneath the transmalleolar axis), and the degree of negative torque (an indication of how far and long the ground reaction force was posterior to the ankle axis). The large standard deviation around the first

peak of Figure 28-4*B* may be indicative of a transitional (immature) pattern since it is not present in curves obtained from adults without disabilities.[3]

The ankle torque data could be interpreted as indicating that the child with DS exhibits a lower peak torque than the child without disability and that the foot orthoses do not change this fact. The first positive peak, however, which is usually lower than the push off peak, is higher (more atypical) when the child with DS is wearing sneakers alone than when she is wearing foot orthoses and sneakers. In addition, the foot orthoses seem to cause these curves to be somewhat smoother, indicating smoother ankle control. Finally, the ankle torque data from the child with DS cross the zero point (the X axis) earlier in stance phase than the data from the child without disability. This indicates that the child with DS did not keep her heel on the ground, during either footwear condition, as long as the child without disabilities. In summary, the data seem to indicate that the foot orthoses cause some aspects of the child's foot movements and ankle torque curves to approximate those of a child without disability. Hence, it was recommended that the child continue to wear the orthoses and that she be reevaluated using gait assessment in 3 months. In this case, the clinician based her clinical decision not only on static measures of foot alignment, as is typically the case, but also on data obtained during dynamic foot and ankle function during gait.

FIGURE 28-4 **A,** Sample three-dimensional ankle torque curve during gait of a child with DS wearing sneakers alone, mean and standard deviation for five trials.

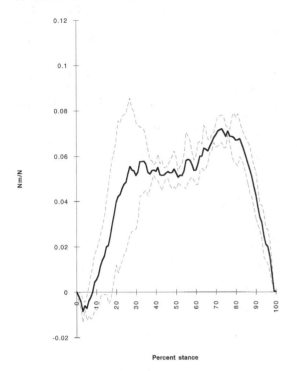

FIGURE 28-4 **B,** Sample three-dimensional ankle torque curve during gait of a child with DS wearing sneakers and foot orthoses, mean and standard deviation for five trials.

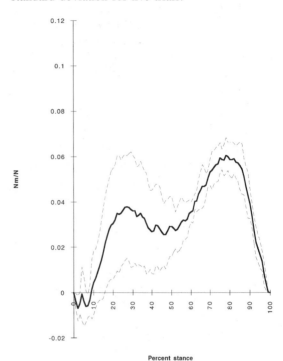

FIGURE 28-4 **C,** Sample three-dimensional ankle torque curve during gait of a child without disability wearing sneakers, mean and standard deviation for five trials.

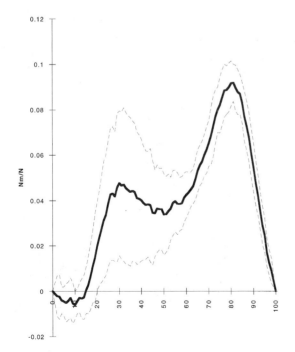

In conclusion, what the clinician should measure is based on what he is trying to understand or modify. Factors that might influence the aspect of gait being studied or be directly affected by the intervention must not be ignored. The clinician or investigator must determine what is feasible, valid, and most important to measure before gait analysis commences and then design the data collection, reduction, and analysis to best represent the behavior being evaluated. Data interpretation and final recommendations should be a team effort, as they are somewhat subjective and influenced by the interpreter's background. Finally, any treatment-induced change should be assessed in light of its relationship to the subject's functional abilities.

Acknowledgment: *The information in this chapter was obtained in partial fulfillment of my Doctor of Philosophy degree and would not have been completed without assistance from the Hahnemann University Doctoral Committee, in particular Robert Palisano, ScD., PT, (Chairman), and Howard Hillstrom, PhD., Director of the Gait Study Center, Pennsylvania College of podiatric Medicine, along with his staff including the podiatric students and Drexel University Engineering students. Financial support was obtained from a*

U.S. Department of Special Education traineeship through Hahnemann University, a research fellowship from the National Institute on Disability Rehabilitation Research, a doctoral scholarship from the Foundation for Physical Therapy, a pilot research grant from the Pediatric Section of the American Physical Therapy Association, and a research grant from the American Podiatric Medical Association. Also thanks to my subjects and their parents.

REFERENCES

1. Andriacchi TP, Ogle JA, Galante JO: Walking speed as a basis for normal and abnormal gait measurements, *J Biomech* 10:261, 1977.

2. Oppenheim AV, Willsky AS, Young IT: *Signals and systems,* Englewood Cliffs, N.J., 1983, Prentice Hall.

3. Perlberg G: *A quantitative diagnostic technique for discriminating between spasticity and contracture at the ankle joint in patients with equinus deformity,* Unpublished Master's Thesis, Philadelphia, 1991, Drexel University.

4. Shores M: Footprint analysis in gait documentation: an instructional sheet format, *Phys Ther* 60:1163, 1980.

5. Silverstein LS: *The effect of neutral position foot orthoses on gait of children with down syndrome,* Doctoral Thesis. Philadelphia, 1993, Hahnemann University.

6. Selby-Silverstein L, Hillstrom H, Palisano R et al: *Efficacy of foot orthoses for children with Down Syndrome.* Unpublished manuscript.

CHAPTER 29

THE USE OF GAIT ANALYSIS TO ENHANCE THE UNDERSTANDING OF RUNNING INJURIES

Irene S. McClay

KEY TERMS

Center of pressure

Closed chain motion

Ground reaction force

Kinematics

Muscle length

Running injuries

Strength

Medical professionals have been faced with a dramatic increase in the number of patients with running-related lower extremity injuries. With the onset of the running boom of the 1970s and 1980s, there has been a great rise in the number of Americans engaged in a running program. Prospective studies have reported that 50 to 65% of runners sustained an injury during a 12-month period[23,48] and 85% sustained one during an 18- to 20-month period.[4] Clement, Taunton, Smart, and McNichol conducted a retrospective study of patients seen by one physician over a 2-year period.[12] They reported that a total of 1650 patients were seen for 1819 running-related injuries. The problem is not always resolved by simply discontinuing running. It may be the threshold of running that precipitates the injury; however, the pain that results often interferes with normal activities such as prolonged standing, walking, and stair climbing. Abnormal mechanics are often implicated as a contributory cause. Because these injuries occur during running, it is imperative that we study patients while they are running. The following discussions will serve to demonstrate the role that gait analysis can play in helping to understand the relationship between mechanics and injury.

Running has long been a topic of scientific interest. Some of the great intellects of our time, from Aristotle (384-322 B.C.) to daVinci (1452-1519), have made contributions that have enhanced our understanding of locomotor mechanics. Aristotle is quoted as saying:

> Further, the forces that which causes movement and of that which remains still must be made equal. . . . For just as the pusher pushes, so the pusher is pushed—i.e., with similar force.[7]

This is an amazing suggestion of the third law of motion nearly two millennia before Newton's time.

We have had the tools to measure objectively running mechanics for about 150 years. Marey (1830-1904), in addition to being a pioneer in the area of photogrammetry, also built one of the first force platforms.[7] In fact, he is credited as being the first to synchronize the data from film and force transducers, which has contributed to the understanding of the relationship between force and kinematics during human locomotion. High-speed film and force plate technology have formed the basis for research in running mechanics for many years. However, analysis of high-speed film is extremely time intensive. Those of us who have spent hours in a darkened room digitizing endless markers will be forever grateful for the development of the newer, automated motion analysis systems that have further facilitated work in this field.

Although an abundance of research has been conducted in the area of running, a large number of the studies are descriptive in nature. Nearly 500 articles on the topic of running were cited in a recent annotated bibliography on gait.[45] However, the majority of these investigations involve normal subjects, and most are not designed with large enough sample sizes to establish normative values. Only a handful of investigations deal specifically with abnormal mechanics and injury. In an extensive review of the literature on running mechanics, Williams notes that "very few systematic investigations have been done which relate structural and functional parameters to injuries. . . ."[49] The study of running injury mechanics continues to remain an area of uncharted waters.

The first major jump that gait analysis made into the clinical arena was in the area of pediatrics and cerebral palsy gait. As we moved into this medical forum, scientists were challenged to provide clinically relevant information. Over a decade ago, Brand and Crowninshield expressed concerns with regards to the efficacy of gait analysis in a letter to the *Journal of Biomechanics*.[5] The ability to use biomechanical tools to diagnose (i.e., distinguish between different pathologies) was questioned. They maintained that measured gait parameters must provide information unattainable via direct observation and that adding precision to the measurement was not enough justification to perform the costly analysis.

Perhaps as an answer to this charge, a study was undertaken to compare visual observation to quantitative gait analysis.[34] The gait pattern of five persons with amputions was visually observed and recorded by experienced medical professionals (i.e., physical therapists, orthopedic surgeons, prosthetists). In addition, the gait was recorded via a video-based motion analysis system. Results were compared and it was determined that the quantitative approach picked up 3.4 times as many deviations as visual observation. The parameters studied were temporal and positional in nature. It is likely that derivatives of position, such as velocity and acceleration would be even more difficult to assess via visual observation.

Thus, it appears that quantitative gait analysis has the potential to provide information not possible through visual observation. The challenge is to establish which parameters provide the most useful information to clinicians and offer the most insight into the etiology of injuries. This may not prove to be an easy task. Running is a repetitive activity of relatively high forces. The runner may strike the ground 5000 times per foot during a typical training run, landing each time with approximately three times body weight. One can readily see how even minor deviations in either structure or mechanics can quickly accumulate into a major problem. These deviations may be at a level of subtlety below which we can accurately measure.

We now have the tools to readily quantify three-dimensional forces and motions. The remainder of this chapter will be focused on how we have used this information, to date, to understand running mechanics. Normal running mechanics will be reviewed followed by a description of documented abnormal mechanics found in runners. Parameters that may hold promise in understanding the etiology of running-related injuries will also be explored. Finally, three case studies will be presented as examples of the use of gait analysis in formulating clinical decisions regarding the etiology and treatment of running injuries. Because the area of injury mechanics is still in its infancy, more questions will be posed here than answers offered with the hope of stimulating further research in this field.

KINEMATICS OF RUNNING

The gait cycle in running is defined as the period of time from foot strike to ipsilateral foot strike and includes both swing and support phases. Unlike walking, running has no period of double support. Secondly, running has a nonsupport phase in which both feet are off the ground. As the majority of injuries occur when the foot is in contact with the ground, the focus of the discussions that follow will be on the support phase of running from foot strike to toe off. This phase can be subdivided further as shown in Table 29-1.

Normal Kinematics

The majority of the literature regarding kinematics focuses on the two-dimensional motion of the hip, knee, and ankle in the sagittal plane* or the rearfoot angle in the frontal plane.[1,6,11] The conventions of these two-dimensional angles and typical angular patterns are illustrated in Figure 29-1.

Motion of the Hip   The true hip angle is measured between the thigh and the trunk. However

---

* Refer to the following sources: 6, 29, 30, 32, 36, 46, 49.

TABLE 29-1   Phases of gait.

Abbrev.	Name	Description
FS	Foot strike	Initial contact
FS-FF	Foot strike-Foot flat	Loading phase
FF-HO	Foot flat-Heel off	Mid stance
HO-TO	Heel off-Toe off	Propulsive phase
TO	Toe off	Pre swing

the majority of studies describe hip motion indirectly by measuring the orientation of the thigh with respect to the vertical (thigh angle).[29,30,49] At foot strike, this thigh angle measures approximately 25 degrees of flexion. The thigh remains fairly fixed from FS to FF, but begins extending with the knee following maximum support phase knee flexion. It reaches a maximum value of approximately 25 degrees of extension near TO and begins to flex again in preparation for swing.

Motion of the Knee   The knee joint actually comprised two articulations: one between the tibia and femur (tibiofemoral joint or TFJ) and the other between the patella and femur (patellofemoral joint or PFJ). Our current knowledge regarding knee joint motion during running is primarily founded in two-dimensional research of the TFJ. The runner strikes the ground with the knee in approximately 10 to 20 degrees of flexion. Flexion continues from FS through FF reaching a peak of approximately 40 degrees. The knee begins to extend at approximately midsupport and peaks at approximately 5 to 10 degrees flexion near TO. McClay reported the three-dimensional motion of the knee during running (Figure 29-2).[24] The motion of knee flexion was found to be consistent with the previously reported findings. In the frontal plane, the knee was found to be slightly abducted at foot strike, moved into adduction of approximately 12 degrees until midsupport and then reversed its motion, moving into abduction again until toe off. In the transverse plane, the knee was in slight internal rotation at foot strike, continued to internally rotate approximately 8 degrees until mid support, and then began to externally rotate through toe off.

Data regarding motion of the patellofemoral joint during running is also scarce. This is a consequence of the difficulty in measuring this motion. External skin markers cannot be used because of the high degree of movement of the

FIGURE 29-1 Angular patterns of sagittal plane motions of the lower extremity during running. Two complete cycles are shown. (Reproduced from *Foot and ankle* with permission of The American Orthopaedic Foot and Ankle Society, Inc.)

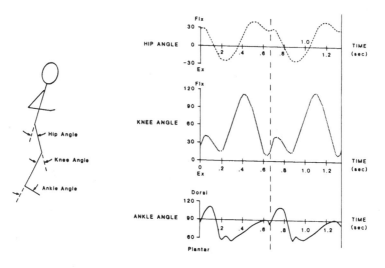

FIGURE 29-2 Three-dimensional angular patterns of the tibiofemoral joint during the contact phase of running. (© 1990 Irene S. McClay)

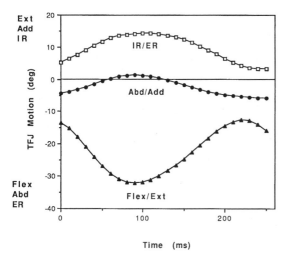

FIGURE 29-3 Three-dimensional angular patterns of the patellofemoral joint during the contact phase of running. (© 1990 Irene S. McClay)

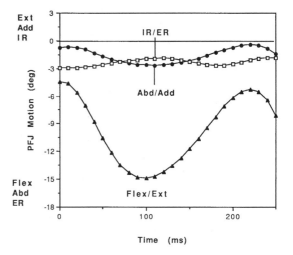

patella with respect to the skin. Two in vivo techniques have been used to monitor patellar motion. Researchers have imbedded tantalum balls into the patella and femur and have collected serial radiographs at various knee angles.[47] In addition, intracortical pins have been inserted into the patella and femur to track motion during walking using three-dimensional cinematography.[22] However, only one study, to date, has examined PFJ motion during running.

Using intracortical pins into the patella and femur, McClay studied the rotations and translations of the patella with respect to the femur in two normal runners (NL) and two runners with PFJ pain (Figure 29-3).[24] PFJ motion is described in the same manner as TFJ motion. Flexion is an anterior rotation of the patella about its mediolateral axis. Abduction is a rotation of the distal pole of the patella medially about an anteroposterior axis. Internal rotation is a medial rotation of the patella about its longitudinal axis. Results suggested that with the exception of motions in flexion/extension and distraction/compression, PFJ patterns were variable between subjects expressing more individuality in this joint compared with the TFJ. In the sagittal plane, the PFJ closely followed the motion of the TFJ. It was slightly extended at FS and remained more extended than the TFJ throughout contact. Total excursion was also less than that of the TFJ. Very little motion was seen in the transverse plane. In the frontal plane, the patella moved into abduction as the knee flexed and adduction as it extended. In general, the patella translated posterior and distally as the knee flexed and anterior and proximally as it extended. Translations along the patella's mediolateral axis in the normal subjects were minimal.

Motion of the Ankle   The ankle is slightly dorsiflexed at FS and continues to dorsiflex, reaching a maximum value of 20 degrees at approximately mid support. The trend then reverses and plantarflexion occurs concurrently with knee extension through TO. Few three-dimensional motion data of the ankle during running are available at this time. However, the ankle joint has primarily a mediolateral axis with the majority of its motion occurring in the sagittal plane.

Motion of the Foot   The foot is one of the body's most versatile skeletal structures. It provides our base of support and serves a number of other functions including mobile adapter to uneven terrain, shock absorber during impact, and rigid lever for propulsion. Of the segments of the lower extremity, it is probably the least understood in terms of kinematics. This is due to the large number of articulations and consequently numerous degrees of freedom of movement a foot can have. In order to fully describe the three-dimensional motion of all of the articulations of the foot, one would have to place at least three noncollinear markers per bone. In order to accurately track foot motion, the markers would have to be imbedded into each of the bones. One can quickly see how difficult this can become. Yet, the foot is the point of contact of the body with the ground and receives the full impact of the ground reaction forces. Abnormalities in the manner in which the foot interacts with the ground can negatively affect joints and segments farther up the kinematic chain. For example, the knee has been cited as the most commonly injured joint in runners, and abnormal foot mechanics are often associated with these knee injuries.[12,19,23]

In order to simplify this complex structure, the foot is often functionally divided into the forefoot, midfoot, and rearfoot. The forefoot is formed by the metatarsal bones, while the midfoot is comprised of the more proximally lying tarsals. The calcaneus and talus together form the subtalar joint and make up the rearfoot. The subtalar joint (STJ) has been the focus of most research in foot mechanics during running (Fig. 29-4).

Model Used to Study the STJ   The STJ axis crosses all three cardinal planes of the body, and therefore is referred to as a triplanar joint.[33] Motion at this joint, then, can be resolved into three components. Dorsiflexion and plantarflexion occur in the sagittal plane; inversion and eversion occur in the frontal plane; and abduction and adduction take place in the transverse plane. The combined triplanar motions are referred to as pronation and supination. During closed chain (foot in contact with the ground) pronation, the calcaneus everts (proximal end tilts inward), the talus adducts (rotates medially), and plantarflexes (rotates downward). During closed chain supination the opposite occurs as the calcaneus inverts and the talus abducts and dorsiflexes. Due to its location between the distal end of the tibia and the calcaneus, the talus is very difficult to monitor with external skin markers. Therefore, motion at this joint is frequently modeled as the motion between the tibia and calcaneus (often referred to as the rearfoot angle depicted in Figure 29-5). The majority of motion at the subtalar joint is in the frontal plane (inversion/eversion), and it is assumed there is relatively little motion in this plane between the tibia and talus.[33] Therefore, this has been the accepted model. When using a two-dimensional, frontal plane analysis, one is assessing the inversion/eversion component of the

FIGURE 29-4   The subtalar joint (articulation between the talus and calcaneus) and its joint axis.

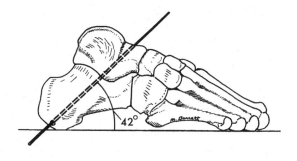

FIGURE 29-5   The measurement of the rearfoot angle.

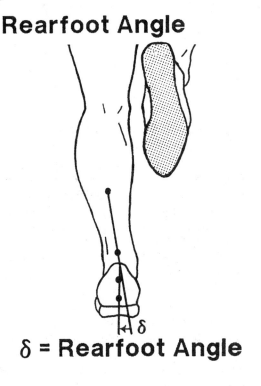

Rearfoot Angle

δ = Rearfoot Angle

triplanar motion of supination/pronation; however, the terms *pronation* and *eversion,* and *supination* and *inversion* are often used interchangeably.

STJ Motion   At distance running speeds (i.e., 3.8m/s), the foot lands in 5 to 10 degrees of inversion. Landing in inversion allows for greater rearfoot excursion and greater time over which to attenuate the peak forces of impact. The foot immediately begins to evert reaching a peak of approximately 8 to 12 degrees at approximately 30% of contact (60 to 90 ms after foot strike). The leg remains relatively fixed in space and the change in angle results from movement of the calcaneus.[6] This eversion is an important component of the gait cycle. As this occurs, it is believed that the oblique and longitudinal midtarsal joint axes become parallel,[15] allowing the foot to become a mobile adapter to whatever surface it comes in contact with. This mobility in the foot also provides cushioning by increasing the time over which the impact forces are applied to the supportive structures of the foot. The foot maintains this pronated posture through mid-support and then begins to invert through toe off. As the foot inverts, the subtalar and midtarsal joint axes are thought to become skewed and the foot be-

comes rigid, providing an effective lever for push off.

Soutas-Little, Beavis, Verstraete, and Markus provide three-dimensional data of rearfoot motion during running.[41] They used a rigid body analysis on the rearfoot model described previously, and their results in the frontal plane (inversion/eversion) were consistent with previously reported values. In the sagittal plane (dorsiflexion/plantarflexion), the rearfoot was slightly plantarflexed at foot strike, then dorsiflexed until mid support, followed by plantarflexion through toe off. In the transverse plane (medial/lateral rotation), the authors reported slight medial rotation at foot strike, followed by lateral rotation until mid support with medial rotation occurring again until toe off.

Abnormal Kinematics
Pronation and Pronation Velocity   The focus of research in abnormal kinematics during running has been on the foot. The rearfoot motion of a runner with normal, excessive pronation and excessive supination are depicted in Figure 29-6. The most commonly noted abnormal behavior during running is excessive pronation. Excessive pronation and pronation velocity are often cited as causes for running related injuries.* Messier and Pittala reported that peak pronation and peak pronation velocity were significant discriminators between injured and noninjured runners.[28] The excessive and/or prolonged pronation places stress on the medial musculoskeletal structures of the foot and ankle. As the foot pronates, the talus rotates inwardly. Therefore, it has been suggested that excessive pronation leads to excessive internal rotation of the tibia and consequently places abnormal rotational stress on the musculoskeletal structures of the knee joint. Increased rotation under loaded conditions may result in excessive torsional stresses experienced by the tibia itself. These ideas have yet to be substantiated. In the one study that examined the effect of pronation on tibial rotation, McClay demonstrated that subjects with excessive rearfoot pronation (26 to 28 degrees) exhibited tibial internal rotation excursions similar to those of their normal counterparts.[24]

Others have suggested that velocity, rather than degree, of pronation may be the more critical parameter. In a study of the effect of foot orthoses on pronation, Smith, Clarke, Hamill, and Santopietro found only a 1-degree change in pronation but

---

* Refer to the following sources: 2, 10, 12, 14, 19, 20, 23, 26, 43, 44.

FIGURE 29-6 The rearfoot motion of a runner with normal, excessive pronation and excessive supination. Only the first 100 ms of contact are shown here. (Reproduced from *Foot and ankle* with permission of The American Orthopaedic Foot and Ankle Society, Inc.)

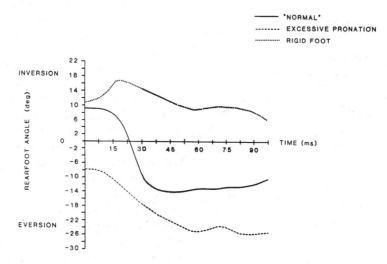

Abnormal Knee Joint Motion Knee joint dysfunction represents 40% of all running injuries seen by sports medicine professionals.[12] Yet, very little attention has been focused on abnormal knee joint mechanics. Most of the knee data that exist in the running literature describe sagittal plane TFJ motion. It has been this author's experience that this motion is often normal in subjects with abnormalities at other joints such as the STJ. As noted earlier, there are few data concerning frontal plane and transverse plane knee motion. Data regarding these motions such as axial rotations may lend more insight into knee joint problems.

Patellofemoral joint disorders make up the largest percent of knee joint problems seen in runners.[12] Conventional wisdom suggests that the etiology of these problems is, in part, due to maltracking of the patella with respect to the femur, and that it is often related to excessive pronation.[13,20,27] For reasons stated previously, this tracking is inherently difficult to measure. In a previously mentioned study by McClay, PFJ motion of two subjects with patellofemoral pain (PFP) and excessive pronation was examined and

compared to two normal subjects (NL).[24] One notable difference was that the PFP subjects' patellae remained more extended than in the NL subjects. This was associated with a more extended TFJ. Maintaining a more extended knee has the biomechanical effect of decreasing the resultant PFJ reaction force, which might be a compensatory strategy to minimize the forces to an already irritated PFJ. Decreased knee flexion may also result in the patella being less well-seated in the femoral trochlea leaving it potentially less stable. It is often suggested that PFJ pain is related to lateral maltracking of the patella. This was not supported in this study. However, total mediolateral excursion of the patella in the PFP group was two to three times that of the normals, suggesting that some instability may have been present.

Gait analysis has great potential for determining the effect of therapeutic intervention. As part of the same investigation, the PFP subjects were prescribed foot orthoses to study their effect on PFJ motion. Both subjects experienced relief of symptoms as a result of this treatment. Figure 29-7 shows that there were measurable changes in PFJ motion of both runners. These subjects received similar orthotic prescriptions that elicited different kinematic responses. The noted changes likely resulted in producing different patellofemoral contact profiles. These results reflected the subjects' individuality in response to identical treatments, which may be related to anatomy, neuromuscular status, or the individual mechanics of the runner.

FIGURE 29-7   Changes noted in patellofemoral joint motion in response to orthotic treatment in two subjects. (© 1990 Irene S. McClay)

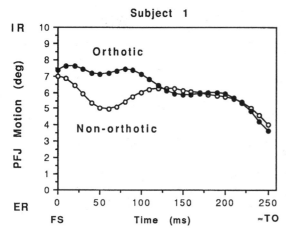

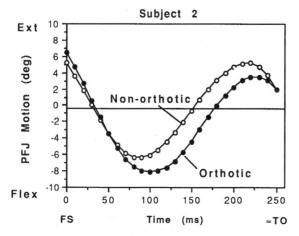

values would occur simultaneously. That is, peak knee flexion and internal rotation would occur with peak STJ pronation so that both joints would be reversing their motion at the same time. Following initial contact, it was noted previously that the knee flexes and internally rotates and the STJ pronates until approximately mid support, and then the trends reverse at both joints. However, there is little information available on the timing of peak values of these three motions.

Bates, Osternig, Mason, and James found no significant difference between time of peak knee flexion and time of peak pronation in either runners with normal mechanics or those who pronated.[3] However, the pronator group demonstrated a mean peak pronation value of only 11 degrees, which would be considered within a normal range.[11] Hamill et al. studied the effect of three shoe types (with different mid-sole durometers) on the timing between pronation and knee flexion.[16] Knee flexion remained unaffected by the shoes. However, peak pronation was greater and occurred sooner in the softer shoes disrupting the normal timing between knee flexion and pronation. McClay found that while the times to peak pronation and peak knee flexion were similar in the normal and pronator subjects (peak pronation of 26 to 28 degrees), those who pronate achieved peak internal rotation 25 ms later than the normals.[24] Therefore, the foot had begun to supinate and the knee had begun to extend while the tibia was still internally rotating. Further research is needed in this area with regard to the degree of nonsynchronicity tolerated between these motions and its clinical significance with regards to injury.

Interrelationship Between Joints   In closed chain motion, such as during the support phase of running, movement at one joint influences that of adjacent joints. This is true of the relationship between STJ motion and knee motion. As the knee flexes, the tibia internally rotates.[24] As previously described, tibial internal rotation is also associated with normal pronation of the STJ. Because the tibia is a functional link between the knee joint and STJ, it is believed that motion between these joints should be synchronous.[1,16] One can easily see the relationship between pronation and tibial internal rotation by pronating the foot in stance and feeling the leg internally rotate. This mechanism can also be driven from proximal to distal, that is, internal rotation of the leg produces pronation of the foot. Ideally, during movement, peak

Foot Position During Contact   Approximately 80% of distance runners strike the ground with the rear portions of their feet.[21] The remaining 20% are either midfoot (flatfoot) or forefoot strikers. This is likely to result in a different pattern of motion of the foot during support, although the lower extremity kinematics of this group of runners have received very little attention in the literature. Investigation into this area is currently under way.

With regards to foot placement during running, it has been suggested that the medial border of the shoe should land along the line of progression established from the midline of the trunk.[37,38] If the foot crosses medial to this line, this is considered crossover (Figure 29-8). Greater than normal calcaneal eversion may be necessary to get the foot plantigrade, which could place greater stress to the medial structures of the foot and perhaps the knee. Conversely, a wide-based gait

Figure 29-8 Crossover foot placement. Foot placement is defined as the distance between the midheel and a perpendicular line drawn from a marker placed at approximately L4-5 level.

DEFINITION OF FOOT PLACEMENT

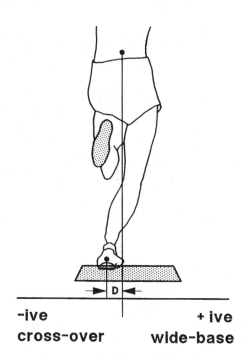

-ive
cross-over

+ ive
wide-base

may predispose one to calcaneal inversion. Normal foot placement in the transverse plane is approximately 9 degrees of abduction.[18] Excessive toe-out or toe-in may also result in potential problems. However, relationships between base of gait or foot placement angles and injury have yet to be established.

As the heel leaves the ground during running, it progresses forward with movement occurring pri-marily in the sagittal plane. Deviations from this typical movement pattern can also be seen. A medial whip is defined as the heel moving in the medial direction (in the frontal plane) as it is being unloaded at the end of stance. This deviation sometimes continues into early swing. Movement of the heel in the opposite direction is a lateral whip. A lateral whip is usually associated with excessive internal rotation of the leg, while a medial whip is associated with excessive external rotation of the leg.

Normal Ground Reaction Forces

The study of ground reaction forces (GRF) helps us to understand the magnitude and pattern of loading experienced by the body while in contact with the ground. In order to make comparisons across a popu-lation of subjects, these force values are typically normalized to bodyweight. The resultant force vec-tor is resolved into a vertical (V), anteroposterior (AP) and mediolateral (ML) components. Differ-ences in GRF patterns have been noted between rearfoot and forefoot strikers.[9] The majority of dis-tance runners are rearfoot strikers.[21] Therefore, this group serves as the source for the current normative database. Typical force patterns from a rearfoot striker can be seen in Figure 29-9. Forces in the vertical (F_z) direction typically have two peaks. An initial peak of short duration associated with the impact of foot strike is followed by a second pro-pulsive peak associated with push-off. For running speeds between 3.0 and 5.0 m/s, the impact peak ranges between 1.6 and 2.3 bw (bodyweight) while the propulsive peak ranges between 2.5 and 2.8 bw.[31] The force pattern is biphasic in the anteroposterior (F_y) direction with a braking phase followed by a propulsive phase. If the runner's velocity is constant, the integral of each of these two phases is about equal and peak forces range between 0.4 and 0.5 bw.

Figure 29-9 Typical ground reaction force patterns. From a runner with a rearfoot strike pattern, the components are vertical: FZ; anteroposterior: FY; and mediolateral: FX. Values are given in bodyweight units.

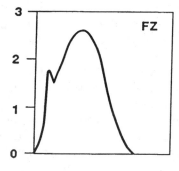
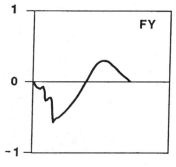
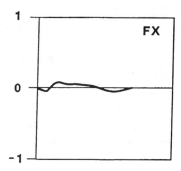

The mediolateral (F_x) component is the smallest and most variable of the three forces. Peak values are between 0.10 and 0.20 bw. They are characterized by multiple peaks and zero crossings and may be different between two feet of the same runner.

It appears that runners with a forefoot strike pattern present with different force-time histories than their rearfoot striker counterparts. This is most notable in the vertical (V) direction as the initial impact peak associated with heel contact is missing. There is some controversy as to whether consistent differences in the anteroposterior (AP) forces exist. A number of authors have noted double or multiple peaks during the braking phase.[9,31] However, Miller disagrees that AP forces are linked in any way to foot strike classification.[29] Harrison, Lees, McCullagh, and Rowe studied the differences in muscle and joint forces between runners with a forefoot strike pattern versus those with a rearfoot strike pattern.[17] They suggested that rearfoot strikers, with lower vertical ground reaction forces and greater contact times, were at lesser risk of injury than forefoot strikers, but they concluded that further study was necessary to determine this.

The center of pressure represents the position of the resultant GRF and can be related to the foot by various methods.[9,31] It is used to determine one's strike index (Figure 29-10) by quantifying its position relative to the foot at initial foot contact.[9] The center of pressure has limited use as it represents the average of the force distribution. In the case of one standing in oxford shoes, the force would be distributed across the forefoot and the heel, and yet the center of pressure would likely be located under the center of the foot where no contact is being made. Plantar pressure measurements provide a more sensitive means of assessing the interaction of the foot with the ground. In-shoe pressure measurements during running are still difficult to obtain due to the problems inherent in the hardware. Commercial products are currently available; however, some problems with breakage, thermosensitivity, and limited sampling rates still remain.

Abnormal Ground Reaction Forces

Abnormalities in ground reaction forces can be apparent in either the magnitudes or the time histories of the component curves. Magnitudes significantly higher than those described for normal running dictate that larger forces must be dissipated by the body. Increased magnitudes may result from inadequate kinematic strategies such as knee flexion to attenuate shock. However, there

Figure 29-10   Calculation of the strike index (SI). The longitudinal axis of the foot is drawn and the location of the initial center of pressure is measured relative to the length of the foot. An SI between 0 and 0.33 = rearfoot striker; between 0.34 and 0.67 = midfoot striker; greater than 0.67 = forefoot striker.

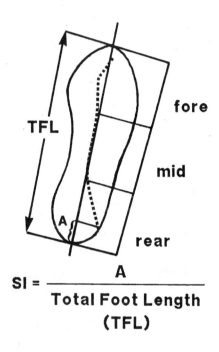

Strike Index

$$SI = \frac{A}{Total\ Foot\ Length\ (TFL)}$$

are no studies, to date, that have examined these relationships during running.

Runners normally strike the ground in some inversion making initial contact on the lateral corner of their shoe. At this time, the vertical GRF (VGRF) falls lateral to the subtalar joint and has a pronatory effect. Initial large VGRFs applied to the foot at contact could result in excessive pronatory moments at the subtalar joint. In addition, with each foot strike, there is a normal amount of vertical oscillation of the body. Cavanagh and colleagues report ranges typically between 6 and 8 cm (as measured from markers placed on the head).[8] Excessively large vertical excursions not associated with adequate shock attenuation strategies (i.e., knee flexion), could also result in larger VGRFs experienced by the body at impact, placing one at greater risk for injury.

As noted previously, mediolateral forces (MLF) are the smallest and display the greatest amount of variability between subjects. In attempt to understand the source of this variability, McClay and Cavanagh investigated the contribution of foot placement with respect to midline on MLF variability.[25] A significant correlation was found between foot placement and mediolateral impulse, but not peak force values. When looking across 40 subjects, only 15% of the mediolateral impulse variance was explained by foot placement. However, the relationship between impulse and foot placement appeared to be stronger at the extremes of wide-based and crossover gaits. Therefore, in a second phase of the study, one runner was trained to run with 5 cm wide-base gait and a 5 cm crossover gait. These results were compared to his normal neutral gait pattern (Figure 29-11). In the crossover gait, the contribution of the lateral impulse to the total impulse was 97%. Similar findings were noted with the medial contribution in the wide-based gait. Finally, the crossover gait resembled the mediolateral force pattern observed during a 45-degree cut to the right (but exhibited

lesser magnitudes), while the wide-base gait was similar to a cut to the left.

These results suggest that variations in mediolateral force patterns may be partly explained by foot placement in relation to midline. The similarity between crossover and wide-base gait patterns and cut maneuvers indicates that these running patterns resemble performing a series of repetitive mini-cuts. This characterization may be helpful in recognizing pathologies in runners associated with different foot placement patterns.

Structural Factors

Human movement is governed by the strength and length of the muscles involved along with the structure and alignment of the joints. One's structure is an important piece of the puzzle in attempting to understand pathomechanics. Therefore, it is incumbent upon those studying abnormal mechanics and running injuries to look at the runner's structural alignment. A number of lower extremity

FIGURE 29-11 The comparison of the mediolateral (ML) ground reaction forces during running with a 5 cm cross-over gait pattern (**A**), a 5 cm wide-based pattern (**B**), and a neutral pattern (**C**). Although magnitudes are less, note the similarity in the loading patterns in the cross-over and wide-based gaits during a cut to the right and left respectively. The unshaded areas in (**A**) and (**B**) correspond to the ML force pattern of a 45° cut to the right (**A**) and to the left (**B**).

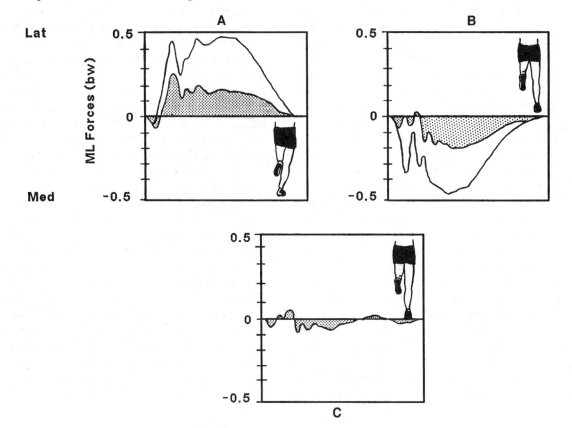

structural factors have been suggested as important indicators in the predilection of abnormal movement and injury.

Beginning proximally, femoral neck anteversion, resulting in internal rotation of the femur, has been noted to predispose one to abnormal locomotor mechanics.[35,42] The increased rotation of the femur can result in compensatory tibial external rotation. If this becomes excessive, the talus may compensate by rotating inwardly, resulting in rearfoot pronation. James et al. described another common set of structural problems, which he named the "miserable malalignment syndrome," and believed it placed one at risk for running-related injuries.[19] These problems include femoral neck anteversion, genu varum, medially deviated patellae, tibial varum, and pronated feet. Various combinations of these malalignments can be seen depending upon each person's structure and the associated compensatory mechanisms.

A number of structural factors have been suggested to place one at risk for excessive foot pronation. In attempt to compensate for the frontal plane deviation of tibial varum, the calcaneus may evert.[19] This calcaneal eversion is a major component of pronation. Structural deviations of the rearfoot and/or forefoot about the foot's long axis (varus/valgus) have also been implicated in the abnormal mechanics of the foot during locomotion. For example, both rearfoot and forefoot varus are thought to predispose one to increased pronation. It is also believed that leg length discrepancies can result in compensatory rearfoot pronation of the longer limb in order to lower the vertical limb length compensatory supination may also be seen on the shorter side.

Motion is also influenced by the orientation of joint axes. In the sagittal plane, the subtalar joint axis is oriented an average of 42 degrees from the horizontal as seen in Figure 29-5.[33] This results in approximately equal amounts of motion in the frontal and transverse planes. As the axis becomes less inclined, a greater component of the motion is in the frontal plane (inversion/eversion). This is due to the fact that motion occurs in the plane that is perpendicular to the joint axis about which the motion takes place. Conversely, as the axis becomes more inclined, a greater component of the motion is in the transverse plane (talar abduction/adduction with resultant tibial internal/external rotation). One might also suppose that a lower inclined STJ axis with greater calcaneal eversion would predispose one to greater injuries of the foot while a higher inclined axis with greater tibial

rotation might result in a stronger predisposition of knee injuries. This correlation, however, has yet to be documented.

Unfortunately, few studies have established these relationships between structure and mechanics. Hamill et al. were unsuccessful in predicting running mechanics from structure[16]; however, some variables thought to be important such as leg length discrepancy, forefoot varus, and rearfoot varus were not included in their model.

Interpretation and Recommendations

Once the structural and biomechanical measures have been collected, one must attempt to piece the puzzle together and determine whether a logical picture unfolds that helps explain the nature of the runner's injury. For example, a weak posterior tibialis muscle (thought to control pronation) detected in the structural assessment might be linked with excessive pronation velocity documented from the gait analysis. From the interpretations that are made, appropriate recommendations may be presented in a number of areas. These might include a directive as simple as a shoe recommendation. Exercises to strengthen weakened muscles or stretch shortened muscles might also be offered. If deemed appropriate, foot orthoses could be prescribed to alter the way in which the foot interacts with the ground. Changes in running style, such as foot strike pattern or base of gait may also be recommended. However, one must proceed with caution when attempting to change mechanics for there is risk of causing further problems. This process must be monitored closely. If results from the gait analysis suggest normal mechanics, a physician may decide to perform other more invasive diagnostic procedures such as a compartment test or arthroscopy. However, surgery is always considered a last resort and is seldom one of the recommendations resulting from a gait analysis of runners.

In dealing with the running population, we have come to realize that each runner has a threshold for injury, which is dependent upon both structure and mechanics. Often a runner will report that the problems consistently begin when a certain mileage is exceeded. The recommendations that are made may only serve to reset that threshold. Once the new threshold is reached, problems may begin to emerge again. At this time, a reassessment may be warranted to determine whether further measures can be taken or whether the runner must maintain a training level below this limit.

CASE HISTORIES

The following case histories serve to illustrate different ways in which gait analysis can be utilized to quantify running mechanics in an objective manner. In the first two cases, injured runners' mechanics have been analyzed with the goal of providing suggestions for therapeutic intervention. The first case study involves a patient who was followed from initial evaluation through treatment and follow-up. The running mechanics of the patient in the second case are presented with suggestions for prospective therapeutic management. In both cases, rationales for treatment based upon information gained from the gait analysis are discussed. The third and final case study involves the use of gait analysis to determine the effect of a knee injury on resultant gait mechanics.

Case 1

The runner was a university track team member. He had been experiencing repetitive spiral stress fractures of the left fibula associated with running. Ground reaction forces in this patient were within normal limits. In assessing his rearfoot kinematics, it was found that he only maximally everted 5 degrees. This is considered low because normal values are typically reported between 8 and 15 degrees. However, this in itself was not enough information to explain the stress fractures. During the lower extremity structural exam, a limitation in left rearfoot eversion (also only 5 degrees) was noted. Therefore, this subject was probably hitting the end of his available range during running. The vertical ground reaction force may have been acting to pronate the foot beyond the time when its maximal available range was reached. It was believed that these forces may have been transmitted more proximally, resulting in the stress fractures.

Based upon this assumption, the treatment was directed at trying to restrict the rearfoot from the end of its range during running. Therefore, foot orthoses were prescribed with a medial rearfoot post in order to limit the pronation excursion. At first glance, this might seem counter-intuitive as dynamic pronation was already decreased. One may not have taken this approach without the information from the structural assessment. However, this proved to be a successful treatment strategy for this subject; he was able to return to competitive running while remaining injury-free. This example emphasizes an important point that structure and function cannot be viewed independently.

FIGURE 29-12   The ground reaction force records of a subject with metatarsal stress fractures. Note the increased vertical force and the extreme anterior strike pattern.

VERTICAL FORCE AND CENTER OF PRESSURE

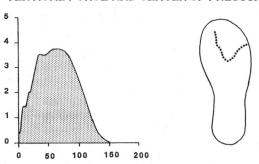

Case 2

A female runner had a right metatarsal stress fracture. Her kinematics were normal; however, Figure 29-12 shows that her peak vertical ground reaction forces were between 3 and 4 bw. This represents a 30 to 40% increase above normal values (2 to 3 bw). In addition, the center of pressure pattern reveals that she is an extreme forefoot striker (strike index = 0.85). The center of pressure moves posteriorly following foot strike; however, all of the force is concentrated in the forefoot region. This runner never makes contact with the rear portion of her foot. This reduces the overall contact area over which the forces are applied. The high forces combined with the smaller contact area results in higher pressures being experienced in the forefoot region.

Visually, it was apparent that this runner did not demonstrate a heel strike pattern. However, neither her extremely high strike index nor the high vertical forces could be determined through observation. The information gleaned from this analysis, therefore, lent insight into the possible mechanism of injury. In this case, a number of recommendations can be made. Shoes with good cushioning would be important. In addition, it might be advantageous to adopt more of a flat-foot strike pattern in order to increase the area over which the forces are distributed. Finally, kinematic adaptations thought to be involved in the cushioning process (such as knee flexion) might be suggested. However, as stated previously, this area still requires further research. It would be requisite that appropriate follow-up be made (i.e., reevaluation of mechanics) following these recommended changes.

Case 3

A young man was struck by an automobile while riding his bicycle and sustained a comminuted fracture of his right patella. A patellar reconstruction was done and the gait assessment was performed 2 years postinjury. Kinematics and ground reaction forces were collected during walking and running. In addition, kinematics during stair descent were measured. The biomechanical effects of this injury can be seen in Fig. 29-13*A, B,* and *C.* The largest effects were evident in the kinematic profiles of his knee. The knee was held in a more extended position for walking, running, and stair descent on the affected side. In Figure 13*B,* it is apparent that the knee remained fairly extended on the affected side during the early loading phase of stair descent. This kinematic adaptation to injury will result in decreasing the patellofemoral joint reaction force on this side as the PFJ force increases with knee flexion.[39] A reduction of this compressive force on the patella would decrease the irritation to an already painful structure.

Because of this injury ground reaction forces during running were also altered—especially in the anteroposterior component. Although the propulsive phase forces are similar, there is a significant difference in the magnitude of the braking phases between the affected and intact sides. A reduction of the braking force applied to the foot results in decreasing the external flexion moment at the knee (Figure 29-14). This, in turn, would decrease the demands placed upon the quadriceps muscle, which was found to be weaker on the affected side. In addition, if less force were required of the quadriceps, the patellofemoral joint reaction force would also be reduced.

SUMMARY

These three cases have illustrated some of the key points brought out in this chapter relating the use of gait analysis in understanding injury. In summary, many variables such as timing and velocity of movement are difficult to visualize. Changes due to therapeutic intervention, such as foot orthoses, may be subtle and therefore difficult to observe. Forces, which are the impetus for movement, are impossible to see. These statements lend support for the additional information gained from objective gait analysis.

A computerized gait analysis results in the generation of literally thousands of numbers. How does one glean meaningful information from the data? Typical presentation of results from such an

FIGURE 29-13 Biomechanical effects of patellar fracture injury. **A,** Comparison between affected and unaffected knee flexion during walking, running, and stair descent in subject. **B,** Comparison of knee flexion pattern during the early phase of stair descent. **C,** Comparison of anteroposterior ground reaction forces during running.

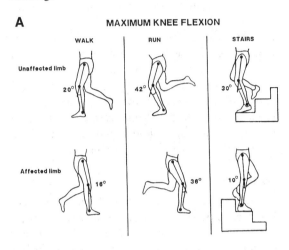

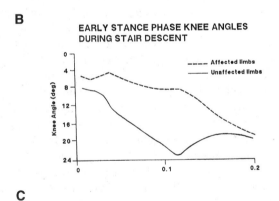

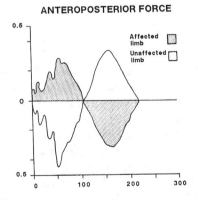

assessment include tri-dimensional angular positions and velocities for all joints of interest. Ground reaction forces are often also included. The combination of kinematics and kinetics yields the estimation of joint forces, moments, and pow-

FIGURE 29-14 Contribution of the braking component of the anteroposterior ground reaction force on the flexion moment of the knee during support.

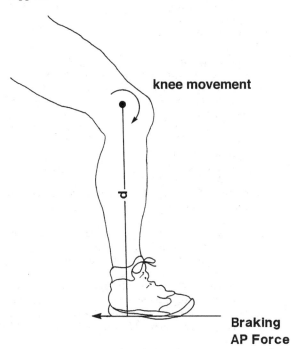

knee movement

d

**Braking
AP Force**

ers. With all this information, the question remains as to why we have not made greater progress in the area of gait analysis for understanding running injuries.

One primary reason is that little running research has focused on runners with a particular disorder or biomechanical problem. Most of the studies in the present literature regarding running mechanics have utilized normal or asymptomatic subjects. As mentioned earlier, the majority of these studies have looked at either sagittal plane knee and ankle motion and/or frontal plane rearfoot motion. We are at the point at which we must delve much deeper. Axial rotations are an important component of all motion and we have essentially ignored this in our running assessments to date. Velocity of motion has been suggested as an important variable, yet normal tridimensional joint angular velocities are not found in the literature. It is well recognized that in closed chain motion, as occurs during support, movement of the distal joints impacts on more proximally located joints in both magnitude and timing of angular motion. Yet, this aspect of kinematics has not been fully investigated. Finally, joint kinetics are rarely mentioned in any of the running injury literature.

Future Directions

As promised, more questions have been posed than answered. But this leaves the topic wide open for further research. Most gait analysis facilities now have three-dimensional capabilities. There is a need for normative data regarding full three-dimensional joint motion during running. Although much conventional wisdom regarding the relationships between structure, mechanics and injury permeate the literature, more objective work must be focused in this direction. Joint interactions, such as those between the foot and knee, require further understanding. Patellofemoral joint pain is common in runners, but unfortunately, in vivo patellofemoral joint motion continues to be difficult to study. Cine-radiography and magnetic resonance imaging may hold promise in this area. These techniques may also assist us in understanding, in more detail, the complexities of foot motion.

Closing

Brand and Crowninshield argued that biomechanical tests are not diagnostic in nature, but are used simply to evaluate (place a value on something).[5] Perhaps we need to consider diagnosis in a different light. It may not be possible to diagnose a disease process such as arthritis from a gait test. However, one may diagnose pathomechanics such as excessive pronation velocity or abnormal ground reaction forces, which are thought to be responsible for injuries. Another important issue that has been raised regarding the efficacy of gait analysis is that it should result in providing information that assists in the clinical decision-making process. Examples demonstrating this principle have been reviewed.

The information in this chapter has attempted to demonstrate the potential use of gait analysis in understanding running injuries and, it is hoped, will serve to stimulate further thought and research in this area. The onus is now on us as clinicians and movement scientists to work together to demonstrate how this information can be used to further understand underlying mechanisms of injury and develop more optimal treatment strategies.

REFERENCES

1. Bates BT, James SL, Osternig LR: Foot function during the support phase of running, *Running* (Fall): 24, 1978.
2. Bates BT, Osternig LR, Mason B et al: Lower extremity function during the support phase of

running. In Asmusen E, Jorgensen K, editors: *Biomechanics VI-B*, Baltimore, 1978, University Park.

3. Bates BT, Osternig LR, Mason BR et al: Functional variability of the lower extremity during the support phase of running, *Med Sci Sports Exerc* 11(4): 328, 1979.

4. Bovens AMJ, Janssen GME, Verstappen FTJ: Occurrence of running injuries in adults following a supervised training program, *Int J Sports Med* 10: S186, 1989.

5. Brand RA, Crowninshield RD: Comment on criteria for patient evaluation tools, *Biomech*: 655, 1981.

6. Cavanagh PR: The biomechanics of lower extremity action in distance running, *Foot Ankle* 7(4):197, 1987.

7. Cavanagh PR: The mechanics of distance running: a historical perspective. In Cavanagh PR, editor: *Biomechanics of distance running,* Champaign, Ill, 1990, Human Kinetics Books.

8. Cavanagh PR, Andrew GC, Kram R et al: An approach to biomechanical profiling of elite distance runners, *Int Sport Biomech* 1:36, 1985.

9. Cavanagh PR, Lafortune MA: Ground reaction forces in distance running, *J Biomech* 13:397, 1980.

10. Clancy WG: Runners' injuries: part one, *Am Sports Med* 8(2):137, 1980.

11. Clarke TE, Frederick EC, Hamill C: The study of rearfoot movement in running. In Frederick EC, editor: *Sport shoes and playing surfaces*, Champaign, Ill, 1984, Human Kinetics Books.

12. Clement DB, Taunton JE, Smart GW et al: A survey of overuse running injuries, *The Physician and Sports Medicine* 9(5):47, 1981.

13. Cox JS: Patellofemoral problems in runners, *Clin Sports Med* 4(4):699, 1985.

14. Donatelli RA: Abnormal biomechanics. In Donatelli RA, editor: *The biomechanics of the foot and ankle,* Philadelphia, 1990, F.A. Davis.

15. Elftman H: The transverse tarsal joint and its control, *Clin Orthop* 16:41, 1960.

16. Hamill J, Bates BT, Holt KG: Timing of lower extremity joint actions during treadmill running, *Med Sci Sports Exerc* 24(7):807, 1992.

17. Harrison RN, Lees A, McCullagh PJ et al: The effects of foot strike on muscle and joint forces generated in the human lower limbs during middle distance running of highly trained athletes. In *Biomechanics in sports,* London, Mechanical Engineering Publications, 1988.

18. Holden JP, Cavanagh PR, Williams KR: Foot angles during walking and running. In Winter DA et al, editors: *Biomechanics IX,* Champaign, Ill, 1985, Human Kinetics Books.

19. James SL, Bates BT, Osternig LR: Injuries to runners, *Am Sports Med* 6(2):40, 1978.

20. Jernick S, Heifitz NM: An investigation into the relationship of foot pronation to chondromalacia patellae. In Rinaldi RR, Sabia ML, editors: *Sports medicine '79,* Mount Kisco, N.Y., 1979, Futura Publishing.

21. Kerr BA, Beauchamp L, Fisher V et al: Footstrike patterns in distance running. In Nigg B, Kerr B, editors: *Biomechanical aspects of sports shoes and playing surfaces,* Calgary, Alberta, 1983, The University of Calgary.

22. Lafortune MA: *The use of intra-cortical pins to measure motion of the knee joint during walking* (Unpublished Doctoral Dissertation), Pennsylvania State University, 1984.

23. Lysholm J, Wiklander J: Injuries in runners, *American Journal of Sports Medicine* 15(2): 168, 1987.

24. McClay IS: *A comparison of tibiofemoral and patellofemoral joint motion in runners with and without patellofemoral pain,* (Unpublished Doctoral Thesis), Pennsylvania State University, 1990.

25. McClay IS, Cavanagh PR: *Mediolateral ground reaction forces in distance running.* Unpublished manuscript.

26. Marshall RN: Foot mechanics and joggers' injuries, *NZ Med J* 88:288, 1978.

27. Messier SP, Davis SE, Curl WW et al: Etiologic factors associated with patellofemoral pain in runners, *Med Sci Sports Exerc* 23(9):1008, 1991.

28. Messier SP, Pittala KA: Etiologic factors associated with selected running injuries, *Med Sci Sports Exerc* 20(5):501, 1988.

29. Miller DI: Ground reaction forces in distance running. In Cavanagh P, editor: *Biomechanics of distance running,* Champaign, Ill, 1990, Human Kinetics Books.

30. Milliron MJ, Cavanagh PR: Sagittal plane kinematics of the lower extremity during distance running. In Cavanagh PR, editor: *Biomechanics of distance running,* Champaign, Ill, 1990, Human Kinetics Books.

31. Munro CF, Miller DI, Fuglevand AJ: Ground reaction forces in running: a reexamination, *J Biomech* 20(2):147, 1987.

32. Nilsson J, Thorstensson A, Halbertsma J: Changes in leg movements and muscle activity with speed of locomotion and mode of progression in humans, *Acta Physiol Scand* 123:457, 1985.

33. Root ML, Orien WP, Weed JHL: *Normal and abnormal function of the foot,* Los Angeles, 1977, Clinical Biomechanics Corporation.

34. Saleh M, Murdoch G: In defense of gait analysis, *J Bone Joint Surg* 67(2):237, 1985.

35. Sikorski JM, Peters J, Watt I: The importance of femoral rotation in chondromalacia patellae as shown by serial radiography, *J Bone Joint Surg* 61-B(4):435, 1979.

36. Sinning WE, Forsyth HL: Lower-limb actions while running at different velocities, *Med Sci Sports Exerc* 2(1):28, 1970.

37. Slocum DB, Bowerman B: The biomechanics of running, *Clin Orthop* 23:39, 1962.

38. Slocum DB, James SL: Biomechanics of running, *JAMA* 205:721, 1968.

39. Smidt GL: Biomechanical analysis of knee flexion and extension, *J Biomech* 6:79, 1973.

40. Smith LS, Clarke TE, Hamill CL et al: The effects of soft and semi-rigid orthoses upon rearfoot movement in running, *J Am Podiatr Med Assoc* 76(4): 227, 1986.

41. Soutas-Little RW, Beavis GC, Verstraete MC et al: Analysis of foot motion during running using a joint coordinate system, *Med Sci Sports Exerc* 19(3):285, 1987.

42. Staheli LT: Medial femoral torsion, *Orthop Clin N Am* 11(1):39, 1988.

43. Taunton JE, McKenzie DC, Clement DB: The role of biomechanics in the epidemiology of injuries, *Sports Med* 6:107, 1988.
44. Tiberio D: The effect of excessive subtalar joint pronation on patellofemoral mechanics: a theoretical model, *J Orthop Sports Phys Ther* 9(4):160, 1987.
45. Vaughan CLV: *Biomechanics of human gait: an annotated bibliography,* Champaign, Ill, 1987, Human Kinetics Books.

46. Vaughan CL: Biomechanics of running gait, *CRC Crit Rev Biomed Eng* 12(1):1, 1985.
47. Veress SA, Lippert FG, Hour MCY et al: Patellar tracking pattern measurement by analytical x-ray photogrammetry, *J Biomech* 21:639, 1979.
48. Walter SD, Hart LE, McIntosh JM et al: The Ontario cohort study of running-related injuries, *Arch Intern Med* 149(11):2561, 1989.
49. Williams KR: Biomechanics of running, *Exerc Sports Sci Rev* 13(5):389, 1985.

GAIT ANALYSIS IN STROKE AND HEAD INJURY

Alberto Esquenazi

Barbara Hirai

KEY TERMS

Abnormal base of support

Abnormal limb stability

Clinical decision making

Equinovarus

Hemiplegia

Heterotopic ossification

Limb clearance

Phenol block

The three main functional goals of human ambulation are: (1) to move from one place to another, (2) To move safely, and (3) to move efficiently.[6] All three goals are frequently compromised in the patient who survives a neurologic event.

Most survivors of a brain insult or a stroke have the potential for return of significant function and resumption of useful lives. The average life expectancy for patients who survive after the first month of a stroke is approximately 6 years.[8] Survival rates for those suffering a traumatic head injury are even longer.[11] Approximately 70% of patients with hemiplegia regain the ability to walk; however, these patients often have problems with ambulation because of inefficient movement strategies, decreased safety and the presence of pain due to abnormal limb postures.

Compensatory movements necessary for ambulation produce abnormal displacement of the center of gravity, resulting in increased energy expenditure. Impaired balance, sensory deficits, inadequate limb clearance, and often pain due to spastic deformity all contribute to loss of balance, falls, and increased anxiety regarding ambulation.[13] Cardiopulmonary fitness is impaired because of decreased intensity and frequency of ambulation.

When a patient with a complex multifactorial gait disfunction presents to us for management, we utilize gait analysis to better understand his/her problem. Gait can be studied through the collection of a wide range of information. The variables that can be recorded can be grouped into four major categories: (a) spatial and temporal measures, (b) kinematics, (c) kinetics, and (d) electromyography.[6] Details of these variables and their actual collection techniques are beyond the scope of this chapter and are reviewed elsewhere in this book.

In this laboratory the initial method of gait analysis is measurement of spatial and temporal measures and recording of kinematic data via video recording, with the ability to view playback in good quality stop motion and slow motion. The use of a special effects generator allows a split screen image with frontal and sagittal views simultaneously. After initial evaluation of the patient's gait pattern, objective kinematic, kinetic and EMG data are measured as deemed necessary. Because there is no standard pre-established evaluation protocol, the patient's specific problems can be addressed in a timely and cost effective manner.

PATHOLOGIC GAIT IN SPASTIC HEMIPLEGIA

In order to properly identify and evaluate the gait problems of the patient with hemiplegia, the clinician must be able to understand *what* the problem is, *where* and *when* it is present, and *why* it occurs. Knowledge of appropriate available interventions as well as a thorough medical, cognitive, and social history are needed to determine the most appropriate intervention.[6]

A comparison of normal gait patterns with those exhibited by individuals with hemiplegia demonstrates differences in temporal, kinetic, and kinematic factors and muscle activation patterns across multiple joints. Although differences occur from patient to patient, some generalities have been demonstrated. These include a decrease in walking velocity with a shorter duration of stance phase, decreased weight bearing, and increased swing time for the involved limb when compared to data from persons without neurological insult.[14] The unaffected limb has increased stance time and decreased step length.

From the functional perspective gait deficiencies can be categorized with respect to the gait cycle. During stance phase an abnormal base of support (i.e., equinovarus, toes flexed) and limb instability (i.e., knee buckling or hyperextension) may make walking unsafe, energy inefficient, and possibly painful. Inadequate limb clearance (i.e., toe drag) and limb advancement (i.e., limited hip or knee flexion) during the swing phase interfere with safety and energy efficiency. In addition to spasticity or weakness as the main causes of limb deformities that interfere with walking, the clinician should be aware of the possibility of joint contractures, new bone formation (heterotopic ossification), undiagnosed fractures, and reflex sympathetic dystrophy as causes for the gait dysfunction.

Treatment interventions may vary based on the specific findings but may include physical therapy, orthoses, shoe modifications, or the use of upper extremity walking aids. For the young or active patient or those who do not respond to noninvasive treatment, other interventions to improve functional ambulation should be considered. The use of intramuscular pharmacological injection with phenol[9] or botulinum toxin for mid-term duration interventions (1 to 10 months) or surgery for long-term improvement should be considered. In the following sections, we will review some of the mechanisms responsible for the most common gait deviations in this population.

Abnormal Base of Support

The lack of adequate base of support results in instability of the whole body. In this population an inadequate base of support is the result of abnormal ankle/foot posture. For this reason, correction of the problem is essential even for limited ambulation.

Equinovarus deformity is the most common pathologic lower limb posture seen in this population. The contact with the ground occurs with the forefoot first. Weight is borne primarily on the lateral border of the foot, often with toe flexion. This position is maintained during the stance phase interfering with weight bearing. Limitation in dorsiflexion prevents forward progression of the tibia over the stationary foot, causing knee hyperextension and interference with terminal stance and pre swing where lack of propulsive phase is noted. During the swing phase there may be sustained plantarflexed and inverted posture of the foot, resulting in a limb clearance problem.

Dynamic poly-EMG recordings are useful in understanding the cause of the deformity and should at least be obtained from the tibialis anterior, tibialis posterior, long toe flexors, gastrocnemius, soleus, extensor hallucis longus, and peroneus longus. The recordings will commonly demonstrate prolonged activation of the gastrocnemius-soleus complex and the long toe flexors as the most frequent cause of plantarflexion. Inversion is the result of the abnormal activities of the tibialis posterior and/or anterior in combination with the gastrocnemius-soleus group and the extensor hallucis longus. In some cases the lack of counterbalancing activity by the peroneal group may be encountered.

Other abnormal base of support problems include toe flexion or extension during stance phase. This can produce interference with weight bearing and significant pain. Abnormal activities of toe flexors or toe extensors can be confirmed with EMG recordings obtained during ambulation. Ankle valgus caused by overactivation of peroneus longus activities is another example of a base of support problem.

An ankle-foot orthosis (AFO) may be used to control the abnormal posture of the ankle during stance and swing phases. An ankle inversion control strap or pad may be used to assist in correcting the inversion deformity. The orthosis can be attached to an orthopedic shoe and should include a plantarflexion stop to prevent ankle plantarflexion. If ankle clonus is triggered during stance phase, a dorsiflexion stop can be used as well to prevent the stretch response. When cognition and sensation are not impaired or adequate social support exists for supervision, the use of a molded plastic ankle-foot orthosis (MAFO) with inversion control buildup is preferred. A long plastic foot plate with soft padding in combination with a toe strap and an extra-depth soft shoe with high toe box can be used to accommodate the abnormal toe posture.

Invasive intervention for a base of support problem may include the use of phenol motor point blocks to the hyperactive musculature. The motor point block provides selective relief of spasticity with decreased deformity and improvement in function for a period ranging from 1 to 10 months.[9]

Correction of equinus posture may require the blocking of the gastrocnemius-soleus complex; varus foot posture may indicate the need for motor point block of the tibialis posterior and/or tibialis anterior and extensor halluces longus. Dynamic poly-EMG will indicate which muscles contribute to the ankle deformity. Inappropriate toe position may be corrected by injection of toe flexor or toe extensor muscles.

Botulism toxin injections to decrease spasticity in selected muscles can be used. This approach has the advantage of permitting the injection of the toxin into any part of the muscle without having to precisely localize the motor point. While the effect of botulism toxin is about the same as for phenol, the botulism toxin costs much more per dose.

Surgical interventions for base of support problems should be considered only after a careful gait analysis in which the dynamic poly-EMG and kinematic data are used for guidance in the selection of appropriate muscles. Selective temporary diagnostic nerve blocks may also be useful to determine appropriate surgical intervention. Surgical options most commonly include Achilles tendon lengthening (TAL) to correct equinus foot posture; split tibiales anterior tendon transfer (SPLATT) or lengthening of the tibialis posterior to correct inversion, lengthening and transfer of the toe flexors and, at times, of the extensor hallucis longus.

Abnormal Limb Stability

Another problem common in this population is limb instability, which can be seen as knee collapse or hyperextension. For example, the normal knee flexion moment evident during early stance phase, coupled with quadriceps weakness, results in limb instability. In persons with stroke or brain injury this problem is more commonly observed in the early phase of recovery, when flaccidity and weakness affect the involved limb. This gait problem may also be the result of over-lengthening of the Achilles tendon. The dynamic poly-EMG of quadriceps demonstrates shortened or out-of-phase activities. Occasionally, increased activities of the knee flexors are also seen.

External means of knee control can be provided through a Knee-Ankle-Foot Orthosis (KAFO), with off-set knee joints; a rigid MAFO set in a few degrees of plantarflexion; or a knee orthosis or a shoe with Solid Ankle-Cushion Heel (a soft wedge in the heel of the shoe), which promotes improved knee stability by positioning the ground reaction force anterior to the knee. It is critical in the early phase of the rehabilitation program to provide and maintain a knee extensor strengthening program, as knee weakness is further promoted by the muscle disuse that the orthotic intervention causes.[5]

Another reason for the presence of knee hyperextension during the stance phase may be spasticity of the ankle plantarflexors or a plantarflexion contracture, or, less likely in the stroke or brain injury population, compensation for knee weakness or impaired proprioception. This abnormal posture of the knee prevents adequate contralateral limb advancement, resulting in decreased step length. Orthotic management includes the use of an AFO with limited plantarflexion or, in the case of ankle plantarflexion contracture, the combination of an AFO and a heel lift. (Figure 30-1) These two options limit the knee hyperextension, while knee collapse is prevented if the orthosis is appropriately aligned. Correction of the knee deformity can also be obtained by decreasing the ankle plantarflexor spasticity, if present, with phenol motor point blocks, surgery, or the use of oral antispasticity agents.

Excessive hip flexion during stance phase is a less common gait deviation. When it occurs, trunk instability and significant interference with ambulation are produced. This problem is common in the early stage of recovery with flaccidity or in patients with significant flexor spasticity. In the latter group, dynamic poly-EMG demonstrates an increase in the activity of the iliopsoas and at times the rectus femoris. The use of a locked or limited motion external hip joint, attached proximally to a pelvic belt and distally to a thigh corset, can be useful to control this gait deviation.[6] Hip hiking and contralateral trunk lean will be needed as a compensation for limb advancement and clearance during swing phase.

Limb Clearance

Limb clearance and advancement occur during the swing phase. When limb clearance is inadequate, limb advancement is usually compromised. In the patient with residual stroke or brain injury the most common causes of limb clearance problems are lack of adequate hip flexion, knee flexion, and ankle dorsiflexion. The clinician needs to recognize the importance of coordinated lower limb motion during the swing phase. Not only the total joint displacement, but also the synchronization of motion between the involved joints is essential to produce adequate limb clearance.

Stiff knee gait pattern is most commonly seen in the patient with spastic hemiplegia (see Figure 3-2). The patient is unable to flex the knee adequately, creating a large moment of inertia, which increases the energy required to initiate the swing phase of the involved limb.[6] This movement requires the patient to utilize ipsilateral hip and trunk and contralateral limb compensatory motions. Even if the ankle-foot has an appropriate position, early swing toe drag is evident and can be corrected only by generating knee and/or hip flexion or increasing the contralateral limb length (i.e., shoe lift).

One explanation for this problem can be found in the dynamic poly-EMG, which demonstrates increased muscular activities for the quadriceps muscles as a group or preferentially in the rectus femoris and vastus intermedius, with or without hamstring co-contraction. Quadriceps percutaneous phenol motor point blocks or surgical intervention may be useful in correcting this problem. Lack of momentum because of decreased walking speed or the lack of hip flexion is another possible cause of this problem. The use of electrical stimulation directly to the hamstrings or in the form of a nociceptive stimulus delivered to the sural nerve in the preswing phase when maximal hip extension occurs has been attempted for research purposes.[3]

Inadequate hip flexion is also a cause of abnormal limb clearance. This problem effectively prevents physiologic "shortening" of the limb, producing a swing-phase toe drag. Compensatory techniques such as hip external rotation and the

FIGURE 30-1 Effect of heel lift or ankle foot orthosis in combination with a heel lift to control knee hyperextension.

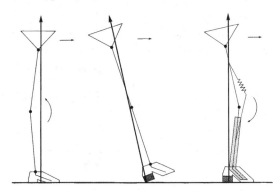

Figure 30-2   Examples of stiff knee and normal slow walking kinematics. Solid lines represent normal; dotted lines represent stiff knee gait pattern.

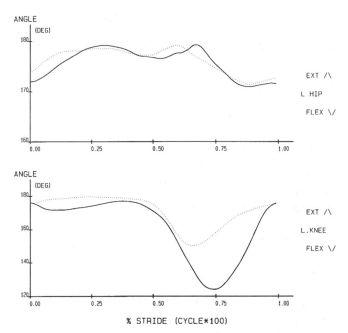

use of the adductors to advance the limb should be attempted. The use of a shoe lift to cause functional lengthening of the contralateral limb or the use of a thigh corset with a waist belt to prevent lengthening of the effected limb by gravity in combination with circumduction can be attempted. The existing technology for electrical stimulation directly to the iliopsoas has many problems. Stimulation of the hamstrings or the sural nerve of the foot to elicit a flexor withdrawal has been attempted for research purposes, with improvement in some cases.

Increased hip adduction can interfere with ipsilateral and contralateral limb advancement and with other activities of daily living. Balance problems caused by a narrow base of support are often also the result of this increased adduction. Overactivity of the adductor musculature or imbalance of the abductor and adductor muscle groups is the main cause of this problem. Because many hemiplegic patients use the adductors to compensate for hip flexion in limb advancement, the clinician needs to be certain that elimination of adductor activities does not result in increased impairment. Percutaneous phenol obturator nerve block is the least invasive approach to this problem. Open phenolization to the obturator nerve and surgery are other available treatment options. The surgical approach may include adductor tenotomy and/or obturator neurectomy.

Another common gait deviation in the hemiplegic population is incomplete knee extension during the late swing and early stance phases resulting from hamstring spasticity. This problem interferes with ipsilateral limb advancement resulting in a shortened step length as the knee is flexed and is unable to easily "reach" the ground. Contralateral limb clearance is also affected, as a decrease in functional height occurs during stance phase for the involved limb, requiring increased hip and knee flexion for the uninvolved limb to avoid foot drag.

Pelvic retraction affecting the involved limb during the gait cycle interferes with limb advancement, resulting in a shortened step. This problem is not amenable to orthotic intervention. Efforts are underway in our laboratory to determine the contribution of the piriformis muscle to this deformity and the possible interventions for it.

In the adult and pediatric traumatic brain injury population, bilateral problems can be evident. Frequently the pattern of abnormality will be common to both legs. In some cases an asymmetrical brain injury may result in extensor spasticity on one side and flexor spasticity on the other, causing complex gait abnormalities.

In our laboratory we have developed simple flow charts to better understand and follow the specific issues that affect the patient with a particular gait problem. An example of this methodology is found in Table 30-1.

TABLE **30-1**   Gait Analysis Decision Chart

Clinical Feature of Problem:

Equinovarus in terminal swing and stance

Generic Issue:

Abnormal base of support

Poor balance

Unstable gait

Inability to transfer full weight bearing to affected limb

Penalties:

Impaired balance and weight bearing

Ankle instability with genu varum and recurvatum thrust

Pain during loading

Shortened stance time, increase loading phase, decreased unloading phase

Increased pressure over the lateral portion of the foot, decreased weight bearing in the heel

Increased energy consumption that interferes with smooth forward progression of the center of gravity and
   increases vertical displacement of center of gravity

Functional leg length discrepancy

Interference with transfers

Shortened contralateral step length

Analysis and Differential Diagnosis:

R/O ankle bony deformity, fracture or heterotopic ossification

R/O soft tissue contracture (static), dynamic deformity, or both

When possible, determine specific muscle causing the deformity, i.e., gastrocnemius, soleus, tibialis anterior and
   posterior, EHL, FDC, peroneus longus

Diagnostic Workup:

Gait Analysis:

   Poly-EMG of gastrocnemius, soleus, tibialis anterior, tibialis posterior, EHL, FDC, peroneus longus

   3-D motion analysis to quantify ankle equinus and ankle varus

   Ground reaction force analysis to quantify anterior/posterior, mediolateral shear, and vertical forces

Passive and active ROM in bed, seated and standing

Sensory examination, including proprioception

Motor control, especially of the proximal joints

R/O ataxia (truncal vs. limb)

Standing balance (if not possible, kneeling balance)

Limb advancement capability determination (standing or kneeling)

Temporary diagnostic percutaneous tibial nerve block to differentiate static/dynamic deformity. May unmask gait
   potential

X-Rays to R/O bony abnormality (heterotopic ossification, fracture, subluxation, or dislocation)

Findings:

Poly EMG

   Gastrocnemius and/or soleus have abnormal activation (out of phase) in swing phase or throughout the gait
      cycle.

   Tibialis anterior demonstrates increased activation in swing and/or abnormal activation in stance phase.

   FHL and FDL demonstrate increased activation in swing and/or abnormal activation in stance phase.

   Tibialis posterior demonstrates abnormal activation in swing and/or prolonged activation in stance phase.

   EHL demonstrates increased activation in swing and/or abnormal activation in stance phase most commonly
      to supplement tibialis anterior or because of increased tone.

   Peroneus longus demonstrates increased activation in stance and/or abnormal activation in swing phase.

Ground reaction force analysis demonstrates abnormal medial-lateral and anterior-posterior shear forces and
   reduction in loading phase and peak vertical force.

Temporary diagnostic percutaneous tibial nerve block results in increased ankle dorsiflexion, indicating a
   dynamic deformity (spasticity) without contracture and an expected increase in ankle dorsiflexion strength.

If varus persists in swing, the most likely cause is tibiales anterior and/or EHL.

No significant change in ROM after a block indicates a static deformity (contracture).

TABLE 30-1—cont'd

Treatment Options:
AFO or MAFO to control the equinus, and with appropriate components, the inversion and toe flexion can be used. If ankle clonus is present articulated braces should not be used but instead a rigid device is used.
If the deformity is dynamic in origin, a percutaneous motor point block with phenol should be considered if injury is early, followed by aggressive ankle plantarflexion stretching and strengthening of ankle dorsiflexors.
Surgical options:
If the deformity is static in origin, tendo-achilles lengthening or intramuscular lengthening is indicated. TFR and transfer to the oscalcis is commonly done to avoid forefoot and toe flexion.
SPLATT is considered if inversion is present and caused by the tibialis anterior.
If inversion is caused preferentially by tibialis posterior, a release is indicated.
If the muscle is found to be active in swing, a tendon transfer to produce ankle dorsiflexion is recommended.
EHL lengthening or transfer may be necessary.
Peroneus longus transfer may be necessary.

FIGURE 30-3   Motion, EMG and force plate data (Information generated with Selspot Multilab).

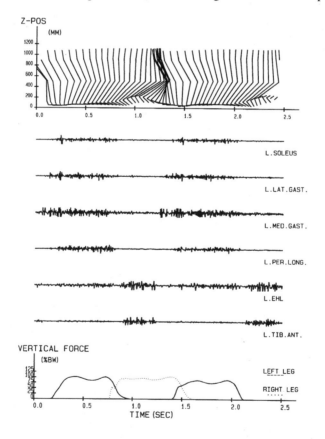

SUMMARY

We have reviewed the basic aspects of ambulation deviations, gait analysis, and interventions as they apply to the patient with hemiplegia and brain injury. The majority of patients surviving a stroke and other brain insults achieve limited ambulation. Gait analysis as presented here is an important clinical tool that allows for optimization of the selection and implementation of treatment interventions. The potential use of surgical and pharmacological intervention has been discussed as has the use of orthoses or other types of interventions to improve their walking capabilities to encourage improved functional level and quality of life.

Acknowledgment: *We thank Rosa Esquenazi for her help with illustrations.*

REFERENCES

1. American Academy of Orthopedic Surgeons: *Atlas of orthotics,* St. Louis, 1985, Mosby.
2. Bampton S: *A guide to the visual examination of pathological gait,* Philadelphia, 1979, Temple University-Moss Rehabilitation Hospital, Rehabilitation Research and Training Center #8.
3. Craik R, Cozzens B, Miyazaki S: *Enhancement of swing phase clearance through sensory stimulation,* Proceedings of the 4th Annual Conference on Rehabilitation Engineering, Rehabilitation Engineering Society of North America, Chicago, 1981.
4. De JB, Saunders MB, Inman VT et al: Major determinants in normal and pathological gait, *J Bone Joint Surg* 35A:543, 1953.
5. Esquenazi A, Wikoff E, Hirai B et al: *Effects of a plantar flexed plastic molded ankle foot orthosis on gait pattern and lower limb muscle strength,* Proceedings of the VI World Congress of the International Society for Prosthetics and Orthotics, 1989.
6. Esquenazi A, Hirai B: Assessment of gait and orthotic prescription, *Phys Med Rehab Clin N Am* 2 3:473, 1991.
7. Finch L, Barbeau H: Hemiplegic gait: new treatment strategies, *Physiotherapy Can* 38:36, 1986.
8. Garraway WM, Whisnant JP, Drury I: The changing pattern of survival following stroke, *Stroke* 14:699, 1983.
9. Glenn MB, Whyte J: Nerve blocks. In *The practical management of spasticity in children and adults,* Malvern, Pa, 1990, Lea & Febiger.
10. Inman VT, Raston HJ, Todd F: *Human walking,* Baltimore, 1981, Williams & Wilkins.
11. Heiden JS, Small R, Canton W et al: Severe head injury and outcome: a prospective study. In Popp AJ, Bourke RS, Nelson LR et al, editors: *Neural trauma,* New York, 1979, Raven Press.
12. Montgomery J: Assessment and treatment of locomotor deficits in stroke. In Duncan W, Badke M, editors: *Stroke rehabilitation: the recovery of motor control,* Chicago, 1987, Year Book Medical Publishers.
13. Olney S, Monga T, Costigan P: Mechanical energy of walking of stroke patients, *Arch Phys Med Rehabil* 67:92, 1986.
14. Peat M, Dubo H, Winter D et al: Electromyographic temporal analysis of gait: hemiplegic locomotion, *Arch Phys Med Rehabil* 57:421, 1976.
15. Redford JB, editor: *Orthotics: physical medicine and rehabilitation: state of the art review,* Philadelphia, 1987, Hanley & Belfus.
16. Winter DA: Pathologic gait diagnosis with computer-averaged electromyographic profiles, *Arch Phys Med Rehabil* 65:393, 1984.

CHAPTER 31

GAIT TRAINING

Clare C. Bassille
Connie Bock

KEY TERMS

Active problem solving

Biomechanical model

Cerebral palsy

Cerebrovascular accident (CVA)

Compensation

Down syndrome

Functional multidimensional perspective

Neurophysiological model

Quality of movement

Quantitative measures of gait

The previous chapters have introduced the reader to gait analysis using a variety of parameters as well as instrumentation. These parameters can be used in the clinical setting to discriminate deviations from normal or to document changes over time. Implicit in the emphasis on measurement is the premise that gait can be improved. The purpose of this chapter is to discuss the treatments used to improve gait known by most clinicians as "gait training."

Clinicians must first be able to document gait improvement, however. We can document improvement in at least four ways: (1) increased success rate for performing the task, (2) decreased time to complete the task, (3) a change in the behavioral strategy used, or (4) a "smooth" movement pattern. Improvement in performance has been demonstrated in clinical populations by an actual increase in the patient's functional abilities (percentage of success/failure) or a reduction in the time to perform the task.[89,122] Such findings are negated by some individuals because an assessment of the quality of movement was not reported. These detractors suggest that improvement in speed or success rate may be at the expense of the quality of movement.[68,123]

Temporal measures that can be used to demonstrate improvement are easily obtainable in the clinical setting without the need of sophisticated equipment. Since clinicians are interested not only in quantitative measures of gait but also in the quality of the movement pattern, another measure has also been advocated. Kinematic analysis can be used to describe the quality of the movement or the smoothness of the movement pattern. However, it is just beginning to be used in the clinic, and data collection and reduction are neither fast nor easy.[68] Therefore, we must ask ourselves whether there is a connection between the quality of the movement and the temporal parameters of gait.

Many learning or relearning studies have demonstrated concomitant changes in temporal, biomechanical, and neurophysiological parameters when subjects are learning "tasks," not movements.[19,97,104,105,111] Each of these parameters does not change in isolation of the other two when a task is learned. The temporal parameters used to document gait function are ideal for assessing both quantitative and qualitative issues. For example, both walking velocity and cadence have been shown to correlate with lower extremity motor recovery in patients with stroke.[18,94] Richards and colleagues also demonstrated that increased muscle activation in both triceps surae and tibialis

anterior (during TA1 and TA2 phases of gait) correlated with increased gait speed and stride length in patients recovering from stroke.[94] Therefore, documentation of improvement in walking speed is not independent of movement and can be viewed as a valuable measure.

Other gait measures more closely linked to quality issues are stance and swing symmetry, double support time, the stance/swing ratio, and temporal and distance phasing measures.[18,29,94] These measures can be used to assess the intralimb and interlimb coordination and are easily derived from temporal data. As the patient's movement pattern improves, there should be a corresponding change in these values as well. For example, the clinician can determine if speed was increased as a result of improving the intralimb or interlimb coordination or at the expense of the movement's quality. Frequency scores can be used for particular gait deviations such as the number of times genu recurvatum was observed to document improvement or detriment with increased speed.

It is our view that there is a connection between the quantitative measures of gait and the quality of movement. Therefore, the therapist can use easily obtainable temporal parameters to document changes both qualitatively and quantitatively. However as stated previously, the focus of this chapter will not be on gait analysis. By using the temporal parameters just discussed, clinicians can document improvement in gait function in a quantitative manner without negating quality issues. This chapter will discuss issues relating to the training of gait and focus on the acquisition of the skill. In doing so, this chapter will review briefly the past and present theoretical models for gait training, identify some factors that affect treatment, discuss some treatment techniques, present examples for treating adult and children with neuromuscular disorders, and end with future clinical research suggestions.

MODELS

Historically, gait training in both adult and pediatric populations with central nervous system (CNS) damage has been based on two models.

The Biomechanical or Components of Gait Model

The therapist identifies, by movement analysis of the gait pattern, those individual components of the gait cycle that are aberrant or missing. Remediation is provided through exercises in a variety of ways including static postures to strengthen weak muscle groups thought to be causing an abnormal gait pattern or the use of orthotic devices to stabilize the joint(s) thereby promoting a more normal movement pattern. The emphasis of this first model is on the movement pattern and has been described in an earlier chapter on observational gait analysis. This model is based on biomechanical principles and has been applied to both pediatric and adult patients with both musculoskeletal and neuromuscular diagnoses.[90,92] However, in the neuromuscular population it has been used primarily as a means of identifying inappropriate temporal firing patterns for lower extremity muscles or as a means of assessing surgical/orthotic intervention.[23,84,93] Therefore, the biomechanical analysis focuses on identifying the neurological cause for the aberrant/-missing gait component. Also, this earlier model analyzes the movement pattern for each joint separately. Only recently has it evolved to analysis of the intralimb coordination pattern and the role of one joint's effect on the motion of other joints during the locomotor cycle.[120] Therefore recent biomechanical analysis is being utilized in the neuromuscular population to identify biomechanical reasons for the aberrant gait patterns. For example, the effect of gait speed on ankle power, weakness in triceps surae, and the effect of ankle power on knee flexion during swing have been recently reported using biomechanical analysis and offer alternative suggestions for clinical intervention.[86,87,88]

The Neurophysiological Model

Treatment using a neurophysiologically based model has been used with patients who have a primary diagnosis of central nervous system damage. This model advocates a prescribed recovery pattern.[21,113] Treatment using this model in both pediatric and adult populations often occurs in a specific progression, e.g., developmental sequencing, or bed mobility, then sitting, then standing, then ambulating.[11,13,21,69,106] Proponents believe the treatment approaches are influencing primarily the nervous system. Although many of the clinicians who developed these techniques have died, the techniques are still being used, and the treatment as well as the theoretical frameworks are continually evolving.[10] Recent publications, however, continue to emphasize the neurophysiological basis for movement.[12,14] When a person is ready for gait training or pregait training, a variety of activities (e.g., weight shifting in a variety of stance positions, cruising, etc.) or components of movement in static postures (e.g., hip flexion

without lateral trunk lean) are practiced to facilitate gait training. Treatment emphasis is on the isolation of a joint's movement, independent of the movement of the other joints in the lower limb segment, e.g., dorsiflexion and eversion of the foot, hip flexion with adduction, hip flexion with knee extension.

An Alternative Model

We are offering an alternative to these two models. While we are hesitant to give our model a name, because we feel clinicians should identify for themselves their own gait training model, we recognize that for the purposes of distinction and ease, a name is required. Therefore, we chose to call our model the *Functional Multidimensional Perspective.*

The four perspectives of motor control were presented earlier in the book: the biomechanical, neurophysiological, motor learning, and dynamical systems perspective. Our model for normal locomotion is an attempt to integrate the four perspectives. However, underlying our model is the assumption that patients are constantly involved in the learning process, which begins the first time the patient attempts to move. In clinical populations what we see behaviorally is determined by the status of the patient *at that moment in time* and the structure of the environment. It is our opinion that the patient is attempting to match the available resources (neurophysiology, morphology, cognition, and motivation) with the demands of the task (biomechanical and regulatory features of the environment).[7,43,56] We view the movement patterns of our patients to be the result of their exploration of various strategies to successfully accomplish the task presented to them. It is the best solution at that time.

As clinicians our treatment intervention (i.e., activities and environment chosen, structure of the practice session, feedback given) impacts on the learning process. Whether we take advantage of this or not, we influence what skills are learned by the patient, how the patient retains the skill over time, and how the patient will deal with new situations that may arise. Therefore, if we wish to influence the patient's learning process in a positive way, we must also be active problem solvers. We must assist the patients in their exploration of strategies and *encourage flexibility* in seeking successful solutions.

Regardless of the theoretical perspective adopted by the clinician, he or she faces treatment issues relevant to gait intervention that need to be addressed. However, we do realize that one's conceptual framework biases evaluation and treatment of the patient.[49,66,98,99] Therefore what follows is the identification of treatment factors and treatment suggestions for gait training in patients with neuromuscular diagnoses as viewed from our integrative perspective.

TREATMENT FACTORS

When to Begin Gait Training

Many changes have occurred over the past 10 years in the treatment of patients with neuromuscular disorders. Pharmacological and surgical advances used currently reduce the effect of an acute insult.[5,63,64,103] For example in the adult, following a cerebrovascular accident (CVA), pharmacological intervention may include resolution of clot formation with heparin, reduction in neurotoxicity with calcium channel blockers, and reduction of intracerebral swelling with steroids.[5,102,103,129] This type of medical intervention may reduce neural shock, diaschisis, and synaptic ineffectiveness. It therefore seems imperative to intervene with treatment as soon as possible to address the rapidly changing neurological status and influence the reorganization that occurs as the patient is emerging from neural shock. Functional reorganization of the CNS has been documented in patients with stroke who have recovered use of their involved upper limb.[28,42,117] Therefore, we are advocating that patients achieve the upright position and ambulate early. If the individuals are *actively* moving and are pushed/stressed to perform tasks in situations similar to their premorbid environment, recruitment of motor neurons and muscle contraction may occur in ways similar to their functioning before the insult, or these individuals may be pushed to functionally reorganize their nervous systems. Early intervention may preserve neuronal integrity at the postsynaptic junction through recruitment of the alpha motor neuron and maintenance of the peripheral component (muscle contraction). Continued active excitation of neurons may prevent retrograde and anterograde loss of cells.[17]

We feel that behavioral compensation should be discouraged, particularly in the early stages of recovery.[71,110,122] *Compensation* is defined as the development of alternative means (behavioral strategies) to accomplish the goal. For example, often the patient's first ambulation experience is on the parallel bars. The parallel bars promote a strategy that incorporates use of the upper extremity primarily in a pulling fashion for postural support and forward progression. This behavior is different from ambulation outside the parallel bars with or without an assistive device. Use of a handheld assistive device requires a pushing strategy in the upper extremity. LeVere suggests that such compensatory strategies, i.e., pushing or pulling by the upper extremity, may become efficient and be difficult for the patient to discard later.[71]

While we are advocating early initiation of gait training we realize that the patient may need more assistance than the therapist can provide safely. Factors to consider include the patient's morphology and ability to handle one or more of the requirements of gait (balance, limb advancement, and limb support).[120] Common options utilized in the clinic are use of an assistive device or one or more therapists manually assisting the patient. An assistive device encourages the patient to find a solution to the problem of gait independent of the therapist. However, the patient may have no stimulus to develop new strategies without the device; in a sense the patient is 'marrying' the device as he/she organizes the movement around it. As the clinician progresses the patient to a device that offers less support, the patient must now learn a new strategy. There appears to be a developmental sequence of devices from parallel bars to quad cane to straight cane commonly employed in the clinic despite the appearance that these devices yield quite different movement patterns. This progression of devices may prolong the progression to independence. It may be more efficient to have the patient practice at the outset with the device we expect him/her to use at home. The alternative solution to use of an assistive device is to allow the clinician to be incorporated into the patient's solution through manual support. The therapist can then gradually remove the support as the patient progresses. In this situation, the therapist helps to provide the gait solution for the patient.

Motor learning requires *active* problem solving. Research using a variety of animal models suggests that active problem solving excites neurons, engages NMDA (N-methyl D-aspartite) receptors and second messenger systems and causes changes in DNA.[2,62] Learning has been demonstrated to induce dendritic arborization and changes in strength of synaptic connections.[61] The remodeling occurs not just in the neonate but has been shown to occur in the limbic system as well as the motor system of adult animals.[58,67,124] As discussed by Higgins and Higgins in the chapter on motor learning, the learning process for a motor task involves many processes, including cognition, perception, sensation, and movement. By asking patients to perform tasks instead of particular movements, we are trying to encourage neuronal remodeling to take place in contextually relevant environments. To make the environment contextually relevant, we ask the subject to perform the task in a safe environment, which is structured so that we are aware of the patient's goal. Also, the features of the environment around which the patient must organize the movements are what would be encountered in the real world.

In summary, we are advocating early initiation of gait training in real life situations. The therapist needs to consider the impact of intervention on the solutions that the patient chooses. Also, we must determine if we should develop criteria for initiation of gait training that incorporates the requirements of gait or develop criteria based on the motivation and morphology of the patient and clinician. For example, is there a threshold amount of limb advancement, balance, or limb support that is necessary before the patient can begin gait training? How does the patient's motivation and size affect this amount?

Influence of the Practice Environment

As we stated in the previous section, we believe that the tasks used for gait training should be contextually relevant. Therefore, the space in which the training occurs should have some relevance to the space in which the patient will function ultimately. Traditional gait training of the adult patient with a stroke takes place in the gym or an empty corridor. Patients get pushed to the gym, or roll themselves with one arm and leg while seated in a wheelchair to then work on gait training. Why don't patients walk the hospital corridors to the gym? Moreover, gait training using obstacles is often contrived and stationary. Patients are rarely asked to step over an electrical cord or a wet spot.[21] Even in the rehabilitation setting, people move out of the patient's way or stop moving to let the patient slowly, taking as much time as needed, move around the person.

Within such a protected environment the patient may not be learning real-world expectations. In an urban setting, people must time their movements with the environment, e.g., crossing a street on a green light, walking along on a busy sidewalk, or avoiding street traffic. This means they need to have flexibility in the speed of gait. When should speed of walking be incorporated into gait training? If there is an interaction between the environment and the performer then the way the environment is structured will directly affect the movement that emerges as well as the learning process.[7,43,54,55] We believe that a patient can be trained in a more complex environment at the same time that the patient is mastering a simple environment. Various gait training activities are not steps or a progression to be administered sequentially but separate entities, each imposing different demands on the performer. Thus, if the goal is to function successfully in an open environment—where people and obstacles are moving and where timing is critical—this should be the environment encountered at the beginning of gait training.

Walking surface is another element of the training environment to be considered. Initiation of gait training in the pediatric population often begins with the child cruising or standing on mats of varying firmness. It is not clear that these surfaces afford the upright position. The rationale for having the child walk on mats of different firmnesses may be to enhance the importance of the sensory information coming from the feet and to reweight the participating sensory systems around the feet.[40,100,101] Investigations by Gibson and Schmuckler have demonstrated that babies choose crawling over walking when the weight-bearing surface is deformable.[48] The therapist therefore should consider that the information the child receives through the feet may determine the transportation strategy and may do more than reshift sensory information within the bipedal position. Therapists can simulate the walking surfaces that the child encounters in the home by the use of rugs of appropriate thicknesses.

The caregiver is also part of the practice environment, particularly for the pediatric population. Therefore, therapists should observe the caregiver playing with the child. The manual assistance that the caregiver provides to the child makes the caregiver part of the regulatory features of the environment. The child's movements will be affected by how the caregiver holds the child. For example, in locomotion, caregivers can be seen holding the child's hands and walking the child across the room. While encouragement of stepping has been advocated as a treatment for children identified as being at risk for neuromotor impairment, minimal attention has been given to the placement of the child's hands.[70,126] If the hands are held in an overhead fashion, the child will tend to pull up, unweight the legs and step along in a digitgrade fashion. In this example the hands have more importance in the execution of the task than the feet. The child may gain forward propulsion by pulling along using the hands. If the caregiver provides the support to the child with the child's hands placed down by the child's sides, increased weight bearing through the legs may force the lower extremities to take a larger role in the task. The child may now be propelling forward by pushing with the feet. In both instances the arms are used for postural support. In the second instance, however, the legs may play a larger postural role along with a propulsive one.

The Effects of Practice on the Ambulation Task

The physical education and motor learning literature has identified the amount of time that a student spends performing a motor task as the best predictor of learning.* Johnson states, "As a general rule, skill in performance increases as a direct function of the amount of practice."† It is assumed that this relationship is also true for our patient populations. The amount of time that a patient spends exercising in a rehabilitation setting is surprisingly short.[65,112,116] The average time spent in both physical and occupational therapy is reported to be between 45 and 62 minutes a day. We believe that practice time should increase both during scheduled treatment sessions and beyond them. We need to provide ways for patients to practice safely on their own and with caregivers. Ada and Canning have offered some creative ideas for structuring independent patient practice.[1] Along with written documentation of the patient's exercise progression, this independent practice time also provides positive reinforcement to the patient and the caregivers. However, there is still no consensus for the types of exercises or tasks that should be practiced in or out of the therapy session.

Since the literature identifies practice of the task as the best predictor of learning, we advocate gait as the task to be practiced if the goal is to improve gait. Clinicians must decide which subtask(s) of the gait cycle is important for the patient to master and develop walking activities for the patient to practice emphasizing this subtask(s). Practice of a subtask outside of the gait cycle, however, may not transfer into the gait cycle. Winstein and colleagues demonstrated in their transfer of training study that an experimental group that practiced standing weight shifting activities in addition to their daily therapy did not improve certain gait parameters any better than the control group.[119] Therefore emphasis on the bal-

ance subtask using static standing activities does not appear to transfer into a better gait behavior. The issue of task specificity should be considered when discussing the presence or absence of gait training effects.

A traditional view of muscle activation would suggest that a muscle is activated in the same manner regardless of the phase of gait or the task being performed. However, this view does not acknowledge that parts of one muscle may be recruited at different times in the gait cycle or during different tasks. Both Loeb and English have documented that motor unit recruitment is not only specific to the task being performed but also to the temporal phasing of the task.[37,73] Therefore, we can not assume that pregait exercises or isolated muscle progressive resistive exercises (PREs) will be activating the same part of the muscle that is needed in gait.

The speed of the movement should also be considered when discussing task specificity of gait. The angular velocities of the hip, knee, and ankle for comfortable paced walking can be as high as 287deg/sec.[120] While a *single* joint's velocity can be reproduced on an isokinetic device it does not mimic the speed relationships among the joints or the motion-dependent forces generated by the multiple moving segments (movement of one segment affecting the motion of adjacent segments).[127] Therefore, the best way to achieve training at these speeds may be to practice the task of gait.

Research from isokinetic studies suggest that strengthening at slow speeds does not transfer to high speed strength.[31,80] The speed of movement also affects the muscles selected and the pattern of firing.[46] Muscle activation patterns are also affected by the motion dependent forces of multiple moving body segments (inertial, centripetal, and Coriolis forces) and speed affects these forces.[97,121,127] It therefore appears that gait training at appropriate speeds and with similar accelerations is essential to activate and strengthen the required muscles. Appropriate speed training may also enable the patient to learn how to utilize or counteract the motion-dependent forces generated during the movements.[7,127]

Since the environment directly affects the learning process and the movement that emerges in our patients, we advocate the practice of gait not only in a realistic environment but with a specific goal in mind.[7,43,55] In the real world an individual rarely if ever simply walks across a room. Also, that individual usually is doing two things at the same time, e.g. walking and talking, walking and

---

*   Refer to the following sources: 16, 26, 32, 60, 83, 85, 118.

†   Johnson P: The acquisition of skill. In Smyth MM, Wing AM (editors): *The Psychology of Human Movement*, New York, 1984, Academic Press, 232.

reaching, walking and carrying something, walking and searching in pockets for something, walking and putting on an item of clothing, etc. We know relatively little about these tasks other than that they can indeed be carried out separately, but how are the two tasks temporally and spatially organized when we link them together? For example, consider the task of walking across a room and carrying a cup of coffee to be placed on a table. The ambulation pattern will change to take into account the impact of the movement on the contents of the cup. The ambulation pattern and the reaching pattern for placement of the cup have to be linked temporally and spatially. This linkage has been demonstrated in patients with Parkinson's disease as they reached for and placed an object while walking.[59] The authors reported that when the patients were on their medication the reaching movement of the arm occurred simultaneously with the walking movement. The two tasks were not discrete time entities. Therefore, as clinicians we should be astute observers of this temporal overlap and facilitate its emergence by presenting dual tasks in gait training.

In summary, we advocate the use of walking tasks to facilitate gait training. The different subcomponents of locomotion should be addressed in locomotor-type activities. The nature of the tasks should easily translate into the daily routine of the patient. In that way patients will be encouraged to perform these activities outside of their scheduled treatment time and thereby increase the amount of time engaged in exercise, learning or practice.

TREATMENT TECHNIQUES

Balance and Strength

Regardless of the gait training model, there appears to be some consensus that there are at least three requirements for gait. Winter has identified three subtasks in gait.[120] They are (1) balance of head, arms, and trunk (HAT), (2) limb support, and (3) limb advancement. Our earlier discussion argued that gait is task specific, therefore the subtasks cannot be isolated and practiced out of the gait cycle. For example, diminished balance is a common problem in adult and pediatric clinical populations. Winstein and colleagues demonstrated that static balance activities in standing do not appear to transfer into a better gait behavior for the adult population with hemiplegia.[119] Since gait is a dynamic activity requiring control over perturbations occurring during both double support and single support phases, perhaps the only way to improve locomotor balance is to practice locomotor-type activities. The activities must have

both double support and single support phases linked together temporally. They must not be discrete, but cyclical and rhythmic. Researchers investigating perturbations during the gait cycle have identified a variety of synergies dependent on the temporal phase of gait.[41,82] Thus, perturbations occurring at heel contact result in a different synergy than those synergies used when the perturbations occur during push off or during swing. Therefore it appears that for balance to be improved during locomotion, the practice of locomotor tasks is essential. The effectiveness of a synergy is dependent on the timing and magnitude of the muscles' activation patterns, in essence the strength of the muscles. Thus, not only is the practice of locomotor tasks essential for improvement in the balance of HAT, but also for improvement in strength of the muscles used during the gait cycle.

Berger and colleagues have reported that children with CP use less muscle activity to walk compared to normal children rather than excessive muscle activity as commonly thought.[6] Some research has documented muscle atrophy in Type I and Type II muscle fibers in children with CP.[25] This lack of muscle power may produce some of the gait deviations observed in these children.[38] Olney and colleagues reported diminished positive ankle plantarflexor work during ambulation in children with hemiplegic CP.[87] Boubonnais and Vanden-Noven in their literature review also identified muscle weakness as a problem in adults with hemiplegia.[17] Furthermore, Olney and colleagues demonstrated that during comfortable-paced walking, adults post-CVA execute minimal positive work at the ankle.[88] Therefore, since the literature identifies muscle weakness as a problem in the locomotor pattern of both children with CP and adults with hemiplegia, how do we as clinicians address strength training in a manner relevant to gait in the neuromuscular patient population?

Sale proposed that "strength performance depends not only on the quantity and quality of the involved muscle but also upon the ability of the nervous system to appropriately activate the muscles. Further the expression of voluntary strength may be likened to a skilled act, in which prime movers must be fully activated and synergists and antagonists appropriately activated."* So strengthening is not just changing the size of the muscle (peripheral unit), it is also learning to

---

* Sale DG: Neural adaptation to resistance training, *Medicine Science Sports Exercise,* 20(5):s135, 1988.

activate the muscles appropriately in the proper sequence and with the proper timing and magnitude. It is specific to the task at hand. The challenge for clinicians is to "strength train" patients within the gait task or some approximation that would transfer into gait. In the adult neuromuscular population this question is being investigated by Guiliani and colleagues who are examining the effects of various strength training regimens on gait.[53,72,95,96] The effects of strengthening programs have not yet been addressed in the pediatric CP population.

Treadmill

Walking on the treadmill has been suggested as a treatment intervention for both pediatric and adult populations with neuromuscular diagnoses.[4,75,96,114,115] There are both advantages and disadvantages to use of the treadmill in gait training. The rationale offered for such an intervention has been to stimulate innate motor patterns by retraining reciprocal stepping motion and by tapping into the central pattern generators (CPG). The use of the treadmill could assist the patients by forcing them to speed up their gait. Fetters hypothesized that faster speeds of locomotion engage the CPG.[38] Therefore, if the patient is matching the treadmill speed then the patient may be strengthening the activated muscles at speeds and in ranges close to overground locomotion. Another reason for training on the treadmill is to gain aerobic endurance without having to handle the requirements of overground locomotion, i.e., person or obstacle avoidance, coordination of assistive device into the lower extremity pattern, or reduction in ankle propulsion for push-off phase of stance.

There are, however, a number of arguments against training on the treadmill. Comparisons in nondisabled individuals during treadmill walking versus overground locomotion have revealed differences for both joint and temporal measures.[3,76,81,107] In the nondisabled individuals, the excursion of knee joint motion is diminished throughout both phases of the gait cycle. There is an increased cadence and decreased stride length at the comfortable walking speed for the treadmill as compared to overground locomotion. EMG activity of the quadriceps muscle is greater during treadmill than during overground walking. Other possible differences not cited in the literature between overground locomotion and treadmill walking are: (1) the speed of walking is being externally driven by the treadmill rather than being internally driven by the patient; (2) the patient is not pushing off to initiate swing but rather lifting up to keep up with the treadmill belt; and (3) the stance limb is pulled backward under the trunk instead of the trunk gliding forward over the stance limb. The animal literature has reported that treadmill walking in cats is mediated by spinal mechanisms.[39,52] The investigators propose that only overground locomotion requires complex visuomotor coordination and cortical modulation of spinal mechanisms.[45]

In a distributed control model of the nervous system, there is not one locus of control of movement. The subsystem that is in control at any given time may be the one with access to the most important information at the time.[44] In the case of treadmill walking, the proprioceptors of the lower extremity may have the most important information since the ground is moving under the patient's feet. Do we want to drive the system from the ground up? Are we now making the patient display a spinally generated pattern? Rather than advocating the use of the treadmill, we suggest visually guided locomotion in simple and complex environments. In summary, therapists should be cognizant of the effects of treadmill walking and question its transferability to overground locomotion.

Casting, Stretching, and Bracing

Many patients have tissue shortenings, which have been implicated as a cause for some of the gait deviations.[6,109] This problem leads to a treatment intervention commonly in use. We ask the patient to reorganize the gait pattern with a new set of biomechanical variables. For example, a patient may have an early heel rise or make initial contact with the forefoot, both of which are believed to be the result of a tight heel cord. Typical intervention would be to stretch the heel cord through casting, stretching, bracing, or passive positioning. Gait training then continues with the lengthened heel cord and the expectation that the gait deviations will disappear.

In adult animals when a muscle is immobilized at a lengthened position the muscle adapts and adds sarcomeres; however, young animal muscle adapts to the stretch by lengthening the tendon, not the muscle.[51] If prolonged stretch on a muscle has different effects across the ages, then clinicians, utilizing immobilization techniques to increase muscle not tendon length, should develop alternative methods for the young population. Also, Tardieu has reported that children with CP have to keep the soleus muscle in the lengthened position for 6 or more hours a day in order to change its length, which suggests that conventional passive ROM exercises may not be adequate to prevent contractures.[109]

Serial casting/splinting has been shown to diminish contractures in the short term.[27,33,77,79,108] The cause of the contracture may be weakness of the muscle put on stretch or weakness of other muscles in the limb. In either case, the ability to recruit the muscles appropriately in the gait cycle is needed in order for the newly lengthened range to be permanent. Therefore, temporarily putting a muscle on stretch may not be sufficient to permanently effect changes in the gait pattern.

Another type of cast whose purpose is often confused with that of the serial cast is the inhibitory cast or the tone-reducing orthosis (TRO).[34] These casts have been advocated to reduce spasticity and alter patterns of muscle activation during the gait cycle.[24,36,57] However, EMG analysis is not usually performed along with the collection of gait parameters. The gait parameter most often reported is stride length. While cadence, gait velocity, and stride length have been positively correlated in the nondisabled population, cadence and gait velocity are not parameters usually reported when increases in stride length are documented during the application of the TROs.[8,57] Therefore, it is unclear if increases in stride length occur as a natural consequence of increased gait speed. In a single-subject design, McGreevy along with Diamond and Ottenbacher were able to document that the application of TROs increased both stride length and gait velocity.[35,77] Although cadence was not reported, we do agree with the investigators that something is changed when the TROs are worn to allow the subject's comfortable-paced ambulation speed to be increased, but without EMG analysis or biomechanical analysis of work/power/-energy the clinician is left to speculate as to the cause of improvement.

The clinician must also keep in mind the long-term goal for the patient. Is he/she to walk eventually without the TRO? Unlike the case study presented earlier in the text of the child with an immobilized foot-shank segment because of fracture, retention of the movement pattern when the cast is removed is not usually demonstrated in a disabled population. The investigations that have looked at retention when the TROs are removed have reported that the positive increases do not remain in the short term.[57,77] Therefore, the new movement pattern is not stable. Whatever caused the improvement (either change in muscle activation patterns or a change in the work or energy biomechanics of the cycle) does not transfer to walking when the TRO is removed. The new movement pattern needs to be as efficient as the old one, otherwise the newly acquired improvements will diminish and the gait pattern will return

to its former state. It is our role as clinicians to determine what causes the positive changes seen with the TROs. Moreover, if a long-term goal is for the patient to ambulate without the TROs, then we must determine what locomotor activities encourage the stability of the movement pattern when the TROs are removed and have the patients perform those activities.

Orthotic devices, without the specific "tone-reducing" foot components, are also often used to help a patient control joint movement. For example, if the patient has a foot drop, a posterior leafspring orthosis is provided, or if the patient has both a foot drop and genu recurvatum, a solid ankle foot orthosis set in 5 degrees of dorsiflexion might be used to control both the ankle and knee. While the orthotic device may successfully prevent the gait deviation, it may also be encouraging disuse atrophy of muscles on either side of the joint.[22,128] The muscle(s) whose activity during the gait cycle is now replaced by the brace has no reason to function because its function has been replaced by the brace. The orthotic device may in essence be encouraging a learned nonuse.[110,122]

In summary, we recognize that there are instances when the only way to change the movement pattern is to change the morphology of the person (e.g., the case study of child in cast) or biomechanics of the foot-shank segment and in effect force the person to come up with a new solution. Therefore casting, prolonged stretching, and orthoses (with or without the tone-reducing component) may be viable treatment options but only if the new solutions are present when the treatment is removed. The new solutions must become skillful and efficient.

PUTTING IT ALL TOGETHER

Although we've stressed functional training in a realistic environment, we realize that a patient may be successful at the task but use a strategy or movement pattern that does not work in all environments or one that leads to biomechanical complications, e.g., contracture or ligamentous injury. What follows are some case studies that highlight some of the movement solutions seen in patients with neuromuscular diagnoses commonly addressed by clinicians.

Consider the person post-CVA beginning ambulation in the gym environment. The patient adducts and flexes the hip of the involved extremity as the limb advances through swing. If we only look at the involved lower extremity, focus is on the adductor muscles and we may say that the individual is flexing the hip with the adductors. The knee position is determined by where the foot lands with reference to the midline. A shortened step length also results from this pattern. However, if we include the other side of the body, we might see that the hip abductors of the uninvolved side are not maintaining a level pelvis during the stance phase, thus dropping the pelvis on the involved side during its preparation for swing. This positions the stance hip in abduction and flexion, a mechanically inefficient position for the hip flexors to work, because the hip flexors are not in a lengthened position. Also, because of the dropped pelvis, the preswing limb has in effect an even larger height it must traverse to lift the limb and effectively get the foot off the floor. Therefore, the individual adducts the swing hip to advance the limb. The adductors are in the lengthened position and are a much larger muscle mass than the hip flexors. The adductors can successfully substitute to advance the limb. The point here is that what we see may have less to do with the involved extremity than with the uninvolved extremity.

How do we treat the problem? Different viewpoints will lead to different treatment approaches. No approach has been demonstrated to be more or less effective, but be aware of your conceptual framework. Some commonly used treatments include:

1. The patient ambulates in free space with an assistive device while the pelvis of the uninvolved side is stabilized with the hands of the therapists.
2. The patient ambulates on the parallel bars and emphasizes true foot abduction.
3. The patient practices weight shifting in static or quasi-dynamic postures (actual stepping) with emphasis on keeping the pelvis level.
4. The patient is taken onto the mat and practices hip abduction with resistance to the uninvolved leg and hip flexion with abduction for the involved leg.

With the exception of the first, all of the suggestions focus on one phase of gait at a time, the limb support phase of the uninvolved leg or the limb advancement phase of the involved leg. The first suggestion addresses both limbs at the same time but eliminates or diminishes the contribution that the perturbation of HAT (two thirds body weight) has on the entire system.[120] Is there an alternative solution more relevant to gait? The most potent reason for a patient to adopt a particular movement pattern may be that the solution works. Rather than verbally telling the patient to move a certain way or focus the patient on the movement pattern, it may be more effective to make the current solution not work. Structure the environment so that the subject's foot placement must be abducted for successful advancement. Perhaps an intermittent obstacle will do. Have the patient ambulate down the corridor with the uninvolved side next to the wall to force limb abduction. Have the patient perform stair climbing with the railing on the uninvolved side emphasizing advancement of the limbs in a step-over-step fashion.

Let's address another common clinical problem. How do clinicians achieve increased step length in their patients? Should attention be focused on gaining a better push off phase in the involved extremity or should the patient get more knee motion throughout the gait cycle?

The following are some standard treatment options:

1. Tell the patient to increase his/her step length.
2. Place a series of obstacles at distances appropriate for that individual's step length and ask the patient to step over the obstacles.[21]

The role of obstacles with reference to their location in space (where in the path they are placed) as well as what types of obstacles should be used needs to be explored. However, the more important question is does ambulation training with obstacles transfer over into increased step length during overground locomotion?

Another solution to the step length problem is possible. The spatial and temporal components of ambulation are gait-speed dependent. Olney and colleagues have demonstrated that temporal, kinematic, and work parameters are also speed dependent in patients post-CVA.[88] If the patient walks faster, the force requirements are greater at the ankle for push off, which translate up to the knee and give greater knee flexion during swing as well as a longer step length. Control issues for the knee during the stance phase must also be met for the increased gait speed as well as faster visual processing with reference to the surroundings and objects (motion and stationary). Thus by increasing the speed of ambulation, which is a functionally relevant task, the desired parameter, step length, can be changed automatically.

Another example can be found in children with a diagnosis of spastic hemiplegia. They may walk with decreased stance time and weight bearing through their involved lower extremity. In addition, they often exhibit little movement of the ankle during locomotion, usually holding the ankle in plantarflexion, which leads to contracture. Many suggestions, which place emphasis on weight shifting and isolation of joint movements either during ambulation or in earlier developmental positions, have been made to address these problems.[30,91] We are suggesting an alternative. Since forced use of the upper extremity has been advocated as an intervention in hemiplegia, why not for the lower extremity?[122] A supervised period of time each day with an AFO on the uninvolved leg while playing, squatting, and walking on various surfaces may force the child to more varied movements of the involved ankle. Thus the uninvolved lower extremity is prevented from compensating for the weakness of the involved lower extremity.

Similarly, children with Down syndrome and children described as "low tone" often perform many of their activities in ring sitting which is sitting on the floor or bed with legs in a circle in front of them. This position does not encourage the use of the lower extremities for weight bearing and may delay the onset of walking. Sometimes, the feet are even used for the manipulation of toys. Having the child instead play while seated in a chair with feet flat on the ground while manipulating toys on the ground will encourage them to get used to pushing on the floor and using their feet for balance. These children may have lower extremity weakness, which may be addressed by supporting some of the child's body weight as they perform stepping for a few minutes a day. This should be carried out in a realistic environment, with the child actually "walking" to a desired toy. In this way, the child will cognitively find meaning in the ambulation task. This may be carried out in conjunction with practice of cruising between two objects next to each other or behind the child to encourage single limb stance.

Children with spastic diplegia display an inflexible gait pattern. Some of this may be due to the environment in which they were trained, namely flat smooth surfaces without obstacles. The children often walk on toes, have an increased lumbar lordosis and lean the entire body forward. By bringing the weight line forward in front of the knees (up on toes) and behind the hip (lordosis) they effectively lock the hip and knee joint. This positioning may enable the children to use the legs as rigid rods. As they lean anteriorly, they fall forward to progress without the need for propulsion at the ankle which they lack[86,87] This solution may be successful on flat barrier-free surfaces; however, a more demanding environment might force the children to come up with a variety of solutions. Having the children walk on a floor with small obstacles such as a towel or piece of laundry or on surfaces of different textures and firmness may force them to be more flexible in their solutions. Activities that force the child to bring

the body's weight line behind their ankle may encourage other combinations of muscle activity, for example squatting to pick up toys behind them. Unexpected objects or people moving in their environment will force them to stop and start their progression quickly, which may also perturb the body's weight line posteriorly.

In summary, our suggestions for treatment offer some common principles:

1. Intervene early.
2. Practice appropriate functional tasks in a realistic environment. The tasks chosen are those that emphasize particular areas of weakness in the patient's strategy or movement pattern.
3. Maximize the amount of practice in and out of the treatment session with the patient actively involved in the solution to the motor problem. By this we mean that the patient is involved in the choice of practiced tasks and the self-monitoring of their performance.
4. Vary the practice in order to promote the patient's ability to perform in a variety of circumstances. However, we feel the functional task practiced must remain the same. For example, if the clinician wishes to emphasize the initial contact phase of locomotion, then *locomotion* on different floor surfaces with obstacles to negotiate around or avoid might be practiced. We are not suggesting that other functional tasks be practiced in place of locomotion. If the strategy or movement pattern the patient chooses will lead to biomechanical complications, we attempt to encourage alternative solutions by varying the environment and making the patient's strategy or movement solution unsuccessful. Thus, a new solution to the task must emerge. If the patient is unable to succeed and we wish to avoid impending frustration, we again would change the environment so that the task would continue to be challenging; however, success would be attainable.
5. Ask continuously "Can the patient retain this new skill?" and "Will the patient be able to generalize the successful solutions to novel situations?" These questions are part of an ongoing assessment strategy by the clinician.

Future Research

In the discussion of our principles underlying gait training and our treatment suggestions, we recognize that there are some clinical questions that are in need of answers. This section discusses those questions in greater detail and grounds them in our theoretical framework.

We advocate early gait training in the patient post-CVA. We recognize, however, that the clinician may need to provide additional postural support for the patient through the use of an assistive device or by the clinician providing the additional postural support. Three questions emerge from these choices: How do these two alternatives affect whether the patient is discharged with or without an assistive device, and how is the level of ambulation independence at discharge affected? Lastly, if the patient is to be discharged with an assistive device, is the choice at discharge dependent on the type of assistive device initially used in ambulation training?

Similarly, the patient may require assistance with the limb support or limb advancement subtasks of gait and the clinician must decide whether to use an orthotic device. We question the use of orthotic devices in a recovering system because it may encourage disuse atrophy and learned non-use. Similar questions as those posed with assistive devices are applicable here. How do the two alternatives of no bracing versus bracing during gait training affect whether the patient is discharged with or without the orthosis, and how is the level of ambulation independence at discharge affected by gait training with or without the orthosis?

If investigators are going to answer the above two sets of questions, they need to control for time postinjury. Since clinicians encounter patients at various times postinjury, research that assesses ambulation treatment techniques should control for this factor. A specific treatment technique may have different effects depending on the time interval postinjury.

In our discussion of the environment and its impact on gait training, we identified research that suggests walking surface may determine transportation mode in the able-bodied pediatric population.[48] We also suggested that children with CNS damage may respond in a similar fashion; however, this result has not been experimentally demonstrated. Therefore clinical investigations are needed to determine how children with CNS damage respond either in movement execution or choice of behavioral strategy to different weight bearing surfaces.

Lastly, the issue of task specificity was discussed with reference to gait training suggestions. We recommended that gait training occur at appropriate ambulation speeds. However, *what* is the appropriate gait speed for training our patients? The able-bodied individual, regardless of age, selects a comfortably paced walking speed that minimizes oxygen consumption.[125] The person 6

months after a stroke has a comfortable walking speed significantly slower than the age-matched normal subject.[18,94] Is the person minimizing oxygen as well, or optimizing a different parameter? Is the slow speed due to the rehabilitation training, or is there a new velocity standard for individuals with stroke that is different from age-matched normal individuals?

We also suggested that the practice of gait tasks would lead to improvements in gait. If practicing the task is the best predictor of learning, then gait training studies should examine the effect of the training of gait. Research studies that examine the efficacy of particular treatment interventions should include a group that practices gait for an equivalent amount of time. If the addition of the gait control group is ignored in the experimental design, then the intervention investigated can only document improvements over time with treatment. The results are confounded because the subjects are also practicing the task of gait. Therefore, the investigation does not identify if the improvement is due to the treatment, the amount of gait practice, or the combination of the two. Some of the literature that confuse the effects of practicing the task of ambulation with a treatment technique specific to ambulation are the treadmill studies and the FES studies.[15,74,75]

We also cannot compare a treatment intervention to a group that does not exercise. This design only demonstrates whether the intervention is better than doing nothing. An additional group that is actually spending an equivalent amount of time practicing ambulation should be added to the comparison. We have yet to document that the amount of time spent practicing gait itself is beneficial for the learning of the task in patients with CNS damage. So when further investigating the efficacy of a particular treatment intervention, a gait control group should be included in the design.*

---

* In a recent study by Richards and colleagues, where an early, intensive gait-focused physical therapy group was compared to two control groups (early, intensive conventional, and later, nonintensive conventional physical therapy), the gait velocity was higher for the experimental group after 6 weeks of treatment. However, no differences were noted between the groups at 6 months. Also, the time spent in "gait training" was correlated to gait velocity after 6 weeks of treatment. One must be cautious, however, because their definition of gait training included the use of tilt table and limb-load monitor, resisted exercises with a Kinetron isokinetic device and a treadmill. The emphasis was on early upright cyclical activities. However, this is not what we mean by a gait control group. We advocate that actual overground locomotor activity be used to establish the gait control group. (Richards CL, et al: Task-specific physical therapy for optimization of gait recovery in acute stroke patients, *Arch Phy Med Rehabil* 74:612, 1993.)

SUMMARY

We have attempted to provide the reader with our conceptual framework, which is the basis for our clinical questions and treatment ideas. Emphasis is placed on early gait intervention with active learning in realistic and relevant environments. We view the patient's movement strategies as the best solution at that time to match the internal and external resources to the task presented to them. In choosing tasks and environments for patients, therapists must be active problem solvers. The patients are exploring a variety of strategies to achieve a successful solution. Therefore, therapists must be aware of this process and build on it. With patients in the early stages of learning, their chosen solutions should not be viewed as right or wrong but rather seen in the broader context of the learning process. We must choose activities that promote flexibility of behavior because no one movement pattern is the perfect solution for a particular task. There is not just one correct way to walk. In this chapter we haven't given specific techniques or formulas for treatment, but rather a glimpse at the process we go through in our attempt to identify problems and intervene therapeutically. We recognize that our model is flexible and may require revision as our knowledge of the motor control of locomotion increases.

REFERENCES

1. Ada L, Canning C: The patient as an active learner. In Ada L, Canning C, editors: *Key issues in neurological physiotherapy,* Oxford, England, 1990, Butterworth Heinemann.
2. Ahissar E et al: Dependence of cortical plasticity on correlated activity of single neurons and on behavioral context, *Science* 257:1412, 1992.
3. Arrants, SL: *Biomechanical and physiological adjustments to treadmill walking by female subjects naive to the treadmill* (Unpublished Master's Thesis), Florida State University, College of Education, 1975.
4. Barbeau H et al: *Impairment of spastic paraparetic gait: implication for new rehabilitation strategies,* Proceedings of the 5th Biennial Conference of the Canadian Society for Biomechanics, Ottawa, Canada, August 16-18, 1988.
5. Barnett JJM et al: *Stroke, volumes 1 & 2,* New York, 1986, Churchill Livingston.
6. Berger W, Quintern J, Dietz V: Pathophysiology of gait in children with cerebral palsy, *Electroencephalogr Clin Neurophysiol* 53:538, 1982.
7. Bernstein N: *The coordination and regulation of movements,* London, 1967, Pergamon Press.
8. Bertoti DB: Effect of short leg casting on ambulation in children with cerebral palsy, *Phys Ther* 66(10):1522, 1986.
9. Biller J et al: Management of aneurysmal subarachnoid hemorrhage, *Stroke* 19(10):1300, 1988.
10. Bly L: A historical and current view of the basis of NDT, *Pediatr Phys Ther* 3(3):131, 1991.
11. Bobath B: *Adult hemiplegia: evaluation and treatment,* London, 1978, William Heinemann.
12. Bobath B: *Abnormal postural reflex activity caused by brain lesions,* ed 3, Rockville, Md, 1985, Aspen Systems.
13. Bobath B, Bobath K: *Motor development in the different types of cerebral palsy,* London, 1975, William Heinemann.
14. Bobath K, Bobath B: Neuro-developmental treatment. In Scrutton D, editor: *Management of the motor disorders in children with cerebral palsy,* Philadelphia, 1984, J. B. Lippincott.
15. Bogataj U et al: Restoration of gait during two to three weeks of therapy with multichannel electrical stimulation, *Phys Ther* 69(5):319, 1989.
16. Borys AH: *Development and evaluation of a training procedure to increase pupil motor engagement time,* (Unpublished Doctoral Dissertation), New York, Teachers College, Columbia University, 1982.
17. Bourbonnais D, Vanden Noven S: Weakness in patients with hemiparesis, *Am J Occup Ther* 43(5):313, 1989.
18. Brandstater ME et al: Hemiplegic gait: analysis of temporal variables, *Arch Phys Med Rehabil* 64:583, 1983.
19. Brooks V: Movement programming depends on understanding of behavioral requirements, *Physiol Behav* 31:561, 1987.
20. Brooks V: How does the limbic system assist motor learning? A limbic comparator hypothesis, *Brain Behav Evol* 29:29, 1986.
21. Brunnstrum S: *Movement therapy in hemiplegia: a neurophysiological approach,* Hagerstown, Md, 1970, Harper & Row.
22. Burdett RG et al: Gait comparison of subjects with hemiplegia walking unbraced, with AFO and with air stirrup brace, *Phys Ther* 68(8):1197, 1988.
23. Cahan LD et al: Instrumented gait analysis post selective dorsal rhizotomy, *Dev Med Child Neurol* 32:1037, 1990.
24. Carlson SJ: A neurophysiological analysis of inhibitive casting, *Phys Occup Ther Pediatr* 4(4):31, 1984.
25. Castle ME, Reymond TA, Schneider M: Pathology of spastic muscle in cerebral palsy, *Clin Orthop* 142:223, 1979.
26. Chao N: *A descriptive study of teaching physical education: pupil motor engagement time in physical education classes in Taipei City,* (Unpublished Doctoral Dissertation), New York, Teachers College, Columbia University, 1987.
27. Cherry DB, Weingand GM: Plaster drop-out casts as a dynamic means to reduce muscle contracture, *Phys Ther* 61(11):1601, 1981.
28. Chollet F et al: The functional anatomy of motor recovery after stroke in humans: a study with positron emission tomography, *Ann Neurol* 29:63, 1991.
29. Clark JE et al: Human interlimb coordination: the first six months of independent walking, *Dev Psychobiol* 21(5):445, 1988.

30. Connor FP, Williamson GG, Siepp JH: *Program guide for infants and toddlers with neuromotor and other developmental disabilities,* New York, 1978, Teachers College Press.

31. Coyle EF et al: Specificity of power improvements through slow and fast isokinetic training, *J Appl Physiol* 51:1437, 1981.

32. Crossman ERFW: A theory of the acquisition of speedskill, *Ergonomics* 2:153, 1959.

33. Cusick B: Splints and casts: managing foot deformity in children with neuromotor disorders, *Phys Ther* 68(12):1903, 1988.

34. Cusick B, Sussman MD: Short leg casts: their role in the management of cerebral palsy, *Phys Occup Ther Pediat* 2(2/3):93, 1982.

35. Diamond MF, Ottenbacher KJ: Effect of a tone-inhibiting dynamic ankle-foot orthosis on stride characteristics of an adult with hemiparesis, *Phys Ther* 70:423, 1990.

36. Embrey DG: Effects of NDT and orthoses on knee flexion during gait: a single-subject design, *Phys Ther* 70:626, 1990.

37. English A et al: *Patterns of EMG activity in the human lateral gastrocnemius muscle during weightbearing and nonweightbearing tasks,* Abstract of 20th Annual Meeting of the Society for Neuroscience, St. Louis, Mo, 1990.

38. Fetters L: Cerebral palsy: contemporary treatment concepts. In *Contemporary management of motor problems: proceedings of the II step conference,* Alexandria, Va, 1991, Foundation for Physical Therapy.

39. Forssberg H: Spinal locomotor functions and descending control. In Sjolund B, Bjorklund A, editors: *Brain stem control of spinal mechanisms,* New York, 1982, Elsevier Biomedical Press.

40. Forssberg H, Nashner L: Ontogenetic development of postural control in man: adaptation to altered support and visual conditions during stance, *J Neurosci* 2:545, 1982.

41. Forssberg H, Hirschfeld H: Phasic modulation of postural activation patterns during human walking, In Pompeiano O, Allum JHJ, editors: *Progress in brain research vol. 76,* New York, 1988, Elsevier Science Publishing.

42. Frackowiak RSJ, Weiller C, Chollet F: The functional anatomy of recovery from brain injury. In *Exploring brain functional anatomy with positron tomography—CIBA Foundation symposium 163,* New York, 1991, John Wiley & Sons.

43. Gentile AM: Skill acquisition: action, movement and neuromotor processes. In Shepherd R, Carr J, editors: *Movement science: foundations for physical therapy in rehabilitation,* Rockville, Md, 1987, Aspen Publishing.

44. Gentile AM: The nature of skill acquisition: therapeutic implications for children with movement disorders. In Forssberg H, Hirschfeld H, editors: *Medicine & sport science: vol. 36. Movement disorders in children,* Basel, Switzerland, 1992, Karger.

45. Georgopoulos AP, Grillner S: Visuomotor coordination in reaching and locomotion, *Science* 245:1209, 1989.

46. Ghez C, Gordon J: Trajectory control in targeted force impulses. I. Role of opposing muscles, *Exp Brain Res* 67(2):225, 1987.

47. Ghez C: Posture voluntary movement: The cerebellum. In Kandel ER, Schwartz JH, Jessell JM, editors: *Principles of neural science,* ed 3, New York, 1992, Elsevier.

48. Gibson E, Schmuckler MA: Going somewhere: an ecological and experimental approach to development of mobility, *Ecol Psych* 1(1):3, 1989.

49. Gordon J: Assumptions underlying physical therapy intervention: theoretical and historical perspective. In Shepherd R, Carr J, editors: *Movement science: foundations for physical therapy in rehabilitation,* Rockville, Md, 1987, Aspen Publishing.

50. Gordon J: Spinal mechanisms of motor coordination. In Kandel ER, Schwartz JH, Jessell JM, editors: *Principles of neural science,* ed 3, New York, 1992, Elsevier.

51. Gossman MR, Sahrmann A, Rose SJ: Review of length associated changes in muscle, *Phys Ther* 62:1799, 1982.

52. Grillner S, Dubuc R: Control of locomotion in vertebrates: spinal and supraspinal mechanisms. In Waxman SG, editor: *Advances in neurology: vol 47. Functional recovery in neurological disease,* New York, 1988, Raven Press.

53. Guiliani CA, Harro CC, Rosecrance JC: The effects of bicycle pedalling on the temporal distance and EMG characteristics of walking in hemiplegic subjects, *Phys Ther* 69(5):367, 1989.

54. Higgins J, Spaeth RK: Relationship between consistency of movement and environmental condition, *Quest* 17:61, 1972.

55. Higgins S: Movement is emergent, *Human Movement Sciences* 4:119, 1985.

56. Higgins S: Motor skill acquisition, *Phys Ther* 71(2):123, 1991.

57. Hinderer KA et al: Effects of 'tone reducing' vs. standard plaster-casts on gait improvement of children with cerebral palsy, *Dev Med Child Neur* 30:370, 1988.

58. Ito M: *The cerebellum and neural control,* New York, 1984, Raven Press.

59. Johnels B et al: Measuring motor function in Parkinson's disease. In Benecke R, Conrad B, Marsden CD, editors: *Motor disturbances I,* New York, 1987, Academic Press.

60. Johnson P: The acquisition of skill, In Smyth MM, Wing AM, editors: *The psychology of human movement,* New York, 1984, Academic Press.

61. Kandel E: Cellular mechanisms of learning and the biological basis of individuality. In Kandel ER, Schwartz JH, Jessell JM, editors: *Principles of neural science,* ed 3, New York, 1992, Elsevier.

62. Kandel ER, O'Dell TJ: Are adult learning mechanisms also used for development? *Science* 258:243, 1992.

63. Kaye AH: *Essential neurosurgery,* New York, 1991, Churchill Livingstone.

64. Kazda S, Morich FJ: Drug treatment of stroke and ischemic brain: From acetylsalicylic acid to new drugs—100 years of pharmacology at Bayer Wuppertal-Elberfeld, *Stroke* 21(12):1990.

65. Keith RA, Cowen KS: Time use of stroke patients in three rehabilitation hospitals, *Soc Sci Med* 34:529, 1987.

66. Keshner EA: How theoretical framework biases evaluation and treatment. In *Contemporary man-*

agement of motor problems: proceedings of the II step conference, Alexandria, Va, 1991, Foundation for Physical Therapy.

67. Kleinschmidt A et al: Blockade of NMDA receptors disrupts experience-dependent plasticity of kitten striate cortex, *Science* 238:355, 1987.

68. Kluzik J, Fetters L, Coryell J: Quantification of control: a preliminary study of the effects of NDT on reaching in children with spastic CP, *Phys Ther* 70:65, 1990.

69. Knott M, Voss DE: *PNF patterns and techniques,* ed 2, New York, 1968, Harper & Row.

70. Leonard EL: Early motor development and control: foundations for independent walking. In Smidt GL, editor: *Clinics in physical therapy: gait in rehabilitation,* New York, 1990, Churchill Livingstone.

71. LeVere TE: Recovery of function after brain damage: a theory of the behavioral deficit, *Physiol Psych* 8(3):297, 1980.

72. Light K, Giuliani CA: *The effect of isokinetic exercise effort on coordinated movement control of spastic hemiparetic subjects.* Final report from the Foundation for Physical Therapy, Alexandria, Va, 1993.

73. Loeb GE: The functional organization of muscles, motor units and tasks. In Binder MD, Mendell LM, editors: *The segmental motor system,* Oxford, England, 1988, Oxford University Press.

74. Malezic M et al: Application of a programmable dual-channel adaptive electrical stimulation system for the control and analysis of gait, *J Rehabil Res Dev* 29(4):41, 1992.

75. Malouin F et al: Use of an intensive task-oriented gait training program in a series of patients with acute cerebrovascular accidents, *Phys Ther* 72(11):781, 1992.

76. Mattson E: *Energy cost of level walking,* Published doctoral dissertation from the Department of Orthopedics, Baromedicine and Physical Therapy, Karolinska Institute, Stockholm, Sweden, 1989.

77. McGreevy M: *The effects of serial casting on one child with diplegia,* (Unpublished Masters Project), New York, Teachers College, Columbia University, 1993.

78. Metzler M: A review of research on time in sport pedagogy, *J Teaching Phys Educ* 1:44, 1989.

79. Mills VM: EMG results of inhibitory splinting, *Phys Ther* 64(2):190, 1984.

80. Moffroid M, Whipple R: Specificity of speed of exercise, *Phys Ther* 50:1629, 1970.

81. Murray MP et al: Treadmill vs. floor walking: kinematics, EMG and heart rate, *J Appl Physiol* 59(1): 87, 1985.

82. Nashner LM, Forssberg H: Phase-dependent organization of postural adjustments associated with arm movements while walking, *J Neurophysiol* 55(6):1382, 1986.

83. Newell A, Rosenbloom PS: Mechanisms of skill acquisition and the law of practice. In Anderson JR, editor: *Cognitive skills and their acquisition,* Hillsdale, N.J., 1980, Erlbaum.

84. Noyes FR et al: Kappa change awards: pre- and postoperative studies of muscle activation in the CP child using dynamic EMG as an aid in planning tendon transfer, *Orthop Rev* 6(12):50, 1977.

85. Ojeda R: *Student motor engagement time in physical education classes in Puerto Rico,* (Unpublished Doctoral Dissertation), New York, Teachers College, Columbia University, 1989.

86. Olney SJ et al: Mechanical energy patterns in gait of cerebral palsied children with hemiplegia, *Phys Ther* 67:1348, 1987.

87. Olney SJ et al: Work and power in the hemiplegic cerebral palsy gait, *Phys Ther* 70(7):431, 1990.

88. Olney SJ et al: Work and power in gait of stroke patients, *Arch Phys Med Rehab* 72:309, 1991.

89. Palmer FB et al: The effects of physical therapy on cerebral palsy, *N Engl J Med* 318:803, 1988.

90. Pathokinesiology Department and Physical Therapy Department, Ranchos Los Amigos Medical Center: *Observational gait analysis handbook,* Downey, Calif, 1989, Professional Staff Association Publishing.

91. Perin B: Physical therapy for the child with CP. In Tecklin JS, editor: *Pediatric physical therapy,* Philadelphia, 1989, J. B. Lippincott.

92. Perry J: *Gait analysis: normal and pathological function,* Thorofare, N. J., 1992, Slack, Inc.

93. Perry J et al: Gait analysis the triceps surae in CP: a preoperative and postoperative clinical and EMG study, *J Bone Joint Surg* 56A:511, 1974.

94. Richards CL et al: *The relationship of gait speed to clinical measures of function and muscle activations during recovery post-stroke,* Proceedings of NACOB II, The Second North American Congress on Biomechanics, Chicago, August 24-28, 1992.

95. Rose DK, Guiliani CA, Light KE: *The immediate effects of isokinetic exercise on temporal-distance characteristics of self-selected and fast hemiplegic gait,* Proceedings of Forum on Physical Therapy Issues Related to CVA., Combined Sections Meeting of APTA, Virginia, 1992.

96. Rose DK, Guiliani CA: *Immediate effects of a short bout of treadmill exercise in patients with TBI.* Abstracts of combined sections meeting 1993 Neurology Report.

97. Schneider K et al: Changes in limb dynamics during the practice of rapid arm movements, J Biomech 22, in press.

98. Shenkman M: Making decisions Part 1: unlock the logic in evaluation. Part 2: putting the logic into action, *PT Magazine* 1(2):57, 1993.

99. Shepard K: *Theory: criteria, importance and impact. Contemporary Management of Motor Problems: Proceedings of the II Step Conference,* Alexandria, Va, Foundation for Physical Therapy, 1991.

100. Shumway-Cook AS, Horak FB: Assessing the influence of sensory interaction on balance: suggestions from the field, *Phys Ther* 66:1548, 1986.

101. Shumway-Cook AS, Woolacott M: The growth of stability: postural control from a developmental perspective, *J Motor Behavior* 17:131, 1985.

102. Siesjo BK, Bengtsson F: Review: calcium fluxes, calcium antagonists, and calcium-related pathology in brain ischemia, hypoglycemia and spreading depression: a unifying hypothesis, *J Cere Blood Flow Metab* 9:127, 1989.

103. Solomon R: *Management of cerebrovascular disease:* Course syllabus given by College of Physicians and Surgeons of Columbia University,

Department of Neurological Surgery & Neurology, New York, 1992.

104. Sparrow WA: The efficiency of skilled performance, *J Motor Behavior* 15(3):237, 1983.

105. Sparrow WA, Irizarry-Lopez VM: Mechanical efficiency and metabolic cost as measures of learning a novel gross motor task, *J Motor Behavior* 19(2):240, 1987.

106. Stockmeyer S: An interpretation of the approach of Rood to the treatment of neuromuscular dysfunction, *Am J Phys Med* 46:900, 1967.

107. Strathy GM, Chao EY, Laughman RK: Changes in knee function associated with treadmill ambulation, *J Biomech* 16(7):517, 1983.

108. Sullivan T et al: Serial casting to prevent equinus in acute traumatic head injury, *Physiother Can* 40(6):346, 1988.

109. Tardieu C et al: Toe walking in children with cerebral palsy: contributions of contracture and excessive contraction of the triceps surae muscle, *Phys Ther* 69(8):656, 1989.

110. Taub E: Somatosensory deafferentation research on monkeys. In Ince L, editor: *Behavioral psychology and rehabilitative medicine,* Baltimore, 1980, Williams & Wilkins.

111. Thelen E et al: The role of intersegmental dynamics in infant neuromotor development. In Stelmach GE, Requin J, editors: *Tutorials in motor behavior II,* Amsterdam, 1992, Elsevier Science Publishing.

112. Tinson DJ: How do stroke patients spend their days? *Int Disabil Stud* 11:45, 1989.

113. Twitchell TE: The restoration of motor function following hemiplegia in man, *Brain* 74:443, 1951.

114. Visitin M, Barbeau H: The effects of body weight support on the locomotor pattern of spastic paretic patients, *Can J Neurol Sci* 16:315, 1989.

115. Waagfjord J et al: Effects of treadmill training on gait in a hemiparetic patient, *Phys Ther* 70(9):549, 1990.

116. Wade DT et al: Therapy after stroke amounts determinants and effects, *Int Rehabil Med* 6:105, 1984.

117. Weiller C et al: Functional reorganization of the brain in recovery from striatocapsular infarction in man, *Ann Neurol* 31:463, 1992.

118. Welford AT: On rates of improvement with practice, *J Motor Behavior* 19(3):401, 1987.

119. Winstein CJ et al: Standing balance training: Effect on balance and locomtion in hemiparetic adults, *Arch Phys Med Rehabil* 70:755, 1989.

120. Winter DA: Biomechanics of normal and pathological gait: implications for understanding human locomotor control, *J Motor Behavior* 21(4):337, 1989.

121. Wisleder D, Zernicke RF, Smith JL: Speed related changes in cat hindlimb interactive and muscular torques during the swing phase of locomotion, *Exp Brain Res* 79:651, 1990.

122. Wolf SL et al: Forced use of hemiplegic upper extremities to reverse the effect of learned non-use among chronic stroke and head-injured patients, *Exp Neurol* 104:125, 1989.

123. Wolfe SL: *A behavioral intervention to enhance motor function among neurologic patients.* Lecture presentation and panel discussion from Neuromotor Processes in Posture and Movement, Motor Learning Conference, Teachers College, Columbia University, New York, April 7, 1990.

124. Yaari Y et al: Development of two types of Ca+2 channels in cultured mammalian hippocampal neurons, *Science* 235:680, 1987.

125. Zarrugh MY, Todd FN, Ralston HJ: Optimization of energy expenditure during level walking, *Eur J Appl Physiol* 33:293, 1974.

126. Zelazo PR, Weiss MJ, Leonard EL: The development of unaided walking: the acquisition of higher order control. In Zelazo P, Barr R, editors: *Challenges to developmental paradigms,* Hillsdale, N.J., 1989, Lawrence Erlbaum Associates.

127. Zernicke RF, Schneider K: Biomechanics and developmental neuromotor control. In Thelen E, Lockman J, editors: *Developmental biodynamics: brains body, and behavior connections* (in press).

128. Zichettella M: *EMG analysis of a functional movement under constrained and unconstrained conditions,* (Unpublished Manuscript), Teachers College, Columbia University, New York, 1992.

129. Zivin JA, Choi DW: Stroke therapy, *Sci Amer* 265:56, 1991.

A FRAMEWORK FOR UNDERSTANDING MOBILITY PROBLEMS IN THE ELDERLY

Aftab E. Patla

KEY TERMS

Accommodation strategy

Avoidance strategy

Classification scheme

Cognitive spatial mapping

Dynamic equilibrium

Effector system

Falls

Locomotor control system

Proactive control

Reactive control

Structural integrity

Visual perception

Nothing epitomizes a level of independence and our perception of a good quality of life more than the ability to travel independently under our own power from one place to another. We celebrate the development of this ability in children and try to nurture and sustain it throughout the lifespan. The sensorimotor apparatus and the control system that make this skill possible clearly have a degree of redundancy built in to be able to withstand some insults to the various components. This overlap in functions is evident in our ability to maintain purposeful travel even though it may be at a reduced level with certain associated costs when a major portion of the motor apparatus or one of the sensory modalities is eliminated. This bodes well when we consider the effects of aging on this important life sustaining and enhancing skill.

Evolution has designed animals to function over a specific lifespan. Ideally one would like to have a life where all systems function at an adequate level till the time of death like the proverbial "one hoss shay" described by Oliver Wendell Holmes in his poem, "The Deacon's Masterpiece; or, The Wonderful 'One Hoss-Shay'." Unfortunately aging, environmental factors, and lifestyle effects currently preclude most of us from realizing such an ideal life. Our life expectancy has increased, although this increase will not all be disability free. Mobility impairments and the corresponding debilitating effects on the activities of daily living constitute a major problem for the elderly.[30] The healthcare costs associated with this decreased mobility are large and will continue to escalate as the elderly population increases. Besides these direct costs, the impact on the quality of life is tremendous.[33] Therefore, diagnosis and rehabilitation of mobility problems in the elderly take on some urgency. The study of age effects on mobility can provide insights into the flexibility and adaptability of the locomotor skill and can help us in treating the effects of disease on this skill.

Characterizing changes in the numerous individual components of the locomotor control system, although useful, has some limitations. Besides being too difficult, costly, and time consuming, a reduction in the capability of one of the sensory systems or parts of the nervous or motor system do not necessarily lead to obvious functional deficits because of the ability of the system to compensate. Standard neuromuscular examination, for example, is unable to reliably predict mobility problems in the elderly because the focus is on assessment of individual components of the locomotor system.[34] Eventually we have to be able to document the effects on mobility.

In this chapter, I use the framework developed to understand the generation and the control of skilled human locomotor behavior to discuss the effects of age on mobility.[20] This framework identifies the factors that influence the expression of skilled locomotor behavior and is shown as a series of nested circles in Figure 32-1.[20] The nested circles representing the layers of locomotor skill include the effector system in the center surrounded by the locomotor control system. In the discussions to follow we examine the effects of aging on the various factors individually following a brief review of the role played by each factor in the expression of skilled locomotor behavior. Such an approach will not only allow us to identify what is known—and, more importantly, not known about the age constraints on mobility—but also assist in the planning and implementation of rehabilitation strategies.

THE EFFECTOR SYSTEM

The effector system, which includes the muscles, tendons, ligaments, and the skeletal structure, has a tremendous influence on locomotor movements. The muscles provide unmatched power-to-weight ratio, flexibility, and range of control when

FIG. 32-1 Schematic diagram. Identifies factors that influence the expression of skilled locomotor behavior. (From Patla AE: The neural control of locomotion. In Spivack BS, editor: *Mobility and gait,* New York, Marcel Dekker [in press].)

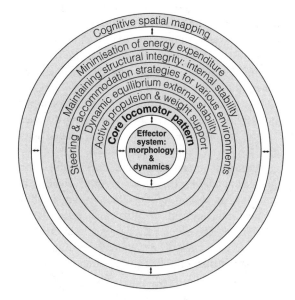

compared to any nonbiological motor currently available. The rich neural interconnections among the muscles, active (due to biarticular configuration of several muscles) and passive (due to nonlinear coupling between segments through Coriolis and centrifugal effects) mechanical interactions, and the highly nonlinear complex muscle actuator are all used by the control system in planning the muscle activation patterns. It therefore occupies the central space in our model. Further details about the role of effector system in the expression of locomotor patterns are provided by Patla.[20]

One of the more ubiquitous findings in the gerontology literature is the fact that strength declines with age.[30] Even though there are problems with how the strength was measured, it is generally believed that a loss of about 25% to 30% in strength occurs over the first six decades of life. This decrement may not necessarily be uniform across all muscle groups. However, such a decline in muscle strength could be detrimental to function if the task requires the full capacity of muscle output. Walking in general does not tax the various lower limb muscle groups to their full capacity. The only muscle group that comes near its maximum during walking is the ankle plantarflexor muscles, which normally provide a major source of propulsive power.[38] But fortunately we can and do use other muscles as sources of propulsive power thereby minimizing any catastrophic effects of limited loss in muscle strength. This shift in locus of propulsive power is evident when there is an insult to a muscle group as in amputation,[39] and can be realized almost instantaneously as seen following an acute reversible ischemic block of the calf muscles,[7] or while walking on a icy surface. When alternate power sources are used, locomotor characteristics such as stride length and velocity are compromised. This was observed when we examined the kinetics of normal walking in the fit and healthy elderly compared to the young; the elderly had a lower push off energy generation at the ankle (0.191 joules/kg vs. 0.296 joules/kg) and a lower stride length (0.808 statures vs. 0.895).[39] Even elite short- and long-distance running records illustrate the reduced speed with age.[18]

Although researchers have concentrated on changes in muscle strength so far, other changes in the effector system of the elderly may have a greater influence on mobility and need to be considered. These considerations include changes in tissue properties of the tendons and ligaments, in mass distribution rather than just an increase or a decrease in the body mass, changes in body

posture due to skeletal changes, and changes in muscle properties such as fatigue resistance. Changes in tendons and ligaments can influence joint stiffness, affect joint range of motion, and limit the ability of otherwise intact muscles to generate power at various speeds over different terrains. For example, Bergstrom et al. showed that subjects with reduced knee joint motion had difficulty using public transportation since many public vehicles have a high first step at the entrance.[3] Increase in mass of the upper body in particular will challenge the already taxed balance control system even further (discussed later). The characteristic stooped posture observed in the elderly will increase the load on the posterior muscles and stress the balance control system because of the apparent anterior shift in the body center of mass. Changes in fatigue resistant properties of the muscles can influence the ability to sustain locomotion over a long period, thereby restricting travel distance. The concomitant changes in the cardiorespiratory system with age can and do influence the functioning of the muscles.

Although it is unlikely that normal age-related changes in the effector system will immobilize a person, they can and do influence the distance travelled, the time it takes to travel, and the types of terrains that can be travelled.

THE LOCOMOTOR CONTROL SYSTEM

The control system is depicted as nested rings around the effector system (Figure 32-1). We divide our discussion into three sections. The first section includes the factors in the four innermost rings that define the essential features for safe locomotion over various terrains. The second section includes the factors listed in the next two rings, which are critical for the long-term integrity and viability of the locomotor apparatus. The last section describes the outermost ring representing cognitive spatial mapping, which makes purposeful goal-directed travel beyond a circumscribed region possible.

Essential Features for Safe Stepping over Various Terrains

Core Locomotor Pattern   The innermost ring is the skeleton pattern around which the locomotor program structure is built. Neuronal circuits in the spinal cord have been shown to be able to produce reasonably complex activation patterns to control near normal inter- and intralimb limb movements observed during locomotion when triggered by a nonspecific input.[10] There is no reason to believe

Figure 32-2 Strategies for maintaining dynamic equilibrium during locomotion. (From Patla AE: Age-related changes in visually guided locomotion over different terrains: major issues. In Stelmach GE, Homberg V, editors: *Sensorimotor impairments in the elderly,* Dordrecht-Nyhoff Publishers [in press].)

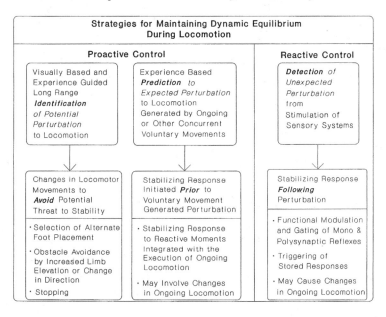

that age has any influence on these rudimentary and necessary spinal neural circuits.

Active Propulsion and Weight Support Animal studies have shown that neuronal structures within the midpontine region in the brainstem modulate the extensor (antigravity) muscle tone to provide weight support and active propulsion not observed in a spinalized preparation.[19] We do not know whether these neuronal structures in the brainstem are changed in any way due to age. Changes with age in active propulsion of the plantarflexors have been discussed in the previous section dealing with the effector system and are probably unrelated to any possible changes in the midbrain structures.

Dynamic Equilibrium: External Stability Maintaining dynamic equilibrium is the *sine qua non* of locomotion. The strategies used to maintain stability are summarized in Figure 32-2, while dangers to stability during locomotion are outlined in Figure 32-3. Note that the reactive control outlined in Figure 32-2 is not purely reactive even though the response occurs after the perturbation. The sensory system is primed proactively such that the reflex gains (and even the polarity) provide functionally appropriate phase and task dependent response.[32]

Figure 32-3 Dangers to stability during walking. The phase of the step cycle in which the danger to stability can occur, along with the locomotor variables that need to be controlled.

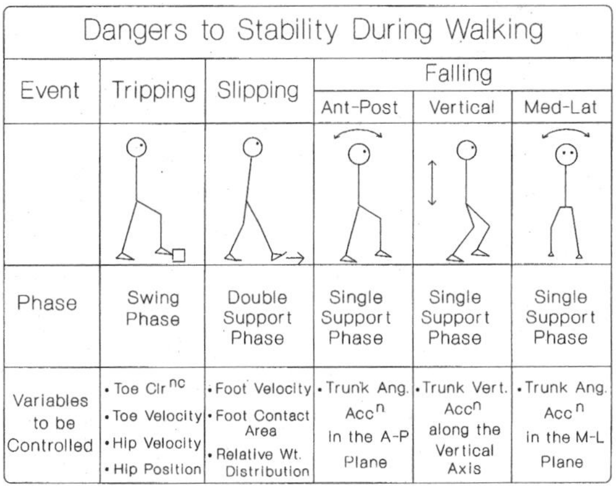

Dangers to Stability During Walking					
Event	Tripping	Slipping	Falling		
			Ant-Post	Vertical	Med-Lat
Phase	Swing Phase	Double Support Phase	Single Support Phase	Single Support Phase	Single Support Phase
Variables to be Controlled	• Toe Clr^{nc} • Toe Velocity • Hip Velocity • Hip Position	• Foot Velocity • Foot Contact Area • Relative Wt. Distribution	• Trunk Ang. Acc^n in the A-P Plane	• Trunk Vert. Acc^n along the Vertical Axis	• Trunk Ang. Acc^n in the M-L Plane

Reactive control relies primarily on detection of the perturbation by the kinesthetic and the vestibular system, which provides a fast corrective response (less than a reaction time) through mono- and/or polysynaptic reflexes or stored responses. These reactive responses are sufficient for smaller magnitudes of perturbations; for larger perturbations a voluntary response may follow these responses to stabilize the body. Voluntary response may also be needed to modify the muscle activation following reflex action to ensure that the next phase of the movement is completed properly. Consider, for example, tripping during the swing phase, which has been identified as a threat to stability in Figure 32-3. In case of an accidental trip, the polysynaptic flexor reflex will be recruited to withdraw the limb.[9] The stretch reflex in the antagonist muscles, which will be stretched due to flexion of the joints (e.g., soleus), is *a priori* reduced to ensure that the limb flexion is not impeded.[32] Following limb withdrawal, the voluntary action of the appropriate muscles will ready the limb for the next landing.[9]

Proactive control, implemented for expected perturbation due to ongoing locomotor movements or other concurrent movements, relies on experience-based prediction of the sign and magnitude of perturbation and is automatically initiated, prior to the onset of movements, less than reaction time in difference between the onset of movements and the proactive stabilizing response. These responses are most likely built in as part of the normal locomotor activation patterns. In Figure 32-3, we have outlined falling of the moving body in any one of the three planes during the single support phase as a major threat to stability. Pitching motion of the trunk with acceleration and deceleration in each step cycle is controlled primarily by the moments about the hip joint. Tipping of the upper body towards the unsupported side (yaw motion) is primarily controlled by the stance limb hip abductors, while the magnitude of destabilization is controlled by the stance limb foot placement in relation to the body center of mass. Collapse of the body in the vertical direction is regulated by the moments about the knee joints. The use of hamstrings to decelerate the limb extension during the end of the swing phase, allows for a gentle foot contact and minimizes chances of slipping. Active limb flexion during the swing phase ensures adequate ground clearance even during normal level walking. The human body is not only able to adequately counter perturbations generated by locomotor movements, but also accommodate additional movement-generated perturbations introduced during locomotion. For example, Patla has shown that subjects are able to proactively control hamstring activation (representing postural stabilizing response) prior to voluntarily raising their arms when visually cued during locomotion.[26]

The most powerful means of ensuring stability is to actively avoid the perturbation altogether. Identification and avoidance of potential threats to stability are made possible by the visual system. Whereas sensory modalities such as the kinesthetic system need physical contact with the external world to transduce and supply relevant information, vision can provide us with information from a distance, which allows us to interpret and take appropriate action before reaching the site of perturbation. We are able to acquire and interpret the information about the environment and to implement changes in the locomotor patterns within a step cycle to avoid a potential threat to stability.[24] These changes as outlined in Figure 32-2 include selecting an alternate foot placement, controlling limb and/or body trajectory to avoid physically contacting an obstacle, changing direction, and stopping. We have documented how the visual system is used during locomotion and determined the rules used to select a particular avoidance strategy. We have also characterized the changes made to the locomotor patterns as the threat is identified and avoided.[20,24]

Dynamic equilibrium is adversely affected by age, according to the fall statistics for the elderly. The high incidence of falls in the elderly, especially during locomotion, has been documented by many researchers.[2] Falls lead to greater injuries, more severe health complications due to these injuries, and even when recovery takes place, falls have an adverse impact on the individual's subsequent lifestyle.[6,33] Falls clearly represent the failure of the balance control system in taking appropriate proactive and/or reactive action when perturbations are encountered during movements such as locomotion.

Consider first the reactive control of stability during locomotion in the elderly. There are no definitive studies that have examined this aspect of balance control in the elderly. Changes in the conduction velocity of the afferent nerves and the reduced sensitivity of the kinesthetic[31] and the vestibular systems[29] are likely to influence the efficacy of this mode of control of stability. The high incidence of falls related to tripping suggests that the reactive responses were inadequate to recover balance in these individuals.[23] Examination of what age-related changes occur in these responses is needed. Is the response organization preserved? Is it delayed? Or is it of insufficient strength? Regardless of the answers, fall statistics do suggest that the elderly cannot rely on this mode of response to maintain balance during locomotion.

Next, let us focus on proactive control dealing with perturbations generated by the movements of the limb segments, whether they are part of the locomotor cycle or represent other concurrent movements. We have examined the changes in proactive control in the fit and healthy elderly dealing with the control of pitching motion of the trunk and the vertical collapse of the body. Winter has identified the high degree of covariance between the hip and the knee joint in young healthy adults during the support phase.[38] He suggests that this represents coupling of regulation of balance along the anterior-posterior and vertical axes. Similar analyses on the elderly revealed an interesting difference. The older subjects had a lower covariance between the hip and the knee joint moments (58% vs. 67%).[39] Recently we have calculated this trade-off between the hip and knee joint at the muscle level using the activity of the two double jointed muscles—rectus femoris and biceps femoris—and found similar results (78% for the young adults versus 70% for the elderly).[21] The covariance at the muscle activity level is understandably higher than at the joint moment level, which is affected by other single-jointed muscles. This reduced covariance between the two joint moments and between the two muscle groups spanning the joints represents impaired coupling of regulation of balance control along the anterior-posterior and vertical axes. Further confirmation is obtained when we examine the energy absorption at the knee during push off, which serves to regulate knee flexion and hence vertical collapse.[40] The elderly showed an increase in the energy absorption at the knee joint (0.087 joules/kg versus 0.047 joules/kg), suggesting a need for better control of knee flexion during push off.[40] The elderly subjects also show a higher horizontal landing velocity at foot contact (0.8 m/s compared to 0.4 m/s for the young), making them more susceptible to slipping—although they landed more flatfooted which could help by increasing the foot-ground surface contact area.[40]

To this point, this analysis has been restricted to subjects travelling over normal level ground, which poses minimal threat to stability. The deterioration in balance control seen over level terrain may lead to an even more disastrous consequence when the elderly subjects are required to travel over more challenging terrains. The ability to accommodate additional perturbations introduced during locomotion is severely affected in the elderly. We have studied responses when subjects were cued visually to raise their arms forcefully

during different phases in the step cycle. Whereas young subjects had a similar response time for the arm muscles during any phase of the locomotion as during standing,[26] the elderly modulated their response time according to the phase of the step cycle.[25] By delaying the response time so that the arm movement coincided with the double support phase, the elderly subjects appeared to minimize any threat to stability caused by the perturbations generated by the arm movement.

Now consider the visually guided strategies used to avoid potential threat to stability. We have begun to examine how visual perception, the basis for selection of specific avoidance strategies, and the implementation of these strategies are influenced by age.[21] Changes in the visual system can affect visual perception. At least 25% of the elderly over the age of 65 years have low vision resulting from macular degeneration. Loss of central field can affect the awareness of exteroceptive information about the environment. We do not know whether these changes in the sensory apparatus result in the elderly relying on different information or a subset of information for the control of the locomotor act. What we do know is that the demands on the visual system to guide locomotion are higher for the elderly. In a recent study we asked elderly subjects to travel over a straight path (9.1 m long) with and without specific foot placement requirements (see Figure 32-4) while wearing liquid crystal glasses that provided a view of the terrain only when they pressed a hand-held switch. When we compare their results with the young, it is evident that the elderly used vision more than the young. This result was achieved not by increasing the number of samples of the terrain but by increasing the duration of viewing the terrain (Figure 32-4). These results suggest that the elderly are not as able to share the visual resources for tasks other than locomotion when the terrain is challenging and requires careful foot placement. The need to pay greater attention is understandable when we examine the success rates of the elderly in changing their step length (by 50%) when cued one or two steps before. The elderly had less than 50% success rate for shortening their step length when cued one step before. This low success rate (compared to over 80% for the young) clearly can have disastrous consequences if the inability to alter step length results in foot placement on an unstable or dangerous surface. It is not surprising therefore that the elderly need to pay more attention to the terrain so that they can plan any required avoidance strategies early.

Figure 32-4 Foot placement data. Data summarizing the number of samples, total visual sample duration, and movement time taken by the elderly (hatched bars) and the young (lightly shaded bars) when travelling over paths that did or did not require specific foot placement.

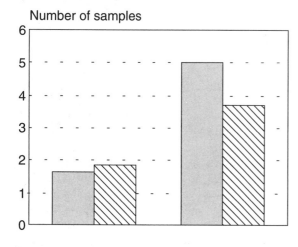

Number of samples

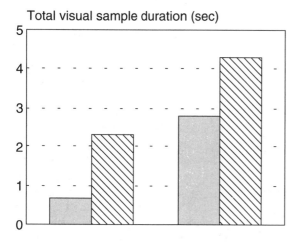

Total visual sample duration (sec)

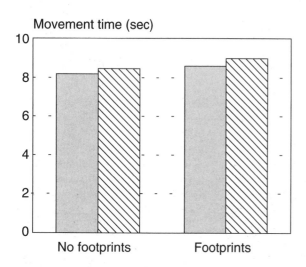

Movement time (sec)

No footprints   Footprints

The bases for selection of an avoidance strategy appear to be reasonably well preserved in the healthy elderly. We have examined this proposition in two sets of experiments. First, we placed obstacles of varying heights in their travel paths giving them the option of going over versus around. Whereas the young subjects showed a lawful transition from going over versus around when the obstacle height reached a proportion of their leg length, the elderly subjects showed more variable results. Most of the elderly (12 out of the 18 subjects tested) chose one or the other strategy for avoiding the obstacle, with more (7 out of the 12) choosing to go around all the obstacles of different heights. This eliminates the decision making during travel, reducing the cognitive demands of the task. The choice of going around is a safer strategy because of the prospect of tripping over the obstacle. One also has to consider the potential of slipping upon landing on a surface that is occluded from view by the obstacle. Similar observations have been made by Konczak et al. in their study on changing affordances (action modes used as a function of stair height) in stair climbing.[12] In contrast to the study of going over versus around obstacles, when we examined the selection of alternate foot placement, the elderly demonstrated similar strategies as the young.[21] As with the young, alternate foot placement in the plane of progression was preferred (Figure 32-5). The alternate foot placement required minimal changes in the ongoing locomotor patterns, maximizing stability while ensuring continued forward progression. In this study, subjects were not given the option of biasing their response (for example stepping around the area where they were not supposed to land). Therefore, given a choice the elderly will select *a priori* strategies and thereby reduce the cognitive demands of the locomotion task.

When we examine the characteristics of the locomotor changes during an avoidance strategy, they appear to be far more conservative in the elderly. Consider, for example, the limb trajectory over obstacles. The elderly show a higher toe clearance, lower horizontal toe velocity, and closer foot placement to the obstacle before going over the obstacle (Figure 32-6). All these changes represent a safer strategy for going over obstacles.

Steering and Accommodation Strategies for Various Environments Different terrains have to be accommodated in our travel path as we move from one place to another. Vision plays a primary

FIGURE 32-5   Foot placement selection. Selection of alternate foot placement when subjects are forced to not step on areas of different proportion and sizes where they would normally land. (From Patla AE: Age-related changes in visually guided locomotion over different terrains: major issues. In Stelmach GE, Homberg V, editors: *Sensorimotor impairments in the elderly,* Dordrecht-Nyhoff Publishers [in press].)

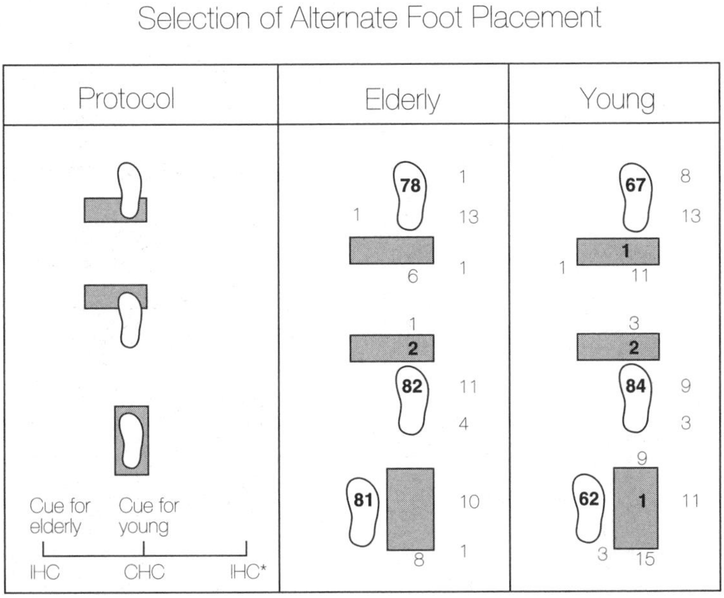

role in mediating the initial adjustments made in the locomotor patterns when we step from a normal level surface to a surface with different geometry or other properties.[22] Knowledge acquired through experience plays an important role in the interpretation of visual information about the altered surface and the strategies used.

As discussed before, the elderly may not be able to travel over certain surfaces such as stairs with high riser heights due to changes in the effector system. It is also likely that deterioration in the visual system may make it difficult for the elderly to accurately perceive small changes in surface properties and therefore will reduce any visually guided proactive adjustments in the locomotor patterns. In a recent study where we examined the ability of subjects with age-related maculopathy to travel over different terrains, we found a greater reliance on haptic exploration for sensing the terrain (unpublished observations).

These results clearly identify deterioration in the control of dynamic balance during locomotion and also highlight the useful adaptive strategies implemented by the elderly. The problems in balance control can restrict a person's travel environment, as well as force the elderly to use assistive devices such as a cane or a walker to improve stability. However, these devices have some drawbacks. Besides lower step length and walking speed achieved when walking with these aids, they impose a load on the arms, which are now used for locomotion.

Factors Critical for Long-Term Integrity and Viability of the Locomotor Apparatus

Maintaining Structural Integrity   Evolution has designed the locomotor apparatus such that during normal operation, the stresses imposed on the structure are well below the stress at which failure occurs.[4] The kinesthetic system plays a vital role in minimizing damage to tissues through protective reflexes such as the flexor reflex and through the variability observed during normal locomotion, which may serve to vary the load on the tissues and hence minimize damage resulting from a constant sustained load.[20] The rotation of load among tissues, even muscles, assumes that these tissues are able to handle larger loads on a short-term basis.

Age-related changes in the skeletal structure clearly reduce the maximum stresses they are able to handle and make them more susceptible to

FIGURE 32-6 Some of the limb kinematics while subjects were going over three different heights of obstacles are shown. Data for elderly subjects are depicted by the hatched bars, while the younger subjects' data are shown by lightly shaded bars.

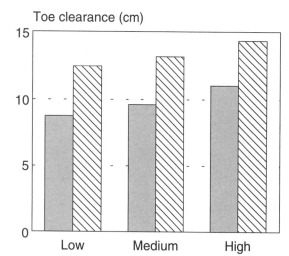

Toe clearance (cm)

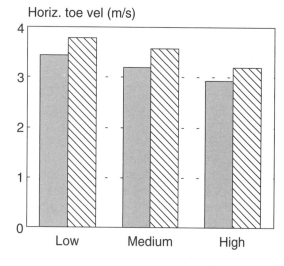

Horiz. toe vel (m/s)

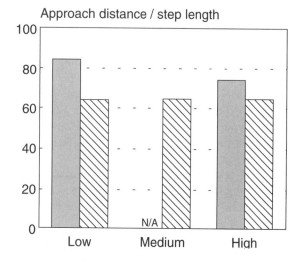

Approach distance / step length

failure. For example, prevalence of osteoarthritis is known to increase with age.[30] Muscular activity generated stresses, which in young subjects have no undesirable consequence, can lead to fractures in the elderly. The large number of hip fractures in the elderly confirm the reduced structural integrity of the locomotor apparatus. In fact, we have found lower variability in the muscle activity patterns in the elderly with a mean coefficient of variation among all major muscles of 34% compared to 44% for the young.[38] This difference was maintained across all muscles. This reduced variability in muscle activity patterns will result in constant (over time) sustained stresses on the locomotor apparatus and is probably undesirable from the point of view of wear and tear.

Minimizing Energy Expenditure Researchers have argued that the animal adopts locomotor patterns that minimize energy expenditure, which is an important evolutionary objective.[1] Any departure from these efficient locomotor patterns has an associated energy cost. For example, at certain speeds walking is more energy consuming than running.[1]

The energy cost for transport increases proportionately for the elderly and is evident in the reduced distance they can travel. This may be due in large part to changes in the cardiorespiratory system, which reduces the maximal energy capacity (lower Vo_2 maximum), resulting in the energy cost of locomotion being proportionately higher in the elderly. The altered locomotor patterns such as the use of assistive devices that require the recruitment of arm muscles will also increase the absolute energy cost of locomotion. Reduced tissue tolerance and associated increased energy costs (relative and absolute) for locomotion in the elderly can and often do have serious consequences by restricting and in some cases curtailing mobility.

Cognitive Spatial Mapping

Purposeful locomotion towards a goal that is not visible from the start is not possible without the aid of stored spatial knowledge.[20,27] These spatial cognitive maps confer greater flexibility in locomotor behavior than would be possible if locomotion were simply triggered and guided by stimuli available in the field of perception. The stored spatial information is allocentric, that is, independent from the subject's location and containing both topological (absolute location of objects and landmarks and their various spatial relationships) and metric representations.[27] Several strategies for navigation to goals that are out of sight have been identified.[8] Some animals such as the desert ants use the strategy of "dead reckoning" to travel to and from their burrows, which relies on the ability to compute the distance and direction traveled, as in the inertial navigational system used in airplanes, and allows the animal to travel without the use of any landmark cues. Researchers have argued that the vestibular system (integrating angular velocity to obtain angular displacement) is a good candidate for the strategy of dead reckoning, although the accumulated integration errors if not corrected (through "visual fixes" of landmarks) can easily lead you off course. Therefore, the strategy of dead reckoning operates over short distances and has a short-term temporal scale.[16] Probably the most common navigational strategy used by humans is piloting. Piloting relies on cognitive spatial maps and the ability to recognize landmarks and use these to travel to a goal. In contrast to piloting's reliance on stimuli that are local and specific, charting used by sailors utilizes global nonspecific stimuli (such as star configuration) as well as a cognitive spatial map to guide travel from one place to another.[8] The topographical knowledge essential for navigation is stored in various parts of the nervous system: the hippocampus and parietal and frontal lobes representing major storage sites.

A general consensus in the literature indicates that an age-related decrement in general cognitive and perceptual-motor abilities occurs.[13] Along with a more general decline, specific tests and measures of spatial aptitude also show a decrement in performance beginning in the fourth or fifth decade of life.[13] The impact of deficits in spatial cognition mobility of older adults is considerable. Disorientation in unfamiliar and sometimes even familiar environments experienced by the elderly can severely constrain their sphere of travel and adversely impact on their quality of life.

Studies reviewed by Kirasic show: (1) the elderly have difficulty placing photographed scenes from their nursing homes in their correct position on a map of the facility; (2) they are less accurate when asked to verbally recall landmarks and in their placement of landmarks on a grid of a familiar urban area; (3) they have difficulty imagining how a specific environment might appear from a different viewing position; (4) they feel more uncomfortable in situations that involve high activity levels (e.g., driving in heavy traffic) and in situations that are uncommon or provide little social support; (5) they perform less accurately and efficiently while shopping in an unfamiliar grocery store compared to the younger subjects.[13] The work of Rabbitt has also shown that as we age

some stored spatial information may become entirely inaccessible, and the information that is retrievable may be accessed in fewer different ways.[28]

A major problem in documenting changes in spatial cognition is the lack of laboratory or field-based tests that are reliable predictors of environmentally based spatial knowledge and mobility performance in large-scale areas. The relationship between standard psychometric tests of visuospatial abilities and spatial cognition for mobility is not always borne out. However, the literature clearly suggests that the aging process does adversely affect our spatial knowledge for travelling to goals not visible from the start. The decrements in spatial cognitive abilities with age are further emphasized by pathologic conditions such as senile dementia of the Alzheimer type.[14,15] It is believed that 9% of the elderly population suffer from moderate to severe cases of dementia. Even mild cases of dementia, which are often difficult to diagnose, can restrict the travel of elderly subjects to familiar environments even though the locomotor system itself may be relatively robust. It is imperative therefore that we pay as much attention to this mobility problem as we do when a person has difficulty walking due to sensorimotor deficits.

STRATEGIES FOR DIAGNOSIS AND REHABILITATION OF MOBILITY PROBLEMS

The framework that I have presented for understanding mobility problems in the elderly can serve to identify factors that limit mobility and point to possible noninvasive rehabilitation programs for correcting these deficits.

Classification Scheme for Characterizing Mobility Performance

There is a lack of consensus in the literature on the most effective and parsimonious way of characterizing decrements in mobility performance. I submit that the two dimensions of space and time are natural candidates for evaluating mobility performance, since mobility involves the transport of body over space in a finite period of time. Traditionally, gait performance is quantified by the speed of walking, which combines space and time dimensions into a single measure. An alternative classification scheme for characterizing mobility performance is provided in Table 32-1.

The magnitude of the spatial dimension defines the area of sphere of travel. Although the magnitude scale is analog and can be quantified at a high level of precision, our ability to use this information probably limits us to categorize the spatial

TABLE 32-1   Classification Scheme for Characterizing Mobility Performance

Dimension	Scale/Qualifier	Levels (with descriptors)
Space	Magnitude	(S) Short (travel within home)
		(M) Medium (travel within neighborhood)
		(L) Large (travel outside neighborhood)
	Type of terrain	(N) Level, unobstructed, normal surface
		(C) Cluttered, uneven, different surface
	End goal:	(V) Visible
	Visibility from the	(NV) Not Visible
	start position	
Time	Magnitude	(NT) Normal travel time
		(LN) Longer than normal travel time
		(NP) Travel not possible within a reasonable time limit

magnitude into three levels. The three levels are short (corresponds to travel within the home or apartment), medium (includes travel within the neighborhood), and large (corresponds to travel outside the neighborhood area). The dimension of space can vary not only in magnitude, but also has two other important qualifiers. The first qualifier of the spatial dimension is the nature of the terrain. We can categorize the terrain into two types: (1) level, unobstructed, and normal travel surface; and (2) cluttered, uneven terrain with surfaces of different properties such as geometry (e.g., staircase), compliance (e.g., carpeted surface), or friction (e.g., icy surface). The second qualifier of the spatial dimension also has two levels that correspond to whether or not the end goal of locomotion is visible from the start position.

Whereas the spatial dimension defines the terrain characteristics, the temporal dimension is what characterizes the decrements in mobility performance. The dimension of time can only vary in magnitude. For a given displacement of the body over particular terrain, we can scale the mobility performance based on the time needed to travel the distance. The less time taken, the better is the level of mobility. Although we can measure time precisely, it is only necessary to classify the time needed to travel a specific distance as one of three levels. It either takes normal time or longer than normal time to travel the distance, or it is not possible to cover the distance within any reasonable finite time period.

Correlating Specific Deficits with Particular Decrements in Mobility Performance

Figure 32-7 contains a flowchart of the process used to determine particular decrements in mobility performance, correlated with specific deficits.

These deficits correspond to the factors involved in the expression of skilled locomotor behavior discussed previously.

The process for diagnosis of specific deficits involves two stages. The first stage is the classification and characterization of mobility performance, which we have discussed in the preceding section. If at this stage our assessment shows that for all terrains subjects take "normal time" to traverse, there is no mobility deficit. The one caveat to this conclusion is of course the definition of normal time for a particular terrain. We need to develop a data base of normal travel times for each terrain and for each age group while factoring out the effects of lifestyle and pathology. It is probably not reasonable to use the times taken by the young subjects as the standard for comparing the older subjects. Even within the older population, we may need to differentiate according to age. Travel time outcome can be any one of the three levels described, but only one output for either LN (longer than normal) or NP (not possible) is shown since this encapsulates any loss in mobility. The other aspect that needs attention is the development of standard travel path(s) with obstacles and different surfaces that can be used for testing subjects. Assuming that we have identified deficits in mobility performance, some diagnostic procedures may be needed in the second step before we can correlate performance with specific deficits.

Any problem with planning a route toward the goal that is not visible from the start clearly suggests deficits in cognitive spatial mapping. This is the easiest deficit to identify as seen in flowchart of Figure 32-7. Limitations in energy capacity will also result in subjects taking longer than normal time to travel even on level, unobstructed normal terrains. Therefore in the flowchart we have used mobility performance outcome only for level, un-

FIGURE 32-7   Mobility deficits flowchart. A flowchart for classifying and characterizing mobility deficits, correlating performance with specific deficits and possible noninvasive rehabilitation programs are shown. The outcome labels in the mobility performance classification are described in Table 32-1.

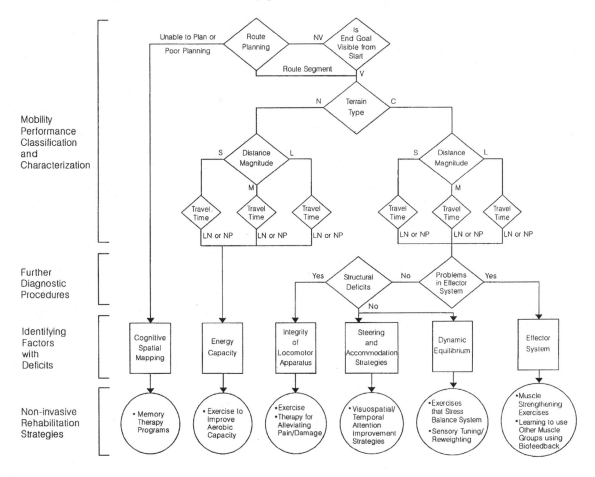

obstructed normal terrain to zero in on energy capacity limitations. Subjects may have no apparent difficulty traveling short distances, but the limitations emerge when larger travel distances are involved.

Decrements in mobility performance over cluttered, uneven terrains with different surfaces may be viewed as a result of poor steering and accommodation strategies, deficits in dynamic equilibrium, poor structural status of the locomotor apparatus, or problems with effector system. To identify the appropriate reason, we need to use diagnostic procedures. Deficits in effector system, in particular muscle strength or mass distribution, are relatively easy to identify. If there are no problems with the effector system, then we need to rule out any defects in structural status of the locomotor apparatus. One of the indications of problems with the integrity of the locomotor apparatus is pain, which usually limits the travel over cluttered, uneven terrain. For example, a degenera-

tive disease such as arthritis makes climbing stairs or going over obstacles difficult, if not impossible. To distinguish between deficits in dynamic equilibrium and poor accommodation strategies, we may also need to test subjects' mobility on terrains with only different surfaces that have to be accommodated in the travel path. It is possible to use results from cluttered terrains of short and medium distance to identify specific deficits. Assessment on long travel paths may not be necessary.

Noninvasive Rehabilitation Strategies for Improving Mobility

Figure 32-7 also contains a list of strategies for improving mobility. Most of these strategies involve specific physical or mental exercise. The basic philosophy behind these exercise intervention programs is encapsulated by the common dictum "use it or lose it." The goals of these intervention programs are ideally to improve mobility performance—if not improve, at least maintain a level of mobility performance or, at a minimum, reduce the rate of decrement of mobility performance.

Two aspects of the exercise need emphasis here. First, the physical exercise needs to be tailored to specific deficits. Exercises that improve aerobic capacity or muscle strength may not improve dynamic stability. Studies examining the effects of physical activity on balance control have shown conflicting results.[5,35] The second aspect of an exercise intervention program is that these exercises do not have to be only physical. Mental exercises can and do improve memory and may be useful in dealing with deficits in cognitive spatial mapping.[36]

Let us examine some of the intervention programs listed in Figure 32-7. Physical exercise has been proposed as a way of reducing fracture risk.[5] Thus exercise and therapy for damaged tissue can be useful in restoring the structural integrity of the locomotor apparatus. Poor steering and accommodation strategies can benefit from teaching subjects to visually scan the environment more often to ensure that appropriate proactive strategies are implemented. As discussed before, the use of reactive strategies (which are the last line of defense) for accommodating different surfaces leaves no room for error.

There is a great deal of interest in improving balance control in the elderly in order to reduce falls. As stated before, the use of standard exercise is not sufficient for improving dynamic stability. The study by Haines suggests that maintenance of muscle strength alone does not guarantee improved balance control.[11] We need to exercise the balance control system and not just its subcomponents. The work by Winstein suggests that exercise of the balance control system in one context (e.g., standing) does not transfer to another context (e.g., gait).[37] This implies that we need to exercise the balance control system in various contexts. The work by Manchester reports that the elderly have greater difficulty resolving sensory conflicts, which results in poorer balance control.[7] Sensory conflicts arise when the visual system is fooled into thinking that posture is affected. We have recently developed and implemented exercise programs that stress the balance control system under different contexts, including sensory conflicts. One specific exercise involves subjects travelling over simulated cluttered terrain, which forces the subjects to proactively change their gait patterns to avoid obstacles and step on different surfaces. This balance exercise program has proven beneficial even in relatively healthy elderly individuals (un-published observation). It is possible therefore to implement intervention programs for improving dynamic equilibrium.

SUMMARY

This framework for understanding mobility problems in the elderly, along with the proposed process of characterizing mobility performance and identifying deficits was devised to be a useful aid in improving the quality of life of older individuals. Aging is not a disease process, and we do not have to accept the age-related deterioration in function and ability. We can and should be able to enjoy a healthy active lifestyle well into our mature years. And as Elizabeth Browning so eloquently penned about the golden years, "The best is yet to be. . . ."

Acknowledgments: *The work in this chapter was supported by grants from Health and Welfare Canada and Natural Science and Engineering Research Council of Canada.*

REFERENCES

1. Alexander R: Optimization and gaits in the locomotion of vertebrates, *Physiol Rev* 69(4):1199, 1989.
2. Baker PS, Harvey H: Fall injuries in the elderly. In Radebough TS, Hadley E, Suzman R, editors: *Clinics in geriatric medicine,* Philadelphia, 1985, W. B. Saunders.
3. Bergstrom G, Aniansson A, Bjelle A et al: Functional consequences of joint impairment at age 79, *Scan J Rehab Med* 17:183, 1985.
4. Biewener AA: Biomechanics of mammalian terrestrial locomotion, *Science* 250:1097, 1990.
5. Buchner DM, Beresford SAA, Larson EB et al: Effects of physical activity on health status in older adults. II: Intervention studies, *Annu Rev Public Health* 13:469, 1992.
6. Cummings SR, Nevitt MC, Kidd S: Forgetting falls: the limited accuracy of recall of falls in the elderly, *J Am Geriatr Soc* 36:613, 1988.
7. Dickey JP, Winter DA: Adaptations in gait resulting from unilateral ischaemic block of the leg, *Clin Biomech* 7:215, 1992.
8. Dusenbery DB: *Sensory ecology,* New York, 1992, W. H. Freeman.
9. Eng J, Winter DA, Patla AE: *Lower limb muscle coordination during the recovery to an unexpected tripping perturbation,* XIVth International Society for Biomechanics Conference Proceedings, Paris, 1993.
10. Grillner S: Neurobiological bases of rhythmic motor acts in vertebrates, *Science* 228:143, 1985.
11. Haines RP: Effect of bed rest and exercise on body balance, *J Appl Physiol* 36:323, 1974.

12. Konczak J, Meeuwsen HJ, Cress ME: Changing affordances in stair climbing: the perception of maximum climbability in young and older adults, *J Exp Psychol* 18(3):691, 1992.

13. Kirasic KC: Acquisition and utilization of spatial information by elderly adults: implications for day-to-day situations. In Poon LW, Rubin DC, Wilson BA, editors: *Everyday cognition in adulthood and late life,* New York, 1989, Cambridge University Press.

14. Leon de MJ, Potegal M, Gurland B: Wandering and parietal signs in senile dementia of Alzheimer's type, *Neuropsychobiology* 11:155, 1984.

15. Liu L, Gauthier L, Gauthier S: Spatial disorientation in persons with early senile dementia of the Alzheimer type, *Am J Occup Ther*:67, 1990.

16. McNaughton BL, Chen LL, Markus EJ: "Dead reckoning," landmark learning, and the sense of direction: a neurophysiological and computational hypotheses, *J Cog Neurosci* 3(2):190, 1991.

17. Manchester D, Woollacott M, Zederbauer-Nylton N et al: Visual, vestibular and somatosensory contributions to balance control in the older adult, *J Gerontol* 44(4):M118, 1989.

18. Moore DH: A study of age group track and field records to relate age and running speed, *Nature* 253:264, 1975.

19. Mori S: Integration of posture and locomotion in acute decerebrate cats and in awake, freely moving cats, *Prog Neurobiol* 28:161, 1987.

20. Patla AE: The neural control of locomotion. In Spivack BS, editor: *Mobility and gait,* New York, Marcel Dekker (in press).

21. Patla AE: Age-related changes in visually guided locomotion over different terrains. In Stelmach GE, Homberg V, editors: *Sensorimotor impairments in the elderly,* Dordrecht-Nyhoff Publishers (in press).

22. Patla AE, Prentice S, Unger-Peters G: Accommodating different compliant surfaces in the travel path during locomotions, *Proceedings of the Fourteenth International Society for Biomechanics Conference* 11:1010, 1993.

23. Patla AE, Frank JS, Winter DA: Assessment of balance control in the elderly: major issues, *Physiother Can* 42(2):89, 1990.

24. Patla AE: Visual control of human locomotion. In Patla AE, editor: *Adaptability of human gait: implications for the control of locomotion,* New York, 1991, Elsevier Publishers.

25. Patla AE, Frank JS, Brown JE: *Postural adaptation to voluntary arm raises during locomotion in the elderly.* Paper presented at XIth International Society for Biomechanics Conference, Amsterdam, 1987.

26. Patla AE: Adaptation of postural responses to voluntary arm raises during locomotion in humans, *Neurosci Lett* 68:334, 1986.

27. Poucet B: Spatial cognitive maps in animals: new hypotheses on their structure and neural mechanisms, *Psychol Rev* 100(2):163, 1993.

28. Rabbitt P: Inner-city decay? Age changes in structure and process in recall of familiar topographical information. In Poon LW, Rubin BC, Wilson BA, editors: *Everyday cognition in adulthood and late life,* New York, 1989, Cambridge University Press.

29. Rosenhall V: Degenerative changes in the aging human vestibular geriatric neuroepithelia, *Act Otolaryngol* 76:208, 1973.

30. Schultz AB: Mobility impairment in the elderly: challenges for biomechanics research, *J Biomech* 25(5):519, 1992.

31. Skinner HB, Barrack RL, Cook SD: Age-related declines in propioception, *Clin Orthop* 184:208, 1984.

32. Stein RB: Reflex modulation during locomotion: functional significance. In Patla AE, editor: *Adaptability of human gait: implications for the control of locomotion,* New York, 1991, Elsevier Publishers.

33. Tinetti ME, Powell L: *Fear of falling and low self-efficacy: a cause of dependence in elderly persons.* Paper presented at the American Society for Gerontology Meeting, 1991.

34. Tinetti ME, Ginter SF: Identifying mobility dysfunctions in elderly patients: standard neuromuscular examination or direct assessment? *JAMA* 259(8):1190, 1988.

35. Wagner EH, La Croix AZ, Buchner DM et al: Effects of physical activity on health status in older adults. I: Observational studies, *Ann Rev Public Health* 13:451, 1992.

36. Wilson BA: Designing memory-therapy programs. In Poon LW, Rubin DC, Wilson BA, editors: *Everyday cognition in adulthood and late life,* New York, 1989, Cambridge University Press.

37. Winstein CJ: Balance retraining: does it transfer? In Duncan P, editor: *Balance,* 1989, American Physical Therapy Association.

38. Winter DA: *The biomechanics and motor control of human gait: normal, elderly, and pathological,* Waterloo, Ontario, 1991, University of Waterloo Press.

39. Winter DA, Olney SJ, Conrad J et al: Adaptability of motor patterns in pathological gait. In Winters JM, Woo SL, editors: *Multiple muscle systems: biomechanics and movement organization,* New York, 1990, Springer-Verlag.

40. Winter DA, Patla AE, Frank JS et al: Biomechanical walking pattern changes in the fit and healthy elderly, *Phys Ther* 70(6):340, 1990.

GLOSSARY

absolute reference frame   A set of three orthogonal axes one of which is parallel with the field of gravity

accelerometer   Analog device that directly measures linear acceleration

accommodation strategy   Different terrains have to be accommodated in our travel path as we move from one place to another. The ability to successfully adapt to different terrains and maintain ongoing locomotion is an accommodation strategy. Knowledge acquired through experience plays an important role in the interpretation of visual information about the altered surface and the strategies used.

accuracy   As commonly defined, a measurement without error. Refer to Strube and Delitto for additional definitions.

aliasing   Sampling error that results from sampling at less than twice the highest frequency component of the signal

ambulation profiles   In general, assessments of time-distance (foot contact) parameters and information about walking skill. There are several ambulation profiles that have been developed for clinical gait assessment. Some profiles provide a global score summing the performance from a series of tests each graded on an ordinal scale. Others use variables such as time and distance that provide a measure of performance on an interval scale.

angular acceleration   The rate of change of angular velocity, usually expressed as radians per second squared or degrees per second squared.

angular displacement   The rotational component of a body's motion.

angular momentum   The vector cross product of a body's position vector and its linear velocity vector.

angular velocity   The rate of change of angular displacement, usually expressed as radians per second or degrees per second.

anterior cruciate ligament (ACL)   The ligament attached to the medial portion of the intercondylar area of the tibia. Passes upwards, backwards, and laterally to attach to the medial surface of the lateral condyle of the femur.

attractor   In the dynamical systems perspective, the system under study is a stable dynamical system. In this system all the trajectories of the system will be attracted to a specific region of the state space. When this occurs, it is called an attractor, which is a low dimensional subset of state space to which all the nearby trajectories converge. There are three types of attractors: point, periodic, and chaotic.

available resources   Term used in motor learning to identify the intrinsic (morphological and perceptual/sensory) and extrinsic (physical world) variables that will effect the solution to the execution of a task. Available resources include body size, torque-producing capacity, degrees of freedom, vision, and gravity.

avoidance strategy   Identification and avoidance of potential threats to stability. Avoidance strategies can occur readily through the visual system. This allows interpretation and action before reaching the site of perturbation.

azimuth   The horizontal angle an object makes about a vertical axis.

base of support   A single definition for base of support has not been standardized. It has been defined as the lateral distance between the heels and the angle of foot placement in relation to the line of progression. **Base of support** has also been defined as the perpendicular distance separating the midpoints of consecutive heel contacts. It has also been defined as the mediolateral distance between either the medial or lateral malleoli during double support.

biomechanical model of treatment In this model, the clinician identifies, by movement analysis of the gait pattern, the individual components of the gait cycle which are aberrant or missing. Remediation is provided through exercises designed to strengthen weak muscle groups or the use of orthotic devices to stabilize the joints promoting a more normal movement pattern.

bode plot A graph of the magnitude of the output of a system such as knee range of motion against frequency.

body segment parameters The inertial properties of an object that define its response to an external force. These parameters include mass, density, and moment of inertia.

body-fixed reference frame Local reference frame. A Cartesian coordinate system that is fixed in and moves with the body.

cadence The rhythm of the walking pattern, defined as the number of steps or strides per unit time.

canalized development In the theory of epigenetic development, characteristics that are tightly constrained, species typical processes are those that undergo canalized development. The development of locomotion is viewed by some as canalized development.

center of mass The point in a body at which the body's mass can be said to act.

center of pressure The point of application of the ground reaction force.

central pattern generator (CPG) A collection of neurons contained within the spinal cord identified in nonhuman vertebrates as being able to generate the locomotor stepping pattern autonomously. The network is not invariant. The CPG has the ability to change output depending on speed requirements and in response to obstacle avoidance. The CPG can be constantly modified by available supraspinal or sensory input.

centroid The two-dimensional coordinates of the center of an area.

closed chain motion Motion of a limb while the distal end of the limb is in contact with a stationary object.

cocontraction Simultaneous activation of the agonist and antagonist musculature to maintain joint stability. An example would be cocontraction of the quadriceps femoris and the hamstring musculature in the stance phase to stabilize the knee joint as weight shifting between limbs occurs.

cognitive spatial mapping Purposeful locomotion requires stored spatial knowledge. Spatial cognitive maps are independent of the subject's location and contain both topological and metric representations.

common mode rejection ratio The measure of how well an amplifier minimizes signal noise and amplifies the true signal.

compensation The development of alternative means, behavioral strategies, to accomplish the goal.

concentric contraction Muscle contraction with simultaneous muscle shortening.

context-conditioned variability The same movement command does not always result in the same movement because of context-conditioned variability. The neuromuscular system must be coordinated within ever-varying anatomical, mechanical, and physiological contexts.

control parameters In the dynamical systems perspective, control parameters are the constraints that when scaled in magnitude move the system from one state to another. For example, an increase in walking velocity may change walking to running as a form (state) of locomotion. Usually, control parameters are sought that have positive effects on behavior are sought.

convergence Refers to multiple afferent input affecting single neuron or nucleus.

critical features   The aspects of the observable movement that are essential for success of the behavior and are least modifiable. A suggested critical feature of walking is control of the center of gravity.

cross talk   The intermingling of signals from neighboring measurement devices.

cutaneous electrodes   Electrodes that are placed on the skin over a superficial nerve site or motor point to produce muscle contraction through electrical stimulation.

deformable body   A body whose particles can move with respect to one another.

detector   The portion of an imaging device that identifies the two-dimensional location of an object.

disability   There are several different definitions for *disability*. The International Classification of Impairments, Disabilities and Handicaps defines disability as any restriction or lack of ability to perform a task or an activity in the manner considered normal for a human being.

disease   The organic abnormality or pathological process leading to impairment.

divergence   Refers to the multiple outputs of a neuron or nucleus.

DLT (direct linear transformation)   The common mathematical approach to constructing the three-dimensional location of an object from multiple two-dimensional images

double support   The stance phase of one limb overlaps the stance phase of the contralateral limb creating a period in which both limbs are in contact with the ground. The overlapping period of time is known as *double support*.

dynamic equilibrium   The ability to maintain upright balance during the on-going task of ambulation.

dynamical systems perspective   A theory about systems that change. Causality is multidimensional and multilevel.

dynamics   The branch of mechanics dealing with bodies in motion with non zero acceleration, that is, time-dependent.

eccentric contraction   Muscle contraction with simultaneous muscle lengthening.

effector system   Includes the muscles, tendons, ligaments, and the skeleton. Torque-producing ability is a function of this system, as well as the mass of tissue, tissue properties of tendons and ligaments, body posture, and fatigue resistance.

electromyogram   A reading or tracing of the electrical signal elicited by a muscle during contraction.

emergent behavior   In the dynamical systems perspective, motor behavior is not prescribed or directed by the brain but emerges from the constraints that surround the goal-directed action.

EMG   Abbreviation for *electromyogram*.

ensemble average   The time averaged EMG of repeated activities.

environmental constraints   In the dynamical systems perspective, environmental constraints refer to the environment that surrounds the mover. Gravity, surface texture, and culture are examples of environmental constraints.

epigenetic development   The manner in which phenotypic characteristics arise during development through a complex series of interactions between genetic programs and environmental signals.

equations of motion   The equations that, when solved, completely describe a body's motion.

equinovarus posture   This deformity is manifested by a lower extremity which comes into contact with the ground with the forefoot first. Weight is borne primarily on the lateral border of the foot, often with toe flexion. The position is maintained during the stance phase and interferes with weight bearing.

error   The positive or negative score increments arising in a particular measurement that are unrelated to the characteristics of interest.

euler angles   The three angles that completely describe the position of one coordinate system with respect to another.

FES   Abbreviation for *functional electrical stimulation*.

field height   Measurement of the short side of the image taken orthogonally with respect to the optical axis.

field of view Measurement of the long side of the image taken orthogonally with respect to the optical axis.

filtering The process of manipulating the frequencies of a signal through analog or digital processing.

flexed-knee gait pattern A pattern that involves increased stance phase knee flexion and external knee flexion moments balanced by increased quadriceps femoris muscle activity. A hypothesis is that this gait pattern minimizes anterior shear forces at the knee.

flexor reflex afferents The afferents included in this reflex pathway include mechanoreceptors, cutaneous afferents, nocioceptors, joint afferents, and muscle afferents. Flexor reflex afferents refer to the interneuronal reflex system that has been suggested to be partially responsible for the generation of locomotion.

focal length Distance between the principal focus and the optical center of the lens.

foot angle Describes the degree of intoeing or outtoeing of the foot relative to the forward line of progression during the stance phase. It is described by the angle formed between a hypothetical line corresponding with the direction of walking and the long axis of the foot, a line drawn longitudinally from mid-heel to the area somewhere near the second and third toes.

foot contact index The ratio between the length of the footprint and the actual length of the shoe.

force plate An analog device to measure directly the ground reaction force.

free body diagram A diagram of an object showing all of the forces on that object.

frequency spectrum The representation of a signal in the frequency domain.

functional electrical stimulation (FES) The direct electrical stimulation to peripheral nerves or motor points to produce a muscle contraction during a functional movement. During ambulation, FES works peripherally to produce normal movement patterns.

functional multidimensional perspective of treatment Underlying this model is the assumption that clients are constantly involved in the learning process. Movement patterns are the result of the exploration of various strategies to successfully accomplish the task presented. The role of the clinician is to assist the client in the exploration of strategies and to encourage flexibility in seeking successful solution.

gage factor The strain gage's sensitivity.

gait The particular manner or style of moving on foot. Human forms of gait include walking, skipping, jogging and running.

gait cycle The fundamental unit of locomotion. The gait cycle is defined as the sequence of events that begin with one extremity and continue until that event is repeated by the same extremity.

gait deviation A gait deviation is defined as a departure from the nondisabled reference. For example, as seen from the frontal view, the normal reference for the pelvis during swing is that the pelvis drops slightly on the side of the swinging extremity. This angular displacement from neutral is approximately 5 degrees. A deviation would be the pelvis lifting on the side of the swinging extremity. This deviation is known as a pelvic hike.

generalizability theory Theory that attempts to model the multidimensional and systematic nature of error. The assumption is that many error sources exert systematic influence that can be estimated and separated from the random error component. Generalizability theory requires measurement on an interval scale.

global reference frame See *absolute reference frame.*

golgi tendon organ A sensory receptor found in series with muscle fibers, located at the musculotendinous junction, which is a muscle contraction-sensitive mechanoreceptor. Golgi tendon afferent information is transmitted via Ib afferents.

ground reaction forces The algebraic sum of the mass-acceleration products of all body segments while the body is in contact with the ground.

handicap The inability to function within society resulting from disability.

heterotopic ossification   The formation of new bone which is manifested clinically as a joint contracture.

H-reflexes   The Hoffman (H) reflex is a technique that selectively stimulates electrically large-diameter afferent fibers and provides the opportunity for the investigator to indirectly measure the excitability of alpha motoneurons. The latency between electrical stimulation and the motor response and the amplitude of the motor response detected by EMG electrodes are the variables measured.

hybrid systems   Combination of functional electrical stimulation with an orthotic device is considered a hybrid system because each system alone improves functional performance and the principles for application of each separate system are different.

impairment   There are several different definitions for impairment. The International Classification of Impairments, Disabilities and Handicaps defines impairment as a loss or abnormality at the tissue, organ, or body system level. Impairments include loss of range of motion, decreased torque, pronated foot, etc.

implanted electrodes   Electrodes implanted into the muscle or over nerves to produce muscle contraction or a reflex withdrawal response through electrical stimulation.

impulse   The integral of the dot product of force times time.

inferred parameter   An inferred or a derived parameter is not directly measured but derived from direct measurement of other variables. For example, some investigators measure average walking velocity (v) and cadence (c) and use a formula to determine step length (l): $l = c/v$.

initial swing   The period of swing that occurs from lift of the foot off the ground to maximum knee flexion.

initial contact   Contact that occurs the instant the previously swinging foot contacts the ground. Initial contact is considered an event rather than a phase of walking because it is instantaneous.

inverse dynamics   The calculation of joint kinetics from the mass–acceleration relationship of a body.

joint moment   The sum of the external moments applied to a joint. This sum is equal and opposite the moment generated internally by muscles and other soft tissue.

joint power   The dot product of the joint moment and the joint's angular velocity.

joint reaction force   The internal reaction force acting at the contact surfaces when that joint is subjected to external forces.

joint reference frame   A set of three axes, not necessarily orthogonal, fixed in a joint and having anatomical meaning.

kinematics   The branch of mechanics that deals with the motion of a body, disregarding force and mass.

kinetic energy (linear)   One half the product of mass and its linear velocity squared.

lens   The portion of an imaging device that collects and focuses light.

linear acceleration   The rate of change of linear velocity, usually expressed as meters per second squared.

linear displacement   The translational component of a body's movement.

linear velocity   The rate of change of linear displacement, usually expressed as meters per second.

loading response   Loading response occurs immediately following initial contact to lift of the contralateral extremity.

local reference frame   See *body fixed reference frame.*

locomotion   An action involving the change in position of the body and limbs in space and time (Higgins and Higgins). Reciprocal activations of muscles and coordinated multi-joint movement (Leonard). To look at locomotion from a dynamical systems perspective is to see locomotor behavior emerge from the constraints embodied in the individual, surrounding the action, and manifested in the task (Clark).

maximum voluntary isometric contraction   Maximum voluntary muscle contraction without an associated visible change in muscle length.

mean EMG   The time average of the full-wave rectified EMG over a given time period.

mesencephalic locomotor region (MLR)   A collection of neurons in the midbrain of nonhuman vertebrates that produces rhythmic, coordinated locomotor movements when stimulated electrically.

mid stance   This occurs from lift of the contralateral extremity to a position in which the body is directly over the stationary foot.

mid swing   This is the period of swing immediately following maximum knee flexion to the time when the tibia is in a vertical position.

modeling   The process of representing a system or phenomenon in an idealized way.

moment   The vector cross product of a position vector and the corresponding

moment of force   The turning effect of a force about a point, calculated as the cross product of the force and its distance from the point of rotation.

moment of inertia   The attribute of a body representing resistance to angular acceleration.force.

motion artifact   The signal noise resulting from motion of the recording electrode or the attached lead.

motor control   The system that guides the selective allocation of muscular tension across the appropriate joint-segment relationships in the body. A controlled motor response should exhibit task appropriate, differential allocation of tension, integrated with the use of external forces. Allocation of tension is specific to the problem being solved (Higgins and Higgins).

motor skill   The acquired ability to consistently solve a movement problem under a variety of conditions. Skill, a product of genetic potential and experiential history, is expressed by some level of control over goal-directed movement.

motor unit   The functional unit of striated unit comprised of the alpha motor neuron and its associated muscle fibers.

motor unit action potential   The detected waveform made up of the spatial and temporal summation of the muscle fiber action potentials within a single motor unit.

moving average   The mean EMG over the period of a window of time recalculated as the window of time moves.

muscle fiber action potential   The depolarization and repolarization of a muscle fiber.

muscle spindle   A sensory receptor found in parallel with muscle fibers that is sensitive to changes in muscle length during some types of movement. Spindles are innervated by the gamma motoneuron, and the beta fiber from the alpha motoneum. Spindle discharge is transmitted via Ia and II afferents.

neurophysiological model of treatment   Model that advocates a prescribed recovery pattern. Treatment using this model often occurs in a specific progression, e.g., developmental sequencing, or bed mobility, then sitting, standing and finally ambulating.

Nyquist frequency   The minimum sampling frequency to prevent aliasing. It corresponds to twice the highest frequency component of the signal.

observational gait analysis   This is a qualitative approach to gait analysis which identifies gait deviations in patients from visual observations. Both the identification and the grading of gait deviations depend on the observer's judgments.

ontogenetic development   Changes in the neural substrates subserving movement change during development. For example, in the cat, a reflex known as low threshold placing is initially controlled by the spinal cord but as development proceeds, the reflex becomes dependent on an intact sensorimotor cerebral cortex.

optical axis   Axis normal to the lens of the imaging device.

organism constraints   In the dynamical systems perspective, organism constraints are the constraints that are part of the mover. These constraints include the physical attributes of the mover and the psychological characteristics.

particle   An object that, for the purpose of analysis, can be treated as a dimensionless point mass.

photogrammetry   The process of obtaining three-dimensional measures of an object from two-dimensional images.

piezoelectric crystal   A crystal that when deformed gives off an electrical charge.

pixel   The basic element of a digital array or image. The digital array consists of a matrix of row and column indices that identify a point in the image.

positron emission transaxial tomography (PETT)   A technique that allows the examiner to view the brain as it produces movement. PETT scans monitor the metabolic activity of cortical areas and thus provide insight into what areas of the brain are active during various tasks.

potential energy   The energy of a mass or spring related to its position or configuration. The gravitational potential energy is a product of a body's weight and its height from some reference level.

power spectral density   The plot of the squared magnitude components of a signal.

precision   As commonly defined: the degree of exactness or discrimination with which a quantity is stated. Refer to Strube and Delitto for additional definitions.

prerequisites for control   Resources available to the learner for engaging in complex movement. Prerequisites are the minimum necessary conditions and include knowledge base, perceptual skill, motor control, training or fitness, and emotional security.

pressure   Force per unit area. A scalar quantity.

proactive control   Proactive control implies that the nervous system anticipates a perturbation and is prepared to respond. Proactive control relies on experience-based prediction of the sign and magnitude of the perturbation and is automatically initiated prior to the onset of movement.

pronation-supination index   This measure was developed to describe the relative amount of pronation or supination of the foot when the distal third of the foot is in contact with the ground. The value is computed by dividing the distance between the center of pressure to the medial footprint border by the distance from the medial to the lateral footprint borders at the distal third of the footprint.

quadriceps avoidance gait   The total absence of the external knee flexion moment during the stance phase of the involved extremity during gait.

range of motion   The angular excursion through which a limb can be moved.

reactive control   Reactive control implies that the nervous system must first sense the perturbation and then respond to it. Reactive control of dynamic equilibrium, for example, relies primarily on the detection of the perturbation by the kinesthetic and the vestibular system and provides a fast corrective response.

reciprocating gait orthosis   Orthosis consisting of an ankle-foot (AFO) plastic splint, a lockable knee joint, and a free hip joint. Lateral aluminum uprights connect the AFO with the knee and hip and extend upward to the mid-thoracic level. The two hip joints are connected with cables so that hip flexion of one leg will produce hip extension of the opposite leg.

reliability   Measures of reliability provide an index of how dependably a measure is correlated with the underlying characteristic being assessed. Reliability represents the ratio of true score variance to observed score variance. As measures approach the status of being error-free, reliability coefficients approach a value of 1.0. A reliable measure is expected to repeat the same score on two different occasions, provided the characteristic of interest does not change.

resolution   The smallest amount of a unit or fixed unit by which two measurements differ. If the measurement technique uses fixed units, the resolution is limited by the size of the fixed unit.

rigid body   A nondeformable body. The distance between the particles of the body remains fixed.

RMS   Root mean square. The effective value of the quantity of an alternating signal.

scalar   A quantity defined only by magnitude.

segmental Reference frame   Anatomical reference frame. A Cartesian coordinate system fixed in a body segment and having anatomical meaning.

self-organization   In the dynamical systems perspective, the property of a system in which system components organize themselves into spatial and temporal patterns.

sensitivity   The proportion of times that a measure correctly identifies a disorder or condition when the disorder or condition is present.

signal to noise ratio   The ratio of the true signal to the random, undesired signal unrelated to the true signal.

single limb support   Single limb support is one of three basic locomotor tasks, weight acceptance, single limb support, and swing limb advancement. The period during the gait cycle when one limb is in contact with the ground is defined as single limb support.

spatial footfall parameters   A measure, in centimeters or inches, of foot contact performance. Stride length, step length, and base of support are spatial foot contact measures.

specificity   The proportion of times that a measure correctly identifies a disorder or condition as being absent when the disorder or condition is absent.

stance phase   The time in which the limb is in contact with the walking surface. A gait cycle has two stance phases, a left and a right. Right stance phase begins with initial contact of the right limb and ends with take-off of the right limb. The elapsed time that a limb is in contact with the walking surface is known as stance time.

standard error of measure   A measure that represents the standard deviation of error scores. The indication of error magnitude is scaled in the original score units. As reliability increases, the standard deviation of error decreases.

state space   In the dynamical systems perspective, the state of the system is the behavior captured in an instant. Continuing to map the system as it evolves in time is referred to as the system's trajectory. The state of the system and its trajectory are mapped in *state space,* which is the map of all possible states of the system.

statics   The branch of mechanics dealing with bodies at rest or in uniform motion—that is, unaffected by time.

step length   Step length is the linear distance between two consecutive contralateral contacts of the lower extremities. Step time is the temporal variable associated with step length.

strain gage   An analog device capable of measuring external forces applied to it.

strength   The ability of a muscle to generate force, which is often measured as torque.

stride length   Stride length is the distance traveled by the limb from initial contact of one foot to initial contact of the same foot.

substrates for control   Tools or resources available to engage in increasingly complex movement behavior. Prerequisites can be identified based on the substrates. For example, a substrate category for identifiying prerequisite skills is postural control. The prerequisites for achieving this substrate include knowledge, perceptual skill, motor control, training or fitness, and emotional security.

subthalamic locomotor region (SLR)   A collection of neurons in the brainstem in nonhuman vertebrates that produces rhythmic, coordinated locomotor movements when stimulated electrically.

support moment   The sum of the moments at the hip, knee and ankle during ground contact.

swing phase   The portion of the gait cycle when the lower extremity is in the air is the swing phase. The swing phase begins as the limb ends contact with the walking surface and ends the moment the same limb makes contact with the surface again. The temporal component of the swing phase is the swing time.

swing limb advancement   Swing limb advancement is one of three basic locomotor tasks, weight acceptance, single limb support, and swing limb advancement. The period during the gait cycle where the swinging limb traverses a distance is known as swing limb advancement.

task analysis A method of problem solving used in motor learning research. The method requires systematic data gathering about the subject and the environment. Data collection surrounds performance of a particular task. The task analysis includes planning, practice, observation, intervention, and evaluation.

task constraints In the dynamical systems perspective, task contraints refer to the constraints inherent in the task at hand.

taxonomy of motor skill A taxonomy developed by Gentile and Higgins in the early 1970s. The taxonomy is a classification scheme for motor skills. Skill is classified using two dimensions. The types of environmental conditions that directly affect the organization of the movement is one dimension. For example, the environment is very different for the person walking alone down an empty corridor with a linoleum floor than for the person walking down a hallway that is filled with people moving in both directions and has a floor with an uneven floor surface. The nature of movement—i.e., the body remains in one place or the body is being transported—is the second dimension.

temporal foot fall parameters A measure in time (s or ms) of foot contact performance. Swing time, stance time, gait cycle time, single support time, and double support time are temporal foot contact measures.

terminal stance This occurs immediately following the position in which the body is directly over the stationary foot to a point just prior to initial contact of the contralateral extremity.

terminal swing Terminal swing is defined as the period following a vertical tibial position to a point just prior to ground contact.

total body response In a learned motor task, the total body response is the movement executed to complete a task. In motor learning literature, the total body response is used to indicate that the motor behavior is executed with the knowledge of the relationships between the individual and the environment. The total body response is not any motor behavior, it is behavior directed toward a particular purpose or goal.

transfer function The filtering action of a mechanical or electrical system.

transformation The process of moving one coordinate system to another.

validity The interpretation of scores based on a gold standard.

vector A quantity defined by two values, magnitude and location.

walking velocity The measurement of distance traveled per unit time.

weight acceptance Weight acceptance is one of three basic locomotor tasks, weight acceptance, single limb support, and swing limb advancement. Weight acceptance occurs during the gait cycle when weight is accepted onto a limb that was swinging previously.

work The integral of the force–displacement vector dot product.

INDEX

Note: Page numbers in *italics* refer to figures. Page numbers followed by t refer to tables.